ERNEST AEGERTER, M.D.

Emeritus Professor of Pathology
Temple University Health Sciences Center
Philadelphia, Pennsylvania

JOHN A. KIRKPATRICK, JR., M.D.

Radiologist-in-Chief, The Children's Hospital Medical Center;
Professor of Radiology, Harvard Medical School
Boston, Massachusetts

ORTHOPEDIC DISEASES

Physiology • Pathology • Radiology

FOURTH EDITION

W. B. SAUNDERS COMPANY

Philadelphia • London • Toronto

W. B. Saunders Company: West Washington Square
Philadelphia, PA 19105

1 St. Anne's Road
Eastbourne, East Sussex BN21 3UN, England

1 Goldthorne Avenue
Toronto, Ontario M8Z 5T9, Canada

Listed here is the latest translated edition of this book together
with the language of the translation and the publisher.

Spanish — Editorial Medica Panamericana,
   Buenos Aires, Argentina

Library of Congress Cataloging in Publication Data

Aegerter, Ernest Emil, 1906–

Orthopedic diseases.

Includes index.

1. Bones — Diseases.   2. Orthopedia.   3. Bones — Radiography.   I. Kirkpatrick, John Arthur, 1926– joint author.
   II. Title. [DNLM: 1. Bone diseases. WE140 A247o]

RC930.A32 1975   616.7′1   74–4551

ISBN 0–7216–1062–5

Orthopedic Diseases:
Physiology, Pathology, Radiology   ISBN 0-7216-1062-5

Last digit is the print number: 9   8   7   6

PREFACE TO THE FOURTH EDITION

The "BASIC SCIENCE" aspect of bone disease has lagged behind that of other systems, not from lack of need or interest, but largely because of the very nature of bone, which until recently has defied investigation on the cellular and intracellular level. The rigors of salt removal by acid so distort the fine morphologic detail of cytoplasm and nucleus that conclusions have depended, to a degree, on interpretation of artifacts. Abnormal variations in mineralization were impossible to appreciate when the mineral had to be removed before the tissue could be examined. Knowledge of the healing of human bone was derived by animal experimentation because even today we are denied serial sampling of the process as it occurs in our patients. Biopsies are usually relatively difficult and taxing to the donor so that the course of a disease process must be extrapolated from one or two known points in time.

Today there is feverish activity in the fields of bone morphology and physiology. New techniques and tools have become available. Histochemistry, immunologic chemistry and radioactive isotopes have allowed us to probe within the cell membrane. The ability to section undemineralized bone, microradiography and x-ray diffraction are telling us something of the tissue in its natural state. Phase, ultraviolet and electron microscopy reveal aspects of cell composition that heretofore were undreamed of. These new tools have set the anatomists, the chemists, the physicists and the physiologists to work hacking out new trails that will eventually converge in precise knowledge of the skeletal tissue cells, what they are and what they are doing in health and disease.

All this sound and fury have bewildered the busy physician who must correlate the new material with one hand while he administers his knowledge with the other. It will take many books to sift the facts, to concentrate the verbiage, to reduce the product to the level of practicability. This book is meant as a starter. It looks at bone disease from the standpoint of its altered morphology and physiology, yet it tries to interpret these in terms of symptomatology and roentgenography. Diseases must be understood if they are to be successfully treated. This book is concerned with the understanding of the diseases that affect the musculoskeletal system. The diagnosis of orthopedic diseases necessitates an understanding of the pathology and physiology of bone; from these disciplines arise the clinical manifestations and the radiographic and laboratory findings.

Very little original material is recorded here. Almost all of it can be found in published papers if the searcher will spend the time and energy. The virtue of this volume, if such it has, is in the availability of this material. A consuming interest in the subject for more than 30 years has given us the opportunity of selecting what we think the physician should know. There is no pretense at completeness, for such would remove it from the field of practical usage. It is intended for the clinician who wants to increase his diagnostic efficiency, for the radiologist who is perplexed by the meaning of an overwhelming array of radiographic nuances, for the pathologist who is distraught by his inability to interpret what he sees through his microscope, for the young specialist who wants to pass his board examinations and for the medical student who must acquire a certain amount of knowledge of orthopedic diseases in order to graduate.

The first three chapters are intended as a review of the complicated anatomy and physiology of the tissues of the skeleton. It is difficult to imagine how one can understand the disease process until one understands the normal. The fourth chapter is a simple histology of the tissues involved in orthopedic diseases. It is meant for the orthopedist and the radiologist who have forgotten rudimentary structural components of bone. It is not meant for the pathologist who reviews these basic principles in the first month of his residency. Chapter Five is a primer of bone radiology intended for the pathologist and the orthopedist who must know the fundamentals of radiology if they are to appreciate gross bone pathology. The remaining chapters are divided into five sections, each section grouping the musculoskeletal diseases in a manner that should make them easier to find and to remember. Classification is stressed, perhaps overstressed, with the deliberate intention of presenting a concept of the whole before attempting the specific. There is no truer maxim in diagnostic medicine than "Before one can name the entity, one must know the possibilities."

When one attempts to acknowledge the help that is so important in writing any medical book, it is difficult to know where to start and where to end. First, perhaps, there were all our colleagues in other fields who unselfishly supplied cases and patiently instructed us in the fundamentals of their specialties. Many of the radiographs are from the Department of Radiology of Temple University Health Sciences Center and St. Christopher's Hospital for Children. Many of the microscopic illustrations are derived from the vast amount of consultation material that arrives at our desk daily. We are grateful to our colleagues all over the world who have contributed these cases.

Finally, we owe a debt of gratitude to those wonderful institutions that housed us, nourished us, taught us and endured us while we worked, Temple University Health Sciences Center and its pediatric unit, St. Christopher's Hospital for Children. If any good comes of this labor let it reflect bountifully upon them.

ERNEST AEGERTER
JOHN A. KIRKPATRICK, JR.

CONTENTS

SECTION ONE • **A GENERAL CONSIDERATION OF CONNECTIVE TISSUES**

Chapter 1
CELLULAR COMPONENTS OF CONNECTIVE TISSUES 3

Chapter 2
INTERCELLULAR COMPONENTS OF CONNECTIVE TISSUES 9

Chapter 3
SKELETAL EMBRYOLOGY AND PHYSIOLOGY 17

Chapter 4
HISTOLOGY OF THE MUSCULOSKELETAL SYSTEM.............................. 37

Chapter 5
RADIOLOGY OF THE SKELETAL SYSTEM... 74

SECTION TWO • **DISTURBANCES IN SKELETAL DEVELOPMENT**

Chapter 6
THE SKELETAL DYSPLASIAS.. 87

Chapter 7
FUNCTIONAL DISTURBANCES OF THE RETICULOENDOTHELIAL
SYSTEM 201

SECTION THREE • **DISTURBANCES IN THE NORMALLY FORMED SKELETON**

Chapter 8
THE REPAIR OF FRACTURES... 231

Chapter 9
INFECTIOUS DISEASES OF BONE 251

Chapter 10
CIRCULATORY DISTURBANCES 289

Chapter 11

METABOLIC DISEASES OF BONE 331

Chapter 12

DISTURBANCES DUE TO ENDOCRINE DYSFUNCTION 376

Chapter 13

MISCELLANEOUS DISEASES OF THE SKELETON 407

SECTION FOUR • **TUMORS AND TUMOR-LIKE PROCESSES**

Chapter 14

GENERAL CONSIDERATION OF TUMORS 461

Chapter 15

TUMOR-LIKE PROCESSES 478

Chapter 16

OSTEOGENIC TUMORS 510

Chapter 17

CHONDROGENIC TUMORS 538

Chapter 18

COLLAGENIC TUMORS 562

Chapter 19

MYELOGENIC TUMORS 572

Chapter 20

OSTEOCLASTOMA 607

SECTION FIVE • **DISEASES OF JOINTS AND MUSCLES;
  SOFT PART TUMORS**

Chapter 21

ARTHRITIS 623

Chapter 22

DISEASES OF SKELETAL MUSCLE 687

Chapter 23

TUMORS OF SOFT PARTS 721

INDEX 777

A GENERAL CONSIDERATION OF CONNECTIVE TISSUES

Chapter 1

CELLULAR COMPONENTS OF CONNECTIVE TISSUES

FACTORS IN CELL DIFFERENTIATION

The various components of the connective tissues, i.e., fat, fibrous tissue, cartilage and bone, arise as differentiated elements from the primitive mesoderm. Differentiation of a cell from those of the multipotent cell mass to become the highly specialized unit of tissue structure is the result of a number of influencing factors some of which are as yet poorly understood. It is now believed that the mechanism by which a mature cell reproduces by mitotic division resides in the chromatin constituents of the nucleus. This substance, largely desoxyribosenucleic acid, is supplied by the cytoplasm and, therefore, conditioned by enzymatic processes which take place in the cytoplasm of the cell. As long as the cytoplasmic metabolic processes are stable it may be assumed that the nuclear hereditary constituents will remain constant and reproduction may continue indefinitely, each cell a faithful duplicate, in both morphology and function, of its predecessor. We may call the combined agents which govern this exact duplication the primary heredity factor.

Obviously this type of exact reproduction can take place only among cells that are completely differentiated, i.e., cells whose enzymatic constituents are mature and stable, and in an environment that is absolutely unchanging. Thus the chondroblast may give rise to identical chondroblasts, osteoblasts to identical osteoblasts, and so on, as long as the medium in which they exist remains the same. If we introduce new elements into the cell environment, we may force the cytoplasmic metabolism to change and conceivably produce a change in the molecular constituency or arrangement of the nuclear heredity apparatus. We may designate the environmental influence on a cell as its secondary or somatic heredity factor.

This latter factor is probably a potent agent in what we know as cell differentiation. It is obvious that in the development of a multicellular organism the environment of cells must change until a stage of stable maturity is reached. When the embryonic form consists of a single cell or a small group of cells each with at least some free surface, the cell may choose from its environment what it needs and discharge its metabolic refuse as it likes. As the organism grows and the early cells become surrounded by other cells (Fig. 1–1) the resources of the deep cells become more and more limited, since the environmental substances must penetrate between surrounding cells to reach them and in doing so must be conditioned by the catabolic products of the surrounding cells. So the environment of the deep cell is changed and thus its metabolic pattern must change if the cell is to survive. Changes in the intracytoplasmic chemistry may result in changes in the nuclear hereditary apparatus and thus, by means of the somatic hereditary factor, differentiation and specialization are achieved to the point of stable maturity.

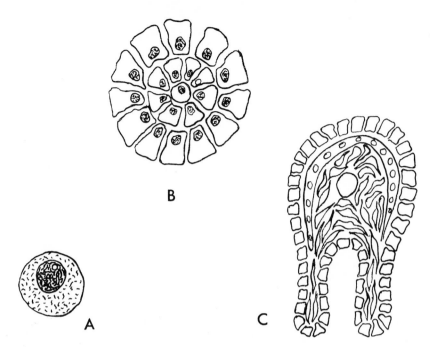

Figure 1-1 Schematic drawing to illustrate cell differentiation. *A,* The unicellular organism ingests what it needs from its environment, processes it to form the plasmagenes in the cytoplasm and passes on the refined product, mostly desoxyribosenucleic acid, to the nucleus. It discharges its wastes into its environment. *B,* In the multicellular organism the surface cells still have access to environmental resources but the central cells must accommodate their metabolism to the materials that can penetrate between the surface cells. These materials are contaminated by the catabolic products of the surrounding cells. *C,* The more complex the organism becomes, the greater the possibilities for differentiation. This drawing illustrates the effects of the secondary heredity factor upon the deep cells.

When the state of maturation is complete we may expect a cell faithfully to reproduce its kind in the normal, physiologic repair of necrobiosis. However, if its environmental resources are altered by changes in blood supply or changes in the selective dispersion of its surrounding, intercellular supportive components, one may find alterations in its heredity mechanism which result in offspring that differ from the mother cell. These differences may be forecalculated when the environmental changes are known. When the heredity alteration is reversible we call this change in morphology and function "metaplasia," a physiologic or near-physiologic process. Disturbances in cell health and growth patterns sufficient to induce tissue changes constitute the lesions of disease. It is the understanding of these lesions, a recognition of their morphologic and functional characteristics, that is the field of interest of the pathologist.

THE DEVELOPMENT OF CELLS

The primitive mesoderm is a pleomorphic tissue substance which arises in the very early stages of embryologic development. As one examines it through the microscope one sees a mound of stellate and reticulated cells in a gel matrix (Fig. 1-2). As the celomic cavity develops, the cells on the cavity surface, and thus the cells that come to line the cavity, swell and line up in a single layer. Their rounded free surfaces characterize their cell type which we may designate as primitive mesothelium. It is of interest that wherever mesodermal tissue or one of its derivatives borders on a natural space or cavity, such as the lumina of blood vessels, the pericardial, pleural or peritoneal cavities or the joint or tendon spaces, they tend to take this shape. These are known generally in their mature, differentiated state as endothelial or simply mesothelial cells. In the vessels they retain their name of endothelial cells. Lining the major body cavities they are called serosal cells and when they face joint and tendon spaces they are designated synovial cells (Fig. 4–39, page 73).

The reticulated portion of the mesoderm forms a syncytium. Deposits of this syncytium are best seen in the mature organism in the spleen, the lymph nodes and scattered lymph follicles, and in the bone marrow. Apparently the differences of environment condition its morphology and function, for though there are similarities, the functions particularly of marrow, spleen and lymph node reticulum appear to differ. One of the functions of reticulum is the production of motile cells. Those of the myelogenous reticulum, that of the bone marrow, concern the orthopedic pathologist (Fig. 4–34, page 69).

From the reticulated cells of the primitive mesoderm comes a multipotent cell which gives rise to derivatives other than the mesothelium and reticulum (Fig. 1–3). These cells form a primitive, reticulated, widely disseminated tissue which we may designate mesenchyme. Its cells soon differentiate, depending upon their position and environment, into a variety of forms and these, the mesenchymal derivatives — that is, bone, cartilage, connective tissue, muscle and fat — make up the bulk of tissue which concerns those interested in orthopedic pathology.

The metabolic processes of some of these cells result in the accumulation of respiratory pigment known as myoglobin. The cells elongate and form intercellular fibrils. Some develop cross striations and form skeletal muscle cells while others mature into involuntary muscle.

Others of this same stem cell type begin to accumulate droplets of lipid material. These droplets coalesce to form a solid accumulation which distends the cell membrane and pushes the nucleus to one side, eventually flattening it against the cell wall. These cells usually form in aggregates and eventually the cytoplasmic membranes of many rupture and lakes of neutral fat are formed between the cells. Thus fat deposits are formed throughout

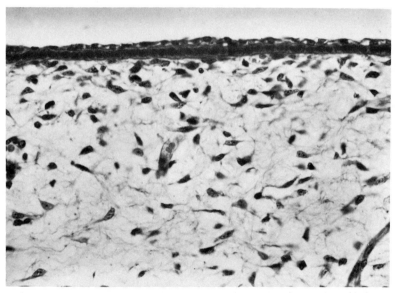

Figure 1–2 Section through the wall of the celomic cavity of an early embryo. The clear area above represents celomic cavity. There is a mound of primitive mesodermal cells. They are spindled and stellate, connected by a cobweb tracery of fibrils in a gel ground substance. This substance condenses and the cells differentiate into the various mesenchymal derivatives. The cells that abut on an enclosed space (the celomic cavity in this illustration) thicken and flatten to form mesothelial cells. Depending upon the space that they enclose they become endothelial (vessel), serosal (peritoneum and pleura) or synovial (joint) cells. In an edematous (myxomatous) environment the various derivatives in postnatal life may revert to the primitive mesenchyme morphology.

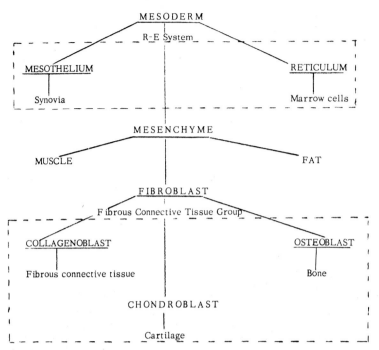

Figure 1–3 Diagram illustrating the origins of various mesenchymal derivatives. From the mesoderm comes the mesothelium which, depending upon its environment, differentiates into endothelium, serosa or synovial lining cells (Fig. 1–2). From it also comes the reticulum which persists in postnatal life in most body tissues but is concentrated in certain stations—the bone marrow and the lymph nodes, spleen and intestinal lymph follicles. The specialization of other forms depends upon their locations. Marrow reticulum gives rise to the myelogenous series of cells producing principally leukocytes and red cells. Mesenchyme comes from the primitive mesoderm and differentiates to produce a number of forms: muscle, both striated and nonstriated, fat and a group, the intercellular matrix of which is composed largely of fibers. This group evolves by way of a cell which, because of this matrix, is best called the fibroblast. The morphology of the mature cell is related to the type of matrix, the collagenoblast (usually called fibroblast) in collagen, the chondroblast in chondroid and the osteoblast in osteoid.

the body, these deposits acting as storehouses of energy. These aggregates of fat cells fill in the angles and crevices, especially of moving parts such as muscles and tendons. Within the medullary areas of bone the fat cells take over the regions previously occupied by the marrow as it progressively shrinks during the aging process. Within the long bones, however, these fat cells retain their conversion potentialities and, under certain conditions of functional marrow destruction, may supply the bed for new marrow proliferation. The available, unneeded neutral fat of the dietary intake certainly plays an important role in the aggregate number of the lipoblasts (eventually, the lipocytes) but the distribution of the fat deposits is controlled, apparently to some extent, by endocrine influence.

THE FIBROBLAST AND ITS DERIVATIVES

A more differentiated form of the mesenchyme remains throughout the life of the organism. The cells of this stage of mesenchymal development seem to have no generally recognized name though the name best suited to them is "fibroblast." This term suggests that they are fiber-producing and, indeed, this is the most important character common to each of the three mature cell types, the collagen-producing fibrocyte (collagenoblast), the bone-producing osteocyte and the chondroid-producing chondrocyte, which come from them. This cell, the fibroblast, is a remarkably labile form which apparently differentiates into any one of three directions, each of the three resultant specialized forms constituting one of the components of what we know as connective tissue. These are fibrous connective tissue, cartilage and bone. It is of great importance that any one of the early or blast forms of these cell types may, upon alteration of its environmental circumstance, undergo conversion to any of the other forms within the fibrous tissue group, and perhaps outside the group they may change to fat, reticular and mesothelial forms and possibly even to nonstriated muscle, though conversion to fat and especially muscle is denied by many histologists.

The cells of this basic fiber-producing group vary considerably in size but their average diameter is about that of the ordinary macrophage (Fig. 4–11), page 45). Their nuclei resemble those of macrophages and they, too, are motile in a liquid medium. They may phagocytize particulate matter. Indeed, but for the degree of their motility and phagocytic activity it is doubtful that they can be differentiated from macrophages, and there is reason to believe that any differences that exist are those of environmental influence rather than genetic components.

The collagenoblast, i.e., the collagen-producing cell usually called fibroblast, can be differentiated from the fibrous tissue blast form only when there is production of collagen about it. As this cell ages it elongates to a thin spindle with pointed ends to each of which is attached a long, fine argentophilic fibril (Fig. 4–11, page 45). As it multiplies and matures it comes to lie in a more or less homogeneous (at ordinary microscope magnification) matrix (Fig. 4–12, page 45). Its growth pattern suggests either that the matrix is formed by the maturing fibroblasts or at least that these cells are instrumental in its production. The nucleus becomes elongated and pyknotic until eventually it becomes a thick, short black line with hematoxylin staining (Fig. 4–13, page 45). The cytoplasmic borders are lost in the collagen matrix. The latter stains a buff to a strong pink with eosin, brown with colloidal silver, green with trichrome and blue with Mallory's stain. It should be emphasized that the mature collagenocyte is a fully differentiated, distinctive form

but that its young, blast form cannot be differentiated from the young forms of the chondroblast and osteoblast except by the presence of collagen.

The chondroblast separates itself from the pool of undifferentiated fibroblasts and can be identified at first only by the chondroid which is laid down in its proximity and by the blue-gray tint it acquires with hematoxylin staining. The nature of this staining reaction has been investigated by Lillie,[1] who has shown that it is probably due to the presence of considerable amounts of ribosenucleic acid. As the cell matures it swells and comes to lie in a space (the lacuna) within the chondroid matrix. The space is actually an artifact since the cell is so exceedingly fragile that ordinary processing for microscopic examination causes it to shrink away from the more durable chondroid walls. The microscopist rarely has an opportunity of studying the detail of the chondrocyte because of this distortion. As the chondroid is being laid down, the cell multiplies so that clusters of two, three, four or more cells are found caught in the matrix (Fig. 4–18, page 53). Chondroid with ordinary magnification has a glassy or powdery, homogeneous appearance with a pale to medium blue color when stained with hematoxylin. The blue color with hematoxylin is apparently due to its chief constituent, chondroitin sulfate.

The osteoblast in the resting stage likewise cannot be differentiated from the young forms of the other two types of connective tissue (Fig. 4–22, page 57). In enchondral bone formation the cells line up in a single row along the face of a calcified chondroid bar and then usually become cuboidal in shape (Fig. 4–23, page 57). As they swell their cytoplasm takes on a gray-blue tint with hematoxylin. Follis[2] has investigated this phenomenon and by special staining technique has concluded that it is due to an unusually high component of ribosenucleic acid. He points out that since chondroblasts and osteoblasts are involved in the production of the intercellular substances, chondroid and osteoid, that are composed largely of proteins, the cytoplasmic ribosenucleic acid may be significant and vital to this function. He has noted that this staining reaction disappears in scurvy[3] and osteogenesis imperfecta, conditions in which there is failure of osteoid production.

A band of homogeneous material appears between the chondroid bar and the row of cells. This is osteoid, called an osteoid seam, and but for its tendency to take a somewhat deeper eosin stain its appearance by light microscopy is that of collagen until it is mineralized.

From these cell descriptions it might be assumed that the blast cell of connective tissue, the fibroblast, is merely the resting form of the young collagenocyte, chondrocyte and osteocyte, and perhaps the lipocyte and reticulocyte, and that it awaits only the proper environmental stimulus to start it on its path of differentiation. Such may well be the case for it is unlikely, since these cells are interchangeable, that their eventual functional differences depend on specific enzymatic constituents. In examining a callus the microscopist gets the impression that these cells originally form collagen; as the callus

matures they form chondroid and eventually osteoid. These three physically different intercellular materials appear to be chemically akin and coextensive with each other.

Bassett[4] has experimented with cultures of these cells. He believes that stress and the level of oxygen tension on a colony of primitive "fibroblasts" dictate the activity, i.e., the identity and function of the mature cell. He states that stress plus a high oxygen tension causes these cells to elaborate osteoid. Stress in a low oxygen tension causes them to form chondroid, whereas tension plus a rich oxygen supply results in the production of collagen. These aspects of cell activity and differentiation have analogues in physiologic callus formation of bone repair.

References

1. Lillie, R. D.: Anat. Rec., *103*:611, 1949.
2. Follis, R. H.: Bull. Johns Hopkins Hosp., *85*:281, 1949.
3. Follis, R. H.: Bull. Johns Hopkins Hosp., *89*:9, 1951.
4. Bassett, A.: J. Bone Joint Surg., *44A*:1217, 1962.

Chapter 2

INTERCELLULAR COMPONENTS
OF CONNECTIVE TISSUES

The cells that make up the connective tissues of the body are morphologically identical in their young forms. As they mature and differentiate, each of the three types of cells is identified by the intercellular substance that is laid down in its proximity. The collagenoblast (fibroblast) is identified with collagen, the chondroblast with chondroid and the osteoblast with osteoid.

In their early stages the intercellular substances are quite similar in appearance with ordinary magnification, and their chemical components are almost the same with some variation in the relative amounts of various constituents. But, owing to certain factors in the maturation process, the physical characteristics of the three substances become quite different. Collagen is firm, fibrous and pliable. Chondroid is hard, resilient and usually not pliable. Mineralized osteoid is stony hard and rigid.

COLLAGEN

When examined by the electron microscope, collagen is found to be composed of four constituents: collagen fibers (Fig. 2–1), which make up the preponderant part, reticulin, elastin and ground substance.

The collagen fibers occur in bundles of parallel fibrils which can be seen with the ordinary microscope. With electronic magnification the fibrils are found to be long, slender and nonbranching with periodic cross bars spaced at about 640 Ångström units.[1] The substance of collagen fibers is considered to be a fibrous protein; i.e., it is composed of an arrangement of extended parallel polypeptide chains.[2] When heated in water it becomes soluble and forms a gel, in contrast to the corpuscular proteins found in serum albumin and globulin and hemoglobin that are denatured by heat and become less soluble. It is digested by collagenase such as that extracted from cultures of Type A *Clostridium welchii* but is not digested by trypsin and other proteolytic enzymes.

The reticulin components of collagen are much finer fibrils than the collagen fibers. In young collagen they appear as a network of wavy, branching argentophilic threads that are cross banded in approximately the same periodicity as collagen fibers. X-ray diffraction studies fail to reveal any essential chemical differences between reticulin and collagen fibers. Reticulin is abundant in young collagen but becomes increasingly more difficult to demonstrate as collagen ages. It has been suggested that reticulin is but the first stage of collagen fiber formation and that the former merges to form the latter.

The exact chemical properties of elastin, the third fibrillar constituent of collagen, are unknown. It is thought to have a molecular structure similar to that of rubber, and with the electron microscope it is found to appear as coarse filaments without periodic banding, supporting this theory.

The ground substance of collagen is

9

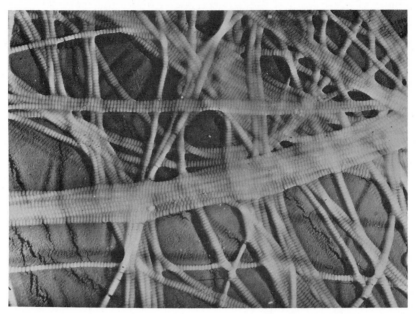

Figure 2–1   Collagen fibrils taken with the electron microscope. They have been shadowed with chromium. (× 18,300.) (Courtesy of Drs. Gross and Schmitt, Massachusetts Institute of Technology.)

composed of a group of mucopolysaccharides. These are made up principally of hexosamine and hexuronic acid. Of the three known mucopolysaccharides, chondroitin sulfate, hyaluronate and heparin, the first two have been identified in the ground substance. Of the several types of chondroitin sulfate perhaps four are found in various types of connective tissue. Chondroitin sulfate and hyaluronate are sugars in which a hydroxyl group is replaced by an amine group. They are chemically similar except that chondroitin sulfate contains ester sulfate groups, whereas hyaluronate contains only the carboxyl group. The various types of mucopolysaccharides depend upon the type of sugar of which they are composed; for example, hyaluronate is a glucosamine and chondroitin sulfate, a galactosamine. The connective tissue mucopolysaccharides exist in a highly polymerized state. Hyaluronidase causes depolymerization.

The periodic acid–fuchsin reaction is currently regarded as the most practical, if not the most accurate, method of demonstrating the presence of mucopolysaccharide in tissues. This test is sometimes referred to as the Hotchkiss-McManus stain or the periodic-Schiff reaction. This staining method depends upon the oxidation of a polysaccharide with periodic acid to yield an aldehyde. The product then gives a red to purple color when treated with the basic fuchsin reagent. Starch and glycogen may first be removed from the tissue by treating with amylase. Unfortunately, this reaction is apparently not specific for mucopolysaccharides, and some tissues which are known to contain mucopolysaccharides do not stain with these reagents.

The phenomenon of metachromasia has also been used to indicate the presence of mucopolysaccharides, and particularly to define their state of polymerization. The test is essentially a change in color of certain absorbed dyes of the thiazine group from blue through violet to red. Basic fuchsin is often used just as it is in the last part of the Hotchkiss-McManus method and other commonly used stains are toluidine blue, methylene blue and crystal violet. The term metachromatic is applied to the property of a tissue which causes this color change. Mucopolysaccharides are more metachromatic in the polymerized state than when depolymerized. As the chondroid of the enchondral plate is depolymerized at the provisional line of calcification it loses its metachromatic staining quality.

The Hale reaction is considered by some to be a more specific test than the two mentioned previously. It depends upon the use of dialyzed iron which is bound to the amino acid groups. This iron gives the Prussian blue reaction.

The ground substance of collagen varies considerably in its physical properties. It may take the form of a rather firm cement, a gel or a liquid. These states apparently depend upon its water-binding properties. It appears that some portions of collagen ground substance may be in the gel state and other portions liquid but it is probable that the two are coextensive.[3] The mucopolysaccharides form the matrix substance that fills in the spaces between the various types of fibers.

Until relatively recent years the principal function ascribed to the connective tissues was that of support. With advances in our knowledge of the physical and chemical nature of collagen a completely new concept of collagen physiology evolves. The interest has been fired by the recognition of a group of clinical entities that have been called the connective tissue or collagen diseases. Out of the research related to these diseases has come much of our knowledge concerning the normal anatomy and activity of collagen.

Certainly one of its most important functions is that of dispersion. It must be remembered that almost all of our so-called parenchymal cells are supported and surrounded by collagen. Although much attention has been paid to the condition of the finer ramifications of the vessels, capillary permeability, and the like, in considering the metabolic resources of parenchymal cells, little has been said about the collagen through which metabolic substances must pass before they reach these cells. It appears, without much factual evidence to support the thesis, that the ground substance is the dispersing agent that selectively protects and supplies the parenchymal cells it supports. Thus it becomes one of the important water-binding (and dispersing) agents in the body. Likewise it probably acts as an ion exchange resin that plays an important part in the control of electrolyte flow.

When the calcium and phosphorus ions are considered it is apparent that collagen physiology is of utmost importance in the mineral metabolism of bone.

CHONDROID

Chondroid, like collagen, is made up of collagen fibrils and elastin in a ground substance (Fig. 2–2). The principal differences between hyalin cartilage, fibrocartilage and elastic cartilage depend upon the relative amounts of these various components. Since hyalin cartilage is found almost exclusively in relation to bone growth and joint surfaces, the term cartilage or chondroid without qualification refers to hyalin cartilage.

The matrix of hyalin cartilage is seen most typically in the growth plate of the unossified epiphysis. With the light microscope it is seen as a homogeneous, translucent matrix substance taking a pale blue stain with hematoxylin. With the electron microscope it is found to have a feltwork of fibers. The proportion of mucopolysaccharide ground substance is said to be much greater than in either collagen or osteoid. There are at least two types of chondroitin sulfate in chondroid.

The chondroid of articular cartilage and that at some distance from the epiphyseal line of the growth plate is highly polymerized. As the epiphyseal line is approached the chondroid becomes depolymerized and loses its metachromasia. This is the area of provisional calcification and it is thought that the calcium salt molecules have inactivated the bonds which formerly captured the dye.

OSTEOID

Through the ordinary microscope, osteoid is an eosin-staining, homogeneous substance which is morphologically identical to collagen. It is only its relationship to its osteoblasts or the advent of mineralization that distinguishes it with ordinary hematoxylin and eosin staining. Progress in the study of osteoid is much less advanced than for collagen and chondroid since mineralization follows close on

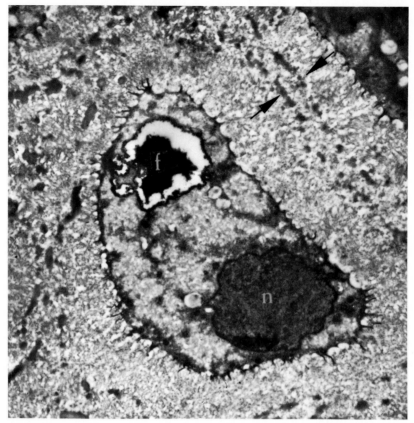

Figure 2–2 Electron micrograph of cartilage. The ovoid structure in the center is a chondrocyte with nucleus marked "n." Around this cell the cartilage matrix consists of a fine feltwork. Between the chondrocytes (the band between the two arrows) is a network of more dense substance. (× 5000.) (Courtesy of H. Sheldon and R. A. Robinson, Johns Hopkins University Medical School.)

the heels of normal osteoid production, thus interfering with study preparation. The demineralization processes are so rigorous that the application of data concerning decalcified bone to bone in its natural state is hazardous.

By piecing together the fragments of knowledge concerning the chemical and physical properties of osteoid we may assume that they are much like those of chondroid and collagen, that is, that osteoid is made up of a feltwork of fibers in a ground substance (Fig. 2–3). It is reported that the ground substance is relatively less in amount and there is disagreement as to the presence of reticulin and especially elastin fibers.

Two other methods in addition to electron microscopy are being used to study the constituents of bone and the manner

in which bone is laid down and mineralized. One of these, x-ray diffraction (Fig. 2–4), is a method whereby a beam of x-rays of less than 1 millimeter in diameter is passed through an object or solution and the pattern of diffraction recorded on a film. These patterns are highly characteristic within certain chemical groups when the spacings of the atoms are such as those seen in crystalline substances. Under these circumstances the diffraction pattern is characteristic of the chemical components of the material examined and offers a means of analysis of solid tissues without disruption of tissue structure.

The other method is known as microradiography. A fine beam of x-rays is passed through a section of undemineralized bone. These sections are cut on a special micromilling machine[4] or ground

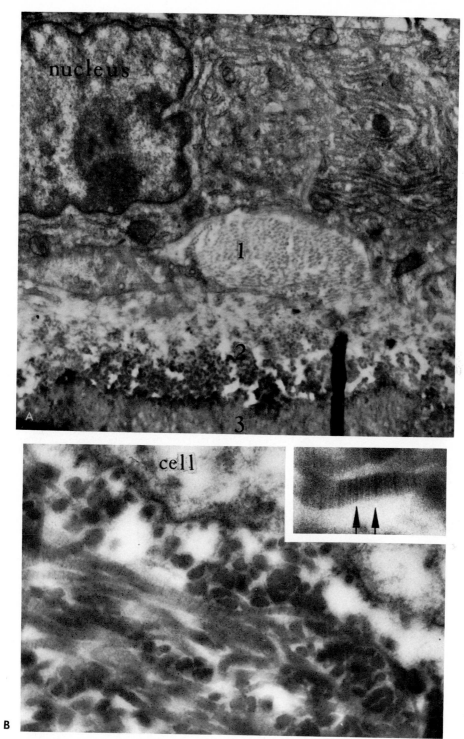

Figure 2–3 *A*, Electron micrograph of a section of bone. The upper half of the photograph is an osteoblast with nucleus and cytoplasm. At 1 there is a bundle of collagen fibrils cut in cross section. At 2 the collagen fibrils are vested with an opaque coating which probably represents the earliest stage of accumulation of inorganic ions during calcification. This is the area of physiological osteoid. At 3 the osteoid is calcified. (× 18,500.) (From Sheldon, H., and Robinson, R. A.: J. Biophys. & Biochem Cytol., vol. 13.) *B*, An electron micrograph of a section of osteoid from a rachitic rat. At the upper right is an osteoblast. Collagen fibrils are seen in the lower portion of the micrograph. The insert shows a greater magnification of a collagen fibril illustrating its periodic banding. The space between the arrows is about 640 Ångström units. Seven subbandings may be seen within the unit. (× 60,000; inset × 100,000.) (Courtesy of H. Sheldon and R. A. Robinson, Johns Hopkins University Medical School.)

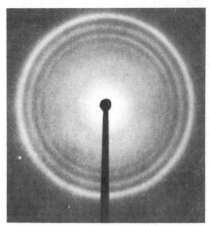

Figure 2–4 X-ray diffraction pattern of a piece of lamb bone. A very fine beam (less than 1 mm. in diameter) of x-rays is passed through an undemineralized section of bone. When the atomic constituents are arranged in space as they are in crystalline substances the chemical components can be read by the pattern of diffraction recorded on a film. (Courtesy of Drs. M. Spiegel-Adolf and G. Henny, Temple University Medical School.)

to a thinness which permits transmission of light by rubbing the specimen, necessarily of small size and usually unfixed, against an abrasive surface.[5] The films are then examined through the ordinary light microscope (Fig. 2–5) and when adjacent sections are used, one prepared for microradiography and the other for routine staining, the variations in opacity in the former reveal the pattern of lamellar formation. By this method, relative densities can be appreciated that are not demonstrable by transmitted light.

THE FORMATION OF INTERCELLULAR SUBSTANCE

Concerning the formation of connective tissue intercellular substance much has been written and little proven. Earlier writers, noting that intercellular substance is found only in the presence of connective tissue cells, concluded that this material was produced and spun out by the cells just as the substance of its web is secreted by the spider. It is probable that these early concepts may be very near the truth. Recently, Welsh[6] showed that the collagen precursors are synthesized in the rough endoplasmic reticulum but fibril formation does not occur until this substance reaches the Golgi apparatus. The latter contributes something that initiates

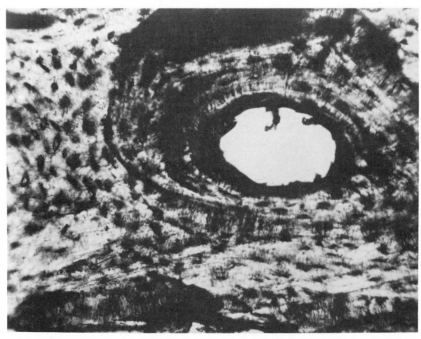

Figure 2–5 Microradiograph of an undemineralized bone section cut at about 70 microns. Lamellae are seen encircling the haversian canal with lacunae between them. The dark areas represent concentrations of opaque calcium salts. This method may be utilized to study relative mineral concentrations at the cellular level. (× 680.)

fibrillogenesis. Golgi vesicles containing molecular collagen eventually discharge their contents by reverse pinocytosis onto the outer surface of the cell membrane. These membrane foci probably represent the "template" for fibrillogenesis on the cell surface.

The various components of the intercellular substances are built up as the result of molecular combinations which can occur only in the substrate provided by certain chemical constituents perfusing from the blood and mingling with the products secreted by the cells involved. By means of the electron microscope, collagenoblasts have been seen synthesizing short rod-shaped structures within their cytoplasm. These later appear on the outer surface of the cell and join end-to-end with others to form the elongated structure that ultimately becomes the collagen fiber. Higgenbotham believes that the fibroblasts ingest various mucopolysaccharides and then elaborate certain constituents of the ground substance. Intensive research is being carried on in this area at the present time and it is hoped that within a short period definite information will be available.

THE DEPOSITION OF BONE SALTS

The mineral deposited in chondroid at the line of provisional calcification and in osteoid is not a simple chemical compound nor are the chemical constituents constant in kind or amount. There appear to be species differences, differences between members of the same species, between bones of the same organism and even between areas of the same bone. The chemical formula also differs with age and in bone disease. Whatever these differences may be, however, bone mineral exists in a crystal form and, according to Mellors,[7] an amorphous form, calcium carbonate. The crystal/amorphous ratio apparently increases with age.

In the apatite form the ions are arranged in units, each unit having the components of the whole; yet because these units are shared by contiguous units, they are not distinct. Thus, if we attempt to write the formula for the crystal structure of

bone it would compare in a sense to the formula of a single room in a large building composed of numerous identical rooms. Four walls plus one ceiling plus one floor equals one room. However, this is not an independent structure, for if one were able to remove a single room one would leave the six surrounding rooms incomplete. Thus, the structure of the crystals of bone mineral is made up of a lattice of ions in which one might find a representative area, but the removal of this area would destroy the integrity of the whole. A concept of this lattice structure is important in understanding the physiology of mineral metabolism.

Bone mineral is laid down in crystal form and the crystals maintain their individuality just as do the components of a brick wall. The crystals are thought to be flat and thin, approximating the shape of a hexagonal playing card. Though the exact relation of the mineral crystals to the various factors of the organic substance of bone is not definitely known as yet, it is thought now that they are laid down about or perhaps within the collagen fibrils.

The formula for bone salt can best be approximated by that of a hydroxy apatite, thus: $3Ca_3(PO_4)_2 \cdot Ca(OH)_2$. It consists largely of Ca^{++}, $PO_4^{\equiv}$ and OH^- together with carbon dioxide, citrate and water. Other ions in trace amounts are Na^+, Mg^{++}, K^+, Cl^- and F^-.

The crystal configuration has been reviewed by Neuman and Neuman.[8] The constant and rapid turnover in normal bone explains the variability in composition at any given time. There appears to be a continuous interchange of ions between the crystal lattice and the fluid that bathes it. At times this may mean substitution of one mineral ion for another. Thus it becomes necessary to think of the rigid and seemingly permanent structure of bone as a dynamic system in a state of constant flux and, therefore, less static and fixed than the soft tissues which surround it.

In order to account for the facility with which ions are exchanged it is necessary to take into consideration the surface chemistry of the crystal lattice. If one chooses an area within the lattice in which all the ions are represented in the proportions of the whole, we may call this area a unit. The crystal of bone salt is so thin that it is only a few of these units thick. A unit may exist within the depths of the lattice or in the surface and apparently the majority are in the latter position. Because of the unit structure of the crystalline component of bone, it has an immense surface area. Someone has estimated that the surface area of the mineral crystals in the skeleton of an average man probably exceeds a hundred acres. Since ions are apparently adsorbed on these surfaces and since the amount of fluid that bathes them is so relatively small that it must be a very thin layer indeed, it becomes easier to understand the remarkable facility with which the ionic composition of the lattice is kept in constant motion.

Of great importance to those interested in bone disease is the mechanism by which mineral salts are deposited in the organic matrix. Though the matter has been of major concern to a number of very able research workers, information which satisfies all of the known facts is still not available. Apparently several factors play a role in the mineralization of normal cartilage and bone. Much of the work has been done on in vitro specimens using the area of provisional calcification and the subchondral area of unmineralized osteoid of experimental rickets.

The pH of the area of mineral deposit is apparently of some importance. Mineralization will take place within the wide pH range of 6 to 8.5. On the alkaline side of pH 7.3 little is achieved by raising this figure. Change of the hydrogen ion concentration causes an increase in the phosphate ions but calcification in vitro is not enhanced, indicating that the pH itself is not critical.

The ion product of calcium and phosphate seems also of importance. However, the fact that it is not critical is shown by the same experiment and also by the fact that the ion concentration is considerably higher in the infant than in the adult, although, under proper conditions in the latter, mineral deposition proceeds unimpaired.

It was Robison[9] who first set forth the hypothesis that the alkaline phosphatase found in chondroblasts and osteoblasts is the local factor which results in the precipitation of calcium salt through the liberation of inorganic phosphate by the hydrolysis of phosphate ester. It is known that alkaline phosphatase brings about this result in the test tube. The idea was further enhanced by the description of the enzymatic degradation glycogenolysis that occurs in the mature chondrocytes as they approach the line of provisional calcification. It was necessary to abandon this theory when it was shown that glycogenolysis could not produce a substrate for the action of alkaline phosphatase and with the failure to demonstrate phosphate ester even in the absence of glycogenolysis. Then it was shown that calcification takes place in vitro, though apparently at a much slower rate, when all enzymes, including phosphatase, are inactivated. At present it is assumed that glycogenolysis must play some part in the process, though it may be no more specific than supplying the necessary energy. If phosphatase plays a role it may be in the production of the ground substance. Very little more of a definitive nature can be added at this time.

References

1. Gross, J.: Structure and Biological Reactivity of Connective Tissue. *In* Ashford, M., Ed.: The Musculoskeletal System. New York, The Macmillan Co., 1952.
2. Shubert, M.: Chemistry of Connective Tissue. *In* Ashford, M., Ed.: The Musculoskeletal System. New York, The Macmillan Co., 1952.
3. McLean, F. C., and Urist, M. R.: Bone. Chicago, University of Chicago Press, 1955.
4. Jowsey, J., Kelly, P., Riggs, B., Bianco, A., Scholz, D., and Gershon-Cohen, J.: J. Bone Joint Surg., 47A:785, 1965.
5. Frost, H. M.: Stain Technol., 33:273, 1958.
6. Welsh, R.: Am. J. Path., 49:515, 1966.
7. Mellors, R.: Clin. Orthop., 45:157, 1966.
8. Neuman, W., and Neuman, M.: Chem. Rev., 53:1, 1953.
9. Robison, R.: Biochem. J., 17:256, 1923.

Chapter 3

SKELETAL EMBRYOLOGY AND PHYSIOLOGY

At a very early time in embryonic development, fields of mesenchyme undergo condensation in the pattern of a model of the skeleton that is to be formed. The intercellular substance of the reticulated cell mass becomes increasingly more opaque until a skeletal pattern develops within the surrounding mesenchyme. The cells of this condensed mesenchyme then begin to swell and in a remarkably short time the whole apparatus takes on the appearance of a hyalin cartilage matrix in which are embedded young cartilage cells.

Transverse lines of division occur at intervals dividing the apparatus into bars, each of which represents the anlage of a future bone. The divisional lines represent the areas where joints will develop. At a certain period in the development of each bone a group of reticulated mesenchymal cells approximating the masses of primitive cartilage mature into fibroblasts. In the case of long bones this occurs as a collar about the middle of the cartilage (Fig. 3–1). Capillary buds from nearby vessels grow into this collar of fibroblasts and thus set up a focus of what is known as

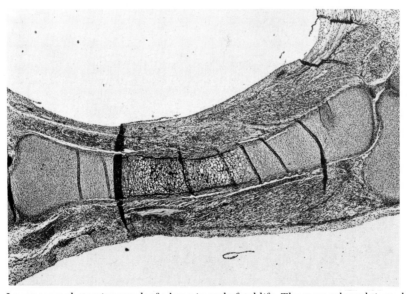

Figure 3–1   Low power photomicrograph of a bone in early fetal life. The mesenchymal tissue has thickened to form a cuff of periosteum about the mid-portion of the cartilaginous bar. The underlying cartilage cells have become swollen with glycogen in preparation for lysis and replacement with primitive fiberbone. (× 30.)

17

granulation tissue. Wherever an area of fibroblastic tissue becomes laced with a network of newly forming capillaries, whether it be in embryonic development or in the later repair of tissue injury, the resulting tissue is called granulation.

Granulation is simply highly vascularized young connective tissue. Wherever this highly vascularized tissue comes in contact with cartilage or bone, whether it be embryonic or quite mature, the cartilage and bone melt away before it. The mechanism of this important phenomenon has been poorly understood, but recently Sledge and Dingle[1] have shown that high concentrations of oxygen may facilitate liberation of hydrolases from the lysosomes within the cells. These hydrolases appear to break down the organic matrix of cartilage and perhaps bone. Thus when there is a proliferation of new vessels in the vicinity of these tissues, the increased blood supply raises the oxygen tension with lysis of cartilage and bone to form an opening into which the vessels may penetrate.

With the formation of a collar of granulation about the waist of the cartilage bar, the latter undergoes lysis and the granulation penetrates the bar from all points of its circumference until it forms a nucleus of fibroblasts and capillaries within its center. Even before completion of this activity the interfibroblastic substance in the wake of the advancing wedge becomes more dense and more eosinophilic and soon undergoes impregnation with bone salt. The fibroblasts of the vicinity take on the characteristics of osteoblasts and thus a cuff-like sheath of bone is laid down about the mid-portion of the cartilage bar. This sheath thickens and widens, extending out over the adjacent cartilage surfaces at either side. Thus is established the primary center of ossification (Fig. 3–2). At the same time the nucleus of vascularized fibroblastic tissue within the core is transformed into marrow reticulum. The structure now consists of a napkin-ring-like circle of bone, the diaphysis, surrounding a nucleus of marrow separating two masses of cartilage, the epiphyses. About the whole structure the mesenchymal cells condense to form a thin fibrous capsule. Over the bone this fibrous tissue is called periosteum; over cartilage it is known as perichondrium.

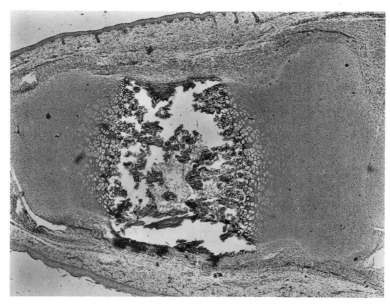

Figure 3–2   Primary center of ossification. The mid-portion of the cartilage bar has ossified. A sphere of cartilage, the epiphysis, remains at each end. At the chondro-osseous junction an epiphyseal line has formed. In the center of the bony portion, the diaphysis, the bone is undergoing lysis and a few marrow cells are beginning to appear. This embryonic bone now has all its component parts. (× 30.)

INTRAMEMBRANOUS OSSIFICATION

The periosteal tissue soon differentiates into two layers (Fig. 4–29, page 63). The outer and thicker layer is more dense and coarsely fibrillar; the inner layer is loose and more cellular. Where the cells of the inner layer, called the cambium, lie in contact with bone and cartilage, they soon become separated from them by a layer of pink-staining homogeneous substance which, because it soon becomes infiltrated with bone salt, one may call osteoid. Here and there these cells become caught in and surrounded by osteoid and then shrink to compact little cells with pyknotic nuclei within their cell spaces, the lacunae. They are now known as osteocytes. Successive layers of bone are laid down in concentric circles, each layer forming a lamina. Thus the compacta or the cortex of the diaphysis is formed. This manner of bone production, i.e., the formation of osteoid without a preformed cartilage scaffolding to shape the resultant osteoid mass, is known as intramembranous ossification. Since, in the mature skeleton, almost all of the compact bone of the shaft of long bones and nearly all of the flat bones have eventually come to be formed by this method, and since worn-out bone is so replaced in skeletal maintenance, intramembranous ossification accounts for the great bulk of the body's bone tissue.

It should be noted here that osteoblasts rarely if ever elaborate normal osteoid except in the presence of and upon pre-existing osteoid or chondroid. It appears that the presence of bone or chondroid is necessary for the metaplasia of osteoblasts from the more primitive fibroblasts. When osteoid is produced directly from fibroblasts without the presence of preformed bone or cartilage (fibro-osseous metaplasia as in fibrous dysplasia), the osteoid is not normal. In contrast, chondroid can be formed by direct metaplasia of chondroblasts from fibroblasts as in the primary ossification centers. Once chondroid is formed, normal intramembranous ossification can proceed.

ENCHONDRAL OSSIFICATION

The other manner of bone formation is known as enchondral ossification. Actually, it is essentially the same process, i.e., the transformation of fibroblasts (that in turn may have been derived from small vessel endothelial lining cells) into osteoblasts about which accumulates an intercellular organic matrix of osteoid. But in enchondral bone formation the osteoid production is always guided by a pattern of preformed, calcified chondroid. Because the steps in the production of this chondroid scaffolding are numerous, enchondral ossification is much more complex.

In general it appears that bone mass is largely the result of intramembranous ossification whereas directional bone growth is accomplished principally by enchondral bone formation. The length growth of cylindrical bones comes about through the latter and the width or strength growth through the former.

Although similar, the two processes should be kept distinct. The configuration of the skeleton, and thereby the conformation of the body, are governed by the relative amounts of each type of growth. Moreover, some of the various diseases which affect skeletal formation, growth and maintenance affect only the elaboration of normal chondroid and therefore affect only enchondral ossification; others are related to the production of osteoid by osteoblasts and thus must affect both enchondral and intramembranous ossification. There is also reason to believe that some of the various governing factors in bone formation, particularly within the endocrine group, may affect one or the other but not both mechanisms.

While the bone collar of primary ossification is forming, a frontier of advancement is set up at either pole of the nucleus of marrow tissue. This line is established at the junction of the marrow and the spheroid masses of cartilage at either end of the structure. These cartilage masses are now called the epiphyses, the line of junction is called the epiphyseal line, the connecting cylinder of bone is known as the diaphysis and the regions at either end of the diaphysis where enchondral bone formation takes place to form cancellous tissue are called the metaphyses.

The epiphysis is at first composed of a homogeneous body of cartilage, with single chondroblasts, each in its lacuna, evenly dispersed in a matrix of chondroid. Then the chondroblasts in the vicinity of the epiphyseal line begin to enlarge, the lacuna is expanded, the cytoplasm takes on a basophilic staining quality with hematoxylin and in it accumulates a substance which takes the glycogen stain. The nucleus appears to imbibe water which breaks up the chromatin and pushes it to the periphery beneath the nuclear membrane. In maturation the cytoplasm accumulates small globules of lipid. In enlarging, the cell becomes flattened, its axis parallel to the epiphyseal line.

This widening of the cells and their surrounding lacunae appears to occur at either side, in the direction of the nearest cells. The result is that the cells interdigitate and come to lie in columns the axes of which are perpendicular to the epiphyseal line (Fig. 4–17, page 51). Between the columns the unaffected chondroid remains as an acellular bar which separates or actually, in three dimensions, surrounds the columns.

Special techniques will now reveal the presence of enzymes, including alkaline phosphatase and succinic dehydrogenase,[2] within the cells, and at a certain point of maturation of the cartilage cells, i.e., at a certain level of the cell columns, bone salts begin to appear in the intervening chondroid bars. This is known as the line of provisional calcification. Each of the greatly enlarged cells, now known as mature chondrocytes, is separated from its neighbor cells on either side by a thin partition of chondroid. The distant margins of the cells at the ends of the columns, nearest the metaphysis, establish the position of the epiphyseal line. The metaphyseal sides of these cells are now exposed to the highly vascularized granulation at either pole of the marrow nucleus. The chondroid wall of the cells gives way, perhaps by the lytic activity of hydrolases released from lysosomes within the cells under the influence of an elevated oxygen tension. The budding

vessel grows into the hiatus thus formed. The multiplying endothelial cells of this structure are pressed against the chondroid wall of the newly formed chamber. One can often find that these cells have joined to form a giant cell which presumably is an osteoclast. One must pose the question, "Are osteoclasts formed at the advancing tip of each vessel and are these cells instrumental in chondroid lysis?" These observations are also important support for the hypothesis that osteoblasts of enchondral bone formation are derived from endothelial vessel lining cells perhaps through mediation of fibroblasts.

Thus the granulation works its way up the column, cell after cell, the last intact cell establishing the level of the epiphyseal line. So the epiphyseal frontier advances, leaving in its wake in the metaphyseal area the intact calcified bars of chondroid which formerly separated (surrounded) the cellular columns, protruding into the granulation like parallel docks extending into a harbor. The single layer of cells which appears to be derived from the endothelial cells previously described, or transitional cells (fibroblasts) of the same origin, now elaborate a seam of osteoid over the calcified chondroid core. The entire process is known as enchondral ossification.

It is apparent that unless fresh cartilage cells were added to the epiphysis, the advancing epiphyseal line would soon spend the available supply and epiphyseal advancement would necessarily cease. New chondroblasts are supplied by division of the young chondroblasts in the depths of the epiphysis—interstitial proliferation—and by metaplasia of the fibroblasts in the deep layers of the surrounding perichondrium—appositional proliferation. As they mature they go through the same cycle as their predecessors. They swell with glycogen and take on enzymatic activity, their cytoplasm develops a blue color with hematoxylin and they columnate and apparently cause mineralization of the surrounding chondroid. Thus the epiphysis is continuously being replenished at one pole and dissipated at the other and length growth of the bone is accomplished by the chondroblastic addition.

The bone of the primary spicules is

coarsely fibrillar; the fibrils run in undisciplined, patternless directions, and the numerous cells that are caught within their ramifications are young and plump. This material is known as primitive bone, coarse fiberbone or "woven" bone (Fig. 4–25, page 59). As these spicules age they appear to dissolve, perhaps because of the lack of a stress stimulus which appears to be necessary for the persistence and health of all bone tissue. The resolving fragments, however, serve as the nidi for a new coat of osteoid laid down by more mature osteoblasts. This time the fibrillar structure is finer; the fibrils are longer and run in parallel bundles in the trajectory lines of stress (Fig. 4–26, page 61). Fewer cells are trapped and they are smaller and more mature, now called osteocytes. These spicules form the secondary spongiosa.

Where the mass of bone necessary to withstand the stress to which it is exposed is greater than a few lamellae in thickness, the lamellae are laid down in concentric rings about a blood vessel, thus insuring a supply of blood to the contained osteocytes. The larger vessels travel in a longitudinal direction and thus their surrounding bone sheaths are oriented in the same direction except where a branch passes horizontally to connect two longitudinal vessels. The spaces carrying vessels (and accompanying nerves and supportive collagenous tissue) are known as haversian canals, and the concentric laminae of bone, oriented with them, make up a haversian system. The tunnels carrying the connecting vessels are known as Volkmann's canals.

A cross section through the full thickness of the cortex (compacta) reveals numerous haversian canals (Fig. 4–30, page 65), circular hiatuses bearing the blood vessels and running longitudinally, parallel to the periosteal surface. These canals are formed by sheaths of bone appearing in cross section as circles and crescents. Each canal and its multilayered sheath of lamellae form a haversian system. The irregular areas which fill in the regions between the haversian systems are also composed of lamellar bone but the concentric arrangement is lacking. These are known as interstitial lamellae. Most adult bone is ensheathed by several lamellae

which encircle the entire circumference of the shaft beneath the periosteum. In some bones one may find a sheath of several lamellae lining the inner cortical surface about the medullary canal.

At a certain period in the development and maturation of each bone a column of granulation invades the spheroid cartilaginous mass of the epiphysis from the perichondrium and penetrates into its very center. Here an aggregate of proliferating connective tissue cells is established just as in the wedge of granulation that resulted in the primary center of ossification. And in a like manner a nucleus of marrow cells surrounded by a shell of mineralized bone is formed.

The chondroblasts in the overlying zone of cartilage, the articular plate, but not those of the enchondral or growth plate, which are now adjacent to bone respond in the same manner as those along the epiphyseal line. They enlarge, flatten and columnate and set up a new zone of provisional calcification which in this case is a spheroid shell rather than a flat plate. This nucleus of bone is called the secondary center of ossification or the epiphyseal ossification center or, in practical usage, simply the center of ossification since the primary ossification center has long since disappeared.

Radiologists are apt to refer to the secondary center of ossification as "the epiphysis." This center grows by the addition of crescent-shaped laminae of osteoid applied by the cells of the concave face of the articular plate. Thus the osseous nucleus is provided solely by activity of the cells of the epiphyseal line between it and the articular plate and is not a function of the growth plate.[3] The latter is responsible for the much more rapid length growth of the diaphysis. These facts become of great importance in analyzing the various types of growth deformity which characterize the skeletal dysplasias.

The time of the appearance of the secondary center of ossification is specific for each bone. It is present in the distal femoral epiphysis at birth but does not appear in some other bones until much later in skeletal growth.

Length growth of the cylindrical bones is thus accomplished by the apposition of new bone at the ends of the diaphysis. Frequently the rate of growth is not equal at both ends. The femur acquires most of its length growth by bone apposition at the distal end. The ulna and radius do the same. The proximal end is that of major growth in the humerus whereas the tibia has approximately equal growth at both ends.

As the time of completion of length growth is approached, the proliferation of chondroblasts in the growth plate slows and eventually ceases. Thus in a short time the chondrocytes of the growth plate are exhausted and the epiphyseal line advances to the diaphyseal surface of the osseous nucleus. When no cartilage remains separating the diaphysis from the bony portion of the epiphysis the center of ossification is said to be closed, fused or ossified. From this point hence, normal length growth is at an end. In certain instances (hyperpituitarism) the cells at persisting cartilage bone junctions, i.e., the opposed interfaces of the articular plate and ossified epiphysis, may be reactivated. Under this condition length growth may be resumed after skeletal maturation. Normally, a line of junction can be discerned on the roentgenogram for a considerable time but eventually this is obliterated by bony union. The articular plate remains as a cap of hyalin cartilage covering the end of the bone. The time of closure for each epiphysis is specific. The condylar cartilage of the mandible is the last to ossify, normally in the late twenties. Thus, by mapping the time of appearance and ossification of the various secondary centers throughout the skeleton one can often calculate its age, if it be under 25 years, to within a few months.

In a general way it may be stated that the human organism, in the course of his development, has three types of skeletons and that he changes these skeletons with growth just as does the crustacean that wears its skeleton on the outside. The first skeleton is composed of flexible cartilage, adequate in situations in which coordinated movement is unimportant and in which support is provided by the surrounding uterine walls. Since the skeleton is still moderately flexible at parturition, this flexibility lessens the danger of traumatic injury in the passage of the fetus through the narrow birth canal.

The second skeleton is composed of primitive fiberbone and this type of bone predominates thoughout the first 18 months of life. It is more rigid than cartilage and more resilient than adult bone. This type of bone makes "green stick" fracture possible in childhood. This type of bone is found in the marine vertebrates which must have coordinated movement but are supported by their environment. It is adequate for the infant who spends much of his time in the supine position.

When both support and movement are essential to the organism the primitive bone must be replaced by a more rigid structure laid down in the trajectory lines of stress. Thus, there is a gradual replacement of coarse fiberbone by the finer grained, oriented adult bone which is constructed along the pathways of greatest stress. In a sense, these changes in skeleton type constitute a phylogenetic recapitulation of the species.

Empirically, it may be said that the preponderance of bone mass and the cortical thickness of long bones are produced by intramembranous ossification. The length and shape of long bones are governed by enchondral ossification and the forces of stress. It is interesting that in certain skeletal diseases these two processes appear to rely upon different governing mechanisms. Thus in some developmental disturbances, such as achondroplasia, intramembranous bone formation is normal, but because there is faulty cartilage production the normal progression of the steps in enchondral ossification is interrupted. Likewise, cartilage formation may progress normally, as in osteogenesis imperfecta, but there is an inability to form an adequate amount of normal bone. In either instance the effects of stress are compromised, making it difficult or impossible to determine the exact point at which the physiologic chain of events is broken.

The interesting phenomenon of growth arrest lines or Harris' lines depends upon the activity, or rather the lack of it, in the chondroblastic cells of the growth plate. In the starved experimental animal and in a number of disease states in the human, growth plate chondroblasts cease to proliferate. When this happens a dome formed of a solid plate of bone is laid down across the metaphysis. When growth is reestablished this horizontal line persists and appears on the radiograph.

FACTORS IN NORMAL BONE PRODUCTION

Though enchondral bone formation is a continuing process, the various steps, which merge imperceptibly one into another often with considerable chronologic overlap, may be listed as follows:

1. Proliferation of epiphyseal chondroblasts at the junction of the cartilaginous and osseous portions of the epiphysis to maintain normal thickness of the growth plate.

2. The formation of intercellular chondroid.

3. Maturation of chondroblasts with the acquisition of glycogen and enzymatic activity, enlargement and rearrangement into columns.

4. Mineralization of the chondroid bars to form the line of provisional calcification.

5. Invasion of the bases of the cartilage cell columns by metaphyseal new vessel growth.

6. Metaplasia of endothelial lining cells to osteoblasts (through fibroblasts?).

7. The production of the organic matrix of bone, osteoid.

8. The deposition of mineral salts within the osteoid.

9. The resolution of the chondroid cores of the spicules of the primary spongiosa.

10. The conversion of coarse fiberbone to adult bone to form the secondary spongiosa.

11. Modeling of young bones to attain the shape of the adult structure.

12. Bone maintenance, i.e., the replacement of bone which is being constantly eroded by normal catabolic activity.

It is apparent that these steps form a continuing chronologic chain and that a deviation at any link may result in an abnormal skeletal structure which one associates with bone disease. A great many of the factors which control normal skeleton formation, growth and maintenance are unknown, but it is evident that if one is to successfully prevent these deviations or to reverse them, once they are diagnosed, to a state of bone health an understanding of these factors is essential. The following is a résumé of what is known and what is assumed concerning some of these factors.

The discussion may be presented under three broad headings:

1. Factors related to the formation of the organic matrix of normal cartilage and bone.

2. Factors related to the deposition of mineral salt in the organic matrix of cartilage and bone.

3. Factors related to the normal lysis of cartilage and bone to allow for conversion from primitive to adult bone, modeling of young to mature bone and maintenance of adult bone to compensate for physiologic erosion.

Factors Related to the Formation of the Organic Matrix

Diet. It has long been known that the level of the dietary caloric intake influences the ultimate skeletal stature. Presumptive evidence may be drawn from a comparison of averages of skeletal size in a race which is known to exist on a bare subsistence diet, such as those in certain parts of China and India, with a race whose caloric intake is adequate and more than sufficient, such as the American. It is not inferred that an inadequate caloric intake affects only the skeleton. Skeletal growth is probably inhibited as a part of the general low metabolic state of all tissues. One can cause the complete cessation of growth plate chondroblastic replication and/or maturation by starving the experimental animal. This results in cessation of length growth of long bones, and on recovery the scar, a horizontal plate of bone appearing as the growth arrest line on the roentgenogram, marks the site of the epiphyseal line at the time food was withheld.

In more specific instances the diet may lack certain essential foodstuffs which are required for normal bone growth and maintenance. Among these, certain proteins probably head the list. It is interesting that the "essential amino acids" listed by the physiologic chemists as necessary for a state of body health have not been identified in cartilage and bone analysis. The amino acids which are involved in bone structure are abundant in ordinary diets. Nevertheless it is thought by most that the fastidious and often whimsical diets of the aged may constitute a factor in senile osteoporosis, and the leaching of skeletons of war populations in a state of chronic starvation (Fig. 3–3) may be due, at least in part, to qualitative dietary deficiencies.

Wolbach[4] in 1947 postulated that a certain amount of vitamin A in one of its forms is necessary for normal epiphyseal cartilage cell growth, maturation, degeneration and bone modeling. It now appears that vitamin A probably relates to chondroblast replication and that once formed these cells are able to mature in the deficiency state. It has been stated[4] that with inadequate amounts of this vitamin there is failure of normal resolution of bone, though surface apposition of bone is not impaired, so that normal modeling cannot take place.

In the experimental animal an ascorbic acid deficiency results in metabolic disturbances in the tissues of mesenchymal derivation. In the human the bleeding phenomena, inadequate scar formation in wound healing and deficiencies in organic bone matrix formation with low ascorbic acid blood levels suggest that this substance is essential for the formation of normal collagen and osteoid. The manifestations of childhood scurvy as seen in the skeleton can all be ascribed to hemorrhage and an inability of the osteoblasts to lay down osteoid (Fig. 3–4). The defect appears to be caused

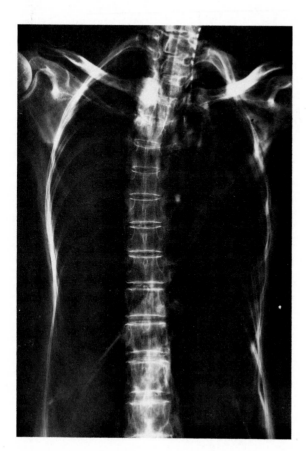

Figure 3–3 Roentgenogram of a patient showing severe starvation osteoporosis. This patient lived for months before her death on a daily ration of a few soda crackers and a cup of tea.

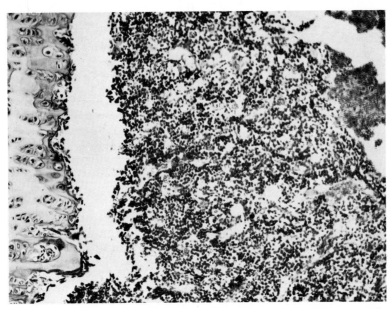

Figure 3–4 Photomicrograph of a section taken across the epiphyseal line in a patient with scurvy. There is a complete lack of osteoid production and, therefore, no cancellous bone in the metaphysis. (× 200.)

by an inability residing within the osteoblastic cytoplasm to synthesize the triple polypeptide chain that constitutes the collagen fibril of osteoid.

Hormonal Disturbances. Disturbances in endocrine hormone secretion quite certainly can be incriminated in certain abnormal skeletal conditions. It has long been known that atrophy and destruction of the anterior lobe of the pituitary are frequently associated with various types of dwarfism, and an abnormal proliferation of eosinophilic cells (eosinophilic adenoma) has been seen in states of skeletal overgrowth, giantism and acromegaly. More recently a growth hormone has been isolated from the glandular portion of the hypophysis cerebri. This is known as the somatotropic growth hormone or human growth hormone (HGH).

It is known that there is cessation of bone growth without closure of the ossification centers in the hypophysectomized animal and that growth may be restored with the growth hormone. It appears also that closure of the ossification centers may be delayed beyond the normal period with this hormone, the epiphyseal plate retaining its normal thickness. The exact point of influence is not known

but it would seem at this writing that the growth hormone governs chondroblastic activity essentially though probably not exclusively and, therefore, registers its effect on enchondral bone growth. HGH elaboration is apparently correlated with serum sugar levels and therefore with insulin secretion. High insulin, low sugar levels stimulate HGH synthesis or release.

It is not anticipated that therapeutic use of the pituitary growth hormone will greatly reduce the distressing consequences of all cases of pituitary dysfunction, since in many cases aberrations in eosinophilic cell secretion are accompanied by perversions of other pituitary hormone production.

Children born with inadequate thyroid secretory function fail to develop a normal skeletal stature and in cases of excessive thyroid secretion there is abnormal deossification of the bone that has already been formed. Again it is not known at which link in the complicated chain of bone growth the inadequacy is registered but the effect appears to be predominantly upon enchondral bone formation so that the stature is dwarfed. The result of inadequate thyroid function appears to be quite similar or identical to that of deficient pituitary hormone secretion. It has been postulated that the subnormal skeletal growth seen in the thyroid deficient state is caused by inadequate human growth hormone secretion by the pituitary, and that the latter is somehow dependent upon a stimulating factor elaborated by the thyroid perhaps to convert the neutral chromophobe to eosinophilic cells. The skeletal leaching which occurs in the severe and prolonged thyrotoxic state has been ascribed to a squandering of the essential proteins necessary for bone maintenance by the exaggerated basal metabolic rate. This explanation appears to be based largely upon assumption.

Concerning the steroid hormones elaborated by the gonads and the adrenal cortex, there is even less factual information and one is apt to find that a perusal of the reports available leads to contradictory findings. It is probably true that gonadal androgen stimulates both enchondral and intramembranous bone growth, i.e., it causes the osteoblast to elaborate organic matrix. Such has been ascribed to be the reason why the male skeleton is usually larger and heavier than that of the female.[5] The results of some studies suggest that the period of skeletal growth at which the abnormal gonadal function occurs is an important factor. If castration in the male occurs before puberty there may be an increase in long bone growth. In general, it is probably true that gonadal androgen supports osteoblastic elaboration of osteoid and therefore stimulates both length and width growth in the bones of animals and the adolescent human but it also influences the enchondral growth centers to close by increasing the osteoid production rate over the rate of chondroblast proliferation so that the growth plate is diminished in depth with premature fusion of the ossification center. If this hormone is deficient

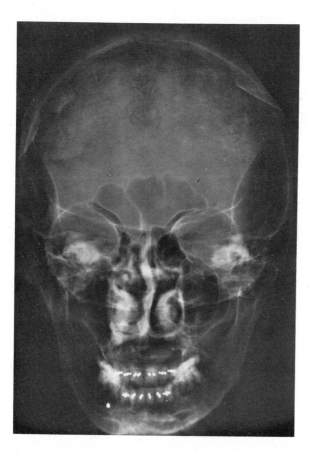

Figure 3–5 Roentgenogram of the skull of a patient with postmenopausal osteoporosis. The degree of osteoporosis is as severe in the skull as in other bones in contrast to the deossification consequent to disuse atrophy.

in childhood, closure of growth centers is delayed, the growth period is prolonged and the eventual result is abnormal bone length (eunichoid giantism).

The adrenal cortical androgen or so-called N hormone is generally regarded as the anabolic hormone for all protein-rich tissues. It has a potent anabolic action but a weak masculinizing effect. The effects of the sugar active hormones from the adrenal cortex which are supposed to produce deossification similar to that seen in Cushing's syndrome are thought by some to rob the stores of amino acids for neoglycogenesis, thus counteracting the effects of cortical androgen. Again these statements are largely hypothetical.

The so-called gonadotropic hormones from the trophoblastic cells of the placenta are said to have an androgenic effect upon bone growth when injected into the experimental animal. It is uncertain whether this effect is a direct action or mediated through the gonads or adrenal cortex or both.

Concerning the granulosa cell secretion from the ovary (estrogen) there seems to be more conclusive evidence, at least on an experimental ground. It has been well established by a number of investigators that certain birds, principally pigeons, and some mammals develop a measurable increase in the calcified spongiosa under the influence of high estrogen levels. This increase may be reversed by reducing the estrogen to normal. Atrophy of the ovaries and, therefore, presumably a low estrogen level have been thought to contribute to the cause of post-menopausal osteoporosis (Fig. 3–5). This may be true but therapy consisting of estrogen alone in an attempt to build up the osteoporotic skeleton is apt to be disappointing probably because other factors, osteomalacia and osteolysis as well as osteopenia, may be concerned in this disease. The effect of estrogen and the androgens on osteoid formation may not be due to direct stimulation of osteoblasts. Conceivably it could be due to an inhibitory action upon a bony lysing agent such as parathormone possibly through a repressive action on the formation of osteoclasts.

Factors Related to the Deposition of Mineral Salt in the Organic Matrix of Cartilage and Bone

Just as there is a critical caloric and protein dietary level for organic matrix production so must there be an adequate supply of calcium and phosphorus available for mineralization. Since both are relatively ubiquitous materials found in a wide range of food substances, dietary inadequacy is almost unheard of in populations of average living standards. In China, where in some areas there is no milk, calcium deficiency may lead to bone disease. At least some of the infantile rickets seen in this country is probably due to a low protein diet and inadequate supplies of phosphorus.

More important to the availability of sufficient quantities of calcium and phosphorus for normal bone formation are factors which influence absorption through the gut wall. Apparently phosphorus absorption is obligatory and if adequate amounts are ingested they reach the blood. The absorption of the calcium ion is more complicated. Insoluble soaps may be formed with large amounts of abnormal lipids produced as a result of celiac disease. Or the bowel wall may be the site of chronic and extensive disease which impairs the absorption function. This coupled with diarrhea may result in an inadequate absorption of calcium.

The Action of Vitamin D. More important than either the dietary amount or the state of the gut wall is the necessity for an adequate amount of vitamin D. It is now widely agreed that vitamin D is the principal governing factor in the absorption of calcium (Fig. 3–6). The actual mechanism of this function is still incompletely understood but recent evidence has been produced to help explain some of the puzzling aspects of calcium metabolism.[6] The prime purpose of vitamin D appears to be to aid the regulation of serum calcium levels; all other actions are of secondary importance. This function is apparently achieved by two different metabolites of vitamin D effective at two

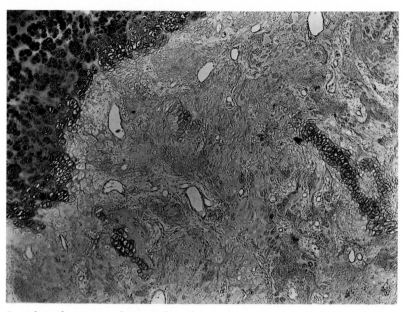

Figure 3–6 In rickets there is ample osteoid production but a paucity of calcium salts for mineralization. At the upper left, one sees the cartilaginous epiphysis. In the metaphysis there are islands of cartilage surrounded by osteoid. This material remains soft and unmineralized. (× 40.)

different tissue sites. It appears that vitamin D_3 is picked up by the liver from the plasma and hydroxylated to 25-hydroxycholecalciferol (25-HCC) and released in the plasma as a hormonal form of the vitamin. This hormone appears to act directly upon bone to release mineral salts. The 25-HCC in the serum reaches the kidney where it is further hydrolized to form 1,25-dihydroxycholecalciferol (1,25-DHCC). This metabolite is necessary for transport of the calcium ion across the gut wall and into the serum.

It is known that in the chronic vitamin D toxic state there is widespread deossification. It is also known that vitamin D in large doses increases the citrate content of bone. It is assumed, therefore, that this citrate acts as a chelating agent to transport calcium ions from bone crystal against the concentration gradient into the serum. Because huge doses of vitamin D over an extended period of time are necessary to elicit this effect, these cases are now rarely encountered. Clinically, these cases may precisely mimic parathyroid adenoma. They usually can be differentiated by a higher serum phosphorus level and, of course, by obtaining the history of excessive vitamin D intake (Fig. 3–7).

Finally, vitamin D in very large amounts apparently causes the kidney to conserve phosphorus. This statement is made with caution since the mechanism of this phosphorus-saving action is not known with certainty. In a small group of cases which are variously known as vitamin D refractory rickets or Fanconi syndrome in children and Milkman's syndrome in adults, abnormal amounts of phosphate, glucose, amino acids, bicarbonate, uric acid and potassium or various combinations of these are lost in the urine owing to a congenital inadequacy in children and usually an acquired disease in adults. The site of dysfunction is apparently the proximal convoluted tubules.[7] The phosphate loss leads to a protracted and severe type of rickets in the skeleton (hypophosphatemic rickets). Several reports by a number of authors[8] indicate that vitamin D in massive doses causes a reversal of this disturbance with phosphate retention. From this it has been assumed that the mode and site of action of vitamin D in this disease are enhancement of phosphate reabsorption by the epithelial lining cells of the tubule.

The Effects of Parathyroid Hormone. Before Mandl first removed an enlarged parathyroid gland for demineralizing

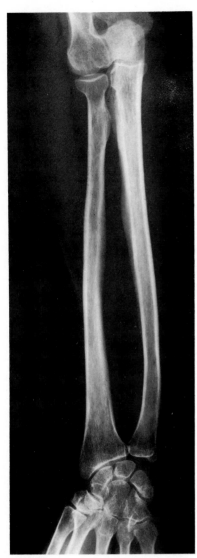

Figure 3–7 Roentgenogram of the forearm of a patient suffering from hypervitaminosis D. The entire skeleton reveals a loss of substance. Here the cortices are abnormally thin.

skeletal disease in 1925, there was considerable speculation concerning the relationship of the parathyroid hormone and bone calcification. Erdheim had postulated that enlargement of the parathyroid glands was the result and not the cause of the high serum calcium levels in demineralizing bone disease. Mandl's operation with like observations made in the United States at about the same time established the causal role of parathyroid enlargement, and therefore presumably the action of its secretion. There remained to be explained the mechanism of the compensatory hyperplasia of the glands in states of chronic low serum calcium levels. Ten years later Castleman and Mallory reviewed the pathology of parathyroid hyperplasia and parathyroid adenoma,[9] but the vagaries of morphology still haunt the pathologist in attempting to differentiate parathyroid adenoma, idiopathic primary hyperplasia (so-called) and secondary hyperplasia on the basis of microscopy.

It is now fairly generally agreed that the parathyroid is not responsible to any other gland secretion for its activity but rather it is governed by the serum calcium level. When the serum calcium content falls below a certain critical level the glands increase their secretory activity. Though high serum phosphate levels have been reported with supposed increased parathormone secretion it appears that the latter is due to lowered calcium levels caused by the influence of pituitary, adrenocortical or islet secretions or combinations of these which also cause high phosphate levels.[10]

Though the multiple target activities of the product of parathyroid secretion have led to the hypothesis that the gland may secrete two or more separate hormones, recent purification techniques have not substantiated this theory. Present evidence indicates that bovine parathyroid hormone is a protein consisting of a single polypeptide chain.[11]

Parathormone apparently has two major sites of activity which have been well documented by numerous workers, and two less important sites of equivocal standing. The last two may be dismissed in a sentence. Parathyroid secretion may enhance absorption of calcium through the bowel wall and inhibit secretion of calcium in breast lactation. The other two actions deserve more discussion. Barnicot[12] and later Chang[13] demonstrated that when parathyroid tissue is placed in direct contact with bone, the latter undergoes deossification. The mechanism of this resorption is not clear but it has been shown both experimentally and in clinical material that parathormone increases the number of osteoclasts in the bone tissue affected. The origin of these osteoclasts is unproved but it is assumed by most that they are formed by osteoblasts. It is common knowledge that osteoclasts are increased in number in hyperparathyroidism.

Though the mechanism of their action is not known, it is generally agreed that osteoclasts are the main, perhaps even the sole, agents of bone dissolution. It is postulated that the increase in the elaboration of citrate, a calcium-chelating substance, due to the influence of parathormone explains the transport of calcium ions from bone salt crystal to the bathing extracellular fluids against the ion concentration gradient. It is probable that the organic matrix, i.e., the osteoid collagen fibril, is dissolved, freeing its contained calcium salts.

Concerning the possibility of another action site of parathormone there has been more controversy, but it is now generally agreed that this hormone acts upon the lining cells of the proximal convolutions of the kidney tubules to cause an increase in the amount of phosphate in the urine and a lowering of the serum phosphate level. Albright and coworkers[14] stated that this action was accomplished by an inhibitory effect upon the reabsorption of phosphates from the glomerular filtrate. Evidence has been published more recently[15] to indicate that parathormone probably increases the secretion of phosphates by these cells, thus producing the "phosphate diuresis" effect.

In hypoparathyroidism there is a failure of utilization of the skeletal calcium stores with lowering of the serum calcium level to cause tetany. Recently, a pseudohypoparathyroidism has been described in which the parathyroid glands are normal in appearance but if the hormone is secreted the skeleton apparently does not undergo the usual resorption.

Kidney Function. Kidney function has been mentioned as a factor in the maintenance of a normal calcium and phosphate balance. In Albright's "tubular-insufficiency-without-glomerular-insufficiency," and in cases of high phosphate renal clearance, other kidney functions such as glomerular filtration are normal so that the principal action is lowering of the serum calcium level, of the serum phosphate level or a combination, and the effect is upon the skeleton. The patient may not manifest a general nephritic symptomatology. However, in kidney disease severe enough to produce an acidosis over a long continued period without killing the patient the serum calcium level is lowered and the parathyroids are stimulated. This effect has been explained in the past as an improvident use of the basic calcium cation to combat the acidosis. More recent evidence[16] suggests that the diseased kidney may be unable to convert vitamin D to the metabolite which governs calcium transport through the gut wall thus lowering the serum calcium level by inadequate supply. Chronic low calcium levels eventually cause a secondary parathyroid hyperplasia and this condition must then be differentiated from parathyroid adenoma. The distinction may be difficult in some cases but usually the impaired kidney tubules are unable to respond to the excessive parathormone level and a failure of phosphorus diuresis results in high serum phosphorus levels. This in conjunction with the serum chemistry and, eventually, the symptoms of chronic uremia usually serves to differentiate renal rickets with secondary parathyroid hyperplasia from parathyroid adenoma.

Finally, it has now been established with reasonable certainty that the acinar cells of the thyroid gland, and probably some interacinar cells, those cells which are derived from the ultimobranchial elements, either elaborate or are related to the elaboration of a polypeptide hormone known as thyrocalcitonin which is concerned with the release of mineral salts from the organic matrix of bone.[16, 17, 18, 19] Its secretion or release appears to be dependent upon serum calcium levels and therefore acts as a counterbalance to parathormone activity which increases this level.[20] There is some evidence that a similar polypeptide with the same function is produced by the parathyroid gland, called calcitonin[21] but convincing data for the existence of this hormone are still wanting. The action of thyrocalcitonin may be mediated by the inhibition of the formation of osteoclasts. There is some evidence for its deossification action in tissue culture, suggesting that it is not due to an antagonistic action on parathormone.

There may be a factor resident in osteoid itself which is concerned with its infiltration by mineral. Glimcher has shown that young fibrous connective tissue collagen (before its three polypeptide chains are cross linked) is soluble in dilute acetic acid. When heated the solution gels; when cooled it expands. The collagen of bone matrix, though identical when evaluated by x-ray diffraction, electron microscopy and even amino acid determination, does neither of these. On the other hand, bone collagen is soluble in potassium thiocyanide solution whereas tendon collagen is not. He states that the polypeptide chains of bone collagen are held together by noncovalent links and that when mineral is deposited in osteoid collagen fibers, it displaces water. The forces involved are not costatic and covalent and so recall the van der Waal explanation. He believes this difference may account for the ability of bone collagen to pick up mineral ions.

Factors Related to the Normal Lysis of Bone and Cartilage

Finally, for normal skeletal growth, maturation and maintenance, the factors that govern conversion of coarse fiberbone to adult bone, modeling and the replenishment of physiologic erosion must be considered.

The stress stimulus is doubtless the most important of these. Throughout the skeleton, mechanical stress is apparently necessary to convert primitive bone to the adult type. Without it the lamellae remain unoriented and pressure causes distortion. These distortion effects are seen in several of the congenital, developmental disturbances in which there is an inability to convert fiberbone to adult bone, perhaps because the fiberbone is abnormal from the beginning.

The effect of the stress stimulus, or rather the lack of it, can be dramatically illustrated by the comparison of the roentgenogram of a normal extremity bone with that of the same bone after it has been im-

mobilized in a cast for several weeks. If immobilization has been complete, severe deossification of the bone is apparent (Fig. 3–8). When considerable portions of the body are put in a cast and the patient is at bed rest, skeletal demineralization may be severe enough to cause a rise in serum calcium levels and even metastatic calcification of soft tissues and nephrolithiasis.[22]

Modeling of bones is almost completely the result of the reorientation of the lamellae into haversian systems laid down in the trajectory lines of mechanical stress. Stress may be a matter of pressure or of tension but apparently either or an alternating of both may cause conversion from fiberbone to adult bone. This conversion results in a reshaping of the bone as a whole and this physiologic reshaping is known as modeling. Bone modeling may be graphically illustrated by superimposing the roentgenogram of an extremity bone of an adult over that of the same bone taken during early childhood (Fig. 3–9). It will be seen that the midportion of the earlier diaphysis has been expanded and thickened whereas the metaphyseal flare has undergone resorption to accommodate the silhouette of the longer shaft of the adult bone.

The principles of modeling can be understood by studying a longitudinal section through the secondary callus of fracture site of a long bone in a case in which alignment has not been good (Fig. 3–10). On the outer cortical surface representing the apex of angulation one finds subperiosteal osteoclastic resorption of bone, and on the inner cortical surface there is a compensatory building up of bone by osteoblastic apposition. At the same level across the bone there is bone absorption from the medullary surface and the laying down of new lamellae beneath the periosteum of the outer surface. Thus, there is accomplished a gradual reduction in angulation so that trajectory lines are straightened by a progressive shifting of the angulation area into a line with the epiphyses without interrupting tubulation.

The mechanism of pressure and tension changes in bone is not entirely clear. It is agreed that stress in physiologic tra-

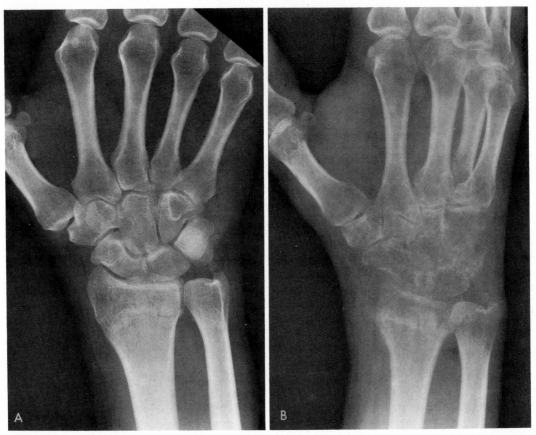

Figure 3-8 *A,* Roentgenogram of the carpal area shortly after fracture of the distal radius. The part was immobilized by a plaster cast. *B,* Roentgenogram of the same area several weeks after immobilization. Note the disuse atrophy of the carpal bones.

jectory lines causes conversion of fiber-bone to adult bone and stimulates osteoblasts to form sufficient osteoid to maintain the cortical thickness which would otherwise be diminished by normal catabolic activity in the mature skeleton. But if pressure is applied at right angles to the long axis of a cylindrical bone quite a different effect is seen. There is apt to be resorption of bone in the path of the stress. The explanation has been offered that the pressure interferes with the blood supply and that the impoverished bone wears away and is not replaced. This could scarcely be called a realistic explanation since elsewhere in the skeleton it is commonly observed that decreasing the vascularity stimulates organic matrix production and mineralization so that the bone becomes more dense.

It has been suggested that a decreased blood supply to bone would allow an increase in citrate concentration at the cell site.[23] This in turn would promote demineralization of the nearby bone matrix. This explanation does not agree with the practical finding that bone tends to become more dense in areas of decreased blood supply. Moreover, the chemical action of citrate may explain the mechanism of decalcification but it does not account for the dissolution of the collagen fibers of the bone matrix which precedes it.

It would seem more logical to suggest that stress stimulates bone in the direction of its trajectory lines, thus causing it to be oriented into haversian systems coursing parallel to these lines. Stress applied perpendicular to the long axes of the haversian systems causes resorption and eventual reorganization with a

90 degree rotation. Such is the fundamental character of bone formation. An explanation of the mechanisms may reside in some observations made by Bassett.[24] In cultures of osteoblastic cells traversed by an electric current he noted a florid cellular activity about the negative pole. Mature bone is said to be a pseudoconductor of electrical current; i.e., at rest it is a nonconductor and when stress is applied it becomes a conductor. It has been noted that a curved or deformed cylindrical bone is electronegative on the concave side and positive on the convex. This may explain the localization of osteoblastic activity in stress lines.

The nature of the biphasic electrical current that is generated during application and release of mechanical force to bone has been investigated by Cochran et al.[25] This complicated subject needs a great deal of clarification to explain how electrical activity caused by stress affects biologic systems.

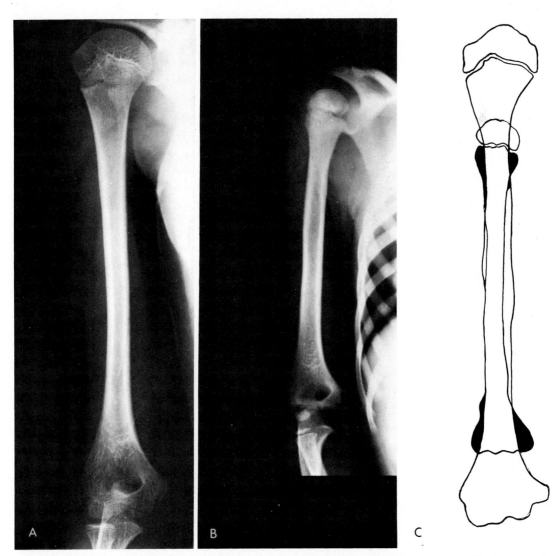

Figure 3-9 *A*, Roentgenogram of the humerus of a 12 year old patient. *B*, Roentgenogram of the humerus of a 5 year old patient. *C*, Line drawing representing the silhouettes of the two bones illustrated in *A* and *B*. The blackened areas are the portions of the younger bone that must undergo lysis to form the shaft of the older bone. This is a part of the process of modeling.

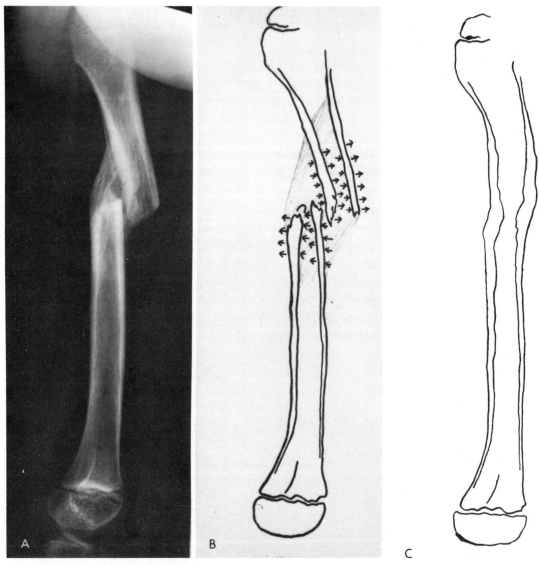

Figure 3–10 *A*, Roentgenogram of a fractured femur showing angulation. *B*, Drawing of the bone shown in *A*. The arrows pointing away from the cortical surface indicate lysis. Those pointing toward the cortical surface indicate apposition. Under the influence of stress there is a gradual shifting and realignment without reducing bone mass or diminishing bone strength. *C*, Eventually alignment may be achieved because of bone shifting into the trajectories of stress.

The Osteoclast. Most observers contend that this cell causes deossification, i.e., the disappearance of both organic matrix and its mineral content. This opinion is based largely on the facts that osteoclasts are usually found in large numbers where bone is undergoing resorption, they are often hard to find at sites where bone is predominantly building, and they

are found in Howship's lacunae, where it is supposed they have nibbled out the bone which they replace.

Some authors contend on the other hand that osteoclasts are merely scavenger cells which come in to phagocytize the debris produced by bone degeneration. But incriminatory evidence of bone fragments and minerals has not been demonstrated within their cytoplasm though other evidence of phagocytic activity has been noted.

The reports of Pommer and von Kollicker in earlier days of bone pathology were fraught with polemics but more recently the controversy has simmered with the admission on the part of most that neither the genesis nor function of the osteoclast is absolutely known.

Some facts and assumptions which are probably related to osteoclastic activity are summarized:

Though osteoid which has never been mineralized can be demonstrated, demineralized organic matrix is probably never seen in tissue section. Apparently the osteoid disintegrates first, thus releasing the mineral, or in the process of demineralization the matrix is simultaneously destroyed. The former seems the more plausible since in the laboratory the mineral may be removed in a variety of ways leaving an intact matrix. Thus the term "decalcified" or "demineralized" osteoid is loosely used. The more exact term is "deossification."

The complete mechanism of calcium salt deposition is not known. It is believed by some that a local factor related to the chemistry of the mucopolysaccharide matrix is necessary. Perhaps a reversal of the change which invokes salt deposition may release it by osteoid lysis.

Chondroid ground substance undergoes depolymerization before mineral is deposited.

The fiber structure of collagen is destroyed by collagenase.

The mucopolysaccharide portion of the matrix is changed by hyaluronidase.

Calcium salts go into solution by a lowering of the pH or are enticed from their crystal lattice by a chelating substance.

Parathormone, vitamin D and probably vitamin A have the ability of destroying bone on contact. It is not known whether this is a direct action, whether mediated by another agent produced by their action or whether they stimulate the production and activity of osteoclasts.

The origin of the osteoclast is not known. Some observers report a conversion of osteoblasts into osteoclasts and back to osteoblasts by raising and then lowering the estrogen level in pigeons and mice. Certain workers have felt that osteoclasts are formed by the simple merging of macrophages or histiocytes. Others have observed their formation from endothelial lining cells of budding capillaries or from fibroblasts which themselves arise from endothelial cells. It is probable that the osteoclast represents a late stage of the cell life span. It has been seen to divide to form two osteoclasts but it probably does not dedifferentiate to produce normal osteoblasts under normal conditions. We believe that it probably originates by a multiplication of the nuclei of the vessel lining endothelial cell or mesenchymal reserve cell without division of the cytoplasm.

The chemistry of intracytoplasmic metabolism of the osteoclast is largely unknown. Under experimental conditions osteoclasts have been observed to cause bone resorption.[26] The direct application of parathormone or of vitamin D to bone results in an increase in the number of osteoclasts in the area. It may be that the action of these substances is not directly upon the cells but is mediated by their resorptive action on bone.[27]

Thus, it appears that if the osteoclast is capable of destroying normal bone it must possess a factor or factors whose action is similar to that of hyaluronidase, collagenase and a calcium salt solvent.

Whether the osteoclast does or does not destroy bone is important to those interested in the physiology of that tissue. To the pathologist large numbers of osteoclasts mean bone destruction though the actual causative agents are varied, including alteration of blood supply, mechanical trauma, parathyroid hormone, vitamin D and a host of unknown forces working through such processes as Paget's disease, solitary cyst and neoplasia.

Additional light may be shed upon the activities of the osteoclast when we know more of its intracellular metabolism. As a working principle it is safe to say that in the presence of large numbers of osteoclasts, bone lysis is taking or has taken place. The reverse is not necessarily true in the absence of osteoclasts since it may be necessary to search numerous sections of normal bone before encountering a single osteoclast. The writing on the subject is an example of the futility and sometimes the damage which can result by the application of presumption dressed in the garb of fact.

References

1. Sledge, C. B., and Dingle, J. T.: Nature (London), *205*:140, 1965.
2. Follis, R., and Berthrong, M.: Bull. Johns Hopkins Hosp., *85*:281, 1949.
3. Collins, D.: Pathology of Bone. London, Butterworth & Co. Ltd., 1966.
4. Wolbach, S.: J. Bone Joint Surg., *29*:171, 1947.
5. Gardner, W., and Pfeiffer, C.: Physiol. Rev., *23*:139, 1943.
6. DeLuca, H.: Trans. Stud. Coll. Physicians Phila., *39*:1, 1971.
7. Wallis, L., and Engle, R.: Am. J. Med., *22*:13, 1957.
8. Zetterstrom, R.: Nature, *167*:409, 1951.
9. Castleman, B., and Mallory, T.: Am. J. Pathol. *11*:1, 1935.
10. Rasmussen, H.: Am. J. Med., *30*:112, 1961.
11. Rasmussen, H.: J. Biol. Chem., *235*:3442, 1960.
12. Barnicot, N.: J. Anat., *82*:233, 1948.
13. Chang, H.: Anat. Rec., *111*:23, 1951.
14. Albright, F., Burnett, C., Parson, W., Reifenstein, E., and Roos, A.: Medicine, *25*:399, 1946.
15. Nicholson, T.: Can. J. Biochem. Physiol., *37*:113, 1959.
16. Hirsch, P., Voelkel, E., and Munson, P.: Science, *146*:412, 1964.
17. Rasmussen, H., and Pecket, M.: Sci. Am. *223*:42, 1970.
18. Arnaud, C., Tsao, H., and Littledike, T.: Mayo Clin. Proc. *45*:125, 1970.
19. Tashjian, A.: N. Engl. J. Med. *283*:593, 1970.
20. Haymovitz, A.: Pediatrics, *45*:133, 1970.
21. Capp, D., and Henze, K.: J. Clin. Endocrinol., *24*:352, 1964.
22. Chiroff, R., and Jowsey, J.: J. Bone Joint Surg. *52A*:1138, 1970.
23. Neuman, W., and Neuman, M.: The Chemical Dynamics of Bone Mineral. Chicago, University of Chicago Press, 1958.
24. Bassett, A.: J. Bone Joint Surg., *44A*:1217, 1962.
25. Cochran, G., Pawluk, R., and Bassett, E.: Clin. Orthop., *58*:249, 1968.
26. Kirby-Smith, H.: Am. J. Anat., *53*:377, 1933.
27. Hancox, N.: Biochemistry and Physiology of Bone. New York, Academic Press, Inc., 1956.

HISTOLOGY OF THE MUSCULOSKELETAL SYSTEM

The chapters of this book subsequent to this one are intended for the clinician who encounters orthopedic diseases, the orthopedic surgeon, the radiologist and the pathologist. If the specialist of any but the last of these categories is interested in the microscopy of the musculoskeletal diseases (the interest of the pathologist is taken as a matter of faith), he may find some help in this, Chapter 4, for it is intended as a primer, of the most rudimentary type, of the histology of the tissue concerned. Since descriptions of cellular morphology make an almost unreadably dry text the material is presented largely in the form of a simple atlas. It is obvious that a much more complete coverage can be found in any histology text, but since this book is devoted to the description of orthopedic diseases only, for the sake of oneness, it seems permissible to include only enough histology to allow the reader to appreciate the more detailed microscopy given later with the description of each disease entity.

It is assumed that the non-pathologist has forgotten most of anything he may have learned while peering through a microscope as a medical student. A considerable experience in teaching clinicians has impressed this fact upon us. Since any concept of morbid microscopic structure rests upon a comparison with normal structure, the following several pages bear illustrations of the latter.

This chapter should be read by the non-pathologist with a set of "bone slides" and a microscope at hand. The pathologist would do better not to read it at all.

Figure 4–1   This represents an organizing hematoma. Soon after blood is extravasated into normal tissue, a network of fibrin is precipitated throughout the clot. Almost immediately, fibroblasts from the surrounding, viable tissue begin to proliferate and the young cells penetrate into the hematoma, climbing among the fibrin strands like sailors on a rigging. These fibroblasts form a network of their fibrils and as they mature they become fixed in this network. Their shape changes from polyhedral to fusiform and then to long spindles. Gradually collagen is laid down about them. In the illustration one can make out the pale, often disintegrating red cells in the background. The darker spindles seen throughout the section represent fibroblasts.

Figure 4–2   This is a section of simple granulation tissue. In a hematoma or in an area where tissue has been injured, concomitant with the proliferation of fibroblasts, the tiny vessels in the contiguous tissue sprout into the affected area. These young vessels, consisting at first of simple tubes of endothelial cells, are supported by the networks of fibrin and fibroblastic fibrils. They penetrate all through the area, bringing the large supply of blood which is necessary for repair. As they age they develop supportive walls of fibrous tissue. About them are the exudative inflammatory cells and the edema which are consequent to the tissue injury. In the illustration one sees the sprouting vessels in an edematous matrix containing exudative inflammatory cells.

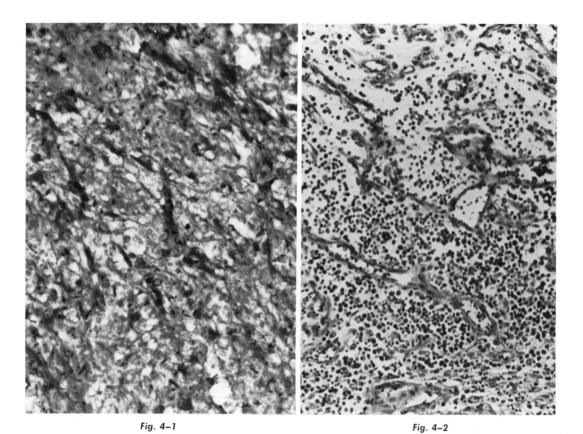

Fig. 4–1   Fig. 4–2

Figure 4–1   Organizing hematoma. (× 260.)

Figure 4–2   Granulation tissue. (× 130.)

Figure 4–3   This is an illustration of a suppurative exudate. The neutrophils are represented by the clusters of two to five small, round, black bodies. Each of these is a multilobed nucleus of a polymorphonuclear leukocyte. The nucleus of all cells contains large quantities of deoxyribosenucleic acid, the main constituent of chromatin. It takes the hematoxylin stain and in sections it is dark blue. The cytoplasm of most cells takes the pink eosin stain in various densities. In sections of tissue the cytoplasmic borders are not usually seen, the nuclei appearing in a more or less homogeneous background of cytoplasm. In exudates the cells are more widely separated so that cytoplasmic borders are usually apparent. In smears of exudate prepared with Wright's stain the various lobes of the nuclei of the neutrophils are seen to be connected by fine filaments of chromatin. In H and E sections these are rarely demonstrable. The more mature the neutrophil the greater the number of lobes in its nucleus. The arrow designates a typical neutrophil.

Figure 4–4   The eosinophil is a type of granulocyte. The cytoplasm is filled with eosin-staining granules which are quite obvious in the section but do not appear in the black and white photograph. The nucleus of the eosinophil is apt to be immature and so usually appears as a single body of irregular outline. The arrow designates the much less common mature eosinophil. Most of the other cells in the illustration are immature eosinophils.

Figure 4–5   The nucleus of the lymphocyte is round or ovoid. Its chromatin is usually heavily condensed so that it appears a solid dark blue or even black in the section. Sometimes the chromatin is irregularly broken, causing clear lines and spaces between the fragments. As the nucleus undergoes degenerative change it takes the hematoxylin less and less heavily and develops a washed-out appearance. The cytoplasm of the lymphocyte is sparse or completely undemonstrable in sectioned tissue. When seen it usually appears as a narrow demilune of a pale gray-blue about one side of the nucleus. All the cells in the illustration are lymphocytes.

Figure 4–6   The nucleus of the plasmacyte is somewhat larger than that of the usual lymphocyte. It, too, is heavily chromatized but more apt to be broken. The fragments are sometimes arranged about the nuclear periphery beneath the nuclear membrane. This may give a clock-face or spokes-of-a-cartwheel appearance. The cytoplasm of the plasmacyte has a peculiar blue-rose color which is very characteristic. In most instances the nucleus is eccentrically placed, sometimes appearing halfway out of the cell and thus giving the cell a piriform outline. The cells in the illustration are typical plasmacytes.

Fig. 4–3

Fig. 4–4

Fig. 4–5

Fig. 4–6

Figure 4–3 Neutrophils. (× 760.)
Figure 4–4 Eosinophils. (× 760.)
Figure 4–5 Lymphocytes. (× 760.)
Figure 4–6 Plasmacytes. (× 760.)

Figure 4–7 The large ovoid structures in this illustration are the nuclei of macrophages. Their magnification is the same as that of the exudative cells on the previous page. Note that they are much larger. Other names for the macrophage are histiocyte, clasmatocyte and mononuclear phagocyte. They are the largest of the mononucleated ameboid cells. Their cytoplasmic borders are demonstrable only if the cell is relatively isolated. The cytoplasm stains pale pink. The large nucleus is usually ovoid and frequently indented or reniform. The chromatin is usually finely divided and evenly dispersed. The nucleolus is often prominent. In this illustration there are also nuclei of lymphocytes and in the lower right corner a neutrophil.

Figure 4–8 When macrophages (or fibroblasts) aggregate to form a granuloma they are called epithelioid cells. The nuclei are often elongated and lie side by side. Early pathologists saw these cells and because of their parallel arrangement compared them to the cells of an epithelial membrane. Realizing, however, that these were not true epithelial cells they devised the descriptive term epithelioid cells. The name has persisted and is applied whether or not the cells have a palisade arrangement. Toward the center of the lesion they may undergo necrosis; toward the periphery they may revert to collagenoblasts.

Figure 4–9 This illustration shows a multinucleated giant cell of inflammation. The nuclei are identical with those of macrophages. The cytoplasm often contains phagocytized particles. This cell probably represents an agglomeration of macrophages or a group of macrophages whose cytoplasm has failed to divide.

Figure 4–10 This picture shows a granuloma giant cell. It is a type of giant cell of inflammation and of the same order as the Langhans giant cell of tuberculosis. These cells are not the same as osteoclasts though they may sometimes resemble them. Another cell which must be differentiated is the megakaryocyte which is found in active marrow and produces blood platelets. The granuloma is a specific type of inflammatory reaction produced by certain agents: lipids, waxes and other foreign body materials, fungi, parasites, and some bacteria, such as the tubercle bacillus. Granulation tissue is a general reparative response to any tissue injury and should not be confused with granuloma. Granulomas are often encountered in granulation tissue.

Fig. 4–7

Fig. 4–8

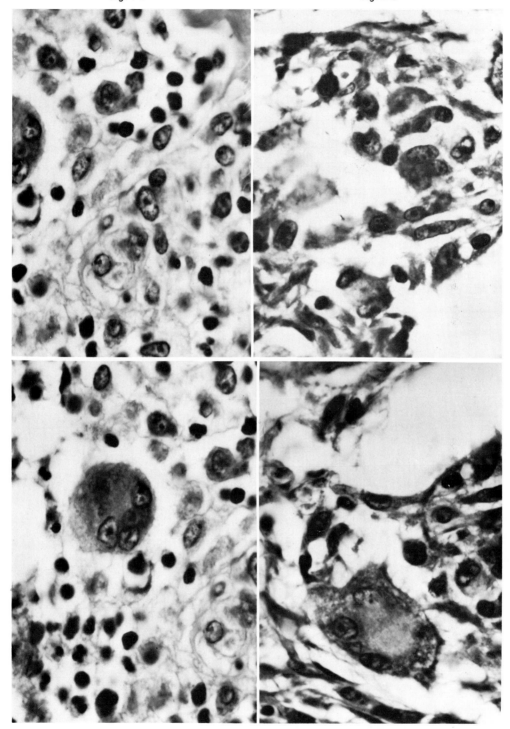

Fig. 4–9

Fig. 4–10

Figure 4–7   Macrophages. (× 760.)
Figure 4–8   Epithelioid cells. (× 760.)
Figure 4–9   Giant cell of inflammation. (× 760.)
Figure 4–10   Giant cell of granuloma. (× 760.)

Figure 4-11 The illustration at high magnification reveals several young fibroblasts. They have passed out of the polyhedral into the fusiform stage. The nuclei are still plump but the ends are tapered. The cytoplasm-nucleus ratio is much smaller than in the polyhedral stage. At the ends of the cell the fibrils emerge and weave throughout the matrix. Most of the cells are bipolar but some are stellate. The arrow designates a stellate form which is deeper in the section than the others and, therefore, slightly out of focus.

The collagenoblast (fibroblast) is found throughout all tissues and areas of the body. It provides the collagenized connective tissue which supports all the functioning parts and binds these parts into a unit. The term collagenoblast is preferred, designating the particular cell which is involved in collagen formation. The term fibroblast is used to designate the forerunner of any of the three cells which form the three types of fibrous matrices, the collagenoblast forming collagen, the osteoblast forming osteoid and the chondroblast forming chondroid. The collagenoblast, the osteoblast and the chondroblast are shaped and identified by their related intercellular substances. The production of the various fibrous substances may be the result of a variety of stimuli acting upon the same cell.

Figure 4-12 This represents an area of a section of collagenous connective tissue at medium magnification. The nuclei are thinner and more compact. The cytoplasm is no longer discernible. The network of fibrils is now filled in with collagen. The nuclei take the usual blue hematoxylin. The matrix takes the eosin lightly, assuming a pale pink to buff color. Collagen has much the same appearance in sections as osteoid but it is never lamellated, and of course there are no lacunae in which the osteocytes are entombed. Collagen stains green with Masson's trichrome, blue with Mallory's and brown with silver. The fibrils of the collagenoblasts stain black with silver stain.

Figure 4-13 This is an area of nearly adult collagenous connective tissue at low magnification. The strands are woven together in such a manner as to give great tensile strength. When completely mature the nuclei appear as hard black lines. The intercellular collagen may hyalinize, obliterating the fibrous character and giving the matrix a homogeneous, glassy appearance.

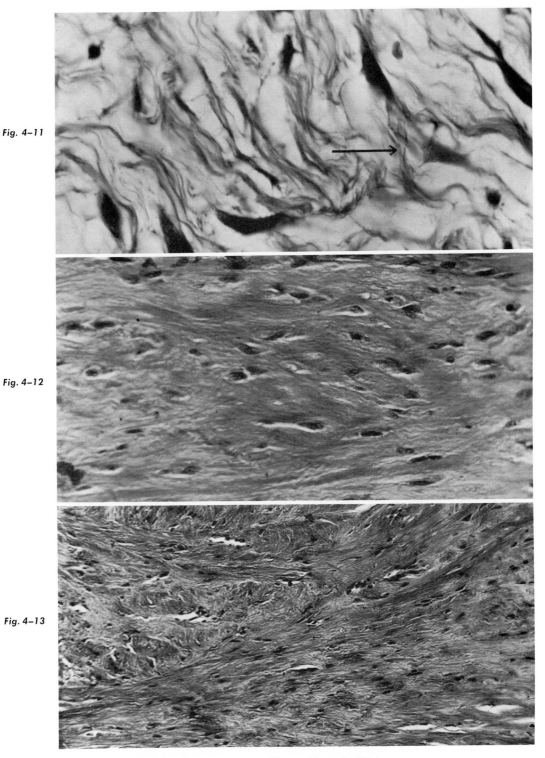

Fig. 4-11

Fig. 4-12

Fig. 4-13

Figure 4-11   Very young collagenoblasts. (× 760.)
Figure 4-12   Young connective tissue. (× 265.)
Figure 4-13   Mature connective tissue. (× 132.)

Figure 4–14   The osteoclast is a huge cell containing from 5 to 20 nuclei in a single plane. The nuclei are usually dispersed throughout the cell but may be arranged about the periphery or clumped in the center. The magnification is high ($\times$ 870).

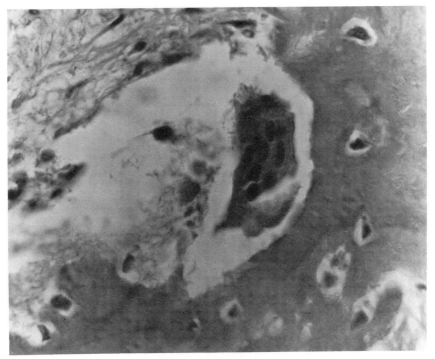

Fig. 4–14
Figure 4–14   Osteoclast. (× 870.)

Figure 4–15   A section of soft tissue illustrating a small artery and its accompanying vein. The artery has a thick wall. Usually the lumen measures slightly less than twice the thickness of its wall. The lumen is lined by a layer of endothelial cells and its supportive areolar tissue which together compose the intima.

Figure 4–16   This is also a section of soft tissue. The cross sections of two arteries are seen embedded in fat. The fat is composed of adult fat cells which in the section appear as large, round spaces surrounded by a delicate membrane. The spaces represent the area that was occupied by neutral fat which has been dissolved by the processing fluids. The nuclei of adult fat cells are small and they are pushed to the periphery by the intracytoplasmic fat. Unless the knife passes through the plane in which they lie they are not seen. Crossing the field from below to the right is a small nerve. Its fibrillar appearance is due to the fibrous supportive tissue. It has a characteristic wavy pattern. A cross section of this nerve can be seen in the upper right.

Fig. 4–15

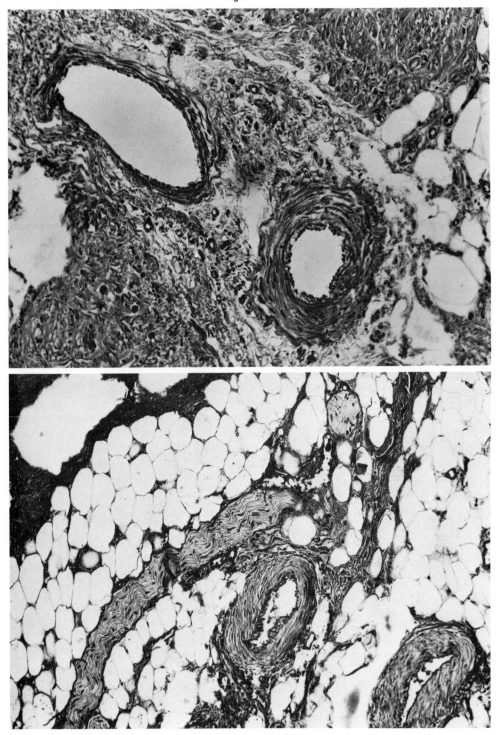

Fig. 4–16

Figure 4–15 Artery and vein. (× 132.)
Figure 4–16 Artery, fat and nerve. (× 115.)

Figure 4–17   This is a very low magnification of a section taken through the epiphyseal line showing the enchondral plate on the left, the epiphyseal line through the center and the subepiphyseal metaphysis on the right. The perichondrium (over cartilage) and the periosteum (over bone) are at the top. The lined rectangle represents the area from which the four following illustrations were taken. Figure 4–18 comes from the extreme left of this rectangle, Figure 4–19 from the area of large, vacuolated, columnated chondrocytes, Figure 4–20 straddles the epiphyseal line and Figure 4–21 comes from the extreme right portion of the area.

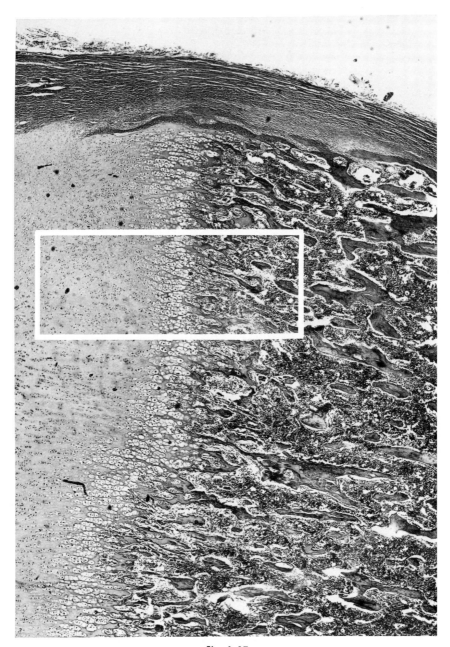

Fig. 4–17

Figure 4–17   The epiphyseal line. (× 12.)

Figure 4–18 This picture is of an area deep within the enchondral plate. The osseous nucleus was to the left and the epiphyseal line to the right. The following three illustrations were taken consecutively from the same section by moving the slide to the left, thereby including fields progressively nearer the diaphysis. The right side of the field in each is nearest the diaphysis; thus if the four illustrations were placed end to end they would represent a nearly continuous progression from the depths of the enchondral plate through the epiphyseal line and into the metaphysis. In Figure 4–18 the cartilage cells are young, small and quite evenly dispersed through the chondroid matrix. The cytoplasm contains little or no glycogen.

Figure 4–19 This area is several fields nearer the epiphyseal line. The chondroblasts are more mature. They are larger and the cytoplasm contains vacuoles from which glycogen was dissolved by the processing fluids. Note that by enlarging in a plane horizontal to the epiphyseal line which is to the right of this picture, the cells have become flattened and have achieved the effect of columnation. Between the columns of maturing chondroblasts remain pillars of chondroid.

Fig. 4–18

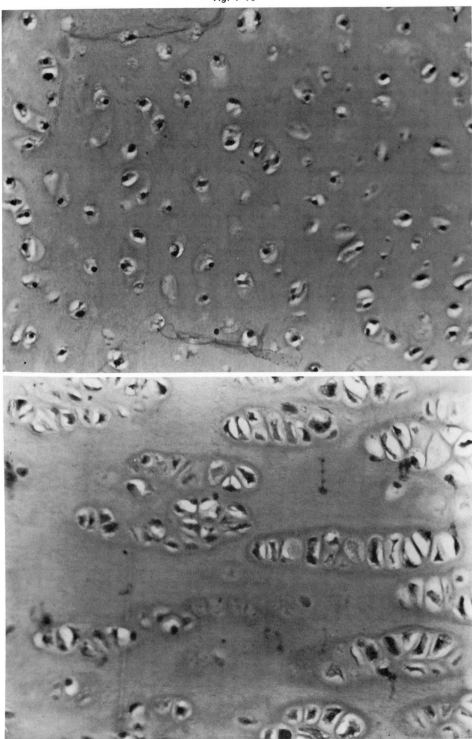

Fig. 4–19

Figure 4–18   Chondroblasts of enchondral plate. (× 266.)
Figure 4–19   Columnation of chondroblasts. (× 266.)

Figure 4–20 This section straddles the epiphyseal line; the epiphysis is to the left, the metaphysis to the right. The cartilage cells are now mature and greatly distended with glycogen. The budding, metaphyseal vessels are breaking into the bases of the columns and the cells are being utilized in the process of mineralization. The pillars of mineralized chondroid now protrude into the metaphysis. Osteoblasts have apparently emerged from the endothelial lining cells of the young vessels which are replacing the used, mature cartilage cells at the foot of the cell columns and are beginning to line up along these pillars and to lay down seams of osteoid.

Figure 4–21 The mineralized chondroid pillars have been largely replaced by osteoid which, toward the left in the younger portion of the area, appears in narrow seams. The entire process is known as enchondral ossification.

Fig. 4–20

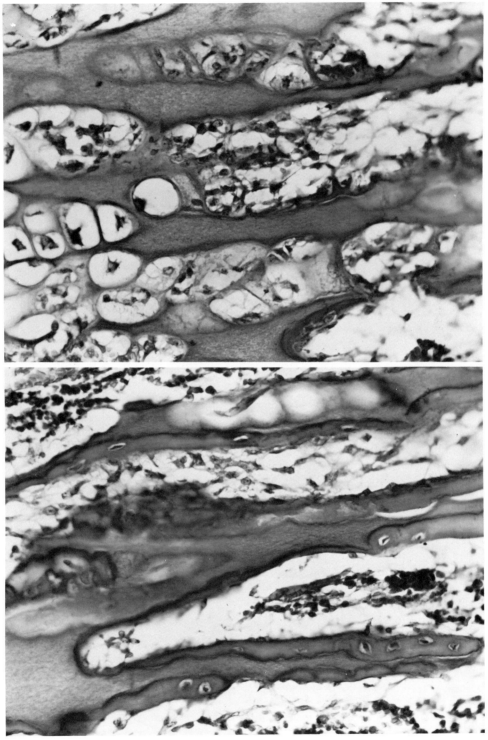

Fig. 4–21

Figure 4–20   Epiphyseal line. (× 266.)
Figure 4–21   Subepiphyseal metaphysis. (× 266.)

Figure 4–22 Though osteoblasts appear to arise from endothelial cells at the epiphyseal line, deeper in the metaphysis they apparently come from transitional primitive fibroblasts. Three types of cells emerge from these primitive fibroblasts: the collagenoblasts illustrated in Figures 4–11, 4–12 and 4–13, the chondroblasts illustrated in Figures 4–18 and 4–19 and the osteoblasts. On the right side of the field in Figure 4–22 one finds an aggregate of round or ovoid nuclei of these fibroblasts. The cytoplasmic outlines, where visualized, are still polyhedral or round. As one progresses left across the field the nuclei become larger and the cell outline elongated. In the lower left portion of the field there is a mass of osteoid. As the undifferentiated cells approach this osteoid they become more rounded or cuboidal in shape. They line up along the margins of the osteoid and enter into the production of that substance. They are now known as osteoblasts. It is interesting that when osteoblasts become neoplastic in nature they are apt to revert to their undifferentiated elongated, fusiform or even stellate shape.

Figure 4–23 This is a section taken from an area of actively forming bone. The osteoblasts are fully differentiated and are now seen as cuboidal cells arranged in rows along the surfaces of immature bone. The core of the latter has already mineralized and thus appears black in the illustration and dark blue in the section. Calcium salts take the hematoxylin stain. Between the row of osteoblasts and the core of mineralized bone one finds a layer, a "seam" of unmineralized osteoid. This stains a rather intense pink with eosin. Normal osteoid mineralizes very rapidly, probably within a matter of hours after it is formed. One can judge the rate at which ossification is proceeding by the amount and width of the osteoid seams. Under normal circumstances one never sees unmineralized osteoid except in forming bone. When bone undergoes lysis the organic matrix (osteoid) apparently disintegrates first, releasing the mineral salts. Nothing is left to indicate where bone has been. When bone is demineralized in the laboratory the calcium salts are removed, leaving the organic matrix. We still do not know what artifacts are induced by this process.

Fig. 4–22

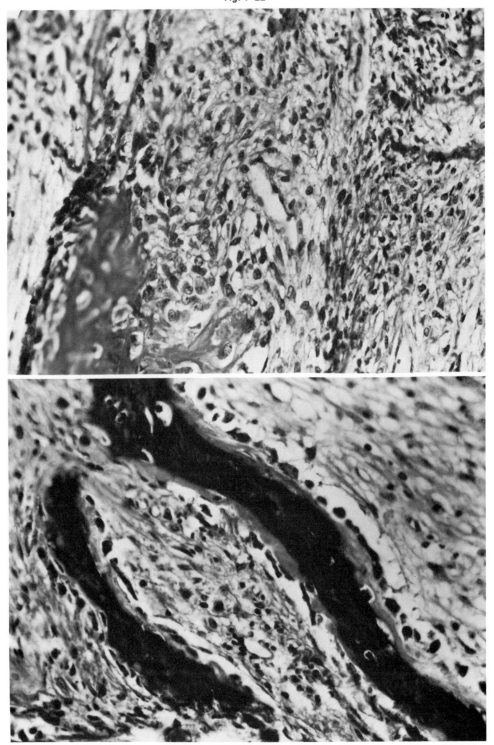

Fig. 4–23

Figure 4–22 Fibroblasts migrating to form osteoblasts. (× 260.)
Figure 4–23 Osteoblasts laying down osteoid. (× 260.)

Figure 4-24   As the mass of bone increases by the apposition of osteoid along its surfaces, some of the osteoblasts disappear and others are caught in the substance which forms around them. The osteoid then mineralizes and these cells become incorporated into the newly formed bone. They are now known as osteocytes and the spaces they occupy are called lacunae. They retain their fibrillar processes which emerge from the lacunae like spider legs and travel through the bone matrix in their minute channels, called canaliculi. These channels appear to constitute the apertures through which nutrients reach and sustain the cell within its lacuna. As the osteocyte matures, the nucleus shrinks and the chromatin condenses and consequently stains more darkly. The cytoplasm which in life fills the lacunar space does not withstand the process of demineralization and so is seen as an amorphous substance condensed around the nucleus. The space which results is an artifact.

Figure 4-25   This picture illustrates at higher magnification a piece of recently formed fiberbone or woven bone. Young fiberbone is easily distinguished from mature bone because the osteocytes are greater in number and larger. The fibers of the matrix are coarser. The bone may be laid down in layers but there is no organization of these layers into a lamellar pattern. Enchondral ossification, producing fiberbone, is responsible for the original shape of the bone. But fiberbone is weak and withstands stress badly. The process of conversion of fiberbone to stronger mature bone is a slow process and results in the modeling of bone to its final shape and in the pattern of cancellous bone in stress trajectories. To accomplish this the fiberbone undergoes a slow, progressive lysis and replacement. Osteoclasts are seen on those surfaces which are receding and osteoblasts on those which are being built up. Thus there is a gradual transition without weakening the area. The bone mass shifts in position as it changes its character.

Fig. 4–24

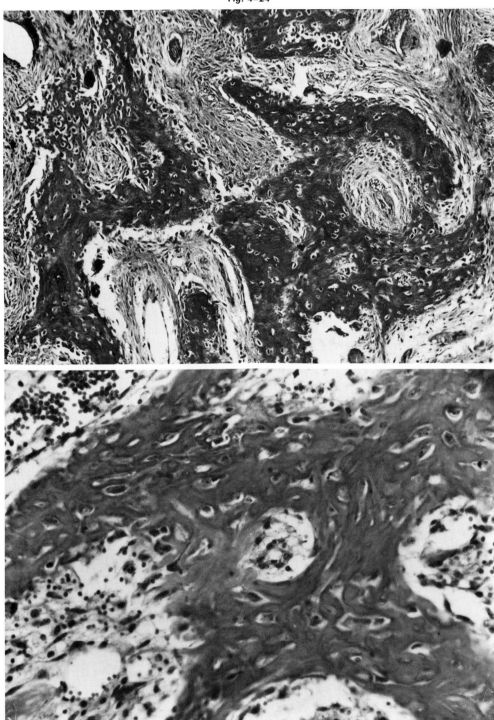

Fig. 4–25

Figure 4–24 Primitive fiberbone. ($\times$ 115.)
Figure 4–25 Primitive fiberbone. ($\times$ 260.)

Figure 4–26   This represents an area of cortical bone from which the mineral salts have been removed in a bath of weak nitric acid. It takes the eosin stain because the salts are no longer present. The striations seen in the illustration represent lamellar bands. The fibrillar structure is much finer than that of fiberbone — too fine to appear at this magnification. Note that the osteocytes are fewer in number. In the center of the field is a haversian system. This system of concentric lamellae is laid down about a haversian canal which appears in the center as a space. A haversian canal is shown at higher magnification in Figure 4–28. The cells are caught in flattened lacunae lying between the lamellae. When a haversian system is cut in cross section it is delineated from neighboring systems by a fine blue line along the surface of the outer lamella. This is known as a *cement line,* and probably represents a narrow crevice or space between the surface of the enclosed system and contiguous systems which have grown independently. There probably is no cement substance which binds the systems together. When osteoblasts lay down an osteoid seam on pre-existing bone no cement line is seen, but when a system is completed and approximated by another system the line of contact appears through the microscope as a black line. The configuration of the lamellae and of the haversian systems is exceedingly important in judging new bone growth and in the diagnosis of several bone diseases. In Paget's disease the pattern is so completely changed that one can frequently make the diagnosis at a glance. Osteopetrosis is another example.

Figure 4–27   This represents an area of cancellous bone which was sectioned without removal of the mineral salts. The bone now stains deep blue because of the presence of calcium. The irregular dark lines represent fractures produced by the passage of the knife. No cellular detail is retained in sections prepared in this fashion. The uninitiated, when looking at undemineralized normal bone, often call it necrotic because of its deep blue color and ragged edges. This mistake can never be made once the microscopist has compared the two types of preparations. There are numerous disturbances in the mineralization of bone. By removing the mineral salts so that the tissue can be sectioned we may efface the character of the disease we are trying to diagnose. For this reason sections of undemineralized bone are sometimes made by a special technique. The procedure is technically difficult and not yet suited to routine diagnosis.

Fig. 4–26

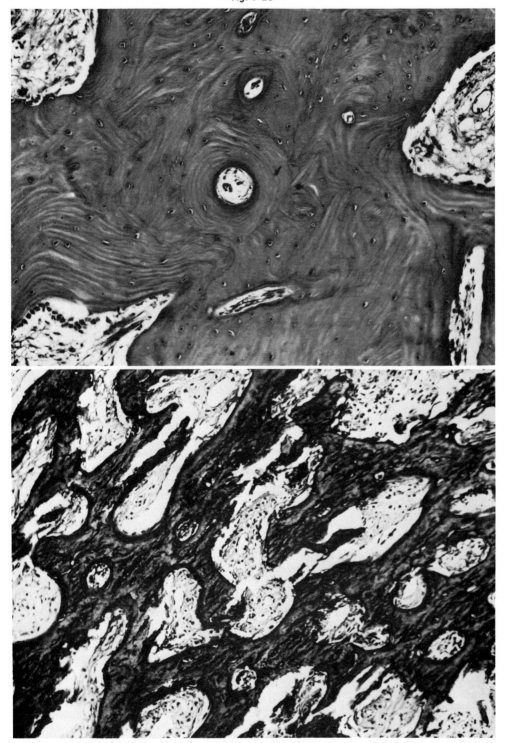

Fig. 4–27

Figure 4–26 Mature bone, demineralized. ($\times$ 115.)
Figure 4–27 Mature bone, undemineralized. ($\times$ 130.)

Figure 4–28   This haversian canal contains an artery and two small veins. Nerve fibrils have been demonstrated in haversian canals by special technique. These structures are supported by loosely arranged collagenoblasts which form what is called areolar tissue. In preparation, this areolar tissue shrinks away from the rigid walls of the canal so that an artifactual space appears. This space is lined by a layer of cuboidal osteoblasts in this picture, suggesting that osteogenesis is still progressing. In the lower right corner there is another haversian canal the contents of which has dropped out of the section. It is surrounded by concentric lamellae to form a haversian system. Note that the lamellae about the larger canal are not concentric. Apparently the systems are built from without inward so that the same lamella may be involved in the outer structure of more than one system as illustrated in this picture. The haversian system cannot be considered as a unit except in relation to the vasculature pattern. Since the mature bone is laid down around the vessels, the canals run parallel to the trajectories of stress. Thus the lamellar pattern in any given area is the same as that of the same area in any other bone of the same type. In disease processes these patterns are disturbed and they change as stress trajectories are altered.

Figure 4–29   This is a picture of a section taken through the cortex of the shaft of a fetal bone. It beautifully illustrates the components of periosteum. The periosteal membrane covers the upper (outer) surface of the portion of cortex seen in the lower portion of the field. Periosteum is composed of two layers which merge and are coextensive with each other. The outer half is made up of spindled collagenoblasts which are quite compactly arranged. A small amount of collagen appears between the cells. Collagenation increases with age. The inner half of the membrane is composed of elongated or fusiform cells which are much more loosely arranged. This layer is called the cambium. It is composed of cells which are in the process of differentiating into osteoblasts. A layer of more cuboidal osteoblasts can be seen approximated to the cortical surface. Bone is added by apposition in seams just as in enchondral ossification. The only difference is that here there is no intermediary stage of cartilage. The cambium has the ability to produce cartilage under abnormal circumstances. One frequently encounters casual reference to an endosteum, which is supposed to be a membrane like the periosteum applied to the inner surface of the cortex. We have examined many sections of cortex without finding any such membrane. In actively forming bone a single layer of osteoblasts may be seen but this can hardly be construed to compose a collagenic membrane.

Fig. 4-28

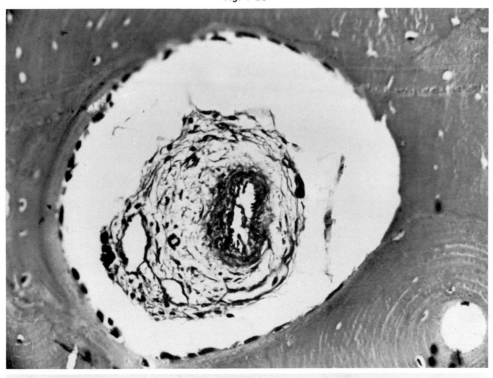

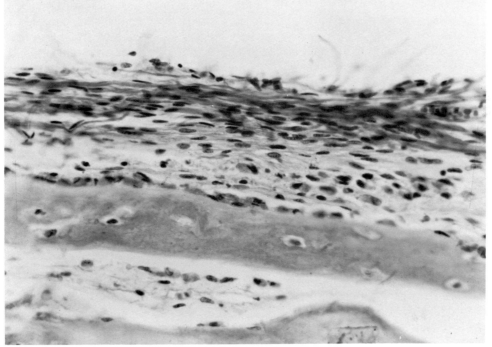

Fig. 4-29

Figure 4-28   A haversian canal. ($\times$ 266.)
Figure 4-29   Young periosteum. ($\times$ 266.)

Figure 4-30   This picture shows an area from a cross section through the diaphysis of a phalanx of an adult. The full thickness of the cortex is represented. Over the upper surface one sees the periosteum. Note that there is no "endosteum" lining the inner surface. Since the section is through the shaft, the periphery of the medullary cavity appears along the lower central margin of the picture. The vertical dark lines which mar the photograph are artifactual folds in the section. A patient technician can tease these out while they are floating on the surface of a water bath. One has the opportunity of studying the pattern of the haversian systems in this illustration. Note that the canals and therefore the lamellar cylinders run parallel to the long axis of the bone. Note also that the canals are not always in the center of the systems and that some lamellae enter into the composition of more than one system. Some bones have an outer and an inner layer of lamellae which contain no haversian systems. The lamellae which constitute the cortical tissue between the systems always parallel those of one or more of the contiguous systems. This suggests that the haversian canals are actually not planned spaces but merely leftover areas where vessels are crowded by the growing bone. Studies of films made by roentgen micrography indicate that the lamellae nearest the canals are the least mineralized and probably the last to be infiltrated with calcium salts.

Figure 4-31   This illustration represents a section through a much thinner cortex at the level of the metaphysis. In the lower half of the field one finds the metaphyseal cancellous tissue. The "spicules" are in reality a continuous membrane of bone just as the partitions which surround the holes in a sea sponge constitute a continuous membrane. The cancellous bone is also continuous with the cortical bone. The spaces and lines in the illustration are artifactual splits and folds. In this bone the metaphysis still contains active marrow. The metaphysis is interposed between the articular plate and the medullary "cavity." It braces and strengthens the thin metaphyseal cortex which surrounds it.

Fig. 4–30

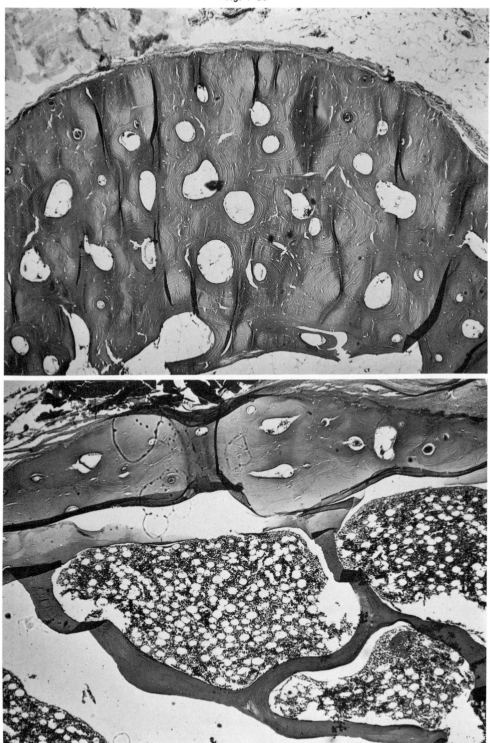

Fig. 4–31

Figure 4–30   Section through diaphyseal cortex. (× 24.)
Figure 4–31   Section through metaphyseal cortex. (× 24.)

Figure 4–32   This picture shows a section through an immature epiphysis. The osseous nucleus occupies the central and greater portion of the field. To the right is the enchondral or growth plate and the epiphyseal line along its right margin. To the left is the articular plate and the articular surface is further left, just out of the field. The time of the appearance of the osseous nucleus is specific for each epiphysis. Vessels reach the center of the epiphysis from the periphery (and sometines through the center) of the enchondral plate. A nidus of bone is formed. An epiphyseal line forms between the overlying articular plate and this nidus. As the epiphysis ages, its chondroblasts in the vicinity of this line mature, a line of provisional calcification is established and enchondral ossification takes place just as it does on the metaphyseal side of the epiphyseal line. As the epiphyseal chondroblasts are used up the osseous nucleus expands to take their place. A thin spherical shell of bone is formed which surrounds a lens-shaped mass of cancellous tissue, its convex surfaces facing the articular plate on one side and the enchondral plate on the other, thus dividing the epiphysis into two parts. As it progresses the ossification line is halted on the articular plate side and an arch of bone seals off the cartilage, thus preserving the articular plate at a constant thickness. On the opposite side of the lens-shaped nucleus chondroblasts are added as the cartilage cells of the enchondral plate are dissipated. Thus enchondral ossification is allowed to proceed until the cylindrical bone has reached its full stature. At another specified time, the chondroblasts cease to proliferate and those of the enchondral plate are used up as the epiphyseal line advances. Eventually the cancellous bone of the metaphysis meets the shell of the nucleus, the enchondral plate is spent and no cartilage intervenes between the two bone masses. At this point growth of the cylindrical bone at this end is completed. Conversion of the fiberbone into adult bone proceeds so that the two bone masses become continuous. Until this time the vasculature of the epiphysis and that of the metaphysis are almost distinct, but now vessels from the more vascular metaphyseal area penetrate the epiphysis and the blood supply becomes continuous and more adequate. Now the only way the bone can increase in length is by reactivation of chondroblasts at the cartilage-bone line of contiguity beneath the articular plate. This may happen in acromegaly in which there is excessive secretion of somatotropic hormone.

Figure 4–33   This illustrates two apposed articular plates in the lower half of the field. The bone arches are complete beneath the plates. The joint space crosses the lower left field. The dark line at the junction of cartilage and bone is caused by a heavy deposition of mineral. It is called the tide line.

Fig. 4–32

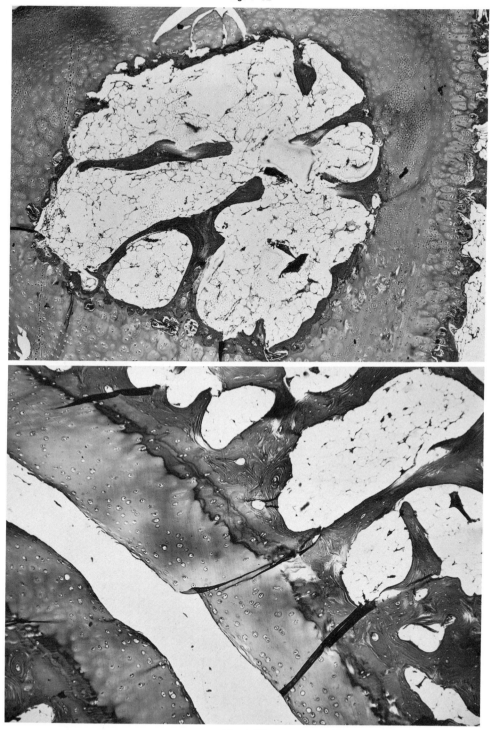

Fig. 4–33

Figure 4–32   Osseous nucleus of the epiphysis. (× 16.)
Figure 4–33   Section across a joint. (× 16.)

Figure 4–34 This is a photograph of a section made through cancellous tissue containing active or hematopoietic bone marrow. No bone "spicules" are included in the field. The microscopist must learn to distinguish hematopoietic marrow from inflammatory exudate and it is not always easy since many of the same cells are involved. The novice is apt to interpret a section such as that illustrated here as chronic osteomyelitis. The difficulty is not eased by the demineralizing process which blurs the detail of all viable cells in the section. One of the most helpful features is the regular dispersion of large round or oval spaces which represent the fat cells. These always appear in normal marrow and are rarely seen in exudate. Also the variety of cell types is usually greater in marrow than in exudates. Normal marrow contains all the cells of the myelogenous series including normoblasts and erythrocytes. One cannot do an analytic count of these cells in demineralized sections because the demineralizing agent destroys the nuclear detail which is necessary for such a count. One can get a fair idea of the cellular constituents, however, in a thinly cut, well stained section. In the illustration one can make out the large, dark nuclei of the young myelogenous forms and the clusters of smaller bodies which represent the nuclei of granulocytes. With the advantage of color in the sections one can distinguish the yellow-pink color of the hemoglobin in erythrocytes. The arrow in the illustration points to a megakaryocyte, a large cell with a multilobulated nucleus which is responsible for the formation of blood platelets. It is rarely mistaken for an osteoclast. Just below the megakaryocyte is a mature fat cell which has been sectioned through the plane of the nucleus. The latter is seen as a line of chromatin at the extreme periphery of the cell. It represents the nucleus which has been flattened to a plate and pushed to one side by the large globule of fat which now distends the cytoplasmic membrane. The fat, of course, has been dissolved out by the processing fluids. It may be demonstrated by doing a frozen section and staining with certain dyes such as Scharlach R which have an affinity for neutral fat.

Figure 4–35 This picture illustrates the fatty marrow which fills the medullary "cavity." Only the cytoplasmic membranes and here and there a flattened nucleus can be seen. This type of marrow is the normal component of the medullary area but in emergency states it may revert to hematopoietic marrow, illustrating the versatility of the mesenchymal derivatives.

Fig. 4–34

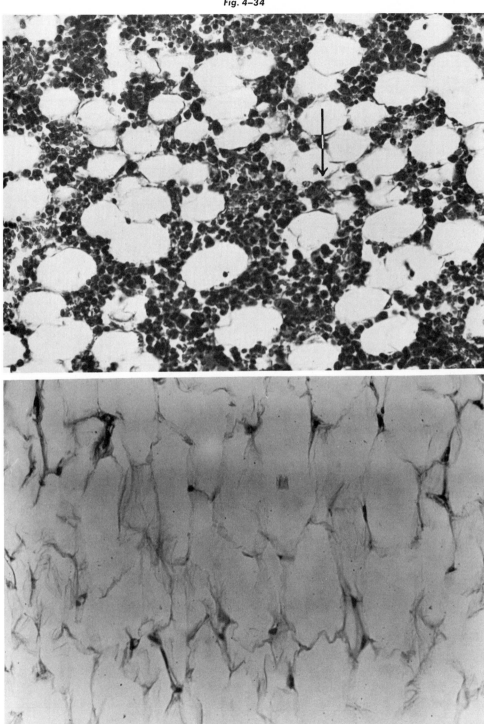

Fig. 4–35

Figure 4–34 Active bone marrow. ($\times$ 275.)
Figure 4–35 Fatty bone marrow. ($\times$ 275.)

Figure 4–36   This is a picture of a rather highly magnified longitudinal section of skeletal or voluntary muscle. Running horizontally through the major portion of the field is a muscle bundle. Each bundle is made up of a group of parallel muscle fibers. Each fiber is a syncytium covered by a cytoplasmic membrane, the sarcolemma, which surrounds a bundle of parallel fibrils, the sarcoplasm, and a number of nuclei which are always located eccentrically beneath the sarcolemma. The sarcoplasm stains a deep rose-pink with eosin. The fibrils are cross-banded and these striations should be seen in a reasonably good preparation if the muscle is healthy. Diseased muscle may show a blurring or loss of its striations. Next the nuclei swell and the chromatin becomes fragmented. Finally the muscle fiber fractures at various levels and may disappear. The products of degeneration elicit an inflammatory reaction and exudative cells may infiltrate into the area. The space occupied by the fibril is taken by fat cells and fibroblasts. Some fibers may atrophy and shrink to a fraction of their normal diameter. The remaining healthy fibers called on to do the work of the whole may hypertrophy to several times the normal diameter. Skeletal muscle is a highly differentiated structure and when injured it attempts to regenerate with but little success. The nuclei divide to produce excessive numbers in long chains but the sarcoplasm is unable to produce new fibrils. One can judge the extent of injury of a muscle field by noting the variation in fiber diameter, the number of nuclei in relation to the amount of sarcoplasm, the inflammatory reaction and the extent of fat and fibrous replacement. It should be remembered, however, that a muscle may reveal severe damage in one area and a short distance away it may appear perfectly healthy. Thus muscle biopsies are notably inaccurate in estimating the extent of disease of the entire structure.

Figure 4–37   This represents a cross section of muscle photographed at the same magnification as the longitudinal section. The ends of the fibrils are seen, surrounded by the sarcoplasm. Here and there an eccentric nucleus is found in the plane of section. The fibrils which stain darkly in the illustration show what appears to be a condensation of their sarcoplasm. Unfortunately, this is an artifact seen in muscle sections prepared by ordinary tissue technique. These dark-staining fibers must not be interpreted as evidence of disease unless one is very sure of the technique.

Fig. 4–36

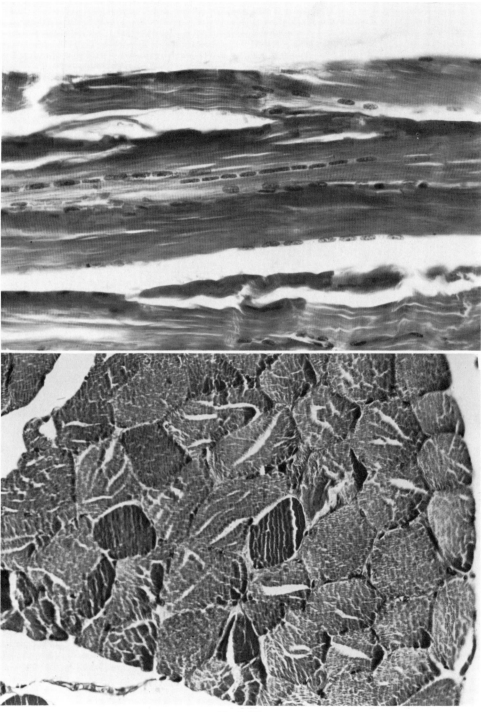

Fig. 4–37

Figure 4–36 Longitudinal section of skeletal muscle. (× 275.)
Figure 4–37 Cross section of skeletal muscle. (× 275.)

Figure 4–38 Tendons, ligaments and fascia are types of collagenous fibrous connective tissue. They are produced by collagenoblasts which lay down a dense matrix of collagen fibrils so arranged as to achieve maximum tensile strength. Tendons are composed of parallel bundles of parallel fibrils. Many fewer cells are caught in this matrix than in ordinary collagen, osteoid or bone, so that the structure is relatively acellular. This material takes the eosin stain and depending upon numerous local factors it may appear pale pink or deep red. When sectioned the fibrils usually assume a wavy pattern such as that seen in the illustration.

Figure 4–39 Synovial membrane lines joint cavities, bursae and tendon sheaths. It consists of a layer (usually single) of cells whose centrally placed nuclei are thicker than the flattened cytoplasm. Thus the membrane in cross section has a cobblestone appearance. Supporting this membrane is a thin layer of fibroblastic cells with a small amount of intercellular collagen. The membrane does not cover weight-bearing surfaces of the articular cartilage. Where the joint capsule is folded the membrane takes a villous configuration. The core of each villous process carries numerous large thin-walled vessels to supply the membrane with an abundance of blood. The joint is lubricated with synovial fluid, a viscous substance composed predominantly of hyaluronate. This fluid is probably secreted largely by the synovial cells. When injured by trauma, infection or impairment of blood supply or when there is alteration of metabolic activity, possibly by change in permeability of the ground substance, the synovial cells may respond by proliferation to form a membrane of several cells' thickness. Exudative inflammatory cells infiltrate the underlying supportive tissue and may penetrate out to the surface where they are caught in the meshwork of fibrin which often forms a covering membrane called a pannus.

Fig. 4–38

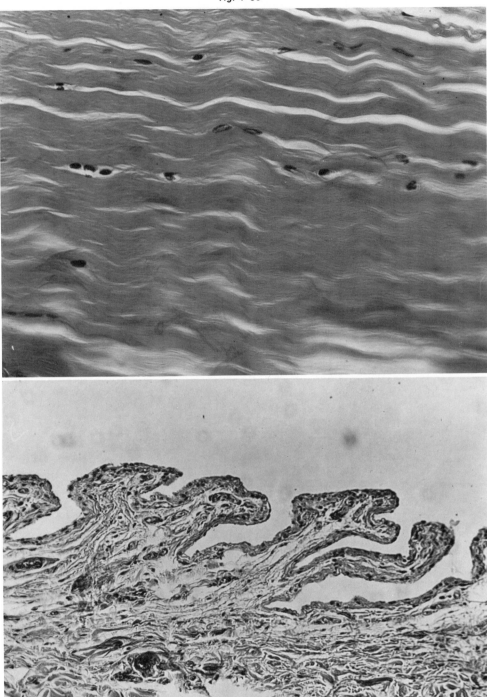

Fig. 4–39

Figure 4–38   Longitudinal section of tendon. (× 275.)
Figure 4–39   Synovial joint lining. (× 125.)

Chapter 5

RADIOLOGY OF THE SKELETAL SYSTEM

Skeletal structures are uniquely suited to radiographic examination. The technical aspects are relatively simple, the facilities are readily available and the results tend to be definitive since bone, because of its physical characteristics, casts a distinct image that is in sharp contrast with the surrounding soft tissues. Of even greater importance, however, is the fact that bone is living tissue, less permanent than the soft tissues attached to it, and so reflects alterations in anatomy and physiology of either a local or systemic nature. It is the recognition and interpretation of these alterations that is significant. To a degree, the radiograph of a diseased bone often substitutes for the gross pathologic specimen. The radiologist is denied specific knowledge of the nature of the abnormal tissue which is present, for pus, blood and neoplastic tissue cast identical shadows. However, the reaction of bone and cartilage to the presence of any one of these might furnish a clue to the underlying abnormality. The examination, therefore, is not an end in itself but is rather a part of the whole that must be evaluated in light of all the known clinical and laboratory data.

It is pertinent to discuss protection of the patient during a radiographic examination. Somatic or tissue damage in the individual from the usual examination need not be considered owing to the nature of present-day equipment. Genetic harm to the individual and the population, though not completely understood, is a consideration but should not act as a deterrent to a study that is necessary for the best care of the patient. Common sense must dictate the rules of gonadal shielding. Radiography of parts distant from the pelvis may be performed utilizing cones of appropriate size and shape to restrict the x-ray beam to the part in question. On an initial study in which a gonadal shield might obscure an abnormality it may be omitted on at least one of the exposures. This is particularly true regarding the female pelvis; in the examination of the pelvis of males it should be employed and be positioned accurately. When follow-up studies of the pelvic structures are indicated, shielding as well as limitation of exposures should be utilized. The best protection, however, is careful consideration of the need for radiographic examination and selection of the optimum exposures to meet the need, followed by efficient processing of the films.

In order to obtain a complete initial examination of a part, it is essential to consider either a single anteroposterior or lateral exposure as inadequate and the combination of both as minimal. In most instances, however, two exposures, one at right angles to the other, are sufficient for diagnosis. If these exposures do not result in definitive information, other projections and roentgen techniques should be utilized.[2] Fluoroscopy, particularly when performed with image intensification, often results in exact localization of a lesion because the part can be visualized in all degrees of obliquity.

This examination is followed by radiographic exposures, made with the part in the best position for the study of the lesion.

To this routine examination may be added other more specialized procedures. However, not to be neglected is the *examination of the entire skeleton*.[5] The presence of other areas of osseous and soft tissue involvement and their location will directly affect the management of the patient as the differential diagnosis is modified. Particularly may this be important in the differential diagnosis of trauma, especially unsuspected trauma, metabolic disease, metastatic malignancy and the osseous dysplasias.

The number and kinds of additional radiologic modalities available for evaluation of bone disease mirror increased understanding of the pathophysiology of the skeleton and increasing technology, particularly in the field of nuclear medicine, arteriography and radiography. Indications for the use of any specialized examination must be predicated on physiologic, anatomic and physical principles and the probability of the examination resulting in usable information relative to the management of the patient.

Stereoscopic examination of a part may be helpful in that it provides a three-dimensional view which allows for visual separation of superimposed structures as occurs in the spine, pelvis or facial bones. *Laminagraphy (tomography)*, or body section radiography, results in a radiograph of a predetermined "layer" of a part; the structures above and below the layer are blurred as the x-ray tube and the cassette move during the exposure (Fig. 5–1). This examination is particularly applicable to abnormalities of the spine and joints as well as their osseous components and to small lesions within the cortex or medullary cavity of a bone. *Radiographic magnification*[5] is achieved by the use of an x-ray tube with a small focal spot and the positioning of the part to be examined at a point between the tube and the x-ray film. This technique is useful for the study of trabecular pattern, especially of the bones of the hands and feet. Tomography may be combined with magnification and therefore may be helpful in delineating subtle fractures, joint disease, and fine detail of calcification, periosteal new bone and destruction.

Arteriography of the skeleton[5] is somewhat different from that of other organs in that there is no need to opacify bone, and, indeed, the normal vascular bed is obscured. However, it may be of value in the assessment of bone tumors, tumors of soft tissue and trauma (Fig. 23–15, p. 734). In the examination of tumors, as the

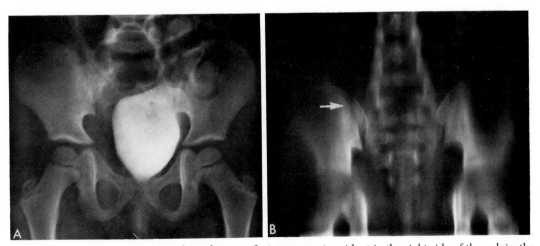

Figure 5–1 Following trauma to the pelvis, a soft tissue mass is evident in the right side of the pelvis; the bladder is displaced to the left (A). Laminagraphy (B) reveals a fracture of the right ilium (arrow) that was not visible on the standard projection.

vessels to and within the lesion are visualized, the extent of involvement of bone and the extent of soft tissue may be seen, as well as the major vessels supplying and draining the lesion. Necrosis may be apparent as a lucent area within the opacified soft tissue, if the lesion is a vascular one. The vascularity of a malignancy is apt to be characterized by the absence of expected tapering of vessels, the irregular course of vessels, the presence of numerous small vascular lakes and rapid arteriovenous shunting. Unfortunately, these findings may be associated with benign tumors and infection. Following trauma, arteriography may be helpful in the management of the patient. Disruption of major vessels may be visualized, although at times the differentiation of vasospasm, vascular obstruction or disruption is not possible. The technique is particularly valuable in the evaluation of arteriovenous fistulae either traumatic in origin or congenital.

Arthrography, particularly double contrast arthrography, is applicable to many joints, but especially to the hip, shoulder and knee. Film studies, either fluoroscopic or conventional, obtained in multiple projections after injections of water soluble contrast material and/or air into the joint reveal the otherwise invisible intra-articular soft tissues (Figs. 5–2 and 5–3). The examination has proved to be of particular value in the delineation of internal derangement of the knee by the demonstration of abnormalities of the menisci and the ligaments.[6]

The use of bone-seeking isotopes, *bone scanning*, is of proved value, particularly in the detection of metastatic disease of the skeleton.[7] The isotopes in general use, strontium (^{87}Sr) and technetium polyphosphate (^{99}Tc-PP), are laid down in areas of bone formation and since all destruction is associated with repair, all types of bone malignancy should be visualized, i.e., primary or metastatic (Fig. 5–4). The technique permits the documentation of lesions not detected by routine radiographic procedures; a focus of destruction of trabeculae must be greater than 1.5 cm.

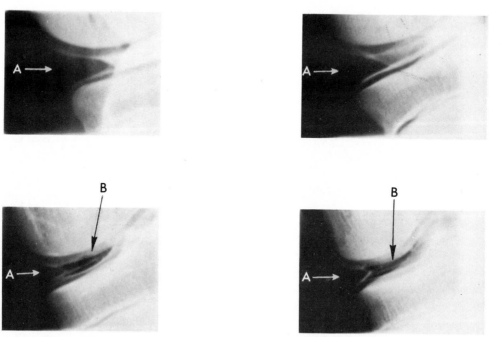

Figure 5–2   Knee, double contrast arthrogram. Four fluoroscopic spot films of the medial meniscus exposed at different degrees of rotation permit visualization of most of this structure (arrow *A*). The thickness and integrity of the articular cartilage is also visible (arrow *B*).

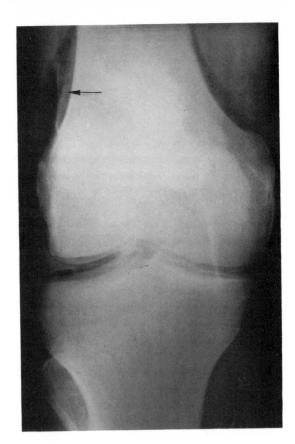

Figure 5–3 Knee, double contrast arthrography. A conventional radiograph, exposed during an arthrogram, demonstrates the extent of the communicating bursa (arrow) as well as the menisci.

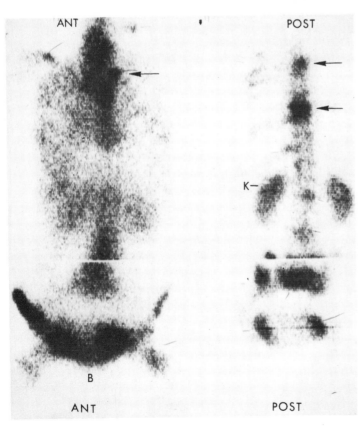

Figure 5–4 Bone scan, ^{99}Tc-PP. Two areas of increased uptake are seen in the spine (arrows); definition is best on the posterior one. The kidneys (*K*) and bladder (*B*) are visualized as well.

in diameter and 50 to 75 per cent of its calcium lost in order to be seen on a radiograph, but such small lesions will be detected by scanning techniques. The interpretation of scans must be tempered by the knowledge that not all areas of increased uptake are abnormal, e.g., the uptake is greater in the epiphyses of growing bones than in the diaphyses. This examination must be correlated with the radiographic examination and utilized only in those instances in which it can add useful information concerning diagnosis, prognosis or management. At the present ^{99}Tc-PP would appear to be a more satisfactory isotope for bone scanning than ^{87}Sr because of the increase in sensitivity and resolution of the scans.

Xerography is an electrostatic process wherein an image is obtained after exposure of the part to x-irradiation.[5] Selenium is deposited on a metal base and exposed to an electric charge. When the plate is struck by radiation the resistance of the selenium drops in proportion to the quantity of the radiation. To make this latent image visible, the surface of the selenium is exposed to a powder that is negatively charged. At that point the image may be recorded on photographic film or transferred to paper. The qualities of xeroradiography that are attractive with respect to diagnosis are excellent resolution, long contrast scale and edge enhancement (Fig. 5–5). Thus, xeroradiography offers bony and soft tissue detail that is beyond the range of usual radiography. At present, the exposure times are long and equipment is in limited supply.

Thermography is a method for the display of surface temperature. In the area of osseous disease and arthritis it is recognized that trauma, inflammation and malignancy increase the temperature of the overlying skin. Thus, this diagnostic modality is another adjunctive examination that may prove useful in the diagnosis of osseous disease.[5]

The value of any radiologic examination depends upon an understanding of anatomy, physiology, pathology and the physical principles of radiography. This understanding permits an interpretation of the findings coupled with a realization of the limitations of the method. Over-

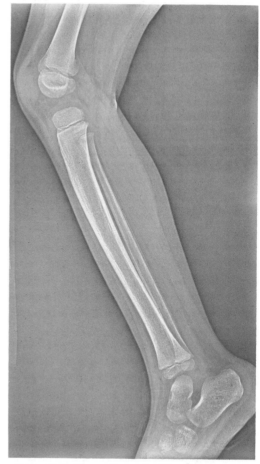

Figure 5–5 Xeroradiograph. The detail, osseous and soft tissue, is excellent and sharply defined. (Courtesy of Dr. John Hughes.)

emphasis and failure to realize the limitations are as much to be avoided as is neglect of the method, resulting from a lack of knowledge of its value. The sections of this book dealing with the radiographic manifestations of orthopedic diseases will attempt to correlate the radiographic appearance with the altered morphology whenever possible. For detailed radiographic description, competent texts and appropriate references are readily available. In many sections, descriptions of the gross pathology are applicable to the radiographic manifestations.

In order to interpret a radiograph and to realize its limitations as well as its value, some understanding of the principles of physics as related to radiography is necessary. Why does bone cast a sharp, opaque and contrasting image? Why do soft tissues, pus and blood cast noncontrasting shadows which do not permit differentiation of these structures? X-rays are electromagnetic in nature. By virtue of their wavelength, which approximates 1 Ångström, they are distinct from other radiations constituting the electromagnetic spectrum. A radiograph results from the differential absorption of the primary x-ray beam as it passes through the tissues to strike the sensitive emulsion of the photographic film. Bone absorbs a significant amount of x-rays as compared with the soft tissues; as a result, few of the rays which strike bone pass through to the film, which after processing is therefore clear or white. Air does not absorb significant amounts of x-rays, so that the emulsion is more affected and after processing the

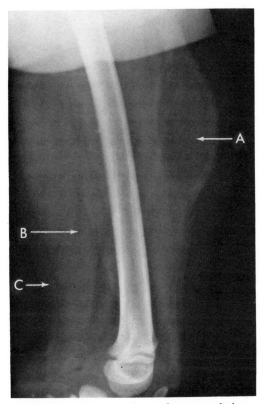

Figure 5–6 A lipoma (A) is evident as a radiolucent structure in contrast to the surrounding muscle. Fat may be seen between muscle groups (B) and beneath the skin (C).

film is black. The soft tissues are intermediate in absorption. The final image is modified by scattered radiation, geometric factors and by the character of the photographic film, of the processing solutions and of the techniques employed in processing the film.

Absorption of x-rays depends upon the atomic number of the irradiated material and upon the wavelength of the radiation employed. An increase in either results in increased absorption. The wavelength of the radiation bears a definite relation to the voltage applied to the x-ray tube and is thus important from the technical standpoint in obtaining radiographs of satisfactory quality. The organic constituents of the body comprising hydrogen, carbon, nitrogen and oxygen have low atomic numbers and the chemical compounds formed by these elements absorb only small amounts of radiation. The inorganic constituents, calcium and phosphorus, have significantly higher atomic numbers, and tissues containing these elements absorb significant amounts of x-rays in contrast with the soft tissues. Differences in density also affect absorption but to a lesser extent. Alterations in the mineral content of bone may be appreciated and under the most favorable circumstances fat may be seen in contrast with muscle. Shades of black and white (or radiolucency and opacity) may thus be distinguished, dependent upon the elements which are present and to a certain extent upon the density of the tissues which are exposed. Gas, air and at times fat are radiolucent, in contrast with soft tissue and body fluids which are intermediate in lucency (Fig. 5–6). These in turn are in contrast to bone and other structures containing calcium salts, which are opaque (Fig. 5–7).

As x-rays pass through matter some of the rays are absorbed, some are scattered by collisions with atoms and some pass through unchanged. Scattered x-rays fog the ultimate image by exposing portions of the film not affected by the primary beam. This may be controlled by the use of cones and grids. The former limit the beam and the latter absorb the scattered radiation before it strikes the film. From the geometric standpoint, an x-ray beam

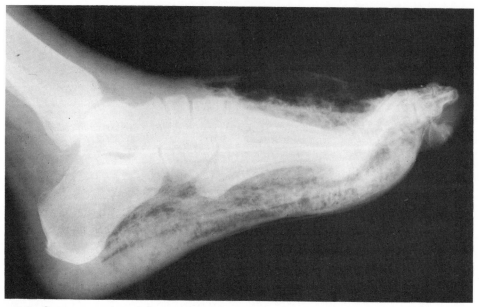

Figure 5–7 Gas gangrene in a diabetic patient 80 years of age. The radiolucent gas is seen in streaks and bubbles throughout the deep and superficial soft tissues of the foot.

is divergent, so that there is an optimal distance from the tube to the film and from the part to be examined to the film. The closer the part to the film and the further the tube from the film, the less magnification and the less distortion. Needless to say, the speed of exposure must be such as to prevent motion being manifest on the radiograph. Processing techniques and the type of film employed in departments of radiology are usually well standardized and will not be considered.

Thus the foundation of radiology is physical. Radiology is not a science of signs but represents the application of physics to anatomy, physiology and pathology. Descriptions of the radiographic appearance of diseased bone are replete with such phrases as "sunburst appearance," "ground-glass appearance of the shaft," "pencil-line cortices" and many others. These signs are only descriptive and are not specific for any disease. They do have a basis in fact, however, and an understanding of the mechanisms responsible for these manifestations is mandatory to the understanding of the disease in question. For example, a long bone of a patient with scurvy may be described as

having "pencil-line cortices" and a "ground-glass-like" shaft. Such descriptions refer to osteopenia in which, because of a lack of organic matrix coupled with continued resorption of bone, the trabeculae become thin and sparse and the cortices become thin. The fine trabeculae absorb less x-rays than do normal ones and thus produce less contrast with the soft tissues of the marrow.

These facts do not lessen the importance of experience. One who sees many osseous lesions recognizes patterns of bone destruction or of formation of reactive new bone. Such experience is rooted in knowledge regarding the reaction of bone as a tissue, the location or distribution of known abnormalities in the skeleton and the lesions most common to different ages and sexes.

The so-called "metabolic" diseases of bone involve the entire skeleton. In the growing skeleton, while involvement is generalized, the abnormalities are first evident and most marked at those sites where growth of bone is most rapid. Lesions that are acquired, or arise *de novo* in bone, result in lysis, bone formation or a combination of the two. These reactions to a lesion are the result of its duration, its rate of growth, its location within a bone and the extent of involvement of the bone. Nelson[3] also notes that the reaction of adjacent tissue must be considered in diagnosis, i.e., the extent of a soft tissue mass, the presence or absence of calcifications and the fact that neoplasm, in contrast to infection, is limited by cartilage.

Regarding neoplasia of bone, Lodwick[4] has defined three basic patterns of bone destruction. *Geographic* destruction is characterized by a uniform area of destruction with a sharp transition between the lesion and intact bone. *Motheaten* destruction is characterized by multiple small areas of lysis which may be confluent. *Permeated* bone destruction results in many minute holes in cortical bone and reflects a very rapidly growing and infiltrating tumor. It is important to note that the tumor extends farther than the visible motheaten or permeated destruction and that the types of destruction reflect the aggressiveness of the tumor. Benign lesions of bone most often have a sclerotic border of reactive bone, medullary, cortical or periosteal, as a reflection of their slow growth.

The manner in which the periosteum reacts to its elevation is a reflection of the nature of the process and its rate of growth. In an aggressive tumor, neoplastic bone or reactive bone is deposited about the vessels and fibers attaching the periosteum to the cortex, causing spiculation or variations of the "sunburst" appearance. In less aggressive tumors there may be layers of new bone secondary to successive elevations of the periosteum. Interruption of periosteal new bone, usually localized, is often associated with malignancy. In benign, slowly growing processes, the periosteal new bone tends to be thick and homogeneous.

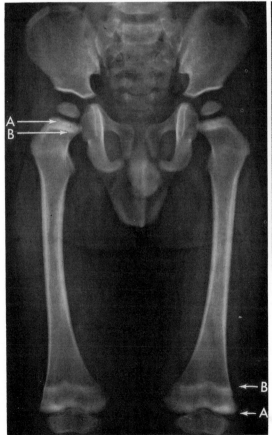

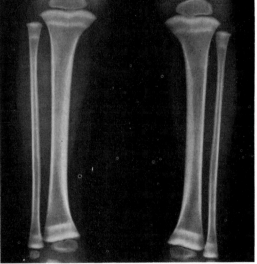

Figure 5–8 The amount of growth at the ends of long bones is demonstrated by these radiographs of a patient in whom there were two episodes of lead poisoning. The dense line in the metaphysis (*B*) marks the first episode, the heavy zone of provisional calcification (*A*) the present one, and the distance between them, growth in the interim.

One must remember that joint spaces are potential spaces and not gross areas of intermediate density as seen by x-ray. The apparent space is in fact cartilage and synovium which have the density of soft tissue and which contrast sharply with subchondral bone. This understanding is essential to the study of joints and particularly to the study of growing bone. The epiphyseal center is a center of bone located within a large mass of cartilage, i.e., the epiphysis. Therefore in diseases involving primarily the joint, cartilaginous destruction must precede destruction of subchondral bone and cartilaginous destruction is manifest by narrowing of the distance between the ossified ends of participating bones. Further, synovial thickening may be seen as well as fluid.

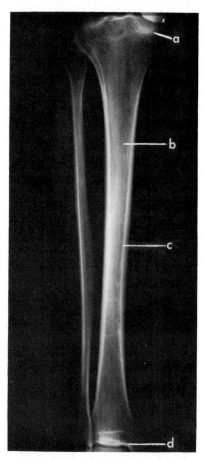

Figure 5-10   Male, 31 years of age. Radiograph of the tibia and fibula: *a*, residual of epiphyseal line; *b*, medullary canal; *c*, cortex; *d*, subchondral bone at ankle joint. (Compare with Figure 5–9.) The epiphyseal centers enlarge and assume a definite configuration as growth occurs. Note the change in the appearance of the ankle joint that occurs when final growth is attained. The amount of epiphyseal cartilage is appreciated.

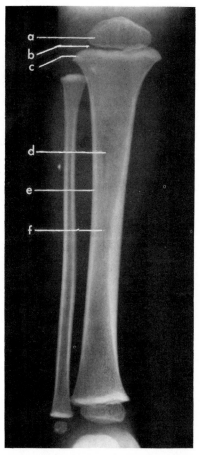

Figure 5-9   Male, 2 years of age. Radiograph of the tibia and fibula: *a*, epiphyseal center; *b*, epiphyseal line; *c*, zone of provisional calcification; *d*, nutrient canal; *e*, cortex; *f*, medullary canal.

From the anatomic standpoint, one must recognize the existence of normal variations. Prominent nutrient foramina are often confused with fracture lines, and irregularities in bone configuration may be confused with periosteal new bone formation. Such variations are usually symmetrical and examination of the "opposite side" for comparison makes their significance evident. Such comparison is especially helpful in growing bones. Bizarre configurations of the bones and joints may be seen as a result of faulty projection or positioning; reexamination

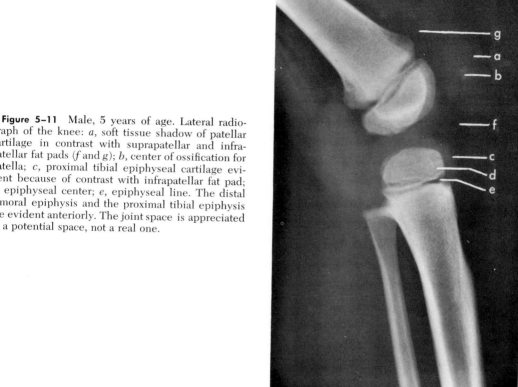

Figure 5-11 Male, 5 years of age. Lateral radiograph of the knee: *a*, soft tissue shadow of patellar cartilage in contrast with suprapatellar and infrapatellar fat pads (*f* and *g*); *b*, center of ossification for patella; *c*, proximal tibial epiphyseal cartilage evident because of contrast with infrapatellar fat pad; *d*, epiphyseal center; *e*, epiphyseal line. The distal femoral epiphysis and the proximal tibial epiphysis are evident anteriorly. The joint space is appreciated as a potential space, not a real one.

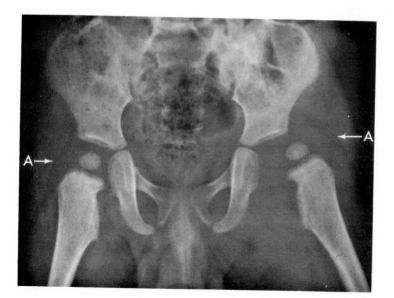

Figure 5-12 The left femur is displaced from the acetabulum and the joint distended by an accumulation of pus within the joint. Fat is evident about the joint capsule on both sides (*A*).

is always indicated when the radiographic appearance of a structure does not correlate with anatomic or pathologic information.

The correlation of physiology and radiology is best illustrated by the changes observed in a growing cylindrical bone. The growing ends of a bone reflect the earliest and most severe changes of metabolic bone disease. The rate of growth of a long bone differs at its proximal and its distal ends, and it is the faster growing of the ends that presents the most apparent alterations (Fig. 5–8). It is for this reason that the wrist and knee are examined when rickets or scurvy is suspected, not because of convenience or for other arbitrary reasons. It is important to note that the epiphyseal center is opaque, not the epiphysis. The zone of provisional calcification, which abuts on the metaphysis, is quite dense and represents the area in which calcium salts are deposited in the cartilaginous intercellular matrix between degenerated cartilage cells. As the blood vessels and osteoblasts invade this zone of degenerated cartilage cells, osteoid is deposited on the surface of the exposed cartilaginous matrix. The metaphysis is that area in which osteoid is being laid down and bone is being formed. With a deficiency of mineral salts, as in rickets, the zone of provisional calcification is the first to be affected and thus disappears early in the course of the disease. When organic matrix is deficient, as in scurvy, new bone is not formed and a radiolucent area is evident adjacent to the zone of provisional calcification, the so-called scorbutic zone. Under normal circumstances the trabecular pattern and the thickness of the cortex are dependent in large part on stress and strain; in bowing of a bone, for example, thickening of the cortex and of the trabeculae along the weight-bearing line is evident.

The soft tissues must not be neglected during the study of bones. They often reflect disease of the underlying bone even when osseous alterations are not apparent. In osteomyelitis, inflammatory exudate in the soft tissues adjacent to the involved bone may distort or obliterate radiolucent muscle planes to indicate the presence of an abnormality before there is evidence of bone destruction. Effusion into a joint may widen the normal radiolucent zone and at times may be associated with dislocation of the participating bones. Fat around the capsule of a joint often outlines the limits of the capsule and reflects its distention by fluid or neoplastic tissue (Fig. 5–12).

The aim of radiographic study is to note the location of disease and the extent to which the skeleton is involved. Objective analysis, based on knowledge of the reactions of bone as a tissue to metabolic, infectious or neoplastic processes, follows. This information correlated with appropriate clinical data (age, sex and duration of symptoms) and laboratory determinations provides the basis for logical radiographic interpretation. The limitations of the method and its worth are evaluated logically, speculation is minimized and specialized examinations are utilized in a way that is most efficacious regarding diagnosis and treatment.

References

1. Glasser, O., Quimby, E. H., Taylor, L. S., Weatherwax, J. L., and Morgan, R. H.: Physical Foundations of Radiology. Ed. 3. New York, Paul B. Hoeber, Inc., 1961.
2. Meschan, I.: Roentgen Signs in Clinical Practice. Philadelphia, W. B. Saunders Co., 1966.
3. Nelson, S. W.: Semin. Roentgenol., 1:244, 1966.
4. Lodwick, G. S.: Semin. Roentgenol., 1:293, 1966.
5. Radiologic Clinics of North America: Diagnostic Radiology of Bone Disease. Vol. 8, No. 2, August 1970. W. B. Saunders Co.
6. Radiologic Clinics of North America: Selected Techniques in Radiology. Vol. 9, No. 1, April 1971. W. B. Saunders Co.
7. Charkes, N. D., Valentine, G., and Crantz, B.: Radiology, 107:563, 1973.

SECTION TWO

DISTURBANCES IN SKELETAL DEVELOPMENT

Chapter 6

THE SKELETAL DYSPLASIAS

In this chapter are collected those disturbances of skeletal growth, found at birth or developing through childhood and adolescence, which have been vaguely classified as the chondrodystrophies. Considered together they compose a confoundingly heterogeneous group, most of which have been inappropriately named to compound the confusion. Some of these conditions are relatively common and therefore important. Others are decidedly uncommon and rarely encountered except in symposia or specialty board examinations.

Since our dictionary informs us that dystrophy implies faulty nutrition whereas dysplasia connotes faulty development, the latter seems to be the more appropriate term to use for these conditions. And since some appear to be due to disturbances in the growth of cartilage, others to the growth of bone and still others to aberrations in the production of both these tissues, it seems better to abandon the prefixes of chondro- and osteo- and to refer to these conditions simply as skeletal dysplasias.

Classification has been the concern of more than one author though Fairbank[1] was probably the one most widely read and quoted until recently. McKusick and Rubin have each written a modern monograph on this subject and though each has its particular emphasis, the one in genetics and the other in radiology, they are more complete and modern and should be consulted for reference.

Whenever we have attempted to better our understanding of any complex subject in medicine, such as the skeletal dysplasias, we have usually found the best approach is by way of a simple definition of the subject and then a comprehensive classification. The definition depends upon one's point of view and area of interest; each writer must therefore compound his own. Our concept of the skeletal dysplasias is more inclusive than that of most, for under this heading we have included the disturbances of skeletal growth, the inherited and the heritable (McKusick makes a good distinction), the congenital, those with no features of genetic alteration and the abiotrophic, those which begin in childhood or adult life and run a progressive and destructive course.

Classification, too, can be approached from a number of aspects. Most have been based on radiographic similarities and differences but since the dysplasias can be expressed in only a limited number of ways, we find that the radiographic expression often encompasses a number of different entities. They have been classified according to their genetic transmission but again there are too few partitions to adequately separate their considerable number. Rubin's classification is the most ingenious to date. He has divided the growing bone into a number of zones. He has included the articular plate and the osseous epiphyseal center in one zone which he calls the epiphysis. This may offend some traditionalists since the enchondral or growth plate has always been included in this region. However, radiologists have always had a tendency to ignore both the articular and growth plates and usually when they speak of the epiphysis in a growing bone they are referring to the osseous nucleus only.

In his second zone which he calls the physis, Rubin designates the growth plate. The terms metaphysis and diaphysis are used with their conventional meanings. He has proposed that most and perhaps all the dysplasias are caused by an alteration in one or more of these zones. This is a fresh and intriguing proposal but we have found it difficult to put into practical usage. For example, he classifies osteogenesis imperfecta as a purely periosteal dysplasia of intramembranous bone formation but we have the same changes in the enchondral-formed bone in patients with this disease and suggest the reason that failure of production of cortical bone appears more dramatic than the length growth production of enchondral bone is because the error registers in the areas in which bone production is more massive. Bone mass of cortex formation is many times greater than that required for length growth. Rubin also places Morquio's disease in the epiphyseal dysplasia category. Very recent work makes it appear that this dysplasia is a disturbance in mucopolysaccharide metabolism of all the bone-forming cartilage cells, not just those of one zone.

Indeed it would seem best to construct a classification on the basis of the morbid physiology of the cells concerned. Collagen is made up of a variety of combinations of amino acid constituents just as hemoglobin is. We believe that eventually it will be shown that improper maturation of the cells from which stem collagenoblasts, chondroblasts and osteoblasts leaves them incapable of combining their amino acids normally. The result of this fault, whether it be too little production, overproduction or abnormal production, is expressed as a dysplasia.

We have tried to construct a classification with this concept in mind. Obviously the result is an unfinished product because of the wide gaps in our knowledge of the physiology of bone. But if parts are sound, they act as piers on which the remaining superstructure may be built. The least that can be said of it is that it is a step in the right direction. Some system, we hold, even a faulty one, is better than no system at all.

As will be noted, we have divided the dysplasias into two principal groups: those related to disturbances in chondroid production and those caused by an inability to elaborate normal or sufficient osteoid.

In the first group, the mucopolysaccharidoses constitute the most definitive class; the metabolic defect is known and we can interpret the microscopic and radiologic alterations in its terms. In the remainder of this group, the metabolic defect is not known; we only assume they, the dysplasias, are caused by failure of normal maturation of growth plate chondroblasts *because* of the microscopic and radiographic picture, the reverse process of the above. As investigation continues, we hope the exact metabolic defect will be defined and then the classification may have to be changed.

In the second group, those dysplasias ascribed to abnormal osteoid production, there are again two main classes: those in which it appears that the osseous nucleus within the epiphysis fails to form normally and a second group in which the fault appears to be abnormal osteoid formation on the chondroid matrix in the metaphysis. The first group is characterized by abnormal articular plates since the osseous nucleus supports these plates and the second by disturbances in length growth and modeling.

In subtypes of these groups there appears to be an inability of the osteoblasts, whether in the epiphyseal nucleus, the metaphysis or the cambium periosteum, to elaborate sufficient or normal osteoid. Thus in osteogenesis imperfecta there is too little, in osteopetrosis there is too much and in fibrous dysplasia the quality is abnormal.

A classification is useful only as long as it offers fixed points of reference. As our knowledge enlarges in the field of the dysplasias these points shift position and our classification will doubtless become obsolete but it will have served its purpose and for the present, that is enough to ask.

I. Dysplasias due to disturbances in chondroid production
   A. Related to abnormal maturation of growth plate chondroblasts
      1. The mucopolysaccharidoses

a. Morquio's disease
b. Hurler's disease
c. Other mucopolysaccharidoses
2. Idiopathic
a. Achondroplasia
b. Cartilage-hair hypoplasia
c. Metaphyseal dysostosis
1. Jansen type
2. Schmid type
3. Spahr type
B. Related to heterotopic proliferation of epiphyseal chondroblasts
1. Enchondromatosis (Ollier)
2. Osteochondromatosis
3. Epiphyseal hyperplasia (Fairbank)
II. Dysplasias due to disturbances in
osteoid production
A. Related to abnormal epiphyseal
ossification
1. Diastrophic dwarfism
2. Spondyloepiphyseal dysplasia
3. Multiple epiphyseal dysplasia
(Fairbank)
4. Stippled epiphyses
B. Related to abnormal metaphyseal
and periosteal ossification
1. Due to deficient osteoid production

a. Osteogenesis imperfecta
2. Due to excessive osteoid production or deficient osteolysis
a. Osteopetrosis (Albers-
Schönberg)
b. Pyknodysostosis
c. Metaphyseal dysplasia
(Pyle)
d. Diaphyseal sclerosis
(Camurati-Engelmann-
Ribbing)
e. Melorrheostosis
f. Osteopathia striata
(Voorhoeve)
g. Osteopoikilosis
3. Related to abnormal osteoid
production
a. Fibrous dysplasia
b. Neurofibromatosis
c. Pseudarthrosis
III. Miscellaneous dysplasias
A. Dyschondrosteosis (Madelung)
B. Marfan's syndrome
C. Apert's syndrome
D. Cleidocranial dysostosis
E. Chondroectodermal dysplasia
(Ellis-van Creveld)
F. Asphyxiating thoracic dystrophy
G. Other affections associated with
dwarfism

DYSPLASIAS CHARACTERIZED BY AN INABILITY TO ELABORATE NORMAL CHONDROID

Those Which Result from Abnormal Maturation of Growth Plate Chondroblasts

There are three varieties of dysplasias in this group. In the first, the mucopoly-saccharidoses, we know there is a meta-bolic fault, an inability to properly metab-olize certain mucopolysaccharides by the fibroblasts and probably the chondro-blasts. Consequently the chondroid scaf-folding is not normally produced and so both epiphyseal and metaphyseal ossi-fication is affected.

In the second variety there is probably a metabolic defect, but as yet we do not know its nature so we have classified these dysplasias as idiopathic.

In the third variety, the disturbance ap-pears to be related to the position of the cells rather than to the quality of the spe-cific maturation defect. In enchondro-matosis the cartilage cells are not used up at the epiphyseal line and so persist in the metaphysis. In osteochondromatosis they are displaced peripherally but con-tinue to function just as they would if they were in the epiphyseal line.

The same applies in the third condition epiphyseal hyperplasia, only the displace-ment is in the epiphysis rather than the metaphysis.

THE MUCOPOLYSACCHARIDOSES

In 1917 Charles Hunter, of Winnipeg, described a curious developmental aberration in two brothers. Hurler[3] described the same or a closely related condition in 1919, and the process acquired the name of Hurler's disease. She recognized it as a hereditary condition and supposed it to be a primary skeletal growth disturbance. Since that time a number of closely related types of this disease have been described, and as our knowledge about it increased, it became apparent that this condition is a group of metabolic diseases involving more than one tissue system, including the skeleton, various fibroblastic derivatives, the reticuloendothelial cells and even nerve and epithelial tissues. Microscopic examination revealed that these cells were crammed with some material that was difficult to analyze.

We had the rare opportunity to autopsy and to study one case.[4] We tried every stain known to us at that time (1938) in a futile attempt to identify the intracellular substance; other workers were no more successful. Because the cells vaguely resembled those of the better known reticuloendothelioses, it was assumed that the substance was a lipid, and the name lipochondrodystrophy was applied. In 1941 Reilly[5] found granules in the blood leukocytes, which stained with Wright's stain, and in 1952 Brante[6] found that this material took the PAS stain and concluded that it was a mucopolysaccharide. Five years later Dorfman and Lorincz[7] found mucopolysaccharides in the urine of these patients. Five types of this metabolic disturbance have been described and Zellweger et al.[8] found Reilly granules in the leukocytes and Pedrini and co-workers[9] found keratosulfates in the urine of patients with Morquio's disease, thus fairly well establishing that this condition also belongs in the mucopolysaccharidosis group.

At present it appears that a genetic aberration results in a failure of normal metabolic maturation of fibroblasts, caused by the presence of abnormal quantities of mucopolysaccharides. It has been suggested[10] that these diseases are in fact protein metabolic defects so that the muco-polysaccharides which are normally complexed by these proteins are left free to be taken up by the affected cells and excreted into the urine.

Several reports have noted lipid rather than mucopolysaccharide in the affected cells in the brain, other than the brain macrophages. This finding is difficult to explain unless one assumes that the same protein involved in complexing the muco-polysaccharides is necessary for the glyco-lipid-protein complexes.

McKusick[11] has divided these conditions into six types according to their mode of genetic transmission, the muco-polysaccharide involved and the clinical and radiologic manifestations. He suggests that eponyms be used for these conditions until further investigation clarifies the point of metabolic breakdown.

Type   I. Hurler's disease
Type   II. Hunter's syndrome
Type III. Sanfilippo's syndrome
Type   IV. Morquio's disease
Type   V. Scheie's syndrome
Type   VI. Syndrome of Maroteaux and Lamy

Morquio's Disease

This condition has been called chondro-osteodystrophy. The eponym "Morquio's" is retained here because it is the one most widely used and because recent knowledge indicates that it is one of the muco-polysaccharidoses, thus making the earlier names obsolete.

The condition is transmitted as an autosomal recessive, often occurring in multiple siblings and causing dwarfism, kyphosis and severe disability. It was incompletely described several times in the years from 1913 to 1928, but in Morquio's report[12] in 1929 it was completely set forth as an entity. In a series of three reports he eventually described four cases in a single family. Brailsford's report[13] of one case was made almost simultaneously, and this dysplasia probably more justly should be called Morquio-Brailsford's disease.

Morquio's is a rare disease. At this writing there are a few less than 100 cases reported in the world literature. It is usually considered to be a disease of childhood, the signs most often appearing between the sixth and eighteenth months. It occurs in both sexes with about equal incidence. Its hereditary nature is now thoroughly established because approximately 50 per cent reveal this characteristic and the majority of these show sibling relationship. The condition has occurred in mother and offspring more than once. There is more than a suggestion that consanguinity plays a role because it appeared five times in 41 families of consanguineous marriage, an incidence of 12 per cent and about 60 times more frequently than might be expected in an average cross section population.

In only a few cases has there been a suggestion of the disease at birth. In almost all, the first symptoms appear at about the time weight-bearing begins by sitting or standing. Since there are no reports of prenatal x-ray studies it is impossible to say whether skeletal changes occur in utero.

The first sign noted is usually a dorsilumbar kyphosis (Fig. 6–1), and as an attempt at weight-bearing continues, a galaxy of skeletal distortions appear. The neck is short so that the head appears to be thrust forward and jammed down into the thorax. The sternum is prominent with a horizontal displacement (Fig. 6–2). The chest is increased in the anteroposterior dimension. The head is normal in size but it appears large because of the lag in growth of the rest of the body, this lag being progressively more apparent as the more caudad parts are approached.

The joints are widened. The wrists and ankles and sometimes larger joints are abnormally mobile owing to muscle and tendon laxity, but extension at the elbows, hips and knees may be incomplete because of an elongated olecranon and epiphyseal distortion. As the patient ages the characteristic stance with kyphotic back and partially flexed hips, knees and elbows develops. The hands are short and trident with thick fingers and ulnar deviation. The feet are short, wide, flat and everted at the ankles. The deciduous teeth are usually well formed but the permanent teeth are distorted both as to position and shape. Since most of the decidual tooth buds develop in utero and the permanent buds after birth, this selectivity in tooth development further suggests that the factor or factors that cause the changes in the skeleton are most effective in late uterine and early postnatal life.

Roentgenographic Manifestations. The roentgenographic manifestations of Morquio's disease reflect abnormal conversion of cartilage to mature bone. Alteration in the size and contour of the vertebral bodies is constant and distinctive. The long bones are affected in most instances, and although the degree of deformity varies, it is the growing ends of the long bones that are most abnormal. There is no disturbance in the density or the architecture of the diaphyses in most instances except when deformity progresses to the degree that disuse osteopenia results.

The vertebral bodies are flat (universal vertebra plana) with rough, irregular

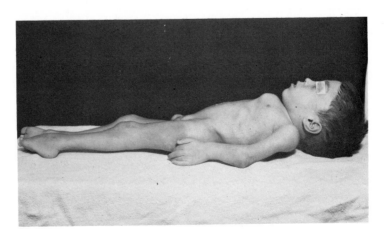

Figure 6–1 In Morquio's disease the caudad portions of the body are poorly developed. The head is relatively large, the neck short. The plastron is bulged forward. The legs are undeveloped. (From Shriners' Hospital, Philadelphia.)

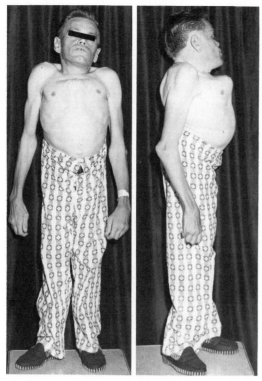

Figure 6–2   Morquio's disease. The head appears to be thrust forward and jammed down into the thorax. The sternum is prominent with a horizontal displacement. (Courtesy of Dr. T. A. Randall.)

contours and an anterior central projection. The intervertebral discs are narrower than is normal. Kyphosis is common and may be aggravated by posterior displacement or wedging of one or more vertebrae. Lumbar vertebral bodies tend to be smaller and more deformed than the dorsal ones. Further, significant deformity of the first and second cervical bodies has been described. The posterior arch of C_1 may lie within the foramen magnum; the odontoid may be absent or hypoplastic and the body of C_2 large such that it encroaches on the neural canal.[14] A small sacrum is common. An increase in the anteroposterior diameter of the chest occurs as a result of kyphosis and a pectus carinatum deformity. The ribs tend to be broad and deformed at both their anterior and posterior ends and the sternum may be short.

The cylindrical bones may be normal in length. In some instances they are short, and it is usually the bones of the upper

extremities that manifest this alteration. The growing ends of the long bones are broad with irregular zones of provisional calcification and irregularly ossified, flattened epiphyseal centers. The proximal femur may show marked deformity, characterized in part by lateral sloping of the proximal tibial metaphysis and epiphysis (Fig. 6–3C). Subluxations at the hip are not uncommon. The acetabula tend to be deep and their osseous roofs coarse in their outline. The ilia flare laterally. The carpal and tarsal bones are irregular in configuration and size. The tubular bones of the hands and feet tend to be short with irregular ossification of the epiphyseal centers. The skull and facial bones are unaffected.

A decrease in muscle mass may be evident about the lower extremities. Knock-knee deformity is extremely common as a result of the relaxation of muscles and tendons about the knees and disturbance in growth at the proximal end of the tibia.

Microscopy. The opportunity of obtaining material for microscopic study has been extremely limited and, consequently, conclusive descriptions cannot as yet be given. Opie and Harrison described a case under the title of "hypertrophic chondrodystrophy" that now appears to be Morquio's disease. They gave a detailed description of the microscopic features of the head of the femur. They reported an abortive and disordered maturation of the epiphyseal chondroblasts with failure to produce an oriented, calcified chondroid scaffolding. There was sealing off of the epiphyseal plate with an irregular vault of bone and islands of cartilage within the metaphysis. We found a similar picture in two cases with repeated biopsies at intervals in one of them (Fig. 6–4). The improper chondroblastic maturation, some chondroblasts collecting material (glycogen or mucopolysaccharide?) in the depths of the epiphyseal plate and others none at all, resulted in a distorted chondroid bar production and irregularities in the epiphyseal line. The line of provisional calcification was broken and distorted and here and there the chondroid matrix showed focal areas of degeneration. The result was a helter-skelter production of primary

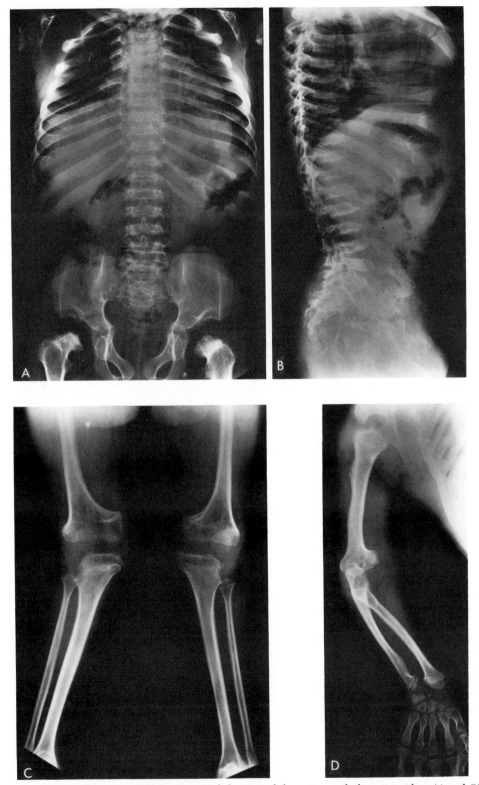

Figure 6–3 Morquio's disease. Characteristic deformity of the spine and chest is evident (*A* and *B*). The acetabula are deep and irregular. The proximal femoral epiphyseal center is poorly formed, and the neck of the femur is short and bent. The bones of the lower extremities are of normal length (*C*); those of the upper extremity are shorter than normal (*D*). Flat, irregular and wide epiphyseal centers are evident. Knockknee deformity is present (*C*).

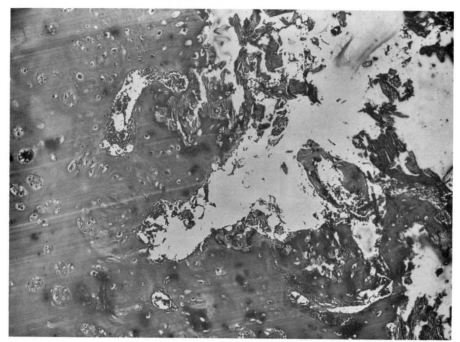

Figure 6–4   Morquio's disease. A section across the epiphyseal line of a growing bone showing a completely chaotic arrangement of the chondrocytes, provisional line of calcification and hyaline scaffolding. The epiphysis is on the left. Note the irregular maturation of the cartilage cells and wandering line which represents the junction of the epiphysis and metaphysis. (× 40.)

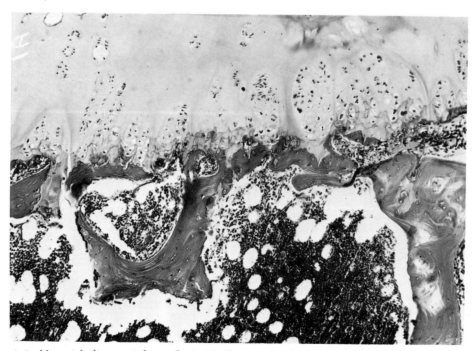

Figure 6–5   Morquio's disease. A dome of primitive bone seals off the epiphyseal cartilage from the metaphysis indicating premature growth cessation. (× 130.)

spongiosa. Lamellated cortex formation appeared to be relatively normal.

Because bone deformity appears on weight-bearing, one might conjecture that there is an inability to convert primitive fiberbone to adult bone. The skeleton, remaining soft, is unprepared for the stress of normal weight-bearing. A single biopsy specimen removed from the shin of a 9 year old patient with Morquio's disease revealed fiberbone where adult bone normally should have been. One must not draw conclusions from such limited material, and it is fortunate for the pathologist that the diagnosis does not depend upon the microscopic appearance. There is also great danger in interpreting the static abnormalities seen in sectioned samples of far advanced cases as one stage of a dynamic process. Rubin points this out in his monograph, "Dynamic Classification of Bone Dysplasias."

It seems to us, however, that Rubin may have erred in his analysis of the radiographic alterations which characterize this disease because he interprets the alterations in the growth plate and metaphysis as a result of stresses that have not been neutralized by a healthy articular plate. He believes that the primary fault in Morquio's disease resides in the chondroblastic cells in the depths of the articular plate and states that in growth plates not normally associated with articular plates, i.e., at the costochondral junction, the growth plate distortions do not occur. We have examined tissue sections of this area in one case and found the same kind of changes as those seen in the weight-bearing areas. Now, since it is almost certain that the dysplasia is the result of an abnormality in the elaboration and storage of heparatin sulfate, it is more reasonable to assume that this abnormality affects all chondroblastic and possibly osteoblastic maturation, function and proliferation.

Differential Diagnosis. Hurler's disease (gargoylism) is the condition most frequently confused with Morquio's disease. The radiologic aspects are so similar in some instances that numerous cases of the former have been reported in series under the title of the latter. Although the two conditions may closely resemble each other clinically, radiologically and pathogenetically, at present it is probably best to consider them distinct clinical entities. Both dysplasias are now considered to belong to the group of mucopolysaccharidoses. In the early stages, differentiation may be impossible on the basis of the radiographs alone. In Morquio's disease the hepatosplenomegaly, brain damage and corneal clouding, if they appear at all, are late and much less severe. On the other hand, the skeletal changes may occur earlier and progress rapidly to a more dramatic stage.

If carefully sought, Reilly granules are often found in both granulocytes and lymphocytes in Morquio's disease. Heparatin sulfate has been found in the urine.

Prognosis. The progress of Morquio's disease usually slows as the patient ages. Some cases seem to be arrested with puberty though a few continue through adolescence and even into adult life. Formes frustes have been described on radiologic evidence alone, but this is hazardous because the radiologic findings in Morquio's disease are not pathognomonic. Whether or not the disease is arrested, the skeletal distortion is usually so marked that woeful crippling is inevitable. Once the progress has come to a halt the patient may live as long as his deformities are compatible with existence.

Hurler's Disease

Classically, Hurler's disease (gargoylism) begins in early childhood, causing skeletal deformity, failure of mental development, blindness, enlargement of the liver and spleen and eventual mitral insufficiency with cardiac decompensation.

The disease is uncommon but not rare, there being more than 200 cases reported. The first symptoms may be noted soon after birth, and it is probable that in most instances the disease begins in utero. Genetic transmission appears to be as an autosomal recessive.

Ellis, Sheldon and Capon[15] coined the term "gargoylism" because of the strikingly repugnant appearance and the fancied resemblance to the well-known architectural device. The condition progresses through early childhood but, because it is not incompatible with life, the patient may live to middle age.

The peculiar facies may be noted soon after birth. The head may be large, the forehead low and covered with fine hair, the nasal bridge sunken and the nostrils flared. The interocular distance is increased; the ears are set low and far back on the head. The distance between the posterior margins of the mandibles may be increased to cause a widening of the lower portion of the face. The tongue is large and thick. Frequently the metopic suture line between the frontal bones is prominently ridged. The teeth are widely separated and poorly formed. A chronic rhinitis is common because of deposits in the nasopharyngeal mucosa. The neck is short. The belly is protuberant because of an enlarged liver and spleen and the intra-abdominal pressure may result in umbilical and inguinal hernias (Fig. 6–6). Peripheral lymph nodes may be enlarged. A dorsolumbar kyphosis usually appears early. The hands are short and thick; the fingers are stubby.

Retardation of sitting, standing, talking and walking is noted in time and some time within the first to third year the cornea may begin to show clouding. At first there may be no impairment of vision but as the clouding increases there is progressive loss of sight. Corneal clouding often masks an accompanying progressive degeneration of the retina.

Mental retardation should be noted early if looked for, and usually development progresses no further than the stage of idiocy.

After six months the disturbances in skeletal growth become more and more apparent. There is failure to attain normal stature with resultant dwarfism. The poorly formed, flattened vertebral bodies and the kyphosis cause collapse of the trunk. Flaccidity of joints has been reported, but usually there is extension disability because of deposits within the tendons and ligaments. The arms may not be lifted above shoulder level nor the forearm completely extended. There is often a flexion deformity at the hips and

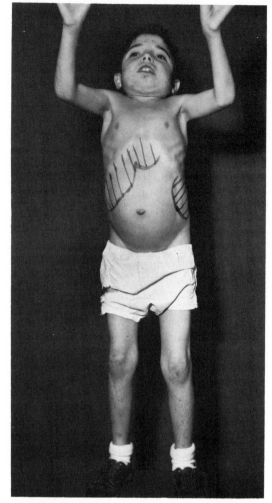

Figure 6–6   Hurler's disease. The liver and spleen margins have been outlined on the skin. There are an umbilical hernia and an enlargement of cervical lymph nodes.

knees with coxa valga, genu valgum, pes planus and talipes equinovarus.

Roentgenographic Manifestations. The skeletal changes in Hurler's disease vary from those of a mild degree to marked severity; they may develop slowly, requiring a considerable period of time. In the typical case, generalized skeletal changes are evident early in life, by two years of age, and are relatively constant. Lesions other than osseous ones are sometimes evident radiographically, such as hepatosplenomegaly and umbilical hernia.

The cranial vault is characteristically enlarged in its anteroposterior dimension and the bones are often thick and dense.

The enlarged vault is often a manifestation of communicating hydrocephalus resulting from involvement of the leptomeninges.[14] Premature closure of the sagittal suture frequently occurs and is responsible for the shape of the head. In many instances, the sella is shallow and elongated anteriorly beneath the anterior clinoids, a reflection of delayed growth of the sphenoid bone. The nasopharynx tends to be small and readily obstructed by lymphoid tissue. The development of the paranasal sinuses and mastoids is retarded.

The mandible is found to be short and broad, and associated with concavity or flattening of the articular surface of the condyle.[16] The latter, too, may be hypoplastic and associated with a deep, irregular mandibular notch and large coronoid process.

The broad ribs narrow at their vertebral ends and are blunt anteriorly. The clavicles are short and thick. There is a char-

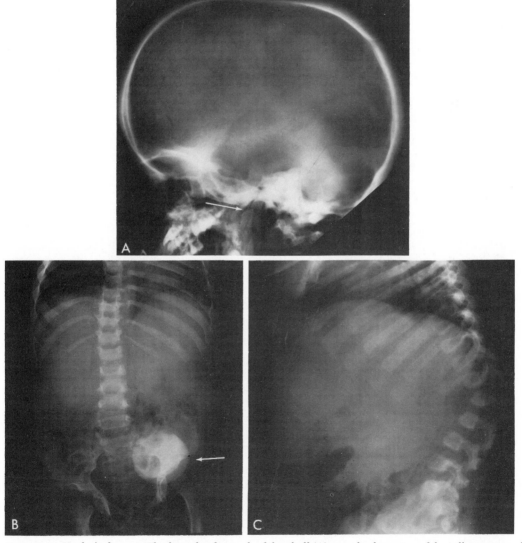

Figure 6–7 Hurler's disease. The lateral radiograph of the skull (A) reveals elongation of the sella turcica and the flat articular surface of the condyle of the mandible (arrow). The vault is prominent in its anteroposterior dimension, the cranial bones are slightly thickened and the nasopharynx is small. B and C demonstrate deformity of the spine and pelvis. An umbilical hernia is evident (arrow). Hepatosplenomegaly is present.

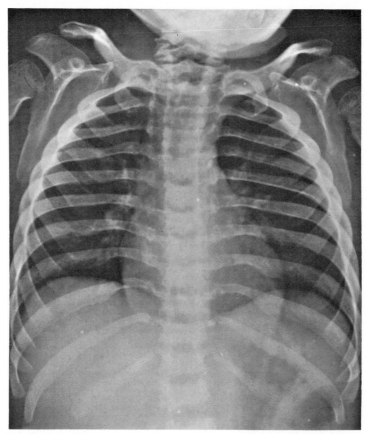

Figure 6-8 Hurler's disease. The ribs are narrow posteriorly and broad anteriorly. The clavicles are large in diameter.

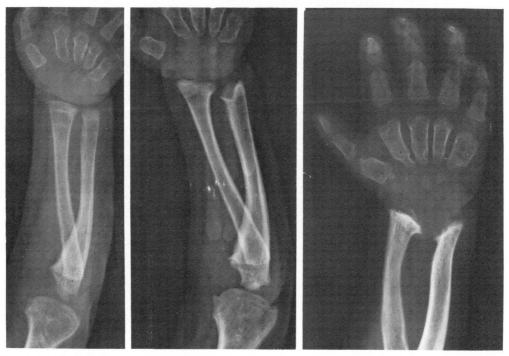

Figure 6-9 Hurler's disease. Progression of deformity of the bones of the forearm and wrist from one year to six years is illustrated.

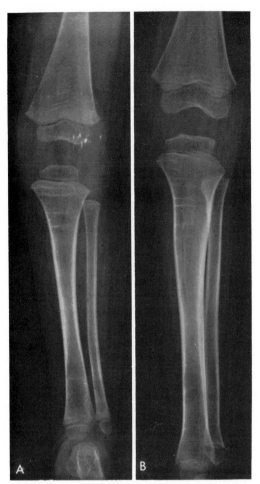

Figure 6–10 Hurler's disease. The bones of the lower extremities are not as abnormal as those of the upper. There is some flattening of the epiphyseal centers and widening of the ends of the bones. *A*, 3 years of age; *B*, 6 years of age.

acteristic gibbus at the low dorsal or high lumbar region occasioned by deformity of one or more vertebrae. The affected vertebral bodies are hypoplastic, have an anterior inferior beak and are displaced posteriorly. The intervertebral disc spaces are maintained.

The bones of the upper extremity are more abnormal than are those of the lower extremity. The medullary canals are widened and the epiphyseal centers are flat and often irregular. The humerus is short and thick, bulges in its midportion and may taper toward its distal end. A concavity develops, with varus angulation, on the medial aspect of the proximal end of the humerus. The radius and ulna too

are short and thick and taper distally where the articular surfaces face one another. The metacarpals tend to be narrow proximally, and the phalanges are short and broad. The bones of the feet show changes similar to those of the hands. The length of the bones of the lower extremity is not affected, but valgus deformity of the femurs and narrow femoral necks are common. The acetabula are shallow, the ilia flared and the ischia thick. Subluxation of the hips may occur.

Although the carpal and tarsal bones are abnormal in contour and may be late in appearing, gross irregularity of the growing ends of the long bones is not as marked as in some other skeletal dysplasias.

In general, ossification of secondary centers is delayed and when it occurs, the centers are apt to be irregular and deformed.

Microscopy. Very little tissue has been available for examination, but in the past two decades all investigators have agreed that deposits of some alien substance or substances are found in both parenchymal and mesenchymal tissues as well as in the urine. These substances have now been identified as chondroitin sulfate B and heparatin sulfate. In our case,[4] an 8½ year old male, the heart was large, pale and firm and the mitral, aortic and tricuspid valves were sites of heavy, yellow-orange deposits with calcification. There was evidence of generalized cardiac insufficiency. The liver was immensely enlarged. There were splenomegaly and an enlarged brain. The cells of the anterior pituitary, the liver (Fig. 6–11) and the adrenal medulla contained globules of what is now known to be a mucopolysaccharide, as did practically all the derivatives of mesenchyme including the cells of the peripheral blood. Brain cells were also distended by some foreign material, causing large round vacuoles in our sections. This substance is now assumed to be a lipid compound.

Dawson,[17] in a later report, expressed the belief that the substance found in the cerebral neurons is a combination of a mucopolysaccharide with a phosphatide and cerebroside, which is insoluble in the usual fixatives. Wolfe et al.[17] reported the presence of a glycolipid in the cells of the brain. They believe that this phe-

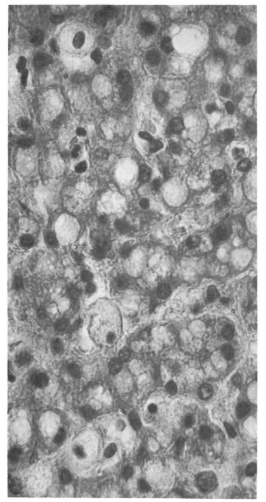

Figure 6–11   Hurler's disease. The offending material, whatever its chemical nature, accumulates in both mesenchymal and epithelial tissue. In the liver it replaces the cytoplasm of the hepatic cells. (× 450.)

chondroitin sulfate B and heparatin sulfate causes clouding of the cornea.

Zellweger and co-workers[19] have found coarse, deeply staining, violet granules (Reilly granules) in the neutrophils, lymphocytes and eosinophilic leukocytes of the peripheral blood with Wright's stain. They believe that these granules may be present in patients without clinical manifestations of the disease and perhaps those who will later develop the disease in an abortive form.

Several authors have examined sections of epiphyseal tissue in cases of Hurler's disease. Apparently some cases (as ours) fail to show significant alterations in morphology, others reveal a lack of chondroblastic activity and presumably stasis of enchondral bone growth, and a third group show irregularity and distortion in the maturation zone and a transverse plate of bone across the metaphysis.

Prognosis. The victims of Hurler's disease may die in childhood or they may live well into adult life, but the appalling skeletal deformity, the mental deficiency and the blindness make them helpless and hopeless members of society.

The offending substances are now known to be chondroitin sulfate B and heparatin sulfate. Normally about 20 milligrams or less of mucopolysaccharides are excreted in the urine per day. In Hurler's disease the amount is usually more than 60 milligrams.

Other Mucopolysaccharidoses

The remaining four mucopolysaccharidoses appear to be variations of Hurler's disease. In Hunter's syndrome the genetic transmission is different because it is sex-linked. Clouding of the cornea does not occur, and mental deterioration is later in onset and slower in progress. It is considerably less common than Hurler's disease, and a gibbus does not occur. Deafness and nodular skin lesions over the back and arms are common. Prognosis is better in this type than in Hurler's disease, with most patients surviving to middle age. There is abnormal excretion of chondroitin sulfate B and heparatin sulfate in the urine just as in Hurler's disease.

nomenon, which supposedly is the cause of the mental deterioration, may or may not accompany the usual mucopolysaccharide storage in the mesenchymal derivatives elsewhere. Foam cells, indicating the latter situation, and glycolipid cells, suggesting the former, infiltrate the rectal mucosa; they advocate biopsy of this area for diagnosis and prognosis. Deposits occurring in the meninges may cause blockage of flow of cerebrospinal fluid and a hydrocephalus. Intracytoplasmic accumulations disturb normal metabolism and function. An infiltration of macrophages containing large quantities of

Sanfilippo's syndrome is autosomal recessive like Hurler's disease, but the somatic changes are much less severe, while the intellectual decay is earlier in onset and more rapid in development. Clouding of the cornea apparently does not occur, hepatosplenomegaly is slight and dwarfing is moderate. Excessive heparatin sulfate excretion in the urine is the major biochemical feature.

Scheie's syndrome is also autosomal recessive, but clouding of the cornea is striking; aortic disease, stiff joints, retinitis pigmentosa and excessive body hair occur but there is no impairment of the intellect. The mucopolysaccharide at fault in this condition appears to be chondroitin sulfate B.

Though the syndrome of Maroteaux and Lamy is autosomal recessive, and the somatic features are the same as those of Hurler's disease, mental deterioration does not occur. As in Scheie's syndrome the chemical fault lies within the chondroitin sulfate B factor.

It begins to appear that the normal organism elaborates and metabolizes a number of related chemical substances—the mucopolysaccharides. Further, normal metabolism of mucopolysaccharides may depend on the synthesis of proteins. We think of these processes as the functions of the intracellular constituents. The cytoplasmic constituents necessary for these functions depend upon a normal genetic composition of the parent cells. An aberrant genetic constitution results in the elaboration of these substances by the wrong cells or by the right cells in the wrong amounts. Eventually there is interference with growth and metabolism of these cells. Because more than one chemical entity are involved and various chemical combinations may affect the cells, several subtypes of this group of dysplasias must occur. It is probable that future accounts will report still other variations.

IDIOPATHIC DISTURBANCES OF GROWTH PLATE CHONDRO-BLAST MATURATION

In the mucopolysaccharidoses the chemical defect appears to lie in the protein complexing of these sugar-linked amines. There are other dysplasias, achondroplasia and metaphyseal dysostosis, in which the microscopic and radiographic features suggest a similar pathogenesis but the chemical defects, if any, are still undetermined.

Actual knowledge of the morbid physiology of these dysplasias is of course lacking but from observations on a limited amount of biopsy material, it appears at present that a disturbance in division and maturation of growth plate chondroblasts, resulting in a deficit of chondroid and eventually a defective chondroid lattice, inhibits normal enchondral growth of long bones. Thus both dysplasias are characterized by micromelia with relatively normal trunk skeletons. These features are more severe in achondroplasia. Less severe is metaphyseal dysostosis that may exhibit only bowing and the degenerative joint disease that is contingent upon abnormal shifts in stress lines because the abnormal metaphysis is unable to support the epiphysis normally.

Achondroplasia

Achondroplasia is a hereditary, congenital, familial disturbance in epiphyseal chondroblastic growth and maturation causing inadequate enchondral bone growth that results in a peculiar type of dwarfism. Some ossification centers appear to be affected more than others, particularly those of the base of the skull and at the ends of long bones. Intramembranous bone formation is normal except as it is secondarily affected by disturbances in length growth. The condition is sometimes called chondrodystrophia fetalis or achondroplastic dwarfism.

The cause of the inadequate cartilage development is entirely unknown. It was long thought to be a disorder of endocrine function, and when certain types of dwarfism were found to be related to pituitary insufficiency, achondroplasia was placed in this group. Failure to find a disturbed function of the pituitary, the thyroid or any other ductless gland has necessitated a reclassification of the condition as a germ plasm defect. This classification may not be entirely beneficial because it tends to close the issue and discourage further investigation. Since the condition is hereditary it is doubtless caused by abnormal genetic components, but no one has shown, as improbable as it may seem on mention, that the failure of cartilage growth and maturation is not due to a lack of response to vitamin A. If some such cause could be identified, the course of the abnormality might be altered just as the prognosis of erythroblastosis fetalis has been bettered, even though its cause is genetic.

There is evidence of the existence of achondroplastic dwarfs as far back as antiquity. Because the condition is not necessarily incompatible with vigorous health and a long life, this peculiar body comformation has always excited a considerable amount of curious interest. Since his mentality is usually not affected, the achondroplastic is faced with the same problems of earning his livelihood as are those of normal physique. Even in ancient times he shrewdly evaluated his assets and turned to the field of entertainment, becoming the clown and jester of those who could afford to keep him. Today one finds a considerable proportion of the world's achondroplastics following their traditional occupation. They are frequently referred to as "circus dwarfs."

Achondroplasia is the most common type of dwarfism. Were it not that more than half of these persons die of a severe form of their malformation in utero and during the first few months of infancy, or during a difficult parturition because of the narrow pelvic outlet of their achondroplastic mothers, the number of cases would be greatly increased because the condition is inherited as an autosomal dominant trait and fertility is not affected. Spontaneous mutations may be responsible for a considerable number of new cases.[14]

Achondroplasia exists in all degrees of advancement. It may be so severe that it is diagnosed in utero and the patient does not survive fetal life. In its usual form the patients are diagnostically obvious as they walk down the street (Fig. 6–12). But there are lesser degrees of involvement in which the stature may be

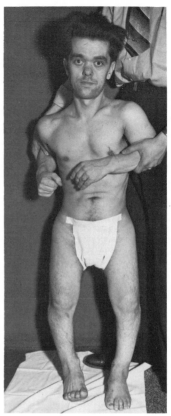

Figure 6–12 Achondroplasia. An adult achondroplastic revealing dwarfism, large head, wide face, saddle nose, prognathism, short extremities and bowed legs.

almost normal and only a roentgenographic skeletal survey demonstrates the stigmata of the condition.

The average achondroplastic attains a height of about 50 inches. His head is apt to be enlarged, though it appears relatively bigger than it is because of his inadequate stature. There is some degree of hydrocephalus in most cases, caused by deficient brain space in the posterior fossa. The hydrocephalus is usually of the communicating type and is rarely severe enough to inhibit mental growth. The failure to provide sufficient space for the brain is due to lack of growth along the inter-sphenoid and spheno-occipital synchondroses. The four principal epiphyseal ossification centers of the base of the skull normally close in early adult life. In the achondroplastic they may ossify in utero or infancy. This accounts for the prominent brachycephaly, the decreased diameter of the foramen magnum and the saddling of the nose. The brain is obliged to grow upward and forward because of the short base, resulting in a characteristic bulging of the forehead and bossing of the frontal bones. The relatively normal growth of the mandible, which enlarges by both enchondral and intramembranous bone formation, makes it look relatively large, resulting in prognathism. These facial features are so constant that most achondroplastics have the appearance of belonging to the same family.

Since only enchondral bone growth is affected, there is less inhibition of trunk growth than of that of the extremities. The vertebral column may achieve normal length resulting in the characteristic disproportion of the stem and the arms and legs. However, vertebral development is usually not normal. The body may be formed in the shape of a wedge and thus be crowded backward to cause angulation. This may happen anywhere along the column, but is most common between the twelfth dorsal and third lumbar vertebrae. Lordosis is usual, resulting in a horizontal

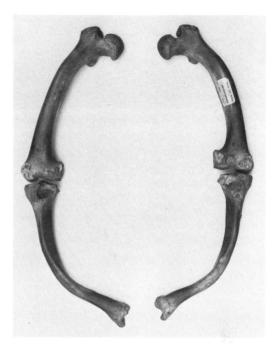

Figure 6–14 The femurs and tibias of an achondroplastic. They are short, thick and heavy. The ends are flared. The shafts are bowed.

tipping of the sacrum. This produces a characteristic prominence of the buttocks (Fig. 6–13). Kyphosis is apt to develop in the thoracic and cervical areas. Sometimes a gibbus is produced. Since there is inadequate growth of the pedicles there is barely sufficient space for the cord and cauda equina without angulation. Distortion and abnormal pressures cause rupture of the intervertebral discs. Pressure upon the cord and nerve roots, particularly in the lower spine, is the most common complication in the adult achondroplastic.[20] This often results in paraplegia and disturbance of bladder function.

The ribs frequently fail to grow to normal length, producing a flattened and narrow chest. All of the long bones are widened at the ends and thus the rib cage may show a prominence of the costochondral junctions.

The long cylindrical bones of the extremities, depending entirely upon enchondral growth for their length, are the most dramatically altered. The finger tips reach only to the hip joint instead of the mid-thigh region and the patient has a

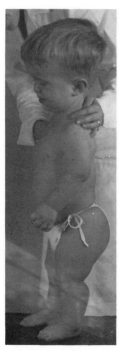

Figure 6–13 Achondroplasia in a child. Note the relatively large head, the saddle nose and brachycephaly, the short extremities and the lordosis with forward tilting of the pelvis.

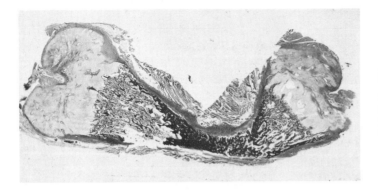

Figure 6–15 Achondroplasia. Longitudinal section of a long bone. The ends of the bone are widened in relation to the diameter of the midshaft. This gives the x-ray appearance of "trumpeting," which is expected in this condition.

duck-legged appearance. The legs are frequently bowed (Fig. 6–14). The fingers are stubby. The trumpeting of the bone ends may cause enlargement of the joint region (Fig. 6–15).

Thanatophoric dwarfism is very closely related to achondroplasia, particularly homozygous achondroplasia in which both parents are dwarfs. It is possible that these two conditions cannot and should not be differentiated. There is a tendency, at least in Europe, to consider them separ-

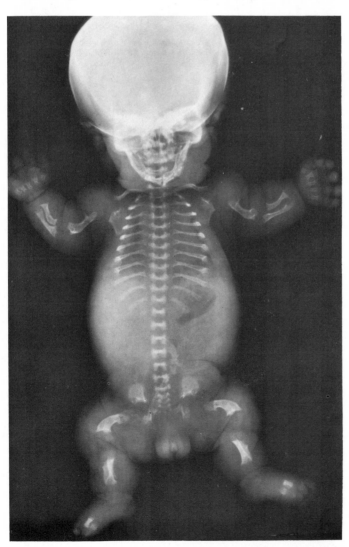

Figure 6–16 Thanatophoric dwarfism. This radiograph of a stillborn fetus demonstrates marked osseous deformities. Particularly there is shortening of the long bones and ribs. The cranial vault is enlarged. The alterations of the lumbar spine and pelvis are as expected in achondroplasia but are more severe.

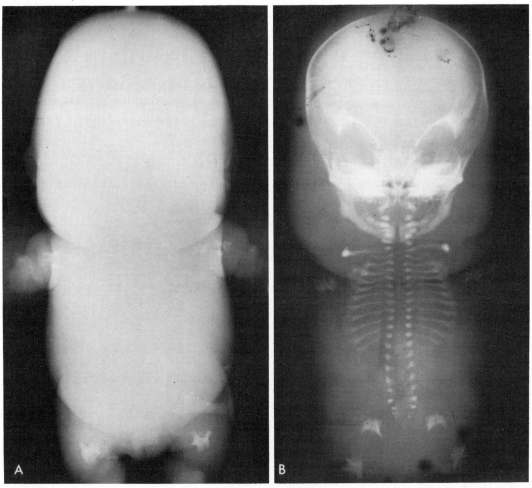

Figure 6-17 Achondrogenesis Type I. The extremities are extremely short, the vertebral bodies are small with intact intervertebral discs and the ribs are short such that the thorax is small. The appearance of the soft tissues (A) may be compared with that of the skeleton (B).

ate entities (Fig. 6–16). In addition, variations on this theme have been described.[20a] For example, achondrogenesis is characterized by extreme osseous deformity, a hydropic appearance, death at or soon after birth and autosomal recessive transmission. This condition has been divided into Type I (Fig. 6–17) and Type II, the major difference being the virtual absence of ossification of the vertebral bodies in Type II.

Metatrophic dwarfism is another condition which is either a subtype or a dysplasia remarkably similar to the less severe types (heterozygous, in which at least one parent is of normal stature) of achondroplasia. At birth the metatrophic dwarf may be impossible to distinguish from the achondroplastic. But as he matures the limbs grow but the trunk shortens because of kyphoscoliosis. Thus, eventually the extremities appear to be disproportionately long for the trunk, quite the opposite of achondroplasia. Because of the changing aspect of the disease as the patient grows, Maroteaux has suggested the name "metatrophic" (Fig. 6–18).

Roentgenographic Manifestations. The roentgenographic manifestations of achondroplasia are to be found in all of the bones of enchondral formation but are most marked in the skull, long bones, spine and pelvis. As the abnormality in this disorder is felt to be located in the proliferating cartilage of the growth plate prior to the stage of cartilaginous maturation, shortening of the bones so derived is to be expected.[21]

Enlargement of the cranial vault with frontal bossing is constant. There is abnormal growth at the synchondrosis between the sphenoid and occipital bones as well as at the cartilaginous segments of the occipital bone. Hence the bones at the base of the skull are small as is the foramen magnum.

The length of the spine approximates the normal. Caffey[22] has documented significant alterations of the vertebrae that are of functional and diagnostic significance. There is progressive diminution in the interpediculate distances from the first lumbar vertebra through the fifth. In the normal individual these distances become greater through the same area. In addition, the pedicles are short and thick throughout and the posterior aspect of the vertebral bodies is concave. Myelography demonstrates the small spinal canal and the protrusion into it of multiple intervertebral discs, a phenomenon that may occur in older children and adults. Deformity in size and shape of the vertebral bodies may be observed, but whether they are thin or wedged in shape, the intervertebral discs are present in normal thickness or, in the former instance, increased in height. Lumbar lordosis becomes evident and marked with weight-bearing.

The bones of the pelvis are affected and their shape is characteristic. Disturbed growth at the lower end of the ilia causes short ilia which result in a flat,

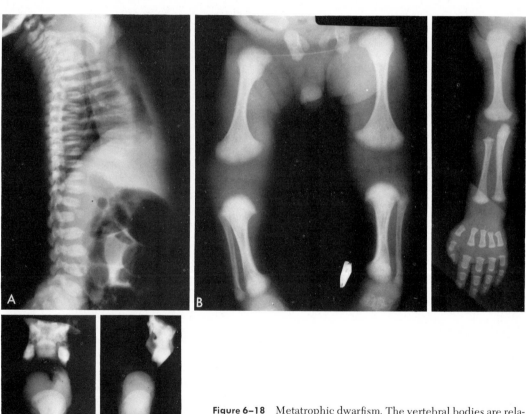

Figure 6–18 Metatrophic dwarfism. The vertebral bodies are relatively flat and elongate (A). The long bones are short with broad metaphyses (B). The amount of cartilage at the ends of the bones can be appreciated in the radiograph of the excised femur (C); the patient expired of respiratory distress secondary to obstruction by large laryngeal cartilages.

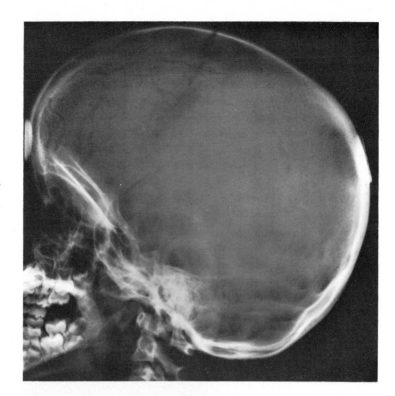

Figure 6–19 Achondroplasia. The base of the skull is short; the vault is enlarged and there is bulging in the frontal region.

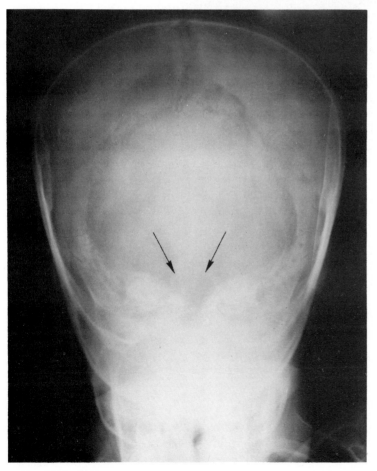

Figure 6–20 Achondroplasia. The foramen magnum is quite small (arrows).

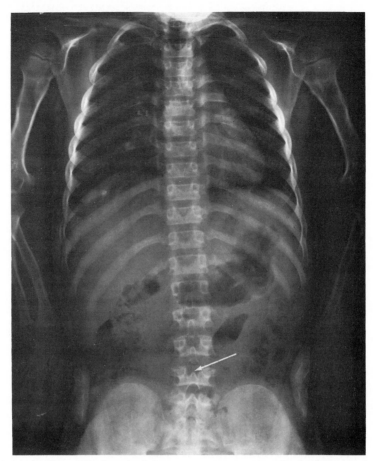

Figure 6–21   Achondroplasia. The length of the upper extremities may be compared with the length of the trunk. The small interpediculate distances of the lumbar vertebrae (arrow) and the narrow sacrum are evident.

often irregular acetabular roof and a small sciatic notch. The sacrum articulates low on the ilia. The ischia and pubic bones are short and broad. Overall, the pelvis is smaller than normal.

Because periosteal osteogenesis is unaffected, the long bones are normal in diameter. They are short and the involvement is such that the proximal ones, humerus and femur, are shorter than the distal ones—rhizomelia. The ends of the bones may flare; the zone of provisional calcification and the epiphyseal center may be relatively smooth in outline, or the epiphyseal line may be irregular and partially enclose the epiphyseal center. Bowing is common as is cortical thickening at the sites of muscle attachment. The fibula is often longer than the tibia causing inversion of the foot. The tubular bones of the hands and feet are short and appear broad. Because the fingers tend to be broader at their proximal ends, a divergence of the fingers occurs when the hand is open, the "trident hand." The fourth and fifth fingers form one group, the second and third another and the thumb another.[14]

In summary, while the severity of the osseous deformities may vary, the nature of the shortening of the long bones and the deformities of the skull, spine and pelvis are constant and diagnostic.

Microscopy. The changes apparent on microscopic examination are best seen in sections made through the epiphyseal plate of a long bone during the growing period (Fig. 6–25). This growth plate is not as thick as normal, but it has a greater circumference to cover the flared end of the diaphysis. This increase in width is probably due to subchondral appositional growth. The decreased thickness appears to be the result of inadequate interstitial chondroblastic division. Not only is there a paucity of chondroblasts but those formed fail to mature properly. They do not acquire their enzymatic and glycogen content as normal cells do and they fail to form definite columns. Thus, the surrounding cylinders of chondroid are not produced, resulting in a failure to produce a normal continuous line of provisory calcification. Without adequate bars of calcified chondroid, the scaffolding of the lattice fails to form (Fig. 6–26). Some bits of mineralized chondroid protrude into the metaphysis and about these there is normal osteoid production, suggesting that the fault is not in osteoblastic activity. But the scaffolding is so irregular and sparse that little osteoid can be laid down in a systematic fashion. Intramembranous, periosteal bone formation appears not to be affected. Compacta is produced and the cortices appear wider and sturdier than normal because of the shortness of the diaphysis. The production of a heavy cylinder of compacta with deficient supporting spongiosa may be the cause of the flaring with stress on the epiphysis. The thin epiphysis and its lack of support by an adequate spongiosa result in sagging, so that the diaphysis appears to surround partially the epiphysis and the epiphyseal line is curved and irregular.

Prognosis. If the achondroplastic survives the trauma of childbirth he stands a good chance of living well into adult life. During late middle age he is apt to be plagued by symptoms caused by pressure upon the cord and the spinal nerves. Thus backache, sciatica, paresthesias and even paraplegia may develop. A herniated disc may add to his difficulties. If he marries a normal spouse he has a 50 per cent chance of fathering normal offspring. If he marries another achondroplastic, he may be fairly sure of helping to perpetuate his kind.

Cartilage-Hair Hypoplasia

McKusick and co-workers have made an intensive study of dwarfism among the Old Order Amish, a religious sect with

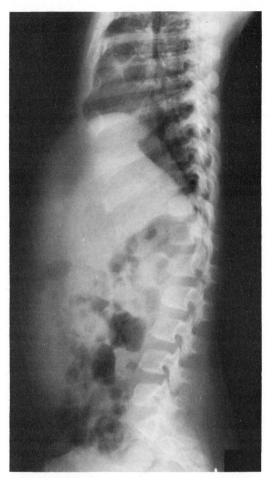

Figure 6–22 Achondroplasia. The lateral radiograph of the spine demonstrates the tendency toward a broad beak anteriorly, particularly in the lower dorsal and upper lumbar segments. The short pedicles and narrow spinal canal are readily appreciated.

large concentrations in eastern Pennsylvania and Canada. The more common type is chondroectodermal dysplasia (Ellis – van Creveld syndrome)[23]; the other is a condition to which they have given the name cartilage-hair hypoplasia.[24] This skeletal dysplasia had been previously described as achondroplasia or metaphyseal dysostosis, but they believe it to be a distinct entity. The genetic pattern is autosomal recessive. Seventy-seven cases were found among 45,000 Old Order Amish or between 1 and 2 per 1000 live births.

The subnormal length of the extremities is noted at birth, and the other features become obvious as the child develops.

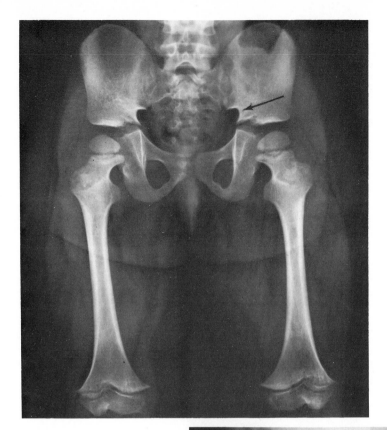

Figure 6–23 Achondroplasia. The sacrum articulates low on the ilia. The sciatic notch is small (arrow) and the roof of the acetabulum is broad and flat. Flaring of the distal end of the short femurs is evident.

Figure 6–24 Achondroplasia. There is marked notching of the midportion of the distal femoral metaphysis within which the epiphyseal center sits.

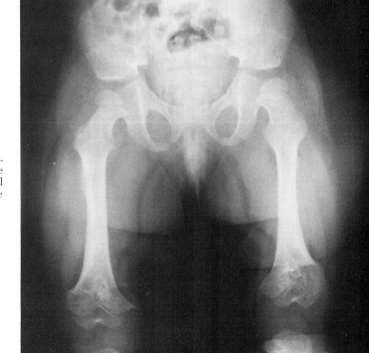

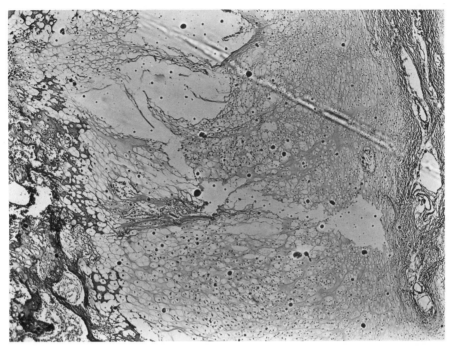

Figure 6–25   Achondroplasia. The enchondral plate is seen on the right side, the epiphyseal line and metaphysis along the left margin. The plate is thin; columnation is extremely irregular if it occurs at all. No scaffolding is formed and there is an incomplete line of provisional calcification. (× 30.)

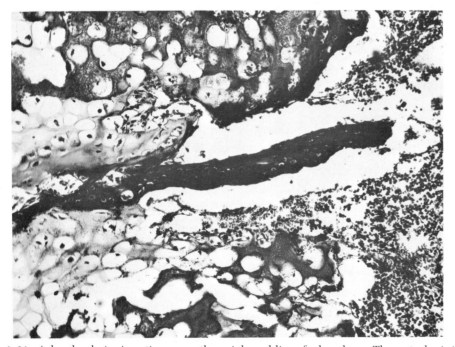

Figure 6–26   Achondroplasia. A section across the epiphyseal line of a long bone. The metaphysis is on the right. There is a failure of orientation and maturation of the chondroblasts which throws all subsequent events in this region into confusion. (× 180.)

Dwarfing is marked; most patients reach a stature of not more than 4 feet at maturity. There may be costochondral beading with Harrison's groove. There is a characteristic deformity of the ankle because of excessive length of the fibula and a loose jointed, flat foot. There is inability to fully extend the elbows and hyperextensibility of the wrist and fingers. The digits are dramatically shortened. The abnormally high upper segment–lower segment ratio gives the appearance of the achondroplastic, but the head in cartilage-hair syndrome, unlike achondroplasia, is always normal, and the epiphyses are radiologically normal. The disturbance in the growth of hair is peculiar to this dysplasia. The hair is fine, sparse, short and brittle.

Intelligence is not impaired, and the urinary excretion of mucopolysaccharides is normal. The findings based on a single costochondral biopsy suggest a deficiency of chondroblastic proliferation and normal columnation like that found in the achondroplastic. Osteoblastic and osteoclastic activity appeared to be normal.

In the minds of many there is considerable doubt that this condition is a dysplastic entity. As its features become more pronounced it becomes impossible to distinguish it from achondroplasia since there are distinct similarities in the pelvis and spine during infancy. However, at the same time, the changes in the long bones are different with mild bowing and cupping of metaphyses.[14] The adult stage of the milder forms seems to be identical with metaphyseal dysostosis. It is probably wiser to study a larger number of cases over a greater period of time before accepting this condition as a separate entity.

Metaphyseal Dysostosis

In 1934 Jansen[25] reported a case of skeletal dysplasia that he called metaphysare dysostosis. Skeletal abnormalities resembled those of achondroplasia except that the head was normal as were the epiphyses of the long bones. There was an elevated serum calcium level. Five cases have been reported since Jansen's case; in one an ample biopsy was taken from the metaphysis of the distal femur.[26] This revealed abnormal masses of "epiphyseal cartilage" mixed with cortical and cancellous bone presenting a similarity to rickets. These findings agreed with those reported by Jansen.

Other cases were described by Gram et al.[27] and Daeshner and co-workers.[28] These showed rachitic rosary, coxa vara, anterior bowing of femurs, genu valgum with distortion of pelvis, clavicles and small bones of the hands and feet. The principal disturbance appeared to be related to the growth plates of cylindrical bones. They were greatly thickened and irregular with what was interpreted on the radiographs as irregular extensions of cartilage into the metaphyseal area. Kidney function was normal and there were no hereditary features. Deformity was severe with loss of function and some cases were fatal. This dysplasia is probably best designated metaphyseal dysostosis, Jansen type.

In 1949 Schmid[29] reported a series of cases in which the skeletal alterations were much less severe; they were not present at birth but appeared with weight-bearing. In most cases the alterations were manifest between the third and fifth year and thereafter underwent repair throughout skeletal growth to maturation. Such cases are relatively common. A series of 18 cases was reported by Stickler et al.[30] (see Fig. 6–29) and another of 21 cases was reported by Miller and Paul.[31] These cases demonstrated autosomal dominance; inhibition of growth was mild, bowing of the legs was marked and a waddling gait was highly characteristic. Schmid believed that his cases were mild instances of Jansen's metaphyseal dysostosis. Most modern writers have conformed with this concept.

Many of these early cases were thought to be achondroplasia. Distinction between these two entities should now be made both clinically and radiologically, but there is still debate as to whether these cases of metaphyseal dysostosis are atypical examples of hypophosphatemic rickets. The radiographs of hypophosphatemic rickets and metaphyseal dysostosis often cannot be distinguished and, moreover,

Peterson[32] and others have reported two cases that responded to massive doses of vitamin D and casting or bed rest. It should be noted that in Peterson's first case there was aminoaciduria, suggesting that it actually may have been atypical hypophosphatemic rickets, and that his second case was successfully treated by bed rest. It has been shown that freedom from stress causes improvement in these cases of rickets.

Typical cases of the Schmid type of metaphyseal dysostosis exhibit inhibition of growth of all cylindrical bones, particularly the large, long bones, bilateral coxa vara and a tendency for slipping of the epiphyses, normal development of the osseous nucleus of the epiphyses and lack of involvement of the head, trunk and carpal and tarsal bones. Kidney function and serum chemistry are normal. Moderate dwarfing, marked bowing and a waddling gait are the outstanding features (Fig. 6–29). Eventually the lesions heal with epiphyseal fusion. The genetic pattern is autosomal dominant.

Spahr and Spahr-Hartmann[33] reported a series with an autosomal recessive genetic pattern. In these cases the only finding was extreme bowing. McKusick[11] has suggested that there may be three types of this condition: (1) the Jansen type, which is rare but most severe and shows no hereditary pattern, (2) the Schmid type, which is milder but more common, with an autosomal dominant pattern and (3) the Spahr type, in which only the bowing occurs and which is autosomal recessive. Others have added to these three, types that have somewhat different manifestations and patterns of inheritance. In all, however, there are degrees of dwarfism with metaphyseal alterations. Of interest is the association of the osseous changes, with pancreatic insufficiency and neutropenia in some and in others with lymphopenic agammaglobulinemia.[14]

We have had the opportunity of seeing tissue samples in only one case. In this case, there was a mass of unidentifiable amorphous material replacing the cancellous tissue immediately beneath the

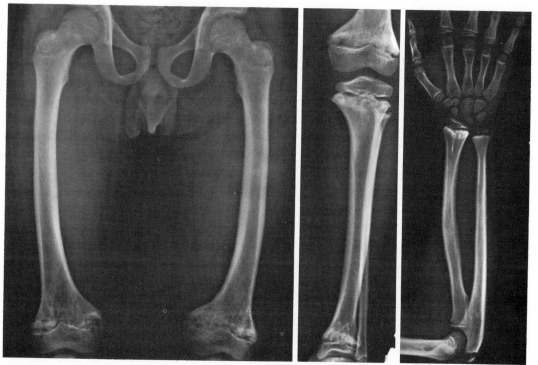

Figure 6–27 Metaphyseal dysostosis. There is bowing of the femurs. Irregular radiolucencies are evident in the metaphyses similar to the alteration in rickets. However, the diaphyses and epiphyseal centers are normal in density and architecture.

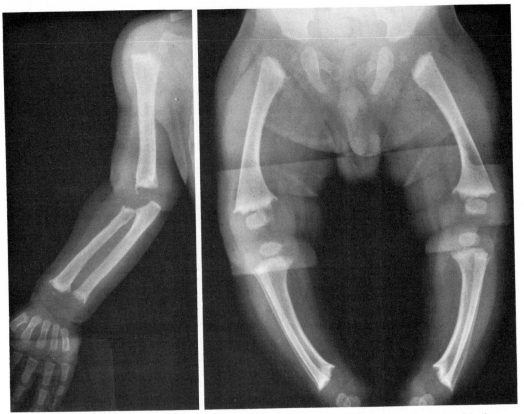

Figure 6–28 Metaphyseal dysostosis. There is marked bowing of the legs. The growing ends of the bones are broad and although the zones of provisional calcification are present, there are linear lucent defects within them causing a fine serrated deformity. The epiphyseal centers are normal.

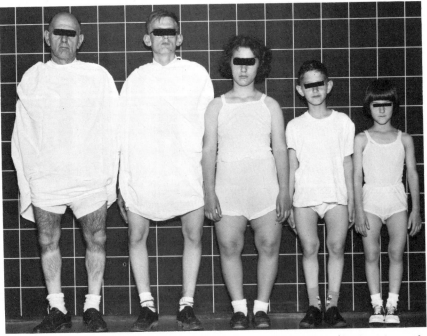

Figure 6–29 Metaphyseal dysostosis. Father, two sons and two daughters all show moderate dwarfing and marked bowing. (Courtesy of Dr. G. Stickler.)

114

enchondral plate. This material may have been degenerating collagen or osteoid. It must have been radiolucent. Whether it was indigenous to the process we cannot say. No chondroid extensions in our sections were in evidence.

Roentgenographic Manifestations. The roentgenographic manifestations of metaphyseal dysostosis vary with the severity of the disease. In general, the metaphysis is affected, and the diaphysis shows normal density and architecture even though a bone may be shorter than normal and bowing may be present. The alterations at the growing end of the bone in the Schmid type resemble rickets and may be impossible to differentiate from those of rickets, although the normal appearance of the diaphysis may be of help in this regard. As noted on page 109, very similar alterations of the skeleton are present in the hair-cartilage syndrome.

The zone of provisional calcification is irregular because of radiolucent masses of what has been reported as cartilage; the metaphyses are broad and at times cup-shaped. If this material is in small linear collections, the result is similar to rickets or, if more marked, it resembles enchondromatosis. Calcification may be present. Unlike rickets, even with severe involvement of the metaphyses, the epiphyseal centers are usually normal. The tubular bones of the hands and feet are similarly involved as are the areas of growth in the pelvic bones. The skull and spine are seldom affected, even in the most severe form of the disease.

Radiographically, then, there are numerous varieties of this dysplasia reported. The more severe the metaphyseal alterations, the more marked is the dwarfism. The metaphyses may be slightly irregular or bulbous, irregularly lucent and show spotty or linear calcification.

Cartilaginous Dysplasias Related to Heterotopic Proliferation of Epiphyseal Chondroblasts

There are three distinct entities in this group, enchondromatosis and osteochondromatosis, both of which are fairly common, and epiphyseal hyperplasia, which is quite rare. Since their patterns of inheritance are completely different (enchondromatosis shows no evidence of genetic transmission whereas osteochondromatosis is a simple autosomal dominant), their apparent dissimilarity is probably valid; yet as large numbers of these cases are compared one finds similarities which make him wonder whether the differences are caused by the areas involved rather than by the basic morbid physiology.

In enchondromatosis it appears that some of the cartilage cells of the growth plate fail to mature. Thus they are not dissipated at the epiphyseal line as enchondral ossification takes place. Left behind in the metaphysis they continue to proliferate, forming large masses of cartilage which have no use and which occupy the area where, normally, metaphyseal cancellous tissue should form and later the medullary tissues should be. These cells mature but fail to columnate. In osteochondromatosis it appears that a fragment of mature, columnated cartilage cells of the growth plate periphery is pinched off by the bone-forming cambium of the periosteum. Isolated in the periosteum outside the metaphysis, like the abandoned cells of enchondromatosis, they continue to grow, forming a new growth plate which produces a cylindrical bone pedicle, a long bone in every way normal except for its direction of growth.

The interesting relationship between these two conditions is that when the enchondroma penetrates the cortex and protrudes out into the surrounding soft tissues, it develops a growth plate and behaves in every way identical to osteochondroma. In these cases the growth period appears to be extended beyond the maturation date of the host bone, posing the question of whether the hamartomatous enchondroma has now become a true neoplasm. We are watching several of these cases in an attempt to answer this problem.

In epiphyseal hyperplasia the heterotopic chondroblasts are related to the osseous nucleus of the epiphysis. A localized area in the periphery of this structure overgrows in a manner similar to an osteochondroma. In this respect it might be considered a subtype of this lesion, an intra-epiphyseal osteochondroma.

ENCHONDROMATOSIS (Ollier)

There were numerous reports of disturbances in enchondral bone formation between 1900 and 1937. It is regrettable that in several papers a variety of entities is grouped under one of several headings, so that it is quite impossible on analyzing certain series to be sure exactly which entities are being reported. The term "dyschondroplasia" has been used by Mahorner[34] to include enchondromatosis, hereditary multiple exostoses, stippled epiphyses and osteopoikilosis, and the same term has been used to report separate series of enchondromatosis and of osteochondromatosis. Apparently Ollier,[35] in reporting four cases of "dyschondroplasia" in 1899, confused the last two conditions but it was he who pointed out the metaphyseal radiolucency which today characterizes enchondromatosis. Since his report the terms "Ollier's disease" and "dyschondroplasia" have been used more or less interchangeably and recently the more exact name of "enchondromatosis" has been largely substituted for both. Since Ollier emphasized the unilaterality of the condition, some writers use the name "Ollier's disease" to designate those cases in which the lesions are entirely or predominantly in one side of the skeleton.

In 1881, Maffucci reported an association of enchondromatosis and multiple cavernous hemangiomas and this rare combination has since been known as "Maffucci's disease." Bean[36] reported 40 such cases in 1958. We have seen one case of combined enchondromatosis and fibrous dysplasia. Biopsy material of the cartilaginous portions displayed such marked nuclear irregularity that we suspect the lesion is undergoing transition to chondrosarcoma.

Enchondromatosis is essentially the hamartomatous proliferation of cartilage cells within the metaphysis of several bones, causing thinning of the overlying cortices and distortion of length growth. It was formerly thought to be hereditary in nature but if, on close scrutiny of the reports, one discards the cases which are probably not true enchondromatosis, the hereditary and familial features of the disease are lacking. In the past it has been difficult to ascertain with certainty whether the condition is congenital but recently we studied material from a case in which lesions were present at birth and proved to be enchondromas by biopsy and x-ray at one week.

The first manifestations of enchondromatosis are usually noted in early childhood. In the more florid instances an obvious impairment of length growth becomes apparent, usually unequal growth of the lower extremities, but in more occult cases the presenting symptom may be pathologic fractures in adolescence or even adult life. Pain is rare unless fracture has occurred or unless there is reactivation in later life with a spurt in growth. This often signifies malignant alteration.

The lesions apparently represent a perversion of enchondral growth and, therefore, are usually confined to cylindrical bones. Occasionally focal masses of cartilage may be found in sites other than the metaphyses, especially in the ribs, combined with the typical metaphyseal lesions of enchondromatosis. These may represent heterotopic islands of cartilage left behind during growth of the bone. The bones of the hands and feet are most frequently involved (Fig. 6–30). Because some cases are limited to these areas there has been a tendency to consider this a special group. At present it appears that this curious localization is but a partial manifestation of the disease as a whole. In those cases with extensive long bone involvement there is almost always at least some evidence of the lesions in the small bones if they are carefully examined. The most vigorous

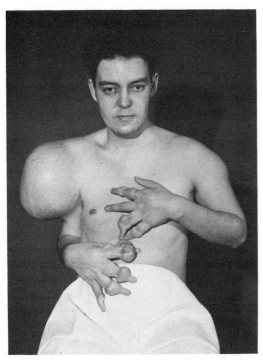

Figure 6-30 Enchondromatosis. The most common site of involvement, the bones of the hands, is here dramatically illustrated. In the large cylindrical bones the enchondroma is more apt to become malignant.

growths are usually seen at the end of greatest activity in the long bones of the extremities.

There can be little doubt that the disturbance seen in enchondromatosis is due to an abnormal proliferation of cartilage cells which arise either from embryologic rests within the metaphysis or from epiphyseal chondroblasts which fail to mature properly and, therefore, migrate into the metaphysis or, more correctly, are overtaken by the advancing epiphyseal line and are left stranded there. The latter appears to us to be the more logical explanation since normal growth may be disturbed, possibly as a result of improper chondroblastic maturation. Retaining their proliferative potency these cells produce masses of useless, disorganized cartilage cells. As such they mimic neoplastic chondromatous growth so closely that the differentiation cannot be made on microscopic examination. The fact that they are not true neoplasms is evident in that they obey, to some extent, the normal growth laws and after

a certain period cease to proliferate. Usually this point in time is about that of the normal cessation of growth of the nearest ossification center of the bone involved.

If during childhood and adolescence the growth is florid, the overlying cortex may be "expanded" producing the "trumpeting" that is characteristically seen. The cortex may be weakened to the point of pathologic fracture. Aggregates of viable cartilage cells protruding through the thin shell of metaphyseal cortex may be pinched off and continue to grow, producing extracortical masses of cartilage and in some instances structures identical with osteochondromas. The lesion of osteochondromatosis or the solitary osteochondroma is actually an example of enchondral bone formation, normal in every respect except for the direction of growth. The cartilage cells of enchondromatosis never fulfill their normal destiny of provoking bone formation while within bone, but once the confining cortex is breached they apparently acquire this capacity.

Eventually, epiphyseal orientation may be regained and normal enchondral bone growth may then proceed beyond the island of cartilage cells. Thus, the abnormal cartilage mass appears to drift into the diaphysis, though in reality the advancing epiphyseal line merely leaves it behind. In large long bones the cartilage masses are always found in the end third or quarter of the bone. In the small bones of the hands and feet they may replace the entire length of the medullary tissues. In some instances the growth is an irregularly lobulated conformation and the roentgenogram has a correspondingly mottled appearance. In other cases there appears to be a semblance of orientation inasmuch as the cells proliferate in a linear pattern producing longitudinal strands of translucency which separate the more opaque bands of normal spongiosa. The streaking of the x-ray film thus produced is highly characteristic of enchondromatosis.

Roentgenographic Manifestations. The roentgenographic manifestations of enchondromatosis reflect a hamartomatous proliferation of cartilage within bone. Because cartilage is lucent as compared

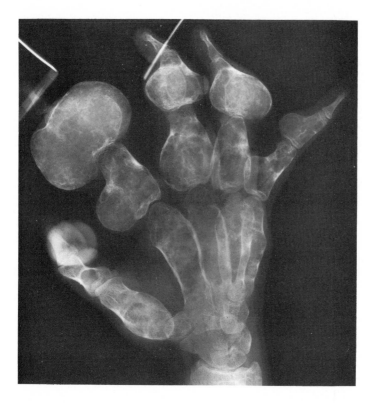

Figure 6–31 Enchondromatosis. There is extensive involvement of the bones of the hand. The lesions have eroded the cortex to a marked degree, but a thin shell of bone covers the cartilaginous masses.

with bone, the masses of cartilage are particularly evident radiographically. Spotty calcification is often present within the cartilage and tends to become more prominent the older the patient. The le-

sions of enchondromatosis may be globular and expand bone, particularly the small bones of the hands and feet. In long bones, the lesions involve the metaphysis and extend into the diaphysis as elongate,

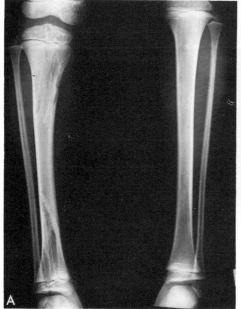

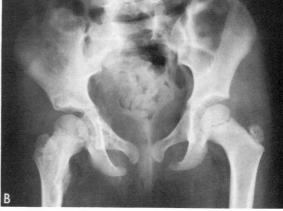

Figure 6–32 Enchondromatosis. There is unilateral involvement of the bones of the lower extremity. Radiolucent streaks are evident in the metaphyses extending into the diaphysis of the right tibia with minimal deformity (*A*). Not only is the femur involved but also the ilium and pubic bone (*B*).

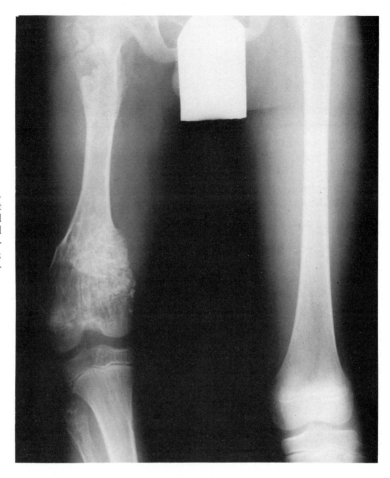

Figure 6–33 Ollier's disease. There is extensive involvement of the right femur characterized by irregular lucent streaks and rounded areas of cartilage; calcification within the cartilage; failure of modeling and shortening.

longitudinal radiolucencies. The most rapidly growing ends of the long bones seem to be most affected. The involved long bone is apt to be short, and in the area of the lesion, broad and often bowed. The epiphyses are spared and involvement of the spine and skull is uncommon.

At times, the only manifestation may be the presence of narrow, radiolucent, longitudinal streaks extending into the shaft from the metaphysis (Fig. 6–32). These streaks are almost pathognomonic of enchondromatosis. In other instances, the cortex is thinned over the proliferating cartilage and may in fact be perforated so that there are external projections of the cartilaginous mass. Pathologic fractures may occur as a consequence of the cortical thinning.

Microscopy. When one sections the curetted material from a lesion of enchondromatosis one finds masses of cartilage cells in a hyalin matrix (Fig. 6–34). These cells range from small chondroblasts to relatively mature, large vacuolated chondrocytes but their pattern is quite disorderly. Areas of "myxomatous degeneration" are common and may dominate the picture. This is probably less a matter of degeneration than an inability to produce normal chondroid with the physical and staining properties of that seen in the epiphysis. The cells are usually irregularly grouped (Fig. 6–35) and it is not always easy for the microscopist to be sure that he is not dealing with chondrosarcoma. The nuances of microscopic differentiation will be dealt with in the chapter concerning chondrosarcoma. On microscopic examination alone the lesions of enchondromatosis and those of solitary enchondroma or even ecchondroma cannot be separated.

As the lesions age they almost always become infiltrated with amorphous calcium salts. That there is a failure of crystal

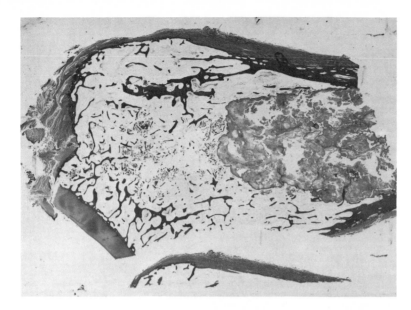

Figure 6-34 Enchondro-
matosis. Very low magnification of the end of a cylindrical
bone with an enchondroma
deep in the metaphysis. Note
that its borders are distinct
and that there is no tendency
to infiltrate like a true neoplasm. (× 4.)

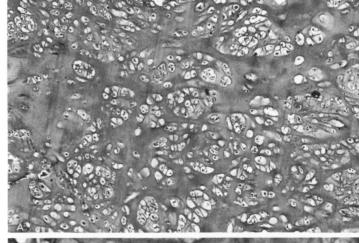

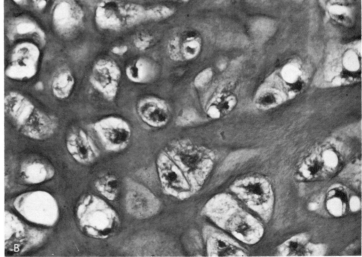

Figure 6-35 A, Section taken
from an enchondroma. The cells
are fairly mature in type but
their arrangement is quite disorganized. The cells are also more
thickly dispersed than those of
normal hyaline cartilage. (× 40.)
B, Higher magnification of an
area from A. The cells are relatively small and there is but one
nucleus to a cell and one cell to
a lacuna. (× 400.)

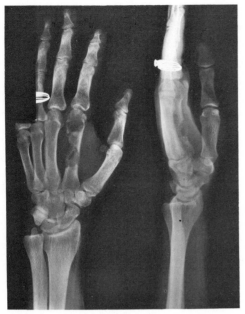 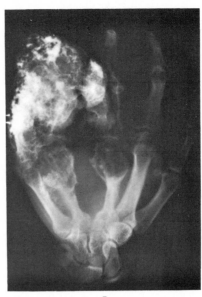

A   **B**

Figure 6–36 *A*, Chondrosarcoma in the midshaft of the second metacarpal. This tumor rarely occurs in the small bones of the hands and feet; osteosarcoma, practically never. *B*, Chondrosarcoma originating in multiple enchondromas of the hand. Most chondrosarcomas of the hands and feet are derived thus.

lattice formation is shown by the lack of rigidity of the calcified areas. The salts are laid down in irregular patches, striations and points which produce the characteristic roentgenograms of these lesions.

Prognosis. Concerning the fate of the patient with enchondromatosis there are almost no factual data on which one may base a valid opinion. It is certain that lesions of enchondromatosis have been discovered in patients of advanced years without evidence of true neoplastic change. It is just as certain that neoplastic growth is the event that leads to the discovery of many of the cases in adult life. Some writers have attempted on the basis of limited series to express the prognosis in percentages, the figures of malignant change ranging from 5 per cent upward. To us, and at the moment this seems unwarranted, the matter had best be left with the statement that the patient with enchondromatosis stands a greater chance of developing a malignant cartilaginous tumor than does the normal individual. Therefore, all known lesions should be periodically surveyed and any reactivation of growth in adult life should be regarded as malignant neoplasm until proven otherwise. Lesions within the large long bones

of the extremities, particularly those in the proximal end of the humerus, are certainly more apt to undergo malignant transition than those in the small bones of the hands and feet, though we have seen two chondrosarcomas in the former (Fig. 6–36) which we believe were preceded by enchondroma.

In recently analyzing our collected cases of chondrosarcoma we found that nearly half of them appeared to originate in preceding lesions. The most common progenitor was osteochondroma, the second most common, enchondroma (Fig. 6–36 *B*). A variety of brain tumors and, less frequently, carcinomas have been reported complicating enchondromatosis. We have encountered a case of the former, a malignant glial tumor of the floor of the third ventricle which eventually killed the patient.

OSTEOCHONDROMATOSIS
(Hereditary Multiple Exostoses)

As the name implies, this is a condition in which multiple bony excrescences grow out from the cortical surfaces, forming tubular extensions roughly transverse to the long axis of the bone involved. This skeletal deformity was known to Virchow, but little was written about it until Ehrenfried reviewed the literature and reported 12 cases in 1917. He suggested the term "hereditary deforming chondrodysplasia." Keith (1920) called it "diaphyseal aclasis," a name which is still preferred by the British. Jaffe[37] proposed the term "hereditary multiple exostoses," which because it is descriptive and simple is the one most widely used today. It is also reported under the titles "cartilaginous exostoses" and "hereditary osteochondromatosis." The latter is eminently descriptive, but has not been used because the same name has been used for a condition characterized by the production of spheroid masses of cartilage within a joint and in the periarticular tissues. Since osteochondromatosis is an inappropriate term for this condition and since the lesion is rare and relatively unimportant, it seems permissible to use the term to designate the disease process of multiple osteochondromas.

The condition is familial and there is a prominent hereditary incidence in the histories of nearly 75 per cent of the cases. The trait is usually passed to his children by the father but there are several well documented cases in which only the mother was afflicted. Several children in one family are not uncommonly involved and the condition has been traced through five consecutive generations. Males are affected almost three times more often than females.

These bony outgrowths are usually discovered some time during childhood or adolescence. None has been reported present at birth. The exostoses themselves are usually symptomless but they may cause pressure upon tendons which must slide over them and thus bursae are formed that may become inflamed. At times they may compress vessels and interfere with blood supply or cause pain by pressure on nerves. Accompanying the osteochondromas there is frequently incomplete length growth of the ulna and fibula. These bones are thus shorter than their paired radius and tibia, with a resultant characteristic curving at the elbow and knee (Fig. 6–37). The wrist is affected

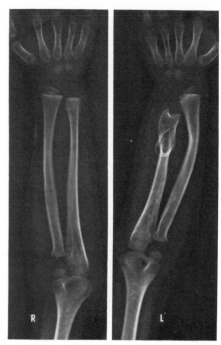

Figure 6–37 Osteochondromatosis. The characteristic deformity of the left radius and ulna is evident. A small lesion involves the distal end of the right ulna.

in about one third of these patients. The short ulna articulates with the radius producing what appears to be a subluxation which must be differentiated from Madelung's deformity.

The lesions of osteochondromatosis most frequently appear on the long bones of the extremities, but the flat bones of the pelvis, the scapula, the ribs and the vertebrae are sometimes involved. Since these exostoses are disturbances in the enchondral growth of bone they are never found in areas resulting from intramembranous formation, though they have been reported arising from portions of skull bones in the vicinity of a cartilaginous ossification center. The small bones of the hands and feet are rarely affected. In long bones the exostoses usually appear at the end of greatest growth, at the knee when they involve the femur or tibia and at the shoulder and wrist when they arise from humerus or ulna.

These lesions probably always begin their growth at the extreme end of the shaft in the vicinity of the periphery of the epiphyseal line. As the latter advances they are left upon the cortical surface and a progressively widening breach separates them from their point of origin. At the same time there is a failure of modeling of the involved metaphysis so that it remains wider than normal. The osteochondromas, the broad metaphyses and the short ulnas and fibulas compose a triad of characteristic features of the disease (Fig. 6–38). One can roughly judge the date of onset of the disturbance by the distance of the osteochondroma from the epiphyseal line and the length of the widened area.

The exostoses are usually bilateral and frequently symmetrical though at times one side is predominantly involved. Several may grow from one metaphyseal area. They are usually flattened transversely, often appearing as a short, high ridge in the long axis of the host bone. They are capped by a layer of hyalin cartilage. This cap frequently extends well down over the pedicle, sometimes approaching the normal cortex (Fig. 6–39). The base is

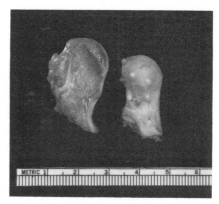

Figure 6–39 An osteochondroma has been sagittally sectioned. The outer surface is shown on the right. The cartilaginous cap comes down over the pedicle. The cut surface is shown on the left; the pedicle of bone is seen at the base.

often wider than the apex so that the growths may be triangular or fin-shaped. They almost always lean in a direction away from the nearest epiphysis and toward the center of the diaphysis. Rarely the pedicle is slender and the distal end bulbous. The cartilaginous surface usually reveals numerous lobular irregularities.

The structure is essentially a cylinder of cortical bone surrounding a core of cancellous tissue and covered with a layer of cartilage which acts as an epiphyseal plate. The cancellous bone is coextensive with that of the host bone and frequently supports hematopoietic marrow. The cartilaginous portion is comparable to the epiphysis of a long bone except that it has no osseous nucleus. It acts as both an epiphyseal and an articular plate. The bone portion is covered with an extension of periosteum from the normal cortex and the cap is covered with perichondrium.

Exostoses are morphologically identical to the solitary lesion which is known as osteochondroma.

The cause of the disturbance that results in osteochondromatosis is unknown. The hereditary incidence, the failure of metaphyseal modeling and the impaired growth of the ulna and fibula suggest an inherent germ plasm defect. Virchow suggested that a piece of the active epiphyseal plate was pinched off and set up independent growth in a direction transverse to the normal long axis. Others have found islands of cartilage cells in the deep layers of the periosteum and

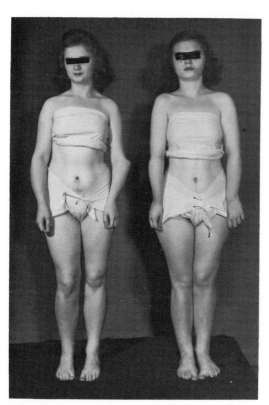

Figure 6–38 Hereditary multiple exostoses. Two sisters show the typical deformity of the elbow and knee. (From Shriners' Hospital, Philadelphia.)

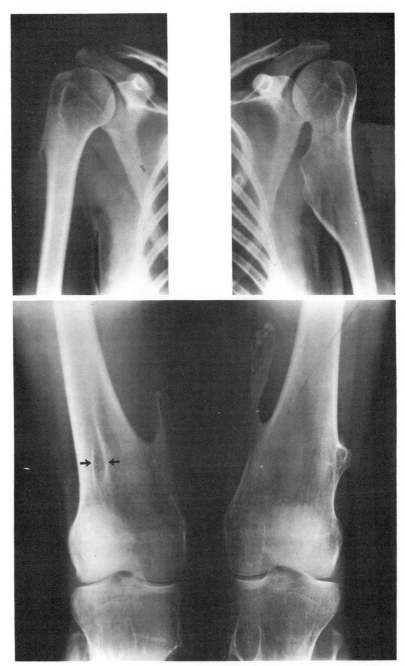

Figure 6–40 Osteochondromatosis. The bony protuberances are evident at the ends of the bones. The end of the diaphysis and the metaphyseal area are broad as a consequence of failure of modeling. The cartilaginous cap on several of the exostoses is irregularly opacified. When seen end-on, the site of origin of the exostosis is visible by virtue of its cortex which casts a dense round or oval shadow (arrows).

have suggested that they are embryonal cell rests or areas of metaplasia which may be activated to produce the osteochondromas. Keith[38] found instances in which the periosteum did not completely reach the epiphyseal line and thought that, lacking the restraining influence which he thought the periosteum exerted on the epiphyseal cartilage, the latter was allowed exuberant growth. Jansen[39] believed that the deformity was the result of an impairment in osteolysis during modeling. Failure of resolution, he believed, left the wide metaphysis and a fragment of the periphery of the epiphysis which continued to proliferate and form an epiphyseal line at right angles to the normal. In the light of present knowledge the original hypothesis offered a century ago by Virchow appears to be the most sensible.

Microscopy. Sections taken through the bone of the pedicle show it to be of the cortical type with normal lamellation and haversian systems. The trabeculae of the cancellous tissue appear normal in all respects. The marrow may be fatty or actively hematopoietic. The appearance of the covering cartilaginous plate varies with the age of the lesion and the stage of its growth. In the depths of the cartilage near the exterior surface the cartilage cells are young, small and evenly dispersed. As the line of junction with cancellous bone, the epiphyseal line, is approached, the chondroblasts are seen to mature. They enlarge, the cytoplasm becomes vacuolated, they flatten transversely and arrange themselves in recognizable though often irregular columns (Fig. 6-41).

The intervening acellular chondroid becomes infiltrated with bone salts to form a provisional line of calcification. The epiphyseal line is usually quite irregular but vascularized tongues of fibrous tissue break into the bases of the cell columns just as in normal enchondral bone formation, and a chondroid lattice is formed. The projecting bars are usually widely separated and run in various directions but seams of osteoid are laid down on their surfaces and bone trabeculae are thus formed (Fig. 6-42). As the lesion matures the cartilage columns become exhausted and an arch of bone seals off the cartilage from the bony portion. When the subchondral trabeculae fail to show cores of chondroid one can be sure that the growth period is approaching its end.

Prognosis. The growth of the osteochondromas apparently begins in childhood and continues until the nearest epiphyseal center ossifies, i.e., its growth period is the same as that of its host bone. Occasionally one finds evidence of activity well into adult life but it is usually

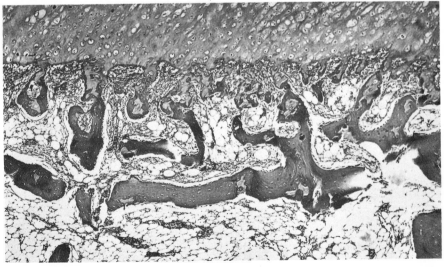

Figure 6-41 Osteochondroma. Low magnification of a section taken through the cartilage cap and adjacent pedicle. The lesion mimics the epiphysis and metaphysis of the growing bone from which it arises. (× 27.)

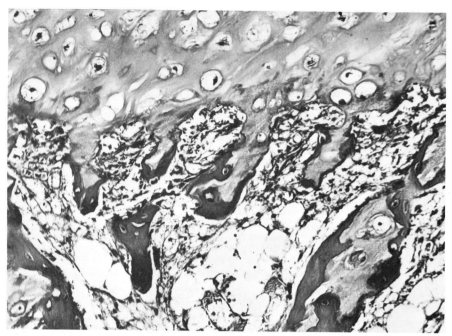

Figure 6–42 Osteochondroma. Section through the epiphyseal line. Chondroblasts mature, form a line of provisional calcification and a hyalin scaffolding for osteoid apposition. (× 290.)

impossible to determine whether this is independent growth or whether there is still activity in the normal epiphysis. Reactivation should always be regarded with suspicion. A diagnosis of malignant change must be presumed until ruled out.

Malignant neoplastic change is encountered frequently enough in hereditary multiple exostoses to make periodic examination mandatory. It is impossible to establish an accurate figure but most authors agree that this unfortunate compli-

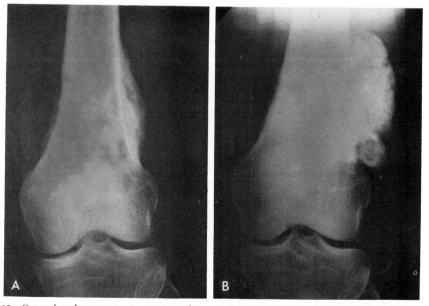

Figure 6–43 Osteochondromatosis. A reactivated exostosis was surgically removed (*A*). A few months later a parosteal sarcoma was found growing at the site (*B*).

cation occurs in about 5 per cent of cases (Fig. 6–43). Trauma, particularly if it causes fracture, should most certainly be watched by x-ray examination.

Parosteal sarcoma is the neoplastic analogue of osteochondroma. It is impos-sible to state what percentage of these tumors arise from the latter though it appears at present that most parosteal sarcomas arise de novo.

Gardner's syndrome is a familial disease characterized by papillary adenomas of

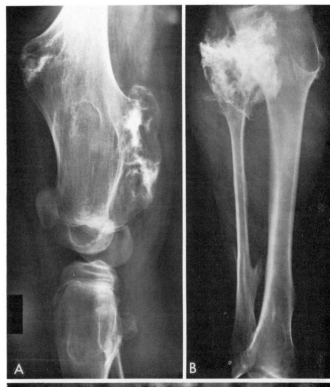

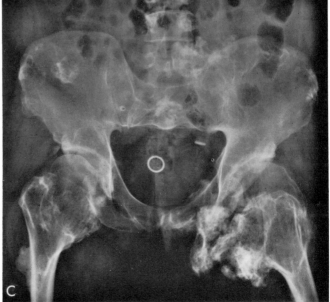

Figure 6–44 Osteochondromatosis. Lesions of the distal femur (A), the proximal fibula (B) and the proximal femurs (C) show rapid and irregular growth suggestive of malignant meta-plasia. This patient is being followed anxiously to learn the outcome of these lesions.

the colon, multiple hamartomatous overgrowths in the soft tissues, such as abdominal desmoids and sebaceous cysts, and localized overgrowths of bone, osteomas and osteochondromas. Osteomas are more common but all patients with one or more osteochondromas should be examined for colon papillary adenomas since they, the adenomas, frequently develop into adenocarcinoma of the bowel.[40]

We have had the opportunity of reviewing several cases of osteochondromatosis and of enchondromatosis in which the intraosseous lesion has penetrated the cortex. Among these are several lesions with such florid growth that they suggest transition to malignant neoplasm (Fig. 6–44). Biopsy of one of them involving the proximal fibula revealed many of the

cellular criteria of chondrosarcoma. Because of the multiplicity of the process it was believed that little could be accomplished in the way of treatment. To date the lesions have been watched for several years without observing notable change. Investigation of other members of the patients' families reveals similar lesions and a history of many years' duration. These cases are being followed with the prognostication that at least some of them almost certainly will develop manifestations of neoplastic behavior.

EPIPHYSEAL HYPERPLASIA
(Dysplasia Epiphysealis Hemimelica)

This bone growth disturbance has the appearance of an overgrowth of a long

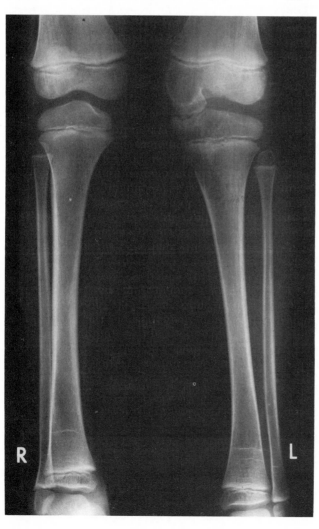

Figure 6–45 Epiphyseal hyperplasia. There is overgrowth of the medial portion of the epiphyseal center of the left femur. Adaptive changes are evident in the tibial epiphyseal center.

bone epiphysis forming an anterior, posterior or side protrusion. It has been described as an osteochondroma which affects the epiphysis instead of the diaphysis, and one might come to this conclusion from its radiographic appearance. This process is not hereditary; it affects but a single epiphysis, in the great majority of instances affecting the talus, the distal femoral or proximal tibial epiphyses, in that order of frequency.

Trevor[41] defined the lesion in 1956 (though it had been described earlier) and gave it the name of tarsoepiphyseal aclasis. Fairbank[42] later reported 14 cases and pointed out that the name was inappropriate since it is probably not an aclasis (such as osteochondroma) and that other than tarsal epiphyses may be involved. He called it dysplasia epiphysealis hemimelica. Keats[43] has written a good review of the subject. Since Fairbank's name for this lesion is cumbersome though accurate we have suggested that this condition be called simply epiphyseal hyperplasia.

The lesion usually presents itself during childhood. It is asymptomatic until the protruding epiphyseal mass interferes with joint function. The process is essentially a disturbance in the formation of the epiphyseal osseous nucleus. There may be excessive growth of this body anteriorly, posteriorly or to one side, or a separate osseous nucleus or several of them may be established in these areas with a hyperplasia of the overlying cartilage zone. Thus the process may appear, in some respects, to resemble stippled epiphysis or epiphyseal dysplasia. When separate epiphyseal centers are formed, as they grow they merge with each other and eventually with the main osseous center. Length growth of the related diaphysis is rarely altered though the associated metaphysis may fail to model and thus be considerably wider than normal.

DYSPLASIAS DUE TO DISTURBANCES IN OSTEOID PRODUCTION

The group of dysplasias discussed to this point appear to stem from an inability to elaborate adequate (achondroplasia) or normal (Hurler's disease) chondroid. Enchondral ossification is affected since in this type of osteogenesis a chondroid matrix is essential for osteoid elaboration. In the next group of dysplasias to be discussed the chondral matrix is formed normally; it is the synthesis of osteoid itself that is at fault. Osteogenesis takes place in three separate locations, in the epiphysis (the osseous nucleus), in the metaphysis (length growth) and along the shaft (periosteal or intramembranous osteogenesis). The dysplasias due to faulty osteoid formation thus can be further divided into types according to the specific areas involved.

Dysplasias Related to Abnormal Epiphyseal Ossification

There is a group of dysplastic deformities of the skeleton in which the formation of the epiphyseal osseous nucleus is abnormal. Of these deformities, four [diastrophic dwarfism, spondyloepiphyseal dysplasia, multiple epiphyseal dysplasia (Fairbank) and stippled epiphyses] appear to be sufficiently distinct to be considered separate entities though there is some evidence to suggest that they may be different forms or even stages of the same process. Until we know more of the morbid physiology of these conditions it is permissible to group them on the basis of certain clinical and radiologic similarities.

Because in diastrophic dwarfism there appears to be an inability to produce any of the three mesenchymal intercellular products (collagen, chondroid or osteoid) normally, among other features, the epiphyseal osseous nucleus cannot be normally formed.

In spondyloepiphyseal dysplasia the fault again appears to be an inability to elaborate the osteoid which constitutes the osseous epiphysis. Both the vertebrae and the cylindrical bones are involved; dwarfing is marked in the severe cases, resembling Morquio's disease or achondroplasia. In the latent cases only the osteoarthritis may be apparent.

In multiple epiphyseal dysplasia there appears to be an inability to form a normal osseous nucleus. The consequent lack of support for the articular plate leads to early osteoarthritis. Growth is stunted rather than dwarfed and since the spine is not involved the skeleton is of the micromelic type.

In stippled epiphyses the cartilaginous epiphysis appears to form normally. Then multiple foci of chondroid calcification appear. These foci may then ossify and finally merge to form a fairly normal epiphyseal center. The fact that collagenous tissues about the joint also may reveal foci of calcium salts suggests that the process may be chiefly a disturbance in calcification rather than osteoid production. Some authors suggest that it may be a disturbance in epiphyseal ossification due to anomalous vascularization or calcification of the arteries which supply the epiphysis.

Osteochondrosis deformans tibiae, Blount's disease, is a disturbance in normal development (sometimes bilateral) of the medial portion of the proximal tibial epiphysis. A failure of enchondral ossification results, causing severe bowing. The condition is sometimes called Blount's disease (because of his original paper) or tibia vara. Some writers have classified this lesion with the series of epiphyseal ischemic necroses. It is probably more appropriately included as a subvariety under the heading of epiphyseal dysplasia, pathogenesis unknown. It is interesting that this condition has the radiographic features of ischemic necrosis

but the pathologic features of an epiphyseal dysplasia. When one examines sections made of the lateral portions of the proximal epiphyseal cartilage it appears normal. Sections of the medial portion reveal a failure of normal chondroblastic proliferation and maturation. The growth plate is thin, misshapen by stress and there is failure of orderly columnation. If Blount's disease is an epiphyseal dysplasia it suggests that this entire group is the result of abnormal congenital epiphyseal vascularization.

DIASTROPHIC DWARFISM

In 1960 Lamy and Maroteaux[44] reported three cases of what they considered to be a dysplastic entity which they named diastrophic dwarfism. Since that time a number of small series have been described,[45, 46] approximately 20 cases accumulating in about five years. The clinical, radiologic and genetic features of this curious skeletal dysplasia appear to be sufficiently unique to cause one to regard it as an entity apart from the other dysplasias.

This skeletal deformity is inherited as an autosomal recessive. There is micromelic dwarfism with little disturbance in the axial development of the skeleton except for occasional cleft palate and lumbar scoliosis. It does not cause death but it may progress to severe loss of function so that some victims have never been able to stand or walk. There is delay in appearance of the osseous nuclei of the epiphyses, particularly of the capital epiphyses of the femur and humerus. When the ossification centers do appear they become flattened and frequently subluxed. Coxa vara is common. Growth of cylindrical bones and thus the extremities is inhibited. The metacarpal and metatarsal bones are short and rectangular causing the typical "hitch-hiker's thumb" and talipes equinovarus. The latter is particularly difficult to treat.

In the majority of cases there is laxity of the tendons and ligaments so that the joints are hyperextensile. In some reports the joints have been excessively rigid. Deformity of one or both ears commonly accompanies the skeletal manifestations. Thus the condition would appear to be related to a disturbance in general cartilage and collagen production. Rubin has suggested that this is a "neuromesodermal defect."

A failure of normal columnation within the enchondral plate has been reported by one observer and a deficit of motor neurons by another. Other than these, no studies of the morphopathology are available. We have not had the opportunity of examining biopsy material. It seems to us, however, that this condition, like those already described in this section, is probably the result of an inability to produce normal chondroid, possibly enzymatic in nature. It differs from these in that the metabolic defect lies back far enough to involve collagen formation also, resulting in weak and ineffective tendons and ligaments. Though the de-

formity of the external ears is accredited to hemangiomas in one report, these lesions were apparently not actually observed by the author. In other reports the deformity appears to be related to the abnormal cartilage component.

Roentgenographic Manifestations. The roentgenographic features of the patient with diastrophic dwarfism depend in some measure on the age of the patient. If dislocations are not present at birth, they soon appear, as is true of flexion contractures. The spine may be straight at birth but scoliosis is soon evident. Hypoplasia of cervical vertebral bodies has been described.[14] Of diagnostic significance are the deformities of the hands and feet associated with a normal skull and vertebral bodies of normal configuration until the latter become distorted as a consequence of scoliosis. The interpediculate distance in the lumbar spine is generally

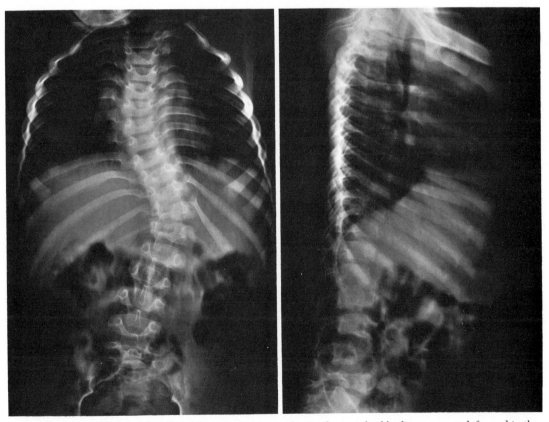

Figure 6–46   Diastrophic dwarfism. There is obvious scoliosis; the vertebral bodies are most deformed in the area of curvature. The ribs are normal. (Courtesy of Dr. H. Steel, Shriners' Hospital for Crippled Children, Philadelphia.)

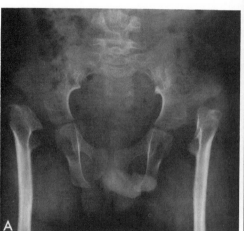
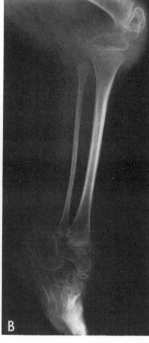
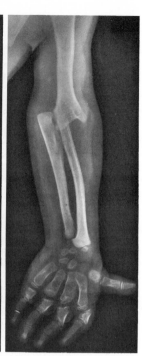

Figure 6–47   Diastrophic dwarfism. The femoral necks are short and broad. The epiphyseal centers are not visible. Both hips are dislocated (*A*). There is a dislocation of the knee and elbow (*B*). Talipes equinus deformity of the feet is marked. Characteristic abnormality of the hand is illustrated; the first metacarpal is diminutive. The phalanges and their centers are short and broad. (Courtesy of Dr. H. Steel, Shriners' Hospital for Crippled Children, Philadelphia.)

described as normal or constant throughout in contrast to the narrowing described in achondroplasia.

The bones of the hands are broad and short with particular shortening of the first metacarpal so that the thumb is at a right angle to the other digits. There is a similar deformity of the great toe and a severe equinovarus deformity. The long bones are short and broad and their epiphyseal centers flat and abnormal in shape. The appearance of the epiphyseal centers of the tubular bones of the hands and feet is delayed; of the centers for the carpus and tarsus, accelerated.

The cartilage of the ear may calcify or, in fact, ossify. Deficiency of tracheal cartilage results in a lack of rigidity which may cause respiratory distress, especially in infants.

SPONDYLOEPIPHYSEAL DYSPLASIA

In Morquio's disease, dwarfing is due largely to failure to attain normal trunk stature; in achondroplasia the major part of the dwarfing is caused by subnormal limb growth. In spondyloepiphyseal dysplasia, poor growth of both vertebrae and extremities makes this condition appear to be a transitional form of these two dysplasias. Actually the principal fault appears to be an inability to normally ossify epiphyseal centers. This causes failure of support of the articular plates which leads to precocious osteoarthritis, the most outstanding feature in adults, and interference with growth plate activity causing dwarfing, the most dramatic feature of the childhood form. The childhood type has been called pseudoachondroplastic spondyloepiphyseal dysplasia; the latent variety is sometimes called spondyloepiphyseal dysplasia tarda. Another type, spondyloepiphyseal metaphyseal dysplasia, is described in which there is micromelic dwarfism with a short trunk.[47] For the well-informed the differentiation of this condition from achondroplasia, as pointed out by Ford et al.,[48] should not be difficult since it manifests itself after birth, head bone features (saddle nose, prognathism) are lacking and the epiphyseal centers are much more irregular and often multiple.

McKusick[11] suggests that there are two hereditary forms of this condition, an autosomal dominant and an x-linked recessive type. Dwarfing of both trunk and extremities may be severe; the hands and feet appear short and pudgy. The appearance of the vertebrae sometimes causes confusion with Morquio's disease. There is vertebra plana. McKusick believes the roentgenographic appearance of the vertebrae is pathognomonic and describes a "heaping up" of the posterior portions of the superior vertebral plates.

Though onset is usually during childhood many cases are not suspected until severe degenerative arthritis begins in early adult life. The hips are probably always involved and the changes here are usually the most severe. These cases usually manifest moderate growth stunt-ing and the characteristic changes in the spine.

Roentgenographic Manifestations. As the name of the disease suggests, the growing ends of the bones of the extremities are abnormal as are the vertebral bodies, but the skull is normal. The epiphyseal centers, particularly of the long bones, are fragmented and ossification is defective, with secondary alterations in the epiphyseal line and, in some instances, in the metaphysis. Appearance of secondary centers is delayed. The outline of the vertebral bodies is irregular with narrowing of the intervertebral discs secondary to a peculiar enlargement of the posterior portions of the bodies. Hypoplasia of the odontoid is said to be absent in spondyloepiphyseal dysplasia and present in Morquio's disease, but this abnormality has been noted in a patient with spondyloepiphyseal dysplasia.

In the adult, the affected joints, particu-

(*Text continued on page 137.*)

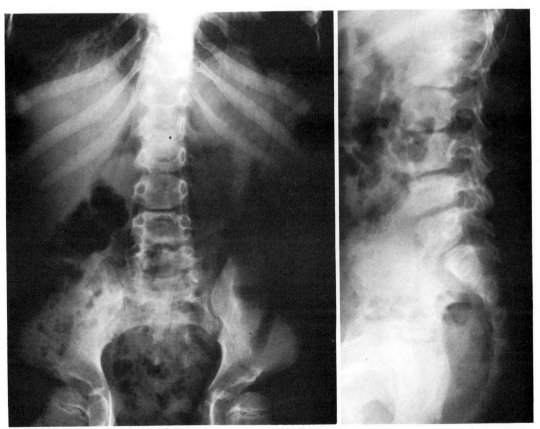

Figure 6–48   Spondyloepiphyseal dysplasia. The vertebral bodies appear thick and irregular; the intervertebral discs are narrow.

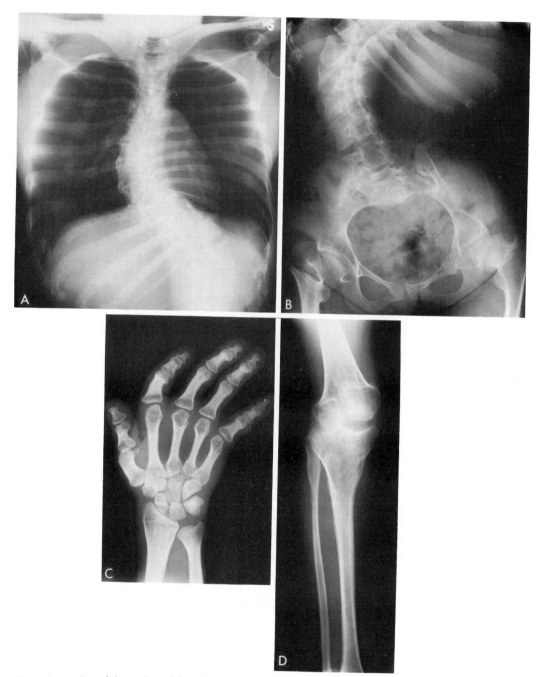

Figure 6–49 Spondyloepiphyseal dysplasia, female, age 25, mother of patient in Figure 6–50. There is marked dorsolumbar scoliosis. Degenerative changes are present in the hips. The bones at the knees are large in relation to the diaphyses and there is mal-alignment. The phalanges are short and the fingers deviate to the ulnar side.

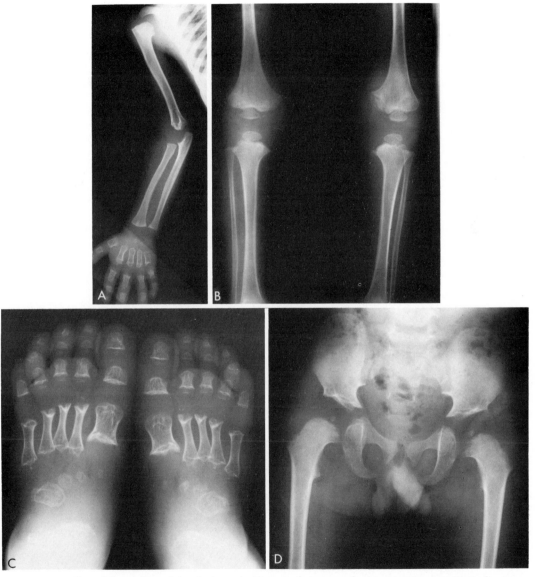

Figure 6–50   Spondyloepiphyseal dysplasia, male, 7 years of age, son of patient in Figure 6–49. Scoliosis was not present. The phalanges are short as are the long bones. The epiphyses are small and ossification is delayed. Epiphyseal lines are irregular.

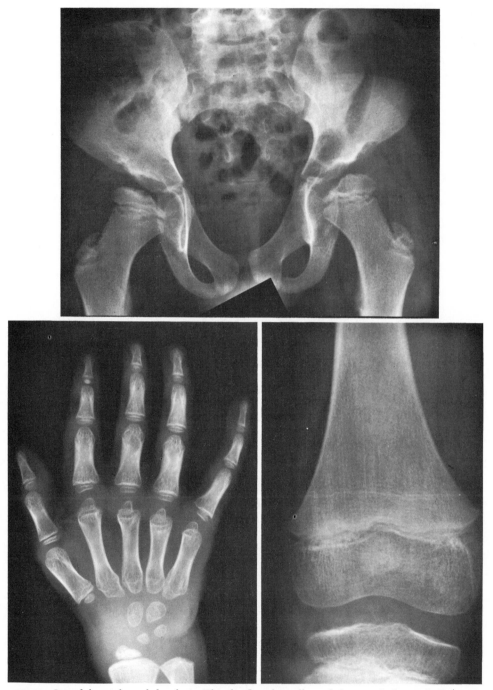

Figure 6–51   Spondyloepiphyseal dysplasia. The ilia flare laterally and the acetabula are shallow. The secondary epiphyseal centers are irregular in outline and moderately flat.

larly the knees and hips, show degenerative changes. The joints are narrow with sclerosis of subchondral bone. The deformity of the vertebral bodies persists and is associated with varying degrees of sclerosis.

MULTIPLE EPIPHYSEAL DYSPLASIA (Fairbank)

This condition, named dysplasia epiphysealis multiplex by Fairbank, is a

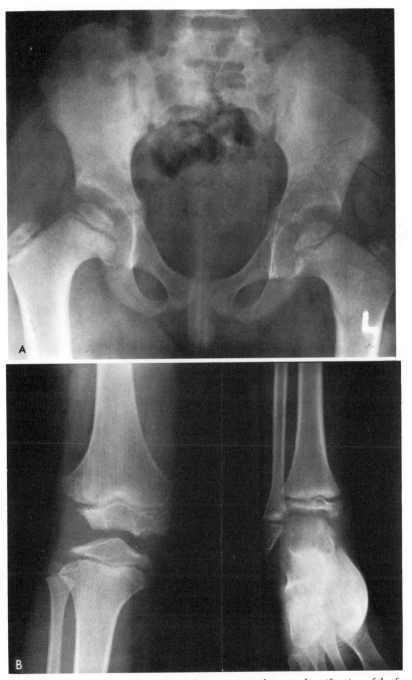

Figure 6–52   Multiple epiphyseal dysplasia. Irregularity in size, shape and ossification of the femoral epiphyseal center is evident (A). There is a superficial similarity to the changes of epiphyseal ischemic necrosis. In the same patient there were other epiphyseal abnormalities; the centers at the knees and ankle (B) are flat and small.

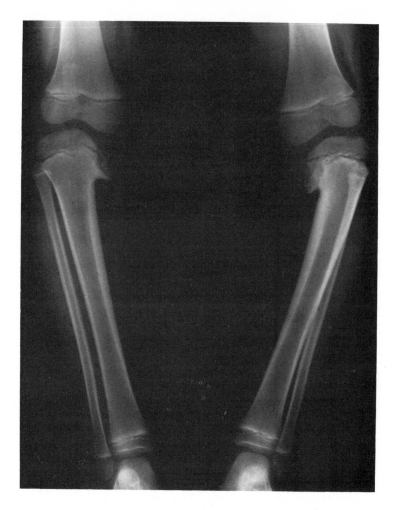

Figure 6–53 Blount's disease. There is obvious bowleg deformity. The medial aspect of the proximal end of each tibia is irregularly ossified and flattened. The tibial epiphyseal center is deformed medially as well.

congenital disturbance in the ossification of the epiphyses. The process rarely comes to the attention of the physician until the child begins to walk, and then it is noted that he has a waddling gait and short stubby digits of the hands and feet. Fairbank originally described the condition in 1935, and reviewed 20 cases in his atlas.[1] Several papers reporting series of these cases have appeared since, suggesting that the condition is not exceedingly rare.[49, 50] In most of the series there has been more than a suggestion of a hereditary and familial incidence. Rubin divides this dysplasia into two types, the pseudoachondroplastic type, which most closely resembles the cases Fairbank reported, and the tarda form. The latter is manifested principally by precocious osteoarthritis, particularly of the hips. One or all epiphyses may be involved and

in the largest series reported to date the affliction was limited to the lower extremities.[49]

Multiple irregular ossification centers cause enlargement of the epiphyses and sometimes flaring of the diaphyseal ends. The tibias are usually curved with knock-knee or bowleg deformity. There is usually some flexion deformity.

As the child develops, a subnormal growth rate becomes more obvious. The vertebrae are usually not affected so that dwarfing is confined to the extremities, resembling achondroplasia. A sloping upward from within outward of the articular surface of the distal tibia is said to occur in about half the cases. The schedule of appearance and fusion of the abnormal ossification centers may be abnormal but is usually not markedly deranged. Fusion of the various centers and of the epiphysis and diaphysis as a whole eventually occurs, but irregularities in the articular plates almost invariably lead to degenerative joint disease by the time the patient reaches middle life.

Other than the difficulties in locomotion consequent to the deformities and arthritis, these patients may lead a fairly normal life of average duration. Because of the difference in prognosis, epiphyseal dysplasia must be differentiated from Morquio's disease. This distinction is certainly not always easy, particularly when the epiphyseal involvement is general.

Blount's Disease. Osteochondrosis deformans tibiae, tibia vara or Blount's disease quite possibly fits into our classification at this point as a clinical subvariety of multiple epiphyseal dysplasia. Why its occurrence is limited to the medial aspect of the proximal tibial epiphysis is unknown. It may be analogous to ischemic necrosis of the head of the femur (coxa plana, Perthes' disease).

It is of considerable interest that though this lesion may be a type of epiphyseal dysplasia, its pathogenesis appears to be that of an epiphyseal ischemic necrosis. This association obviously suggests that the other epiphyseal dysplasias may have the same pathogenesis.

STIPPLED EPIPHYSES
(Chondrodystrophia Fetalis Calcificans, Dysplasia Epiphysealis Punctata)

This is an exceedingly rare condition in which multiple punctate opacities appear in the unossified epiphyseal cartilage, usually at birth. The infants are frequently stillborn or die of associated anomalies or intercurrent disease within the first year. There is a milder form which may not be noted at birth. Dwarfism is lacking in these cases and the stippled areas may merge into normal appearing epiphyseal osseous centers, sometimes as early as two years of age.

In the more severe form the osseous nucleus may fail to appear, the epiphysis remaining as a bulbous mass of stippled

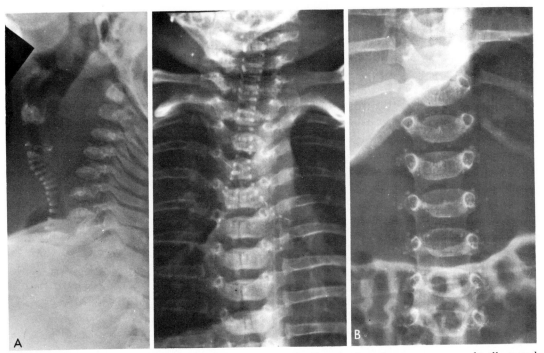

Figure 6–54 Stippled epiphyses. Calcification of laryngeal and tracheal cartilages may occur and is illustrated in A. The x-ray of the spine of the same patient (B) showed many areas of calcification in relation to the vertebral bodies.

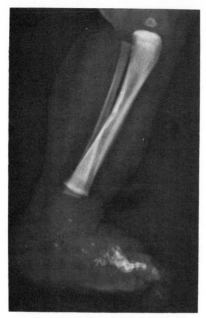

Figure 6-55 Stippled epiphyses. Punctate stippling in relation to primary and secondary epiphyses in the foot is evident. The cylindrical bones are of normal length in this instance.

cartilage. Since there is no growth plate there can be no length growth. Flat bones and vertebrae as well as cylindrical bones are involved.

Microscopic sections show great irregularity in vascularization of the epi-physis and chondroblastic maturation. Areas of ectopic ossification and chondroid mineral deposition are responsible for the stippled appearance on the roentgenogram.[51] Epiphyseal sections of a severe case examined by us revealed irregular areas of amorphous calcification of the chondroid. There was no evidence of ossification of the epiphyseal center.

Though in both stippled epiphyses and epiphyseal dysplasia the dominant feature is multiple abnormal epiphyseal ossification centers, the two diseases are usually considered to be distinct. Rubin,[52] Silverman[53] and McKusick,[11] however, believe that they are variants of the same bone growth disturbance. Stippled epiphyses lacks the hereditary and familial features of epiphyseal dysplasia, and though it may be associated with dwarfing of the extremities and flexion deformities, the patients in addition are apt to develop congenital cataracts, hyperkeratotic dermatoses and failure of proper mental development—features that are lacking in epiphyseal dysplasia. Calcification of soft tissues about the joint and of cartilage elsewhere in the body also sets it apart. The latter has been described in the nasal septum, the trachea and the larynx. The last has been severe enough to cause laryngeal stenosis.

Dysplasias Due to Abnormal Metaphyseal and Periosteal Ossification

There is a rather heterogeneous group of dysplasias that appear to result from too little osteoid production (osteogenesis imperfecta), too little osteolysis (osteopetrosis and others) or the production of defective or immature osteoid (the fibrous dysplasia group). In these, the elaboration of chondroid is normal so that the cartilaginous epiphysis is normal, and enchondral ossification is affected only to the extent to which metaphyseal osteoid production is involved. Thus, dwarfing is not the outstanding feature as it is in most of the dysplasias due to abnormal cartilage growth and metabolism. Instead, we find fragility of bones in cases in which too little osteoid is produced, excessive bone mass or density in those in which there is too little osteolysis and abnormal bone when the osteoblasts are incapable of providing the proper constituents for osteoid elaboration.

The condition osteitis condensans ilii et pubii is not included among the dysplasias because it appears to be a variation in localized bone density within normal limits. Zones of radiopacity are found in relation to the sacral and pubic synchondroses. They are asymptomatic.

DYSPLASIAS RELATED TO DEFICIENT OSTEOID PRODUCTION

Osteogenesis Imperfecta

Osteogenesis imperfecta has been called osteitis fragilitans, fragilitas ossium congenita, osteopsathyrosis idiopathica and brittle bones. It is a hereditary, often congenital and familial disease that is manifested by an inability to produce the adequate and normal intercellular substances of certain mesenchymal derivatives, particularly osteoblasts and fibroblasts, in various body areas. The result is a young patient with a fragile skeleton, thin skin and sclera, poor teeth, a tendency to macular bleeding and hypermotility of joints.

There are two forms of the disease. Osteogenesis imperfecta congenita is noted at birth, and it obviously develops in utero. It is often fatal. Osteogenesis imperfecta tarda starts its course some time in childhood. It may produce symptoms of only one or two system disturbances, and its effects are much less severe than those of the congenital form.

The disease is quite rare, but because of its unique symptomatology it has been recognized as an entity for nearly 200 years. Its peculiar and dramatic expression has resulted in the reporting of more than 2000 cases, and even in the older literature the diagnoses appear to be quite accurate.

Several writers have concerned themselves with the hereditary features of this disease. It apparently occurs as a spontaneous mutation, and once established in the hereditary apparatus it persists as a dominant. Thus, it may appear in a single member of a family and his offspring are apt to inherit the disease, while those of his siblings show no trait. Since the congenital form is severe and affects children before reproductivity, the affected branch soon dies out.

The outstanding characteristic in the full-blown disease is the skeletal fragility and proclivity for fracture on slight trauma. Thus, the case that develops in utero may not survive the rigors of parturition. Some doggedly tenacious writers have recorded thousands of fractures in a single case. If the patient survives the neonatal period or if the disease begins later in childhood, he is haunted for the remainder of his life by the specter of fracture on minor trauma. If the fractures are numerous and the deformity profound (Fig. 6–56) he may literally grow smaller instead of larger as overriding and bending cause loss in stature.

Though the bone is inadequately formed to resist normal stress, the fractures heal, often within a normal time. Callus formation may be frugal or it may be exuberant, but the bone that is formed is of the same

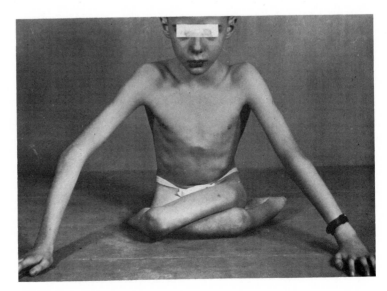

Figure 6–56 In osteogenesis imperfecta the skeleton is normal in length but the cortices are deficient in thickness and strength. The extremities are long and gracile. The fragile bones of the lower extremity often show multiple fractures because they are subjected to stress. (From Shriners' Hospital, Philadelphia.)

poor quality as that it replaces. Ordinary activity may cause partial fractures that eventually result in bending. Manifestations are usually more obvious in the lower extremities because these must bear the stress of the trunk weight and so are more vulnerable to trauma; invalidism is therefore a common sequence of the disease.

In some cases fracture is followed by callus formation of astonishing magnitude (Fig. 6–57). Because of the size of these callus masses, their abrupt onset and rapid growth, they have been misdiagnosed as osteosarcoma. The explanation of this exuberant callus growth is not obvious. To some extent it resembles the bone formation that is the sequence of some cases of traumatic or scorbutic, subperiosteal hemorrhage of massive degree. It is worth noting that the osteoid is apparently produced by cells recently metaplased from chondroblasts that have stemmed from collagenoblasts (see Repair of Fractures, Chapter 8) and as fresh, new cells, may retain the potential for

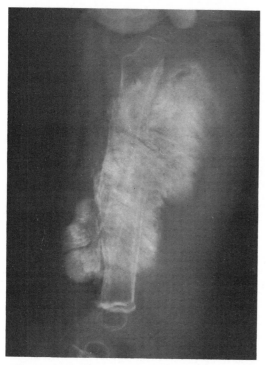

Figure 6–57 Roentgenogram of the femur of a 5 year old child with osteogenesis imperfecta. The radiopaque mass represents exuberant callus which grew rapidly following a fracture.

osteoid production that the native cells do not possess.

Those who have had the opportunity of observing many patients with osteogenesis imperfecta state that bone growth is abnormal apart from the fractures and subsequent deformities.[54] The cylindrical bones of the extremities are apt to be long and gracile, and skeletal muscles are poorly developed. The skull is reported to be misshapen with protrusion of the frontal and parietal regions and a deeply overhanging occiput. The cranial bossing has been explained as a result of a failure of ossification of the membranous skull.

Though pathologic fractures are the most trying features of the condition, the inability to produce normal components of intercellular matrix (collagen fibers?) is manifested elsewhere. The blue sclerotics are probably of this order. The sclera may range from a blue-white tint to a deep sky blue color. Some observers insist that the shade is not constant and that it may vary from time to time within the same patient. Others have described a "Saturn's ring" of white about the cornea. The color is apparently due to the intraocular pigment, which is visible through the sclera. Some writers have reported sclera of subnormal thickness; others contend that the thickness is normal, but that the substance is translucent. The abnormality does not affect vision.

The teeth are often poor because of malformation of the dentin.[55] Both deciduous and permanent teeth are affected. When the teeth alone are involved, the condition has been called "dentinogenesis imperfecta" or "hereditary opalescent dentin." They are usually discolored bluish gray to a yellowish brown, and they often have an opalescent appearance. The enamel, being a product of cells of ectodermal rather than mesenchymal derivation, is normal, but because it rests upon a foundation of poor dentin it chips, and the teeth may be lost by the age of 30. Roentgenograms show short roots and sometimes obliterated pulp canals.

Deafness is frequently mentioned as a characteristic feature of osteogenesis imperfecta tarda during adult life. Some authors believe that this is the result of pressure upon the eighth nerves as they emerge from the cranial vault, but others state that its onset is like that of otosclerosis and is due to abnormal proliferations of cartilage, which becomes calcified and results in sclerosis of the petrous portion of the temporal bone.

The hypermotility of the joints, especially at the wrists and ankles, has been frequently noted. It may be due to a disturbance in the production of the collagen components of tendons and ligaments.

Follis[56] has noted a peculiar appearance of the skin on microscopic examination. By special staining technique he has demonstrated the presence of an immature collagen of the corium and suggests that there is an inability to transform fetal collagen into the mature adult form.

A tendency for macular hemorrhage into the tissues has been noted. The Rumpel-Leede test may be positive. This again may be the result of an inability to produce a normal collagenous substance to support the capillary wall.

There is still controversy concerning whether there is normal scar formation in patients with osteogenesis imperfecta. Scot and Stiris[54] investigated this question and concluded that though healing occurs, and often within a normal time, the resulting scar is broader than normal and the collagen is of poor quality. This is probably analogous to the excessive bone callus formation in fracture healing.

Roentgenographic Manifestations. Osteogenesis imperfecta affects the entire skeleton. Roentgenographic manifestations vary according to the severity of the disease, but in general the bones are of subnormal bone mass and show evidence of old or recent fractures. The osseous changes may not be apparent dur-

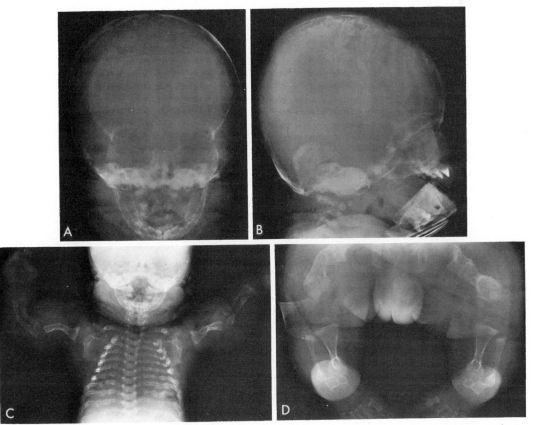

Figure 6–58 Osteogenesis imperfecta. A newborn with the severe form of the disease. In *A* and *B* note the inadequate mineralization of the cranial bones, the wide sutures and multiple centers of ossification. Multiple fractures of the extremities and rib cage are evident in *C* and *D*. The cortices are thin and the spongiosa is markedly deficient.

ing the first years of life, and when they appear, progress rapidly. The osteopenia reflects inadequate osteoblastic activity. The trabeculae are fine and sparse, and the cortex is thin. Because enchondral ossification supplies only a small portion of the total bone mass, the cylindrical bones usually are of normal length. Their diameter, however, tends to be smaller than normal as a consequence of disturbed periosteal osteogenesis. The ends of cylindrical bones appear wide when compared to their shafts, and because the trabeculae are sparse the zone of provisional calcification may appear more opaque than normal. However, in the severe form of the disease encountered in the neonate,

the long bones may be wide and short secondary to multiple fractures, but the cortices are thin. Rarely, cyst-like areas of lucency are encountered within the metaphyses.

In the severe, infantile form of the disease the radiographic appearance of the skull may be striking. Multiple centers of ossification, less opaque than normal, are evident, and as these slowly enlarge the cranial bones exhibit a mosaic pattern. Chipping and crumbling of the teeth may result in radiographic abnormality akin to caries. Compression fractures of the vertebral bodies are common as manifested by a decrease in their stature. Biconcave deformities of the vertebrae are

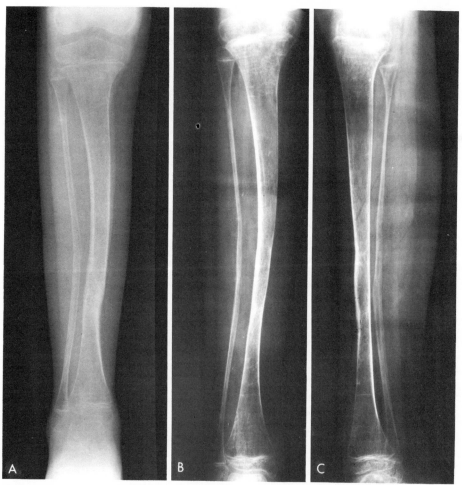

Figure 6–59 Osteogenesis imperfecta. Radiographs of the tibia and fibula of a child exposed at the age of 5 years (A) and 7 years (B and C). Longitudinal growth is evident over the two-year interval but note the change that occurred in the diameter of the bones, particularly the fibula. The cortex is narrow and trabeculae sparse. Healing of the fracture of the shaft of the tibia (A) occurred, but with deformity.

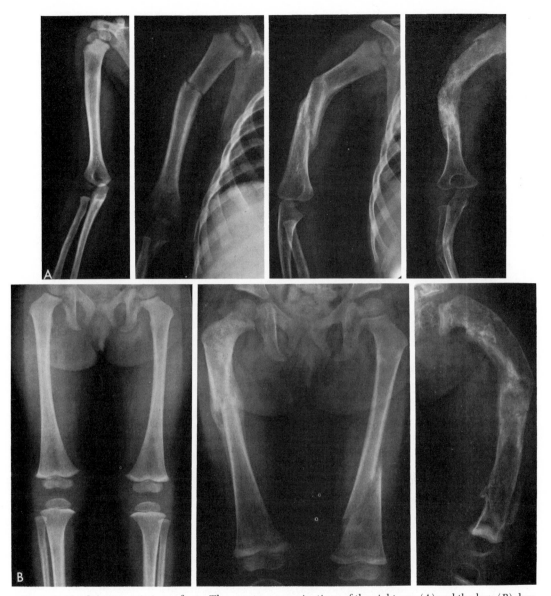

Figure 6–60   Osteogenesis imperfecta. The roentgen examinations of the right arm (A) and the legs (B) demonstrate the progression of the disease over a period of four years. Note the normal appearance of the bones during the first year of life. Abundant callus is evident in relation to fractures.

frequently observed. The epiphyseal centers have a normal configuration but demonstrate a thin cortex and sparse trabeculae.

Fractures and deformity are an integral part of the radiographic appearance. Subnormal stature may result from interference with length growth by multiple small fractures in the metaphysis, as well as being secondary to multiple diaphyseal fractures. Deformity, the result of muscle

pull, may be evident. In the less severe forms of the disease, frequent fractures may be the dominant feature with little recognizable abnormality of the cortex and spongiosa.

Microscopy.   Demineralized sections of bone in osteogenesis imperfecta reveal a disturbance in both enchondral and intramembranous bone formation. The cartilaginous epiphyses are normal, and the secondary ossification centers appear on schedule. Chondroblastic proliferation is present and orderly, and maturation with columnation and glycogen imbibition appears to be undisturbed. Mineral salts are deposited in the line of provisional calcification, and a chondroid lattice is formed (Fig. 6–61). Here, enchondral growth appears to stop. Osteoblasts fail to emerge in proper numbers from the undifferentiated cell mass; consequently, the fingers of calcified chondroid remain naked or inadequately covered because a paucity of osteoid is laid down. Very few osteoclasts appear, but whether because there is no use for them or because of the paucity of osteoblasts from which they emerge is unknown. Thus, the spongiosa is exceedingly scant. It consists of a few thin and often fractured spicules of primitive bone in a relatively large marrow space. Eventually a thin dome of mineralized osteoid seals off the epiphyseal line preventing further osteogenesis. Follis[57] and Weber[58] independently reported wide seams of an unknown substance that takes a deep blue stain with hematoxylin surrounding the fragments of mineralized chondroid lattice.

Osteoid formation by the periosteal osteoblasts is equally deficient. Some primitive fiberbone is laid down, but there is poor transition to adult bone and, therefore, poor lamellation and haversian system formation. The result is a deficient cortex that lacks continuity. The bone that is formed remains in the coarsely fibered state and never becomes arranged in the lines of normal stress. There is apparently no fault in mineralization because the osteoid becomes mineralized promptly and adequately.

These descriptions were made from sections of bone in cases of fatal osteogenesis imperfecta congenita. All degrees of bone production are seen in cases of osteogenesis imperfecta tarda, but the spongiosa almost always appears scant and the compacta inadequate.

Sections of the skin in the fatal congenital form were stained by Follis[56] using the periodic acid–Schiff and silver techniques. He interpreted the persistent metachromasia and argentophilia as evidence that the collagen of the corium was immature.

Some interesting studies have been done by Engfeldt et al.[59] utilizing microradiography, x-ray diffraction and polarized light techniques. These methods demonstrate irregular mineralization of osteoid, which appears to be on the basis of a disturbance in osteoid production rather than in the mineralization itself.

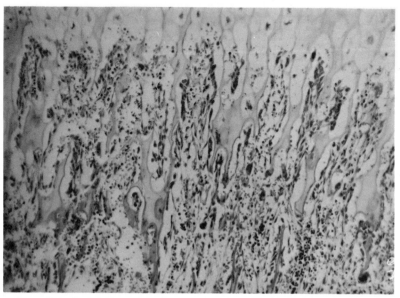

Figure 6–61   Osteogenesis imperfecta. The chondroid lattice is formed but there are no osteoblasts to cover them with seams of osteoid.

The osteoid is of a peculiar fetal character, coarsely fibered and arranged without regard to vasculature. There is consequently no lamellation and no haversian system formation. There is little or no attempt at replacement by secondary or mature osteoid. The defect appears to lie either in an inability of the osteoblasts to differentiate from the multipotent cell mass or in some deficiency that prevents them from providing the normal constituents necessary for osteoid formation. Because presumably there is no inadequacy in the nutrients supplied to the cell, the fault would appear to lie within the cell itself, which is either refractory to normal stimuli or lacking in a normal enzyme equipment.

It is of great interest that in osteogenesis imperfecta there is a dissociation of chondroblastic and osteoblastic activity. Cartilage appears to develop normally and is affected only because of the abnormal mechanical stresses that result from inadequate bone formation.

Another condition in which this dissociation is clearly apparent is scurvy. In ascorbic acid deficiency, there is normal chondroblastic activity, but the osteoblasts fail to develop normal components of phosphatase and cytoplasmic ribosenucleic acid and there is a comparable failure of osteoid and collagen production. Thus, scurvy may be considered a deficiency type of osteopenia, whereas osteogenesis imperfecta is a congenital form of this condition.

Osteogenesis imperfecta now appears to be a systemic inability to produce normal and adequate osteoid, dentin and collagen in sufficient amounts to balance the concomitant bone lysis. This inability is registered in the skeleton, the teeth, the sclera, the joints, the skin and the blood vessels. Rubin has concluded that the disability is confined entirely to periosteal bone formation, but analysis reveals the same deficiency in enchondral growth. It is less obvious in these sites because enchondral osteogenesis supplies only a small proportion of the total bone mass and, thus, its deficiency does not register so dramatically.

Most authors believe that the difficulty lies in an inability to elaborate osteoid at a normal rate, but recently some have contended that the rate of osteoid production is normal but the rate of bone absorption is increased. The evidence presented has not impressed us. We choose to believe that eventually it will be found that there is an inborn inability of the cells that normally elaborate osteoid and collagen to synthesize the normal amino acid constituents of these substances, probably the collagen fibers, that are such important components of both. A variety of abnormal substitutes are produced giving the tissues a shoddy warp and woof.

Prognosis. The patient with severe osteogenesis imperfecta in childhood is almost certain to develop disabling skeletal deformity if indeed he survives to adulthood. At the time of cessation of normal skeletal growth the severity of the condition may subside but the skeleton remains weak, and the patient must continue to avoid trauma of all degrees. The abatement of symptoms at adulthood has led some to consider endocrine dysfunction as a possible cause. There are no facts to substantiate this hypothesis. It appears that the condition is a disturbance in skeleton formation and is, therefore, most manifest at the time skeletal bone is being produced. As the rate of growth diminishes, the demand decreases and the manifestations of the disease become less obvious. If the victim survives to maturity he may learn to live with his affliction.

BONE DYSPLASIAS RELATED TO EXCESSIVE OSTEOID PRODUCTION OR DEFICIENT OSTEOLYSIS

Osteopetrosis (Albers-Schönberg)

Osteopetrosis, also known as Albers-Schönberg disease, osteosclerosis fragilis, marble bones and chalk bones, is a rare hereditary, congenital and familial abnormality in bone growth, the disturbed mechanism of which appears to be a failure or inhibition of resorption of calcified chondroid and primitive bone. Because there is little or no inhibition in the formation of cartilage and primitive bone, growth continues but, lacking resorption, the cores of calcified cartilage and their sheaths of unlamellated osteoid persist, interfering with the formation of adult bone which normally replaces it and crowding the areas in which resorption should occur and the primitive bone be replaced by normal medullary tissues.

Recognizable cases of osteopetrosis have been described since the middle of the eighteenth century under a variety of names but Albers-Schönberg was the first to report a roentgenographic description of the condition in 1907, and it has since borne his name. Karshner[60] introduced the term osteopetrosis in 1926, and since that time numerous papers have appeared ascribing an amusing variety of alterations in physiology to account for the clinical and morphologic findings of the disease.

The terms osteopetrosis and marble bones were suggested because of the density to x-ray and a few descriptions of the bones as harder than normal. Other reports state that a drill sinks into the bone as though it were chalk and call attention to the high incidence of pathologic fractures. These features have inspired the terms chalk bones and osteopetrosis fragilis. It is true that transverse fractures do occur, indicating that the affected bones are brittle rather than soft. In a few instances the bone is eburnated causing the drill to smoke as penetration is attempted, but in most instances the bone is hard but actually of a chalky consistency.

Some writers have contended that the disturbance is due to an excessive deposition of normal calcium salts. For any measured volume of bone, the mineral content is greater than that of normal bone, but if the normal spaces of the latter are taken into consideration the quantitative relation of mineral to organic matrix of osteopetrotic bone remains about that of the normal bone. Others have contended that the mineral in osteopetrosis is abnormal and have compared these bones to those seen in cases of fluorine, strontium and phosphorus toxicity. Chemical analysis of the salts extracted from osteopetrotic bone has not corroborated this hypothesis. Some have thought that the crystalline architecture was altered by an abnormal quantitative variation in the normal constituents. The results of several analyses are conflicting and the facts are not as yet clear, but it is probable that at least in some cases of osteopetrosis the chemical make-up of the bone salts is the same as that of normal bone.

Because of failure to find a cause for the condition in the mineral content it was suggested that the disturbance was due to an abnormal proliferation of bone by the endosteum. Actually, in the sense of a periosteum-like membrane lining the medullary cavity, an endosteum does not exist and in osteopetrosis bone does not grow into the medullary cavity from the inner surface of the cortex. Cortical bone remains from its embryonal inception so that a normal medullary cavity is never formed. It has been stated that only enchondral bone is affected because, grossly, the metaphyseal areas are the most dramatically altered, but actually all bone, both enchondral and intramembranous, is involved. A comparison of large sections of infant and adult osteopetrotic bone with the normal bone of comparable ages bears out this statement.

A careful reading of the admirable paper by Zawisch[61] is infinitely helpful in understanding the process that results in the changes that characterize osteopetrosis. It must be stated that the exact mechanisms of the disease are not known. The most that can be said is that there appears to be a failure or an inhibition of the resorption processes so that primitive chondro-osteoid persists and interferes with its replacement by normal mature bone.

Osteopetrosis is a rare condition, there being less than 200 cases reported in the literature. It has been diagnosed by roentgenograms of the fetus in utero. In most fatal cases death is due to anemia during the second year. The average case is diagnosed some time during adolescence, attention being directed to the condition by fracture, anemia, failing vision or osteomyelitis of the jaw. Rarely, cases are diagnosed in adult life, and at least one instance is recorded in advanced senility. Like most of the congenital diseases of the skeleton, the earlier the manifestations occur, the worse the prognosis is apt to be. Those with the severest type, often placed in a special group, die in utero or, if these patients survive the fetal period, they usually succumb before their second birthday. Those who live through childhood may develop difficulties at any time thereafter with a progressive anemia.

Occasionally one finds a focal area of sclerosis in a single bone of an adult, and biopsy shows the characteristic microscopy of osteopetrosis. Whether these are bona fide instances of solitary, focal osteopetrosis or a variety of some other sclerosing disease is not certain. The incidence of the generalized type suggests that it is inherited as a simple Mendelian recessive. Some have suggested that the more florid type behaves as a Mendelian dominant. There is a higher incidence of consanguinity in the parents than in the average population.

In the cases of osteopetrosis that are manifested early the skull bones are usually quite drastically involved. Because the major cartilaginous growth centers are within the base, this area is most extensively involved. The failure in modeling which characterizes the disease results in the formation of a massive base with improper and inadequate formation of the various fossae. There may be inadequate room for the growth of the pituitary with disturbed function of that gland. Inadequate space for the circulation of the cerebrospinal fluid about the hemisphere results in hydrocephalus in many cases. This may be severe enough to cause widening of the sutures and delayed closure of the fontanelles. Consequently, the head may be enlarged. In the same manner, there is apt to be incomplete formation of the foramina so that there is inadequate room for the passage of the cerebral nerves. Atrophy of the optic nerves causes failing vision, and this may be accompanied by nystagmus and ocular palsy. Many of the juvenile cases progress to complete blindness. Deafness and facial palsies are also common. The teeth are apt to be late in erupting, and severe caries develops early. Caries is followed by infection with eventual osteomyelitis and necrosis of the mandible. These difficulties are attributed to the inadequate bony channels for nutrient circulation.

The vertebrae are usually severely involved, and there may be impingement on the spinal nerves as well. Cylindrical bones develop a highly characteristic conformation. At times, the shaft is widened throughout its entire length, but more often the middle third of the diaphysis is of about normal width. The ends of the diaphysis develop a peculiar bulbous clubbing, which extends to the epiphyseal line. This is due to the failure in absorption of both the calcified chondroid islands and the young bone that is laid down about them. Normally this first product in the formation of bone, osteochondroid, undergoes a slow lysis and replacement with adult, lamellated bone in stress trajectories. Because absorption of the osteochondroid does not occur, modeling cannot take place and the bone elongates, maintaining the diameter of the metaphysis. This elongated "metaphysis" is the hallmark of osteopetrosis, but if a careful examination is made the bone of the shaft laid down by the cambium is seen to be involved also.

Fractures are common in osteopetrosis. They are often characteristically transverse. These have puzzled investigators who have assumed that, because the bones are more massive and opaque, they should be stronger. It has been suggested that the crystalline lattice in osteopetrosis is abnormal and, therefore, lacking in strength. The little investigation that has been done in this field has not substantiated this view. When one examines osteopetrotic bone under the microscope, the reason for its tendency to fracture becomes obvious. Normally, a fine lamellated bone is laid down in lines that are arranged to most effectively resist stress. In osteopetrosis, finely lamellated bone is not formed nor is there organization of the unresolved osteochondroid in trajectory lines. Consequently, though the bone is hard to the touch because it contains large quantities of calcium salts, the alignment and reenforcement is defective and it breaks like chalk, transverse to the long axis.[62] Fractures heal producing a callus that has the same abnormal features as the original bone.

Normal growth is impeded. The skeleton is apt to be moderately stunted. Ossification centers appear and close on schedule

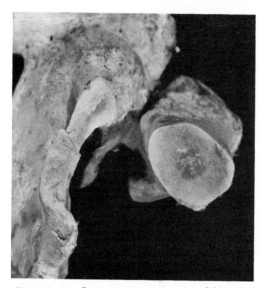

Figure 6-62 Osteopetrosis. A portion of the pelvis and the upper portion of the femur. The latter is tilted to show a cross section through the upper shaft. Note the markedly thickened cortex and obliteration of the medulla by cancellous bone proliferation. The pelvic bones are heavier than normal, the cortical surfaces roughened. The acetabular silhouette is altered because of longstanding, severe degenerative joint disease.

except where there is secondary interference by fracture, abnormal pressures or disuse atrophy.

A myelophthisic anemia is apt to be a most troublesome complication and is frequently the cause of death. In the advanced case one can find no gross evidence of hematopoietic marrow because the spongiosa and the medullary cavity are replaced by porous bony tissue (Fig. 6-62). The spleen and, in children, the lymph nodes and liver attempt to compensate for this lack by myeloid metaplasia. The enlargement of these organs constitutes a part of the clinical expression of osteopetrosis.

Roentgenographic Manifestations. Radiographically, osteopetrosis is manifested by striking opacity of the bones and obliteration of the normal architecture. In many areas the cortex and spongiosa are of the same density, resulting in a homogeneously dense bone. In the growing long bone the zone of provisional calcification is indistinguishable from the adjacent spongiosa. The entire skeleton is affected.

The bones at the base of the skull tend to show the most marked change, but all of the cranial bones may be involved. The mastoid air cells and paranasal sinuses may never develop, and distortion of the cranial fossae and foramina may be evident. Similar alterations may be evident in craniometaphyseal dysplasia, idiopathic hypercalcemia and vitamin D intoxication. The appearance of the remainder of the skeleton, however, is different.

The ends of the long cylindrical bones are widened as a manifestation of failure of modeling. This widening is most marked where bone growth is rapid; particularly do the distal femurs show this alteration (Fig. 6-65). Obliteration of the medullary canal, totally or in part, is a manifestation of failure of normal resorptive processes. Radiolucent striations, vertical or horizontal, in the distal diaphyses of long bones are common. A radiolucent outline of a bone within a bone may be evident These sclerotic masses of bone have been termed endobone.[14] They are noted to have been observed immediately after birth and to have disappeared usually by adult life. This phenomenon is also present in the vertebral bodies, flat bones and ossification centers (Fig. 6-66). Fractures of the skeleton are common and are most often transverse fractures. Rapid healing with abundant callus is said to occur.

The roentgenographic manifestations then are a reflection of the persistence of primitive chondro-osteoid and inhibition of normal resorptive processes.

Microscopy. The morbid microscopy of osteopetrosis can be best appreciated by examination of sections made through the epiphyseal plate and metaphysis of a growing bone. It is seen that chondroblasts multiply quite adequately and follow the normal pattern of maturation. Columnation is poor with crowding at the frontier of provisory calcification. It is impossible to be sure whether this irregularity is due to the essential mechanisms of the disease or whether it is secondary to the more obvious changes that take place within the metaphysis. A lattice of mineralized chondroid bars is formed, and normal appearing primitive osteoid is laid down in wide seams about them. This combination

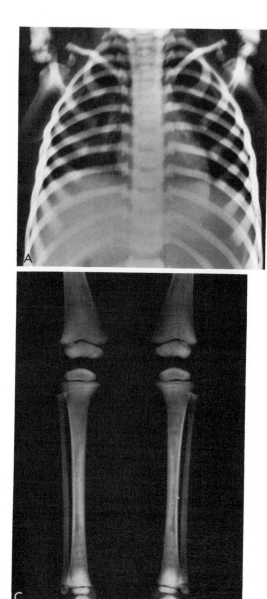

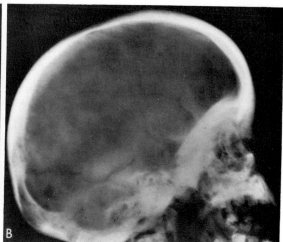

Figure 6–63 Osteopetrosis. The ribs, vertebrae (A) and bones of the skull (B), particularly those at the base of the skull, are thick and uniformly opaque. Widening of the distal femurs (C) is apparent and the medullary canal is almost obliterated in the diaphysis of the tibias. Striations in the diaphyses of the long bones are evident. The epiphyseal centers are involved.

of cartilaginous nucleus with a perimeter of osteoid may be designated as osteochondroid. Under normal circumstances the cartilage portion gradually fades away as the epiphyseal frontier advances beyond it, but in osteopetrosis it persists.

Osteoid continues to pile up about these cartilaginous islands, occupying the space that is normally devoted to the vascular granulation. The latter is gradually squeezed out of existence so that there is little remaining to penetrate the feet of

the cartilage cell columns distally. This may account for the crowding that occurs in this area. Because the osteochondroid persists, new, lamellated osteoid cannot replace it, and the metaphysis gradually increases in length as the bone grows, forming the distal enlargement of the "clubbed diaphysis." The failure of lysis of the osteochondroid also results in an obliteration of the space normally occupied by the medullary "cavity," which is filled with fat, and the areas at either end

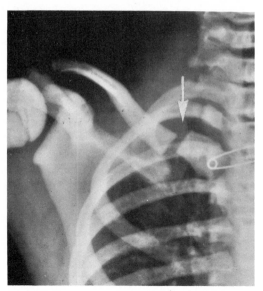

Figure 6–64 Osteopetrosis. There is a transverse fracture of the clavicle; this was associated with minimal trauma.

bands of opacity and translucency that are seen in roentgenograms crossing the clubbed areas of long bones are caused by layered strata of almost solid osteochondroid and more normal appearing bone. One gets the impression from examining these areas that the more normal bands represent periods when the disease process is arrested and the resolution of osteochondroid proceeds normally. Nearer the center of the diaphysis, bands of the same type may be seen running longitudinally, signifying the same activity sequence in the bone that is laid down by the periosteum.

Sections through the diaphysis proximal to the clubbed ends also reveal the presence of cartilage and primitive osteoid. It is unknown whether such sections have represented fortuitous examples of post-fracture callus, remnants of the originally formed metaphyseal cortex or an example of cambium cartilaginous metaplasia.

When one examines a section of osteopetrotic bone, it is difficult to see any normal, organized bone structure. Irregular patches of chondroid containing scattered chondrocytes are embedded in a ragged matrix of coarse fibered bone. The latter is put together in a coarse mosaic, which has a resemblance to that of Paget's disease except that the fragments are larger

in which the spongiosa and hematopoietic marrow should be. The metaphyseal cortices that are normally formed by a combination of the outermost spicules of spongiosa covered with a layer of cambium bone are made up of the same type of primitive bone as that found deeper in the metaphysis. The alternating horizontal

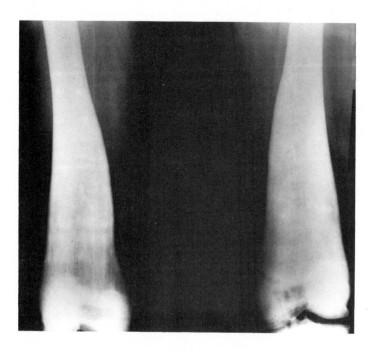

Figure 6–65 Osteopetrosis. Distal femurs of a 61 year old white male. The inhibition of normal modeling and the uniform opacity of the bones are evident.

and their shape conforms to the cartilage islands that they surround (Fig. 6–67). The cement lines are wide and prominent. In the opaque bands there are no forms that even remotely resemble a normal spicule. The translucent bands are made up of connecting trabeculae largely without cartilage remnants and composed in part of adult bone. The haversian spaces are wide and contain loose aggregates of splindled and stellate fibrous cells. Islands of hematopoietic marrow appear here and there.

It is obvious that the regions that normally support cell-forming marrow are deficient. The anemia may be ascribed to this deficiency. In the opinion of some the condition is the result of a depression of the multipotent mesenchyme, which should normally differentiate into the various components of bone, cartilage, fibrous and marrow tissue. From examination of the sections, one gets the impression that all the skeletal elements could be normally formed if only the products of the first stage could be cleared away to give them space. The myeloid metaplasia in the spleen and lymph nodes appears to support this impression.

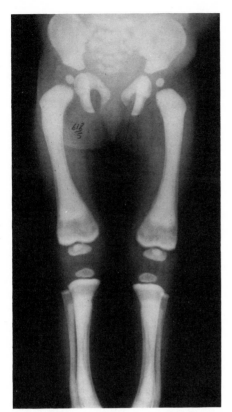

Figure 6–66   Osteopetrosis. Bone within a bone or endobone is seen in the ilia, the long bones and the secondary centers.

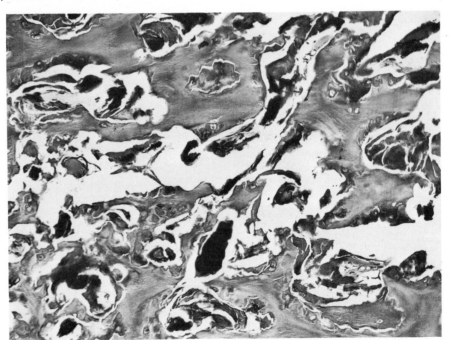

Figure 6–67   Osteopetrosis. Section taken from an area that should normally be cancellous tissue. The bone is laid down about nidi of densely calcified cartilage producing a helter-skelter arrangement without spicule formation.

Prognosis. The symptoms and ultimately the course of osteopetrosis depend largely upon the severity of the involvement and the age at onset. If the patient survives early childhood, he has a fair chance of attaining adulthood. The longer he lives the less likely he is to die of this disease though sarcoma has been reported as a late complication.

Pyknodysostosis

Pyknodysostosis is a curious skeletal dysplasia, which is often confused with osteopetrosis because the bones are denser than normal, with cleidocranial dysostosis because of skull and clavicle abnormalities or with osteogenesis imperfecta because of fracture with minimal trauma. It probably is related to none of these. It is now generally believed that this is the dysplasia that affected Henri de Toulouse-Lautrec.[63]

The condition is not rare; there are probably more than 500 cases described in the literature. It appears to be autosomal recessive, the abnormal chromosome probably being a member of the G-22 pair.[64] Dwarfing occurs in the more severe cases, the height usually not exceeding 5 feet. Some loss of stature (dwarfing) may be due to the numerous fractures that the patient suffers throughout his life.

Consistently there is failure of closure of the cranial sutures with the appearance of numerous wormian bones. The mandibular ramus is hypoplastic, resulting in a receding jaw (Fig. 6–70). The hands are short and stubby (Fig. 6–71) with acro-osteolysis of the terminal phalanges. The nails may show koilonychia (spoon nails). The deciduous teeth may persist with unerupted or malformed permanent teeth (Fig. 6–72), and the clavicles are poorly formed with absence or hypoplasia of the acromial ends. The entire skeleton usually displays increased bone density (Fig. 6–69).[65]

Dr. Stanley Elmore was kind enough to send us material from his published case.[66] The microscopy here (Fig. 6–73) was remarkably similar to that of osteopetrosis.

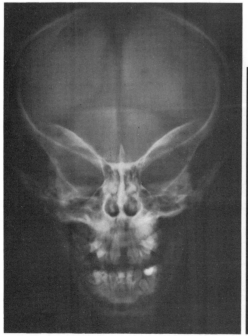
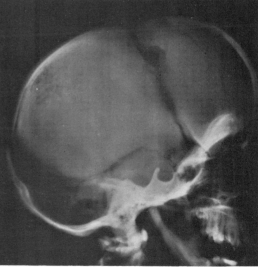

Figure 6–68 Pyknodysostosis. The cranial vault is slightly enlarged, the sutures are wide and the anterior fontanelle is open. The angle of the mandible is flat and deciduous teeth are visible. (Courtesy of Dr. Henry Burko, Vanderbilt University Hospital, Nashville.)

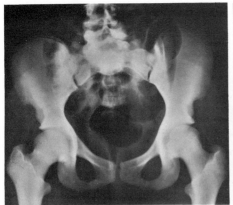

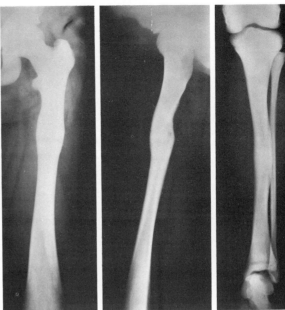

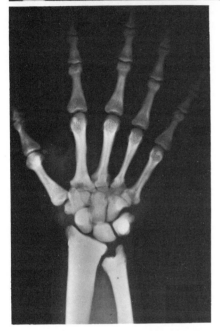

Figure 6–69 Pyknodysostosis. The bones of the extremities are dense and the ends of the bones flare, but the medullary canal is visible. There is evidence of an old fracture of the femur. The tufts of the distal phalanges are absent and these phalanges taper distally. (Courtesy of Dr. Henry Burko, Vanderbilt University Hospital, Nashville.)

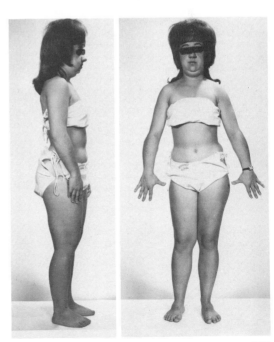

Figure 6–70 Pyknodysostosis. The large head (unclosed sutures), receding chin and stubby fingers are characteristic. (Courtesy of Dr. Stanley Elmore.)

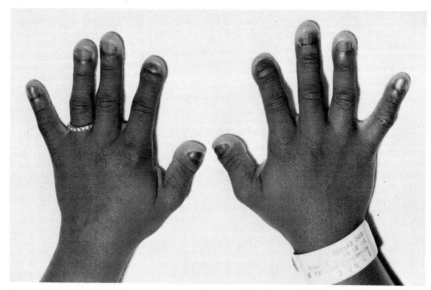

Figure 6–71   Pyknodysostosis showing short, stubby digits. (Courtesy of Dr. Eyering.)

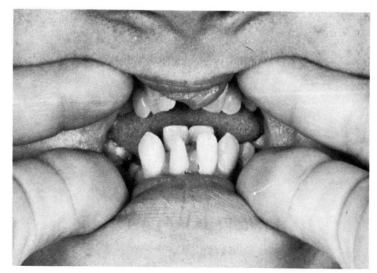

Figure 6–72   Pyknodysostosis. There may be a double set of teeth. (Courtesy of Dr. Eyering.)

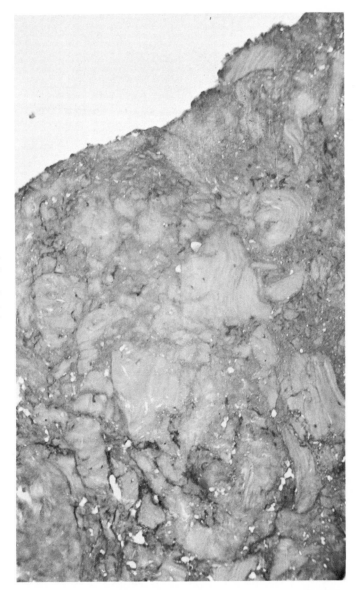

Figure 6–73 Pyknodysostosis. Osteons are strikingly irregular surrounded by prominent cement lines. Interspicular spaces are minimal, the "spicules" massive. Appearance is very similar to osteopetrosis and hyperphosphatasia. (Courtesy of Dr. Stanley Elmore.)

Metaphyseal Dysplasia (Pyle)

Metaphyseal dysplasia or craniometaphyseal dysplasia is a disturbance in enchondral bone growth in which there is failure of modeling of cylindrical bones so that the ends of the shafts remain larger than normal in circumference. Roentgenograms present the Erlenmeyer flask deformity, which has been noted in osteopetrosis. The cortices in these areas remain thinner than normal and are, therefore, more subject to fracture by trauma.

The amount of cancellous tissue, however, is greater. It impinges upon and reduces the extent of the medullary area. Thus, it appears that there is a lack of osteoclastic activity in the metaphyseal and diaphyseal periosteum as in osteopetrosis but, unlike osteopetrosis, there is osteoclastic activity for enchondral bone formation. Because metaphyseal subperiosteal osteoclasis apparently is responsible for modeling, the ends of the long bones remain flared, resembling those of osteopetrosis in which the same mechanism is said to

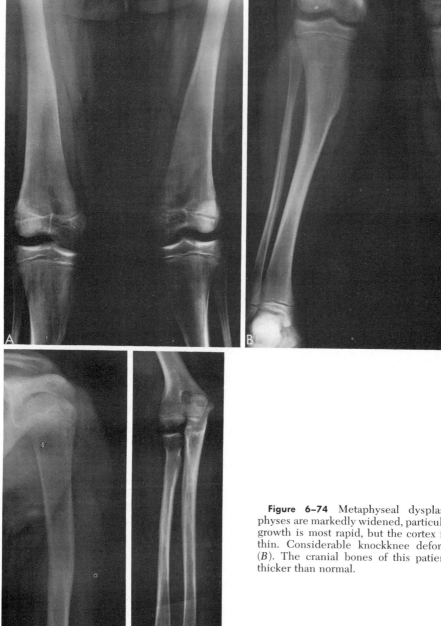

Figure 6–74 Metaphyseal dysplasia. The metaphyses are markedly widened, particularly where bone growth is most rapid, but the cortex in these areas is thin. Considerable knockknee deformity is present (*B*). The cranial bones of this patient were slightly thicker than normal.

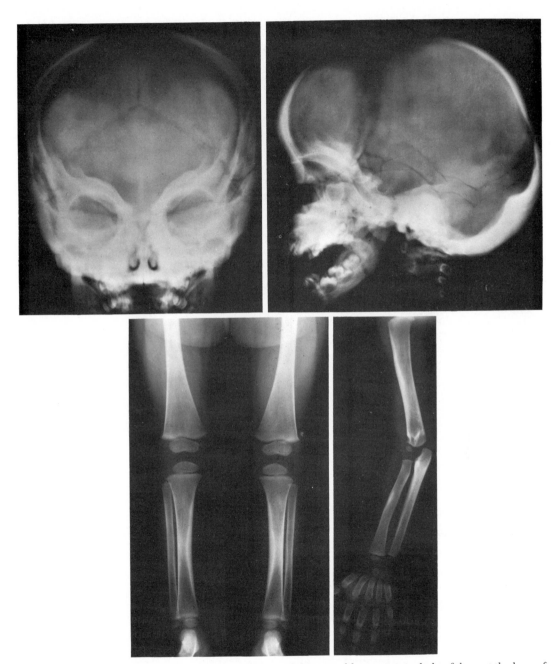

Figure 6–75 Craniometaphyseal dysplasia. Sclerosis of the cranial bones, particularly of those at the base of the skull, and of the facial bones is evident. The long bones of this male, 18 months of age, are broad with slight sclerosis of the mid-portion of the diaphysis. (Courtesy of Dr. J. W. Hope, Children's Hospital of Philadelphia.)

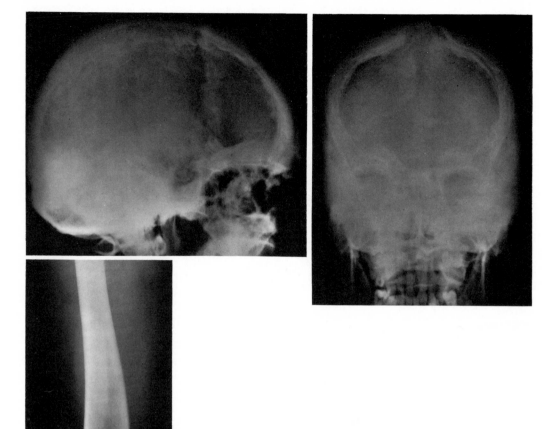

Figure 6–76 Craniometaphyseal dysplasia. This 32 year old male is the father of the patient illustrated in Figure 6–75. (Courtesy of Dr. J. W. Hope, Children's Hospital of Philadelphia.)

pertain. Also like osteopetrosis the shaft cortex is thickened, but unlike it the flared ends are abnormally thin.

Pyle[67] first described this condition in 1931, and since then there have been several reports of small series including an informative analysis by Jackson et al.[68] in 1954.

The disease is familial and apparently hereditary though its incidence is so low that exact mechanisms are still uncertain. Consanguinity probably plays a role.

The epiphyses develop normally so that bone age is not altered. General health is not affected except by a tendency for pathologic fracture, so that life expectancy is not shortened. Normal stature is attained.

The distal femurs and proximal tibias are usually most dramatically involved, but the growth center of any cylindrical bone may show the abnormality and the bones of the hands and feet often present the same changes as those seen in the long cylindrical bones.

Jackson et al.[68] noted that metaphyseal

dysplasia is sometimes associated with an overgrowth of the head bones, leontiasis ossea, and suggested that the combination of these two conditions may represent a variety of the same process. They called this condition craniometaphyseal dysplasia. Since that time, a number of reports have confirmed this observation[69, 70] though others continue to regard head involvement as an entity and call it "craniofacial dysostosis." All of the head bones including those of the face and mandible are involved, presenting a classic leontiasis ossea. There is hypertelorism with overgrowth of the bridge of the nose. Bone overgrowth at nerve foramina may lead to neurologic symptoms, blindness and impairment of hearing.

It has been suggested that the skeleton has a greater than normal avidity for calcium, suggesting a relation to osteomalacia. This aspect needs further investigation.

Diaphyseal Sclerosis (Camurati-Engelmann-Ribbing)

This condition was described by Camurati[71] in 1922 and by Engelmann[72] in 1929. Sear's paper[73] in 1948 provided the eponym "Engelmann's disease" by which this interesting condition has since been known. Ribbing[74] in 1949 described very similar alterations in the skeletons of four siblings under the title of hereditary multiple diaphyseal sclerosis, believing it to be a different entity because of its familial character. Since that time, a considerable number of small series have appeared. A very good review of the literature up to 1961 is supplied by Lennon et al.[75] From our present and incomplete knowledge it appears probable that these are all variations of the same process. We have suggested the simple, descriptive but noncommittal title of diaphyseal sclerosis.

The severity of the condition varies greatly, the most florid cases beginning early in childhood; the mildest cases are often asymptomatic and undiscovered until adult life. This dysplasia is often familial, congenital and probably hereditary.

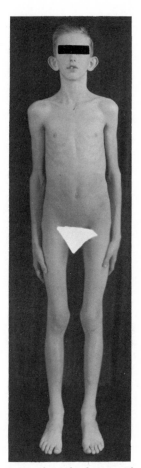

Figure 6–77 Diaphyseal sclerosis. The cylindrical bones of the extremities are longer than normal. The body appears markedly undernourished.

The well-defined case begins in early childhood with difficulty in walking. The gait is described as shuffling or waddling. Movement in some cases is painful, and there may be periods when the limbs are tender. The bones first involved are usually the femur and tibia. There is thickening of the mid-diaphyseal cortex, which progresses toward the metaphyses. The thickening is subperiosteal with failure of absorption from within so that the cortex becomes greatly thickened although the medullary and cancellous areas remain the same size and, thus, appear small when the bones enlarge. There may eventually be inadequate space for hematopoiesis, with the development of anemia and the enlargement of the spleen and liver presumably because of myeloid metaplasia. As the disease progresses over

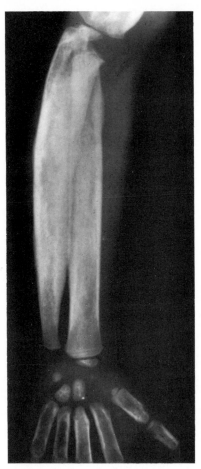

Figure 6–78   Diaphyseal sclerosis. The radiograph of the forearm shows fusiform enlargement of the bones occasioned by new bone formation, endosteal and periosteal. The medullary canal is irregularly narrowed. Sharp demarcation of the process at the distal diaphyses is evident and the metaphyses and epiphyses are spared. Elongation of involved bones is common. (Courtesy of Dr. E. B. D. Neuhauser, Children's Hospital Medical Center, Boston.)

Nutrition is often poor. Severe dental caries is frequently reported. In about a quarter of the reported cases the skin appeared thick and dry and the hair scant. In several of the cases the genitalia failed to develop properly. Eventually there is apt to be thoracic kyphosis, lumbar lordosis, valgus deformities of the knees and ankles, anterior bowing of the tibiae and flat feet (Fig. 6–80).

Only a few descriptions of involved tissue are available. Apparently the new bone is laid down by the periosteum and soon becomes incorporated into the cortex. The bone tissue has a normal microscopic appearance. A complete autopsy description has been reported by Cohen and States.[76]

The pathogenesis of this curious disease is unknown though in material which we have been fortunate enough to examine microscopically we noted a dearth of haversian canals and thus a subnormal number of vessels. We have noted that when oxygen tension is reduced below the optimum there is excessive osteoid production. This observation may have some bearing on the pathogenesis of this disease.

In some cases involvement of the musculature is lacking, and these cases may be exceedingly difficult to differentiate from the childhood form of Caffey's cortical hyperostosis. As one reviews the literature on this dysplasia, one gets the impression that he is dealing with a syndrome of variable manifestations. We have had the opportunity of studying three cases and except for the fusiform enlargement of the diaphyses of cylindrical bones one would scarcely suspect that they are all the same dysplasia.

Melorheostosis

This is a rare condition in which there are curious linear longitudinal thickenings of the shafts of long bones. These irregular streaks of thick bone protrude both internally into the medullary tissues and externally beneath the periosteum. Since they appear to start proximally and progress distally along the entire length of the shaft and epiphysis, involving the

the years, bone after bone becomes involved, the short cylindrical as well as the long and the flat bones of the trunk, skull and face. The cylindrical bones become fusiform. Multiple areas of gross thickening appear in many of the flat bones. The head becomes enlarged, and there is prominent frontal bossing. Neurologic symptoms develop because of impingement upon nerve foramina, proptosis or enophthalmia or optic atrophy or deafness. Later there may be nystagmus and headaches. In typical cases there is improper development of the skeletal musculature. Muscles are small, flabby and weak.

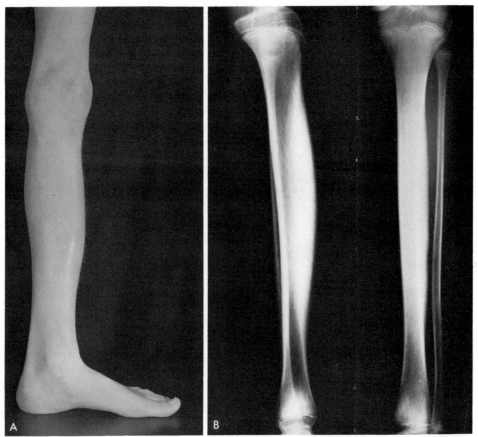

Figure 6-79 Diaphyseal sclerosis. The circumference of the leg is small (*A*). There is cortical thickening in the diaphysis; the metaphyses and epiphyses are not affected. (Courtesy of Drs. Outland and Gross, Pennsylvania State Hospital for Crippled Children, Elizabethtown.)

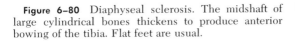

Figure 6-80 Diaphyseal sclerosis. The midshaft of large cylindrical bones thickens to produce anterior bowing of the tibia. Flat feet are usual.

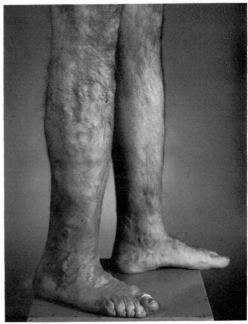

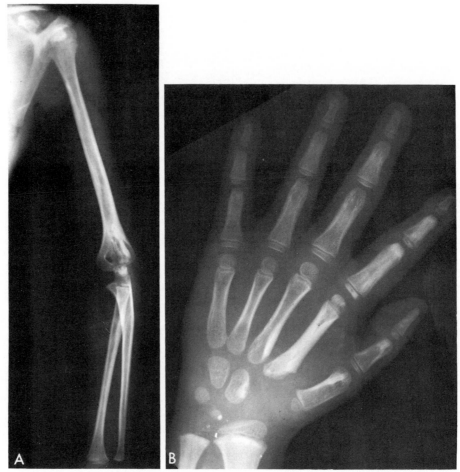

Figure 6–81 Melorheostosis. Cortical thickening is evident in the humerus and radius (*A*). The wavy, dense cortex encroaches on the medullary canal and is most marked in the distal diaphysis of the radius. *B* is a radiograph of the hand and wrist on the same side as *A*. Phalangeal, carpal and metacarpal involvement is present as well as involvement of secondary epiphyseal centers (proximal humerus, capitellum and proximal phalanx of the second digit).

bones of an extremity consecutively, the roentgenograms have the characteristic appearance of a molten substance flowing down one side of the bones of a member. It has been repeatedly likened to melted wax flowing down the side of a lighted candle.

Leri and Joanny were the first to describe this condition in 1922. They suggested the name "melorheostosis," which means flowing member. Since that time less than 50 cases have been reported.

The disease has usually been diagnosed in patients between the ages of 5 and 20 years, but in several instances there has been evidence of onset in infancy. It appears, therefore, that the malformation is congenital in origin. No hereditary features have been reported.

The presenting symptom of melorheostosis is most often pain,[77] which may be severe but difficult of localization because an entire bone or several bones may be involved. More than three quarters of the reported cases have been monomelic, involving the bones of but a single extremity. Usually the side of the pelvis or shoulder girdle corresponding to the involved member is affected. Involvement of one side of the mandible and maxilla has been reported. If the condition is marked and begins early, the epiphysis may close prematurely, causing shortening of the extremity. The hyperostosis may extend in the soft tissues across the joint to cause interference with motion and even ankylosis. The outward protrusion may press upon nerves to cause sensory disturbance or upon the vasculature of the part with consequent edema. At least two cases have been reported in which a thickening and induration of the skin over the bony lesion has resulted in a diagnosis of scleroderma.[78] The correct diagnosis is usually made on the appearance of the roentgenograms.

Microscopy. Complete studies of the skeleton in melorheostosis have not been reported. Only a few biopsy descriptions are available. The substance of the bone is apparently normal, but the mass in the regions involved is increased. There appears to be a condensation of bone at the expense of the haversian and interspicular spaces.

The nature of the physiologic disturbance that accounts for the excessive production of bone in this peculiar pattern is entirely unknown. Numerous theories have been offered, but none of them seems sufficiently plausible to be worthy of listing.

Prognosis. The malformations may advance throughout the years of skeletal growth and cease progression at the age of maturation of the bone involved. Since the bony lesions, once developed, do not regress, the patient must be resigned to his malformations unless they can be altered by surgery. Pain from the lesion itself is troublesome only during the developmental stage.

Osteopathia Striata (Voorhoeve)

Voorhoeve described this condition as a distinct radiologic entity in 1924. The abnormality is characterized by multiple condensations of cancellous bone tissue, which begin at the epiphyseal line and extend into the diaphysis. In the ilium, the striae form a sunburst about the acetabulum and fan out toward the iliac crest (Fig. 6–82). Any or all of the long bones may be involved, and the end of greatest growth is said to be more obviously involved. The condition differs from osteopetrosis, melorheostosis, progressive diaphyseal dysplasia (Engelmann) and

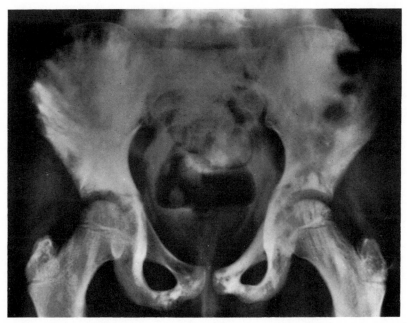

Figure 6–82 Osteopathia striata. Condensation of cancellous bone is manifest by opaque streaks in the ilia (particularly the right ilium) and in the proximal femurs. (Courtesy of Dr. E. B. D. Neuhauser, Children's Hospital Medical Center, Boston.)

hereditary multiple diaphyseal sclerosis (Ribbing) in that only cancellous bone is affected. However, the condition has been described in association with osteopetrosis in other bones[79] and in one instance in the same bone. The lesions are without symptoms and are discovered only on radiologic examination. At least one case showed accompanying punctate opacities in the epiphysis and another an elevated serum alkaline phosphatase.

Osteopoikilosis (Osteopathia Condensans Disseminata)

Spotted bones were described by Stiede in 1905. Since that time more than 100 cases have been reported. Since the condition is without symptoms these cases have been discovered by roentgenologic examination for coincidental disease. The abnormality is characterized by numerous spheroid or lenticular nodules of condensed bone occurring in the spongiosa of the metaphysis or epiphyseal osseous nucleus. Schmorl published a description of the microscopic appearance in 1931. These well-delineated opacites have been described in almost every bone, but they are most commonly encountered in the small bones of the hands and feet,[80] at the ends of the large bones of the extremities or in the pelvic bones about the acetabulum. They are rarely found in the skull.

The condition is apparently congenital because it has been diagnosed in a fetus and also in a newborn. It is familial and hereditary. One report describes the lesions in eight siblings.

It may be accompanied by hereditary, multiple exostoses, by a tendency to form keloids, and more than one case have been associated with dermatofibrosis lenticularis disseminata.[81]

Microscopy. Several biopsy and a few autopsy studies have been done. The nodules are found within the cancellous tissue, sometimes with a peripheral attachment to the inner surface of the cortex. They are not cortical ingrowths. They may be round, lens shaped or elongated, and composed of lamellated bone. They merge with the surrounding spongiosa; i.e., the spicules of cancellous tissue ap-

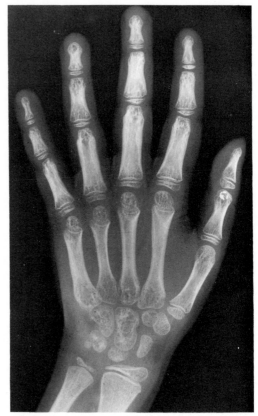

Figure 6–83 Osteopoikilosis. Spheroid opacities are evident in the carpal ossification centers as well as in the epiphyseal centers of the metacarpals. (Courtesy of Dr. E. B. D. Neuhauser, Children's Hospital Medical Center, Boston.)

pear to blend into their substance but their mass has a greater density so that they can be dissected quite easily. Sections show them to have haversian spaces in about the same proportion as dense, cortical bone.

Prognosis. Osteopoikilotic nodules may be present at birth or they may appear and increase in number during the growing period. In some cases they have been periodically checked over a period of years and they are said to grow larger or diminish in size and may even fade away completely. Thus, it appears that they obey the laws of normal bone growth and maintenance. Perhaps their appearance is related to occult alterations in stress lines. One of the many cases in our collection eventually developed typical osteosarcoma which ran the usual course to pulmonary metastasis and death. This complication must be exceedingly rare since we are unable to find a report of a like occurrence.

BONE DYSPLASIAS RELATED TO ABNORMAL OSTEOID PRODUCTION

Fibrous Dysplasia

Fibrous dysplasia of bone is a disturbance in postnatal cancellous bone maintenance. Normal bone undergoing physiologic lysis is replaced by an abnormal proliferation of fibrous tissue. The process is therefore slow, frequently requiring years to cause cortical weakening and to produce clinical lesions. The proliferation of fibrous tissue and abnormal osteoid may eventually extend beyond normal boundaries, thus causing cortical "expansion." Since the inability to produce normal bone involves only the cancellous tissues and never cambium bone formation, the lesions may replace normal cortex, which is eroded from within, but they are always covered with a shell, however thin, of adult compacta.

This condition was first recognized as an entity probably no earlier than 1922 when Weil (quoted from Schlumberger[82]) first reported it in the German literature. Since fibrous dysplasia is a fairly common disease, one wonders how cases were classified prior to this date. Solitary lesions were almost certainly confused with unicameral cyst, ossifying fibroma, non-osteogenic fibroma and subperiosteal cortical defect. At least some cases of multicentric but unilateral involvement were, from our personal knowledge, diagnosed as Ollier's enchondromatosis. Cases with extensive skeletal lesions were categorized as hyperparathyroidism (osteitis fibrosa cystica), neurofibromatosis and, in the older age group, Paget's disease.

Freund and Moffert[83] reviewed the condition in 1936 under the title "fibrous osteodystrophy," and in the following year McCune and Bruch[84] recognized the entity and used the term "osteodystrophia fibrosa." In 1937, Albright and co-workers[85] reported five cases of bone involvement with disturbance of endocrine function and pigmented patches in the skin using the name "osteitis fibrosa disseminata." They noted its similarities to parathyroid adenoma (osteitis fibrosa cystica) and neurofibromatosis but considered it a separate entity. Since this paper the condition has frequently been referred to as "Albright's syndrome." It should be remembered, however, that these writers were concerned as much with the endocrine disturbance as with the bone lesions and, therefore, this eponym should not be used in considering most of the cases, i.e., those with bone involvement only.

In 1938, Lichtenstein[86] reported eight cases with detailed studies of the lesions in bone. He proposed the name "fibrous dysplasia" or "polyostotic fibrous dysplasia" when multiple bones were involved. Since then this has been the name of preference. Lichtenstein and Jaffe[87] added 15 more cases in 1942, and a considerable number have been reported since. Schlumberger[82] was able to collect 67 cases of monostotic fibrous dysplasia from his survey of the army material. He expressed the opinion that ossifying fibroma and non-osteogenic fibroma were variants of this condition. Thannhauser[88] thought that it was a skeletal manifestation of neurofibromatosis.

Sufficient material has been collected to show undeniably that fibrous dysplasia is an entity, though it resembles neurofibromatosis because both are germ plasm defects involving fibroblastic proliferation and maturation and there is some, though not great, overlap in incidence. The microscopy of typical lesions of ossifying fibroma (benign osteoblastoma) and non-osteogenic fibroma appears to be sufficiently unique to separate them from fibrous dysplasia, but in atypical sections the distinction may be difficult or impossible.

Fibrous dysplasia may appear as a solitary lesion or there may be more than one lesion in a single bone. Sometimes several bones of a single extremity may be involved (monomelic) or only the bones of one side may be affected. In severe cases the lesions may be scattered throughout the skeleton.

When one divides the cases into minimal, moderate and severe, the complications of involvement of extraskeletal systems are found to fall into a pattern. Solitary lesions are rarely accompanied by endocrine disturbance, skin patches or irregularities of skeletal growth (monomelic hypertrophy), whereas severe cases usually show one or more of these complications.

Clinical evidence of the bone lesions usually becomes manifest in late childhood though a few severe cases have shown evidence of beginning in infancy. It is not uncommon to discover solitary lesions in the third decade and at times even much later, but the bulk of evidence suggests that most if not all areas of involvement begin during the growing period. All types of bones are affected though there is some slight predilection for the large bones of the extremities. Though any part of the latter may be the site of origin, fibrous dysplasia is apt to begin in the metaphysis and progress toward the mid-diaphysis. It appears to be an inability to maintain cancellous tissue but as the mass of fibrous tissue proliferates, it "erodes" the cortex from within. As mature bone undergoes physiologic lysis it is replaced by solid masses of proliferating collagenoblastic cells. The process suggests an inability to maintain bone in certain focal areas, but it must be admitted that as it progresses it may extend beyond the normal cortical limitations. The original mass usually extends peripherally in projecting lobulations so that the affected area is scalloped and highly irregular in outline. The cortex is "eroded" from within while the periosteum attempts to compensate by laying down a thin shell of normal bone on the outer surface. Cylindrical bones become "expanded" and large elevations appear on the surface of flat bones.

The cortex may be so weakened that pathologic fracture occurs, and this may be the presenting symptom of the disease. The second most common complaint is the deformity that occurs, particularly when bones of the head are involved. These may involve the orbit, to cause exophthalmos, the maxilla or the mandible (Fig. 6–84). Pain is usually not an out-

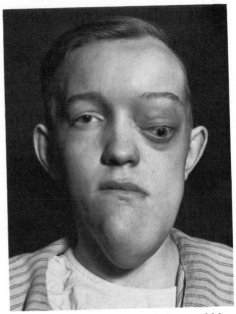

Figure 6–84 Fibrous dysplasia. The mandible and bones of the orbit are common sites of involvement.

standing feature until infractions and deformity make weight-bearing difficult.

When the area is approached surgically it is seen that normal bone has been replaced by irregular masses of pale tissue streaked with brown and red where there has been hemorrhage (Fig. 6–85). This material is usually gritty and has been likened to putty containing granules of sand. On slight magnification the particles are seen to be irregular, spicular masses of bone lying in the fibrous matrix. Small masses of cartilage are often found, and though these never constitute the predominant element of the entire lesion they may be large enough to confuse the issue in biopsy diagnosis. Small irregular regions of fluid have been reported. These are areas of cystic degeneration rather than true cysts, and they are never a prominent part of the picture. The "cysts" reported in roentgenograms are areas of relative translucency resulting from the replacement of bone by fibrous tissue. The only true cysts of bone are found in "solitary cyst" though the cystic degeneration of parathyroid adenoma (osteitis fibrosa cystica) may be difficult to differentiate.

The pigmented, non-elevated skin patches occur in perhaps a third of the

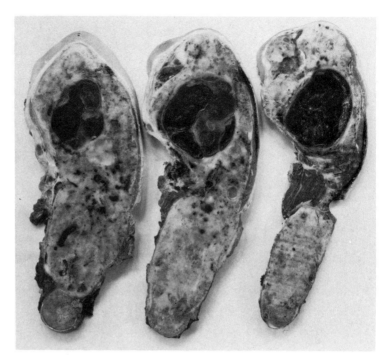

Figure 6–85 Fibrous dysplasia. It became necessary to remove the left arm because of multiple arteriovenous fistulas. Multiple anomalies are seen in many cases of fibrous dysplasia. In the lower portion of the specimen one finds the gritty, gray material that characterizes the condition.

cases of fibrous dysplasia, usually the more extensive. They usually occur on the trunk, have a geographic outline and vary from a few millimeters in diameter to the size of one's palm or larger. They have a café-au-lait or chestnut color. The epidermis and underlying corium are normal in texture and consistency.

Endocrine dysfunction is almost restricted to females though a few cases of hyperthyroidism have been seen in males. Again, the bone involvement is usually severe. The usual complaint is precocious menstruation, which occurs in less than one fifth of the cases. The menarche appears early (it has been reported at 3 years) and the menses are usually irregular in amount and periodicity with a tendency to become regular at the normal age of puberty. Hyperthyroidism is also seen in patients with fibrous dysplasia in a higher incidence than in the normal population. Precocious skeletal growth has been reported in a few cases. There may be abnormally rapid growth during childhood, but premature closure of the epiphyseal centers is apt to occur so that ultimate growth may fall short of average stature.

The precocious menstruation, which is presumably on the basis of premature ovarian stimulation, the hyperthyroidism and the early rapid growth and epiphyseal ossification all suggest the possibility that these disturbances may be the polyglandular effects of a dysfunctioning pituitary. Support is given this hypothesis by the fact that the base of the skull is frequently involved in fibrous dysplasia, and this involvement may affect the pituitary space or the floor of the third ventricle above it. There has been insufficient investigation either to prove or to disprove this theory. Against it is the occasional accompaniment of anomalies in other systems that could hardly be of endocrine origin. Such are reported in rather wide variation.[89]

Roentgenographic Manifestations. The lesions of fibrous dysplasia may be radiolucent or somewhat opaque depending on the amount of irregular, microscopic masses of bone that exist within the fibrous matrix. The individual lesion may not be always sharply outlined. In the advanced lesion the involved areas are lobular and scalloped in outline and the margins tend to be sharply defined. The lesions that erode and expand the cortex are nevertheless covered by a layer of bone because periosteal bone formation is normal.

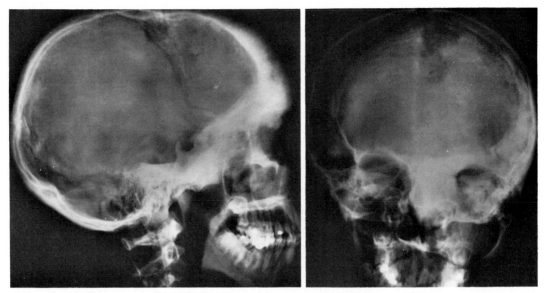

Figure 6–86 Fibrous dysplasia. The bones at the base of the skull are opaque and markedly thickened. The paranasal sinuses, except for the right maxillary sinus, are obliterated and the left orbit is distorted. The patient is 17 years of age.

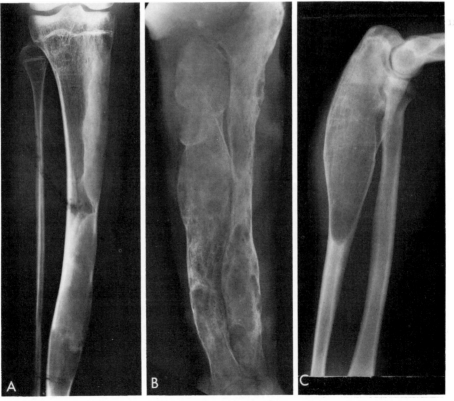

Figure 6–87 Fibrous dysplasia. Representative lesions are illustrated (A and C). The semiopacity of the lesions is evident as well as widening of the diaphysis and thinning of the cortices. Marked involvement with distortion of bone architecture is apparent in (B), the radiograph of a forearm of a young adult.

Abundant periosteal new bone is seen when pathologic fracture occurs through a lesion although cortical thickening, perhaps containing lucent lesions, may be a manifestation of the disease. The lesions are most frequently located in the proximal bones and decrease in severity and extent distally. In view of the fact that intra-osseous arteriovenous malformations are known to exist, some of the lucent defects may be related to this abnormality.

Deformity of the long bones in the form of bending and, in the severe disease, telescoping is common because of the fibrous nature of the lesion.

The manifestations of the disease as it involves the bones of the cranial vault are similar to those elsewhere. However, when the base of the frontal bone, the sphenoid, ethmoid and maxillary bones are involved, the results differ. Here there is marked thickening and opacity of the bones with obliteration of the paranasal sinuses and a decrease in the capacity of the orbits.

Microscopy. Sections taken at random through a lesion of fibrous dysplasia should show a matrix of collagenous tissue in which are embedded sparsely scattered spicules of bone. The character of both the matrix and bone is important in reaching a decision on the basis of microscopy, and the appearance depends greatly upon the age of the lesion. In the mature process the matrix is usually quite dense, the cells (collageno-blasts) are well-spindled and the nuclei are elongated and densely chromatic. There are considerable amounts of intercellular collagen. The cellular pattern is that of organized fibrous connective tissue seen elsewhere in the body. There is a paucity of vessels though the tissue cannot be described as being avascular (Fig. 6–88). Small aggregates of hemosiderin are common though hemorrhage is never a very important feature. In the vicinity of extravasated blood or old blood pigment there may be collections of giant cells. Usually these are sparse and they may be hard to find though at times these collections are large enough to suggest giant cell tumor or brown tumor of parathyroid adenoma. These cells are usually moderate in size and contain from three to twenty nuclei, usually grouped in the central portion of the cell. The giant cells appear to be formed by a merging of the individual matrix cells. Here and there one may find a few pale xanthoid cells, their cytoplasm filled with lipid granules. Typical osteoclasts are found but are never very abundant.

The bone may appear quite normal in the older lesions, but usually it is of the primitive type, coarse-fibered and contains numerous large lacunae with young cells. Mineralization is apt to be uneven. Sometimes the edges of the spicule are quite rough. Many of the spicules show their convex surfaces to be covered with a layer of cells, which are indistinguishable from normal osteoblasts (Fig. 6–89). Frequently a seam of pink-staining osteoid separates them from the mineralized portion of the spicule. Usually there is a highly characteristic pattern to the multiple components of the lesion. These elements vaguely take the form of a spheroid mass with the vessel in the center. A thick zone of collagen-forming spindled cells surrounds the vessel; their long axes are parallel to the circumference. About this zone are curving slender spicules of osteoid forming arcs of irregular length, each a segment of the circumference. These "units" crowd each other to form the lesion.

In younger lesions the matrix is composed of more loosely arranged collageno-blasts. The cells are less spindled, their nuclei are larger and younger and there is less collagen. In these sections fibro-osseous metaplasia is usually prominent. At times the spicules appear to be no more than fibrous condensations with obvious transition of their cells into those of the surrounding matrix (Fig. 6–90). Fibro-osseous metaplasia is probably an important feature of the process, but it quite certainly is not pathognomonic when present nor does its absence rule out the diagnosis. Actually, fibro-osseous metaplasia may be a difficult thing to recognize, and one might reasonably ask the question "Just what is fibro-osseous metaplasia?"[90]

We know that in normal osteogenesis cells emerge from the undifferentiated "fibrous" mass, line up about bars of calcified chondroid and engage in the laying down of an osteoid seam. It is only

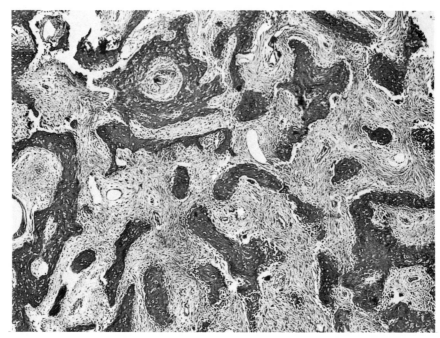

Figure 6–88 Fibrous dysplasia. A section to illustrate the spicules of fiberbone interspersed in a field of fairly mature collagenous tissue. This lesion is well established and probably no longer progressive. (× 40.)

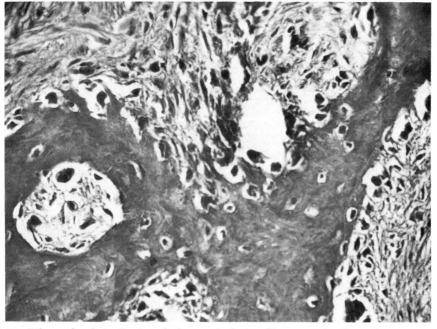

Figure 6–89 Fibrous dysplasia. Section of a bone spicule in a fibrous matrix. Along the upper margin there appears to be osteoblastic osteogenesis. (× 375.)

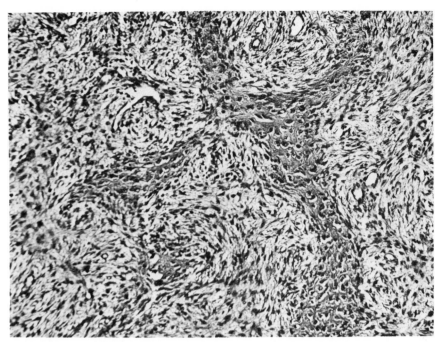

Figure 6–90 Fibrous dysplasia. A section through an immature lesion. Fibro-osseous metaplasia is quite obvious. The bone spicule is vaguely seen in a field of young collagenous tissue. (× 180.)

when the seam emerges that we recognize them as osteoblasts. Before then they cannot be distinguished by any staining method yet devised, from collagenoblasts or, for that matter, from primitive chondroblasts. It is the intercellular product that makes the distinction between these three types of cells. We speak of the periosteum as fibrous, yet physiologically there is osteoblastic metaplasia and the production of normal cortical bone. It is confusing to insist that the metaplasia in fibrous dysplasia is abnormal though admittedly the metaplastic transition is quite obvious. Actually, it is the character of the bone product and its relation to the matrix that are abnormal in fibrous dysplasia.

The islands of cartilage (Fig. 6–91) that are found in this condition have the same microscopic appearance as the cartilage of enchondromatosis, and it is probable that they arise in the same manner, by a failure of normal differentiation of the cells of the primitive cell mass. One might hypothesize that the dysfunction in fibrous metaplasia is only one step further along the normal maturation path than that of enchondromatosis.

McIntosh et al.[91] investigated the circulatory dynamics of six cases of fibrous dysplasia and found that the lesions of this condition contain functioning arteriovenous fistulas that are capable of increasing regional blood flow and occasionally cardiac output. It is as yet undetermined whether all lesions of fibrous dysplasia contain these vascular abnormalities or that they are the cause of the structural changes. Similar vascular alterations have been described in Paget's disease and we have encountered one patient with an advanced case of fibrous dysplasia who developed multiple, large arteriovenous fistulas. These communications caused increased cardiac output and cardiomegaly. Amputation of the extremity bearing the lesions halted the progress of cardiac deterioration.

Prognosis. If the lesions of fibrous dysplasia begin in early childhood, are multiple and progress throughout adolescence, skeletal deformity is apt to be advanced and crippling may be severe. If the lesion is solitary and first noted during adolescence, the patient may escape with scarcely a scar. One may expect the progress of the disease to slow or become

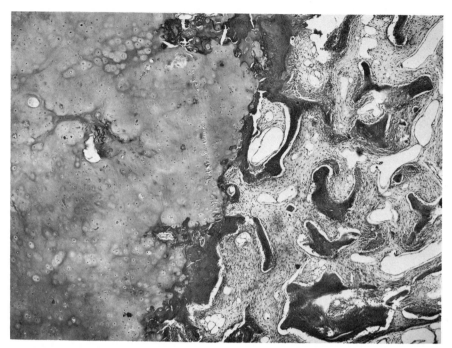

Figure 6–91   Fibrous dysplasia. The section reveals a portion of an island of cartilage on the left and fibrous dysplasia on the right. (× 35.)

completely arrested at the time of skeletal maturation. It is difficult to explain the lesions that make themselves known during adult life. They probably began and developed during the growth period of childhood and adolescence and remained symptomless until circumstances of later life called attention to them. None of these is apt to produce serious skeletal damage, and it is possible that they have not become reactivated but that circumstances of aging such as osteoporosis or changes in stress trajectories point up a lesion that otherwise might have been carried unknown throughout life.

It has been stated that some fibrous dysplasias eventually undergo change to fibrosarcoma. We believe that this is a very unusual event but we have two such cases in our collection.

Neurofibromatosis

Neurofibromatosis or von Recklinghausen's disease is a hereditary, often congenital and sometimes familial disturbance in the supportive tissue of the nervous system, both central and peripher-

al. It usually involves the skin, it may involve the skeleton, and disturbances in other systems such as the endocrine and gastrointestinal tract have been reported.

Ewing states that Kölliker was the first to describe the condition in 1860. In 1882, von Recklinghausen associated the lesions with the nervous system and the disease has since borne his name, though this sometimes leads to confusion because the same eponym is applied to parathyroid adenoma. Verocay (1910) suggested that the masses of proliferating cells arose from the Schwann syncytium rather than the fibrocytes of the nerve sheath. The work of Masson (1926) supported this contention because the nevus cells of the skin are also involved and both as well as the glial supportive cells are derived from the neuroectoderm. Stout and Murray have long contended that the neurilemmoma (sometimes spelled neurilemoma), a solitary, benign, encapsulated hamartoma of nerves, occasionally encountered in neurofibromatosis, is schwannian in origin. They base their opinion on the morphology of cells grown in tissue culture. One might question the validity of such dogmatism and ask how the cells originally selected to establish the criteria were indubitably known to come from the Schwann sheath, because morphology becomes even less trustworthy than usual when the cell environment is changed as radically as is necessary for culture work. However, the matter is highly academic and hardly worth the polemics it has provoked.

Neurofibromatosis, as the name implies, involves principally the nervous system. Masses of spindled cells arise from either the Schwann or fibrous supportive cells or both, along the course of peripheral nerves, in branches of the autonomic nervous system and in the meninges. These masses are pale and moderately firm. They may involve a short segment of a peripheral nerve or extend along the greater portion of the full length, sometimes continuing proximally to involve the substance of the cord. They greatly increase the diameter of the nerve trunk and often cause a tortuosity of its course — plexiform neurofibroma. Pain is not usual but at times it results from pressure on the contiguous nerve fibers. Accompanying meningiomas are not unusual. In a small percentage, glial "tumors" occur within the brain, often involving the floor of the third ventricle.[92] It is debatable whether these proliferations of the supportive cells of neurons are truly neoplastic or simply the product of an unrestrained, hamartomatous growth. The nerve enlargements, often called "neurofibromas," may occur along the cranial or spinal nerve roots (acoustic neuromas and spinal neurofibromas) and here cause bone changes by erosion. The endocrine disturbances that have been reported may result from pressure upon the hypophysis by enlargement at the chiasm.

The skin is almost always affected, not only by the neurofibromas, and less often neurilemmomas, but also because its supportive tissue, its nevus cells and appendages are involved.

Proliferations of melanoblasts may be limited to geographic brown patches within the skin, café-au-lait spots measuring from a few millimeters to several centimeters in diameter, or true benign dermal and compound nevi and even malignant melanomas may develop. The café-au-lait spots or chestnut patches are the commonest skin manifestation of neurofibromatosis. They are also seen sometimes in pseudarthrosis and fibrous dysplasia.

At the dermal nerve endings there are apt to occur poorly delineated proliferations of spindled cells within the corium, that elevate the epidermal surface. Sometimes the epidermal melanin is heavier in these areas, and they may support a thick growth of hair. Some of these elevations may become pedunculated. They may occur singly, in patches or literally cover the skin by the hundreds. These lesions are sometimes called fibroma molluscum (Fig. 6–92). Large areas of skin may become diffusely thickened and redundant so that it hangs in coarse, heavy folds, a condition called elephantiasis. Occasionally there are patches of hypertrophied sebaceous glands (Pringle) and there may be lipomas.

Lesions in the skeleton include bone erosion by the neurofibromas, scolioses, pseudarthrosis, abnormalities in size and areas of demineralization that have been called cysts on the basis of roentgenographic examination (Fig. 6–98 A). The cause and the nature of the scolioses are unrecorded. The vertebrae are often found to be wedged. In pseudarthrosis a segment of diaphysis is known to undergo softening by deossification and replacement by masses of spindled cells similar to those found in the skin. It is probable that the vertebral lesion is analogous to pseudarthrosis in the extremities. The curvatures occur most commonly in the lumbar areas, the angulation is often sharp and as the lesion progresses paraplegia may occur.

Though pseudarthrosis is a relatively common complication it occurs apart from neurofibromatosis and so will be treated in a separate section (p. 184).

Skeletal enlargement or focal giantism is perhaps the most bizarre and fascinating aspect of von Recklinghausen's disease. The hypertrophy may involve a single bone, the bones of a part such as a single digit or those of the entire extremity (Fig. 6–93 and 6–98 B). The bones are usually normal in shape. The associated muscles and joints are proportion-

(Text continued on page 181.)

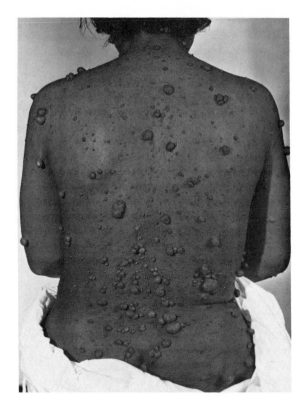

Figure 6–92 Back of a patient showing examples of fibroma molluscum.

Figure 6–93 Focal giantism of neurofibromatosis. *A* shows enlargement of the entire right lower extremity; *B*, enlargement of the right foot.

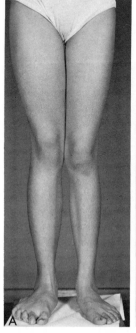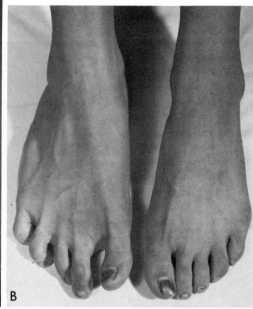

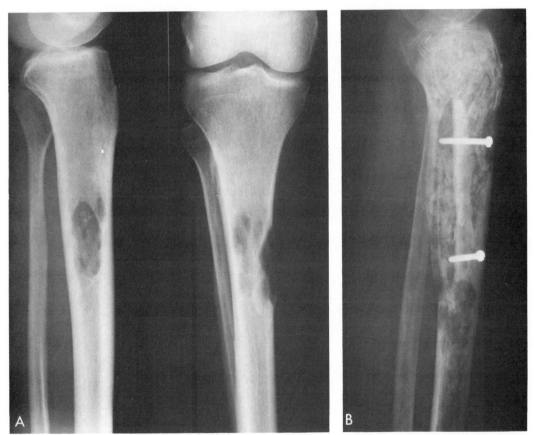

Figure 6-94   Neurofibroma in bone. *A*, Localized area in the proximal tibia. *B*, Postoperative radiograph two and one-half years later showing extension of the lesion.

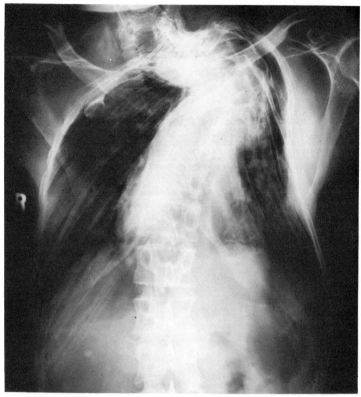

Figure 6–95 Neurofibromatosis. Severe scoliosis with extensive deformity of vertebral bodies is evident in the dorsal spine.

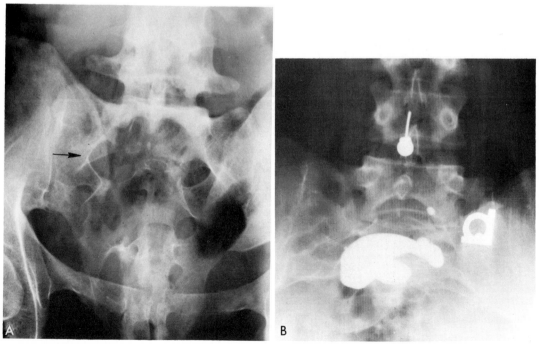

Figure 6–96 Neurofibromatosis. An anterior meningocele is present in the sacrum (A); this fills with opaque material during myelography (B).

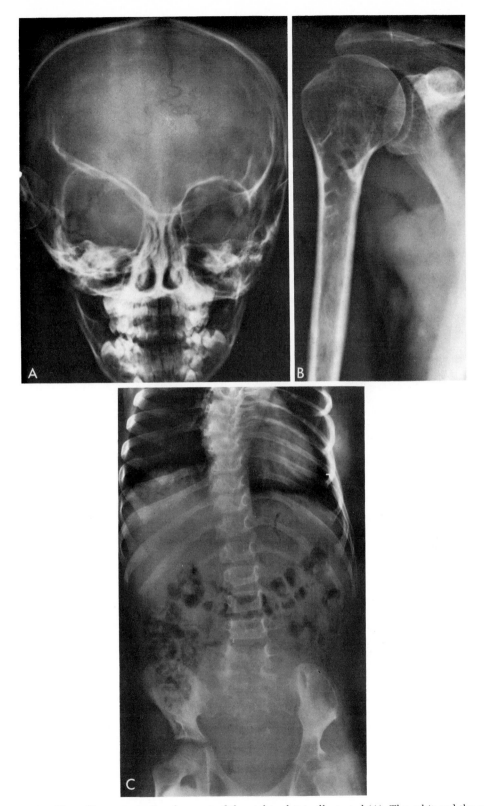

Figure 6–97 Neurofibromatosis. Involvement of the right orbit is illustrated (A). The orbit and the orbital fissure are enlarged; exophthalmos was present. Small, radiolucent cyst-like areas with opaque margins are evident in B, the radiograph of the humerus. In C, a large soft tissue mass fills the pelvis (neurofibroma). Scoliosis and deformity of the pelvis and left femur are present.

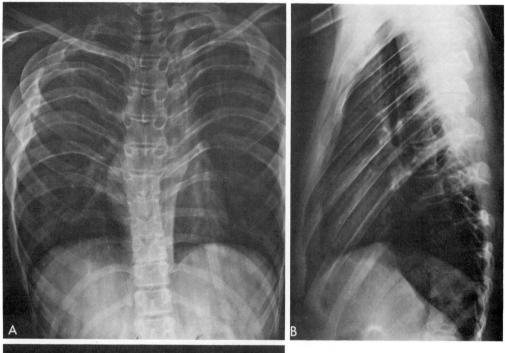

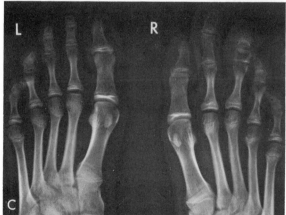

Figure 6–98   Neurofibromatosis. Scoliosis, thoracic lordosis, wedging of the lower thoracic vertebra and rib notching and deformity are evident in *A* and *B*. Enlargement of the second and third digits of the right foot is evident in *C*.

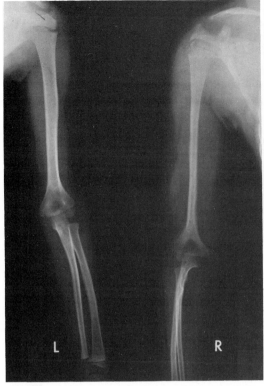

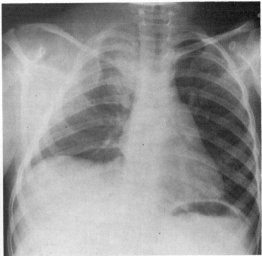

Figure 6–99 Neurofibromatosis. A plexiform neuroma involves the right supraclavicular area, the shoulder and the right upper extremity. A soft tissue mass is evident in the mediastinum on the right. The clavicle is eroded and thin, and the bones of the arm are small in caliber with irregular thickening of soft tissue around the humerus.

ately enlarged. The involved part is usually in the distribution or segment of an affected nerve. At times a well-delineated neurofibroma occurs within the bone during childhood. It causes a focal area of radiolucency. It may progress slowly to destroy a large segment of the host bone (Fig. 6–94).

It would appear in surveying the many facets of this kaleidoscopic disease that the fault lies deeply buried within the germ plasm of one or more germ layers. The neuroectoderm is almost certainly involved judging from the incidence of lesions in the entire nervous system and also its related neuroepithelially derived supportive tissue, melanoblasts and related skin. It has been suggested that the disturbance in the nerve impulse conduction channels results in altered nutritional supplies and growth potentials.[93] Though at present this is nothing more than an unsubstantiated hypothesis, the distribution and character of the extraneural lesion lends some credence to it.

Microscopy. Sections made through an area of bone softening reveal poorly delineated masses of spindled cells resembling rather mature collagenoblasts (Fig. 6–102 *B*). In some areas there is a tendency for trabeculation and palisading, but the major portion of the mass shows no attempt at organization. Considerable amounts of collagen are readily demonstrable with special stains. In some areas there is a rather abortive attempt at fibro-osseous and fibrocartilaginous metaplasia. These sections suggest an inability to maintain and replace normal bone. Instead, fibrous connective tissue is produced and overproduced with some attempt· at bone and cartilage metaplasia. Sections of this tissue in the typical bone lesions of neurofibromatosis cannot be differentiated from those of pseudarthrosis and one may encounter similar sections taken from lesions of fibrous dysplasia which have undergone fracture.

The lesions of the nervous system show a variety of pictures (Fig. 6–100). The neurofibromas are made up of masses of spindle cells, which with ordinary staining methods look much like those of the bone lesions. The occasional neurilem-

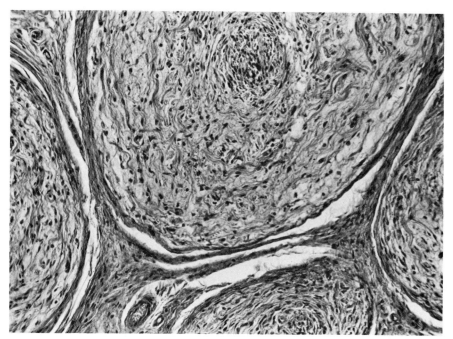

Figure 6–100 Neurofibromatosis. Section through a peripheral nerve showing immense thickening due to proliferation of collagenoblasts of the supportive tissue.

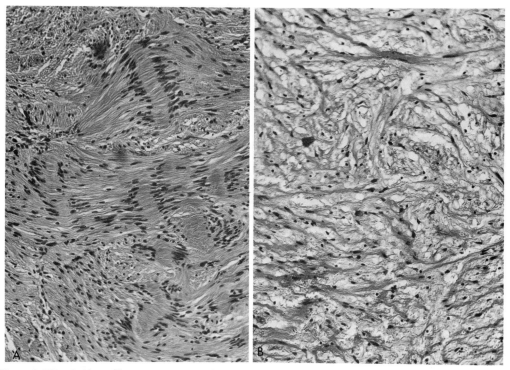

Figure 6–101 *A,* Neurofibromatosis. A neurilemmoma showing the characteristic palisading of cells to form Verocay bodies. This is the Antoni Type A. (× 180.) *B,* A neurilemmoma illustrating the myxomatous character of the Antoni Type B lesion. (× 180.)

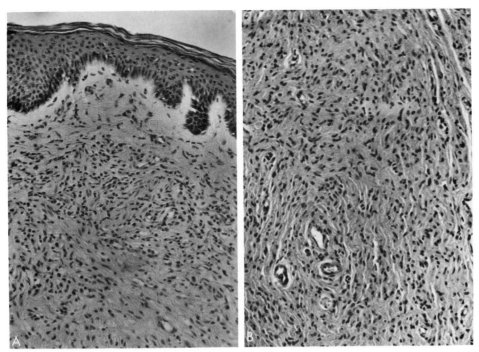

Figure 6–102 *A*, Neurofibromatosis. Section through a fibroma molluscum covered with epiderm. (× 130.) *B*, Section from a lesion in bone. The same collagenoblastic proliferation is seen here as found in the soft tissue lesion. (× 130.)

moma may contain Verocay bodies, aggregates of palisaded nuclei and when this pattern predominates they are classified as Antoni Type A (Fig. 6–101 *A*). When whorls, trabeculation and Verocay bodies are lacking and the tissue appears myxomatous with areas of cystic degeneration, the lesion is said to be of the Antoni Type B (Fig. 6–101 *B*). A variety of gliomas, benign and malignant, have been described in the central nervous system.

The fibroma molluscum in the skin consists of masses of spindled cells, that might be either schwannian or fibrous in origin (Fig. 6–102 *A*). They are smaller and more firmly woven than the components of the usual skin fibroma.

Prognosis.   Neurofibromatosis (von Recklinghausen) may be of any degree of severity. There may be only a few neurofibromas or café-au-lait spots or the process may involve almost every system with hideous skeletal deformity, fantastic skin lesions and death with a glial tumor of the brain. There is a tendency for the progress of the disease to slow and sometimes to stop at about the time of cessation of normal growth. The condition may then

remain latent for the remainder of a normal life span or it may be reactivated at any time and go on to death. Perhaps 10 per cent of the neurofibromas undergo a change to frankly malignant neoplasms. The rate of growth increases, they become more invasive and metastasize by way of the blood. It has been suggested that repeated biopsying of these lesions in the various clinics that these patients eventually enter, seeking help, predisposes to malignant change. Since biopsy is not usually necessary for diagnosis, and assists in no way in therapy, it should not be done for teaching purposes or to illustrate papers written by the clinician.

There is a curious congenital anomalous condition that is usually manifested by the triad of tuberous sclerosis, adenoma sebaceum and epilepsy. It is frequently associated with other anomalies, including rhabdomyomas of the heart, cystic disease of the kidneys and retina, and large collagenous tumor-like masses of the subcutaneous tissues, particularly of the hands, feet and gums. The last may be edentulous. Smaller discrete nodules in the corium of the skin are called shagreen plaques and are said to be pathognomic of this complex condition. The presence of café-au-lait patches in the skin and dramatic osseous growth deformities have caused this condition to be confused with neurofibromatosis. It should be considered a distinct entity because tuberous sclerosis is usually the outstanding feature and the one that leads to a fatal termination.

Congenital generalized fibromatosis [94, 95] is another disease which should probably be differentiated from neurofibromatosis. It is a disorder of fibroelastic derivation with multiple, widespread, infiltrating lesions that may involve any organ or system. It is a disease of children.

Lytic areas appear in cancellous and cortical bone and must be differentiated from the histiocytoses, particularly Letterer-Siwe disease.

Pseudarthrosis

Pseudarthrosis is a pathologic entity characterized by deossification of a weight-bearing long bone, bending, pathologic fracture and inability to form normal callus in healing. Approximately half the cases reveal at least some evidence of an accompanying neurofibromatosis of which café-au-lait spots are the most common. The condition is hereditary, congenital and familial.

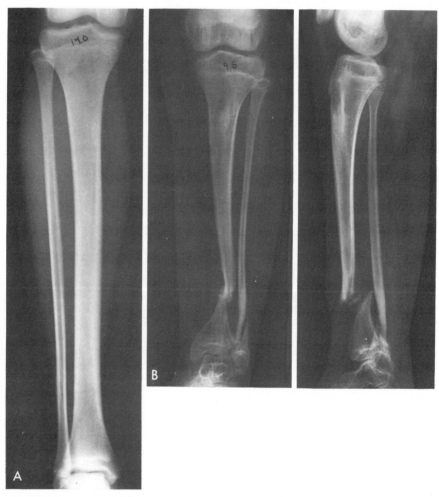

Figure 6–103   Pseudarthrosis. The left tibia and fibula are involved (*B*). There is a discontinuity of these bones which are shorter than the right tibia and fibula (*A*). The bone at the site of the abnormality is tapered and delicate. The cortices are thin and a radiolucent area representing fibrous tissue separates the bones at the site of the pseudarthrosis. Deformity is apparent.

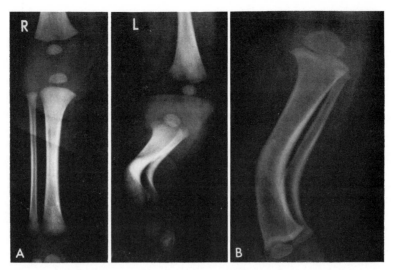

Figure 6–104   Prenatal bowing. There was bowing of the left tibia and fibula associated with localized cortical thickening at birth (*A*). Considerable regression had occurred by the end of the first year (*B*). The localized radiolucency at the site of bowing that is seen in congenital pseudarthrosis is not evident, and the medullary canal is present through the area of bowing.

Ducroquet[96] reported 11 cases of pseudarthrosis in 1937. Of these, nine had accompanying café-au-lait spots including one with neurofibromas. There was evidence of neurofibromatosis in one of the parents of four of this series. Barber[97] was the first to report the condition in the American literature. He emphasized the association with von Recklinghausen's disease. Until the paper of Holt and Wright[93] in 1949, it was generally believed that the pathologic fracture was the result of weakening of the bone due to the presence of a neurilemmoma. This belief was supported by the finding of nerve fibers within cortical bone. Aegerter[98] pointed out that if the clinical aspects of the disease are considered from the beginning it is noted that the fracture site is only a part of a much wider area of diffuse deossification and that the fibro-osseous tissue interposed between the bone ends is the result and not the cause of the fracture.

The early stages of pseudarthrosis, or even fracture, have been noted at birth. More attenuated cases develop during childhood or occasionally in adolescence. Pathologic fracture is the event that usually calls attention to the condition, though roentgenographic studies frequently reveal a more diffuse process than is represented by the fracture site. The tibia in its lower two thirds is the most commonly affected bone, though the fibula is frequently involved and other long bones are not excepted. The softening of the cortices appears to be a gradual lysis, probably physiologic, with an inability to replace the bone that is lost. Instead, there is a fibrous proliferation, which does not accept the calcium salts and, therefore, remains pliable. There is an attempt at callus formation with indifferent success. Usually the bone ends are welded together, but the failure to form rigid bone leaves the region flexible. Sometimes there is sufficient fibro-osseous metaplasia to stimulate normal repair, but when weight-bearing is resumed, the bone that has been formed melts away and "refracture" occurs. This sequence may be repeated indefinitely until the limb becomes distorted beyond functional practicability. The formation of a "false joint" has given rise to the name "pseudarthrosis."

Prenatal bowing is to be differentiated from congenital pseudarthrosis because of the benign course of the former (Fig. 6–104). Prenatal bowing most likely occurs as a result of faulty fetal position and tends to regress over the first years of life.[99] Localized cortical thickening that

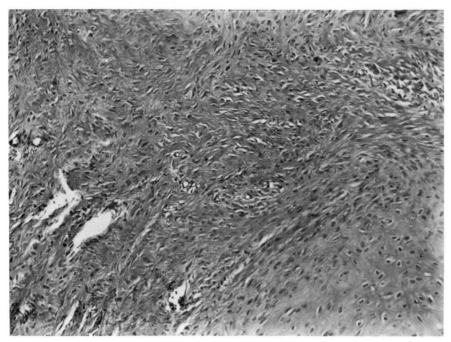

Figure 6–105 Pseudarthrosis. Section made from a lesion in bone. In the lower right corner there is evidence of fibro-osseous metaplasia. (× 130.)

obliterates the medullary canal is seen at the site of bowing, and as regression takes place the medullary canal is established through this area. Congenital pseudarthrosis is associated with a radiolucent defect in the bone through which a fracture occurs.

Microscopy. If tissue is removed from between the bone ends and sectioned, a monotonous pattern of purposeless fibrocytes is seen (Fig. 6–105). The spindled cells are rather small, and there is little evidence of organization into a pattern of trabeculation. Collagen formation is usually ample, but there is no more than a half-hearted attempt to form osteoid. There seems to be no deficiency in mineralization if a normal organic matrix can be produced. Cartilage formation is entirely lacking or very scant. There is often an extension of the fibroblastic proliferation out around the external cortical surfaces of the area. Areas of the same type of aimless spindle cell proliferation often can be found in neurofibromatosis (bone and soft tissue lesions) and fibrous dysplasia with fracture.

It has been suggested that the component cells of the primitive cell mass are incapable of differentiation into normal osteoblasts. This inability is apparently a part of a more generalized mesenchymal derivative defect, and when the manifestation is more florid the other aspects of neurofibromatosis become apparent.

Prognosis. The inability to heal a fracture sustained in childhood may persist throughout life if orthopedic attention is inadequate or unsuccessful. The patient usually has periods of limited function interspersed with longer episodes of complete disability of the part. There is a tendency for the condition to improve upon skeletal maturation, but by this time deformity may be so extensive that complete function is never regained.

MISCELLANEOUS DYSPLASIAS

There is a group of dysplasias in which so little is known of the pathogenesis that classification on this basis is probably unwise. They are grouped here under the noncommittal heading of "Miscellaneous Dysplasias." Some of them, such as Marfan's syndrome and dyschondrosteosis, or its partial expression, Madelung's deformity, are important because of their relatively frequent incidence.

This should be an ever changing group. As our knowledge grows concerning the dysplasias, some of the entities can be removed from this category and properly located in more definitive sections and other newly defined entities take their place. For example, we may be on the threshold of removing Marfan's disease from this category because the finding of hydroxyproline in the urine may eventually lead to knowledge allowing us to properly categorize it. This is as it should be as long as the new entities are not merely variations in expression of the more basic processes. Too much splitting confuses rather than enlightens in this already difficult and complex area.

DYSCHONDROSTEOSIS
(Madelung's Deformity)

In 1929 Leri and Weill described in the French literature a type of dysplasia involving the forearm and shank, calling it dyschondrosteosis. Earlier, the German surgeon Madelung had described the deformity of the wrist, which has since come to be known as Madelung's deformity. Langer, in his splendid paper,[100] gives convincing evidence that they are different stages of the same process. In a review of 17 patients, Felman and Kirkpatrick found that nine had Madelung's deformity without evidence of short stature or other osseous abnormality.[101]

This dysplasia is an autosomal dominant. It is four times more common in males than in females. It is characterized by a moderate shortness of stature due to failure of length growth of the tibia and a short radius, which produces the typical wrist deformity. The latter is often painful.

It appears to be due to a failure of growth at the distal radial growth plate with a backward subluxation of the distal end of the ulna, producing a fork deformity at the wrist. The ulnar subluxation can be reduced but only temporarily. There is usually limitation of motion at the wrist and elbow. This may be accompanied by genu varus because of growth abnormality at the proximal tibial growth plate.

Because this is a disturbance in the balance of growth rate, the condition is most apt to be noted during periods of rapid growth. Most cases are diagnosed during early adolescence. A few cases of the more severe form manifested in early life have been confused with thalidomide embryopathy.

MARFAN'S SYNDROME
(Arachnodactyly)

This is a congenital growth disturbance of the musculoskeletal, cardiovascular and ocular systems. It was first described by Marfan in 1896 and named "arachnodactyly" by Achard in 1902. The name was inspired by the appearance of the hands and feet because the digits are abnormally long and slender, suggesting the appendages of a spider. Whittaker and Sheehan[102] suggest that because the peculiar deformities of the hands and feet constitute only part of the syndrome and, indeed, may be lacking, the name "Marfan's syndrome" be retained as the term of choice.

There are numerous reports of this syndrome in both the foreign and the American literature, and any active orthopedic, cardiovascular or ophthalmologic service is apt to encounter at least one of these patients with one or more of its manifestations from time to time.

There is a strong heredity factor in the incidence of Marfan's syndrome. If the genealogy is carefully searched, perhaps 50 per cent of patients will reveal at least some of the stigmata among their progenitors. It is considered to be a simple mendelian autosomal dominant.

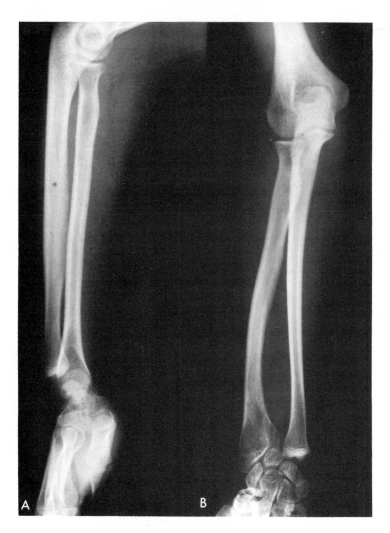

Figure 6–106 Madelung's deformity. The lateral projection (A) reveals radioulnar subluxation at the wrist which is responsible for the clinical deformity of the wrist. In the frontal projection (B) there is medial sloping of the epiphysis and metaphysis of the distal radius associated with lateral bowing of the radius.

All of the cylindrical bones are abnormally long and slender, thus producing the conformation of the hands and feet that has suggested the name of the condition. The patient is tall (Fig. 6–107), the adult usually attaining a height of over six feet. The extremities are long and gracile. The arch of the palate is unusually high and there may be a double row of teeth. The latter are often unusually long and poorly spaced. There is apt to be dolichocephaly. The thorax may be funneled and pectus excavatum is common. The muscles are poorly developed and show poor tone. Hypotonicity of muscles, tendons and ligaments results in hypermobility of the joints with dislocated hips, genu recurvatum, dislocated patella and pes planus. Inguinal and diaphragmatic hernias are common.

Numerous congenital anomalies have been reported in the heart, including dilatation of the ascending aortic segment, aortic insufficiency and less frequently mitral insufficiency and septal defects. Myocardial strain frequently leads to endocarditis just as in other cardiac anomalies that interfere with normal function. The most common and important cardiovascular complication is aneurysm formation. The aneurysms are usually of the dissecting type and often terminate the life of the patient in the early adult period.

Poor vision is a common accompaniment of this condition. It is usually due to dislocation of the lens because of lax or torn suspensory ligaments. A high-pitched voice is said to be highly characteristic of the condition.

It is apparent that arachnodactyly is a

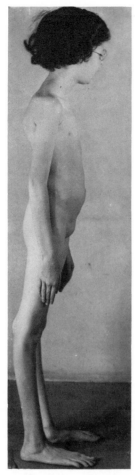

Figure 6–107   Marfan's syndrome. The cylindrical bones are abnormally long and slender. The thorax is funneled; the muscles are of poor tone. There is hypermotility of joints and poor vision due to lens dislocation. This patient died of aortic aneurysm soon after this picture was taken.

disease caused by an inability to manufacture normal collagen or one of the constituents of collagen, i.e., collagen or elastin fibrils. It is of interest that many of the same features are found in the toxic state induced by lathyrogenic substances. Recent experimentation has suggested that in the latter there is interference with normal sulfate (chondroitin sulfate) or zinc ion metabolism.

Sections of bone have shown no departure from the normal microscopy. Sections of the aortic wall reveal an excessive amount of collagen rather than a deficiency. This has led to the hypothesis that the disturbance in collagen is one of quality rather than of quantity. A sparsity

and fragmentation of elastin fibers has been described, leading some to conclude that this rather than poor collagen fiber production is the basic fault. Since collagen contains both collagen and elastin fibrils, which apparently are elaborated by the same cells, it may be that both elements are involved.

An increase in the urinary excretion of hydroxyproline has been reported in at least a few cases. Since this substance is an amino acid unique to collagen, it has been suggested that the inability to properly metabolize this substance is the primary fault in Marfan's syndrome. But many cases do not show this feature, and urinary hydroxyproline has been found in numerous other types of disease.

Roentgenographic Manifestations. The roentgenographic manifestations of Marfan's syndrome are less important than the clinical manifestations. The bones are of normal density and architecture but are elongate, particularly the bones of the lower extremities and of the hands. Scoliosis and pectus excavatum are frequently associated. Radiographically, the associated disease of the heart and aorta may be of primary importance. Relative paucity of subcutaneous fat in the extremities is often evident.

Arachnodactyly, kyphoscoliosis and deformities of the sternum are also associ-

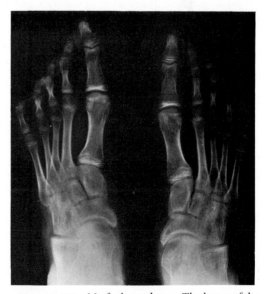

Figure 6–108   Marfan's syndrome. The bones of the feet are elongated, but normal in density and architecture.

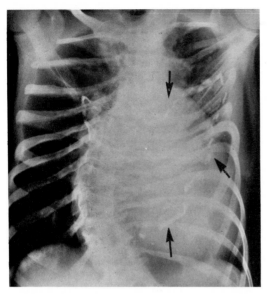

Figure 6–109 Marfan's syndrome. There is scolio-sis to the right. Opaque prosthetic material (arrows) was utilized in the repair of a pectus excavatum de-formity. The heart is enlarged. The patient died as a result of rupture of the aorta.

ated with homocystinuria. The clinical features differ, however, and the diagno-sis is made by demonstrating the presence of homocystine in the urine.

APERT'S SYNDROME
(Acrocephalosyndactylism)

This is an uncommon, congenital dis-turbance in the growth of bone and soft tissue affecting principally the head, the hands and the feet. As the name suggests, the head is elongated and peaked, and the hands and feet show various degrees of syndactylism.

The name "acrocephalosyndactylism" was suggested by Apert in 1906 though several cases had been reported before his paper appeared. The most complete review was published by Park and Pow-ers[103] in 1920. A later review stated that there were at least 49 published cases as of 1955.[104]

The condition is congenital because numerous cases have been described in the newborn. There have been no pub-lished data to indicate that Apert's syn-drome is hereditary though both syndacty-lism and scaphocephaly (usually a part of the syndrome) commonly show a hered-itary incidence. It may be that those with severe involvement do not reach the age of reproductivity or are unable to bear children, thus concealing a heredity factor. There are no data on this phase of the subject.

The peculiar appearance of these pa-tients is such that one might mistake them for members of the same family. It has been stated that the finer facial character-istics and traits of expression are masked by the changes so that there is a species resemblance.

The head is vertically elongated and peaked, the highest point varying between the anterior and posterior fontanelles. The dome slopes sharply, front and back (Fig. 6–110). The face is usually consid-erably widened. The head is shortened in the anteroposterior diameter. The planes of the face and the back of the skull, which is often flush with the neck, are flattened and remarkably parallel (Fig. 6–111). The calvarium appears to have increased in volume chiefly by growth above the level of the face.

The cause of this curious malformation of the head, according to Park and Powers who go with considerable length into the existing theories of mechanism and offer some of their own, is a premature syn-ostosis of the cranial bones due to inade-quacies on the part of the nonossifying mesenchymal tissue to separate the vari-ous ossification centers. The synostoses result in inadequate expansion in certain directions and increased intracranial pres-sure caused by the enlarging brain. The latter undergoes convolutional atrophy. Impaired mental development is reported in a few cases. In some instances an in-ternal hydrocephalus has developed, its cause and association not understood.

The increased intracranial pressure is the cause of the disturbance in vision, which is one of the outstanding symptoms of the condition. The eyes are displaced forward so that their transverse axes di-verge and slant downward. There is often strabismus. The contents of the orbit are pushed forward so that the eyes bulge prominently and may develop staphy-lomas. In severe cases they have been completely displaced. Progressive im-pairment of vision is the usual result.

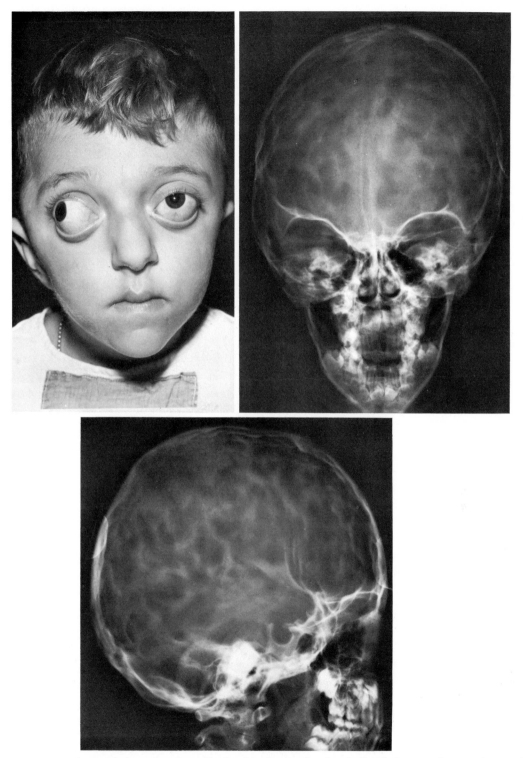

Figure 6–110   Acrocephalosyndactylism. The head is elongated and peaked with sloping sides; it is shortened in the anteroposterior diameter with parallel planes of the face and back of the skull. The eyes are displaced forward with divergence of their axes. (Courtesy of Dr. Michael Scott.)

Fusion defects of the maxilla and mandible occur, particularly notable in the posterior palate, which may be narrow and high-vaulted. There is often interference with the normal development of the teeth. The mandible has been reported to be prognathic in some cases and recessive in others.

The excessively high forehead, often with a prominent horizontal, supraciliary groove, the peaked head flattened posteriorly, the wide-spaced bulging eyes, flat face and short nose constitute the characteristic facies of the acro-scapho-brachycephalic portion of the condition.

Syndactylism is another prominent feature of this malformation (Fig. 6–113). It may be complete or partial. There may be synostoses between metacarpals and between metatarsals. There are often synostoses between the phalanges of different digits, and there may be failure of joint formation between the various units of the same digit.

The syndactylism is apparently due to the same disturbance in growth that causes the malformations of the head

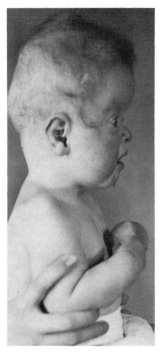

Figure 6–111 Acrocephalosyndactylism. The head is vertically elongated. The planes of the face and the back of the skull are parallel. The calvarium appears increased in volume by growth above the level of the face.

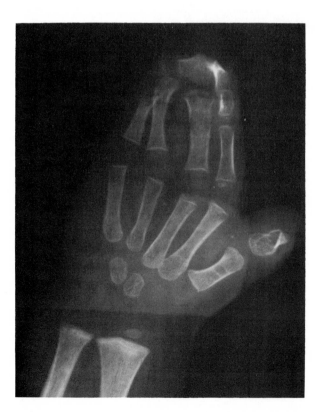

Figure 6–112 Acrocephalosyndactylism in male aged 19 months. Syndactylism is present in the hands, and the bones of the feet may show a similar abnormality.

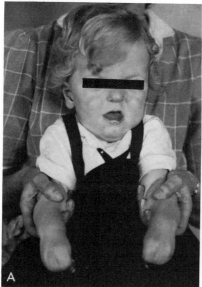
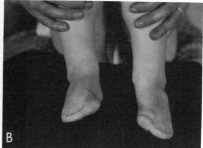

Figure 6–113 Acrocephalosyndactylism. Syndactylism of the hands (A) and feet (B).

bones, a failure of the non-osteogenic mesenchymal tissue to isolate the various ossification centers. It is of interest that in both instances the defects are the result of the failure of a process that normally occurs toward the end of the sequence of events that result in the formation of the skeleton.

Sections of the involved bone, when examined with the aid of the microscope, show only normal bone tissue. The condition is apparently a disturbance in skeleton formation, not in bone tissue production. It appears to be, as Park and Powers insist, the result of a germ plasm defect. The literature is lacking in long term follow-up data. It is known that some of the cases have become progressively worse throughout childhood, but it is not clear what course the disease takes after cessation of skeletal growth.

CLEIDOCRANIAL DYSOSTOSIS

Cleidocranial dysostosis is a developmental disturbance of the skeleton in which a wide variation of deformities occurs involving numerous bones. There is almost always involvement of the skull bones or the clavicles or both.

The first report of such a case (quoted from Soule[105]) was that of Cutter in 1870. Marie and Sainton recognized the condition as an entity, supplied the name of cleidocranial dysostosis and reported two cases in 1897. Since that time approximately 350 cases have been described in the literature. The most complete recent survey is that of Soule[105] who added six cases.

A familial incidence was recorded in approximately two thirds of the reported cases, and the condition was found in as many as five successive generations. The trait is passed on by either the mother or father who manifests the deformities. The condition is congenital. Well-documented sporadic cases have been noted.

Rhinehart suggested that since either, or in rare cases both, the clavicular and/or the cranial deformities may be lacking, the term "cleidocranial dysostosis" should be abandoned and replaced by "mutational dysostosis." This suggestion was supported by Soule.

The typical case is usually a patient with a large head, a small face, drooping shoulders and a narrow chest.

There is a marked brachycephaly with widening of the interparietal diameter above. The skull thus appears excessively

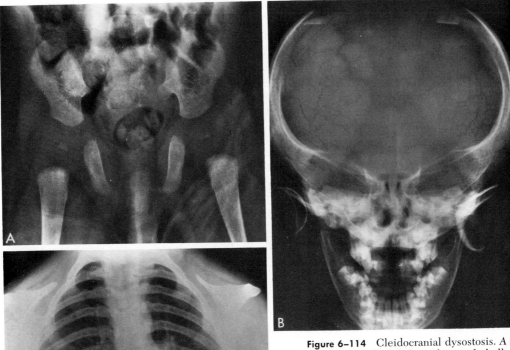

Figure 6–114 Cleidocranial dysostosis. *A* and *B* are radiographs of the pelvis and skull of a male 6 months of age. The pubic bones are underdeveloped; only a small portion of the body of each is evident. The epiphyseal center for the heads of the femurs is tiny. The radiograph of the skull (*B*) shows widely patent sutures and fontanelles, numerous centers of ossification in the cranial bones and an increase in the biparietal diameter. The facial bones are small. This child had no clavicles and the radiograph of his mother's chest (*C*) revealed absence of clavicles.

broad. The foramen magnum is larger than normal and slants forward and downward; the mandible is prognathous. The maxilla appears underdeveloped as do the other bones that compose the face. The malar, lacrimal and nasal bones may be deficient or absent. The palate is narrow, sometimes cleft, and the arch is high. The paranasal sinuses are small. The frontal and parietal bones are prominently bossed. The principal sutures are greatly delayed in closing, giving a "hot cross bun" appearance to the head. The metopic suture may persist throughout life. Wormian bones commonly develop from secondary centers within the suture membranes.

Since the clavicle is produced from three separate centers, great variation occurs in its development. In a small percentage of cases it is absent entirely. Only the sternal third may be present, or the acromial third, or the two ends without the middle, or all three portions without uniting. The scapula is small and often winged. These abnormalities allow great mobility of the shoulders. One or both sides may be involved. In the latter instance the patient may be able to approximate the shoulders until the tips of the acromial processes touch beneath his chin.

The large bones of the arm are less frequently involved but occasionally the radius fails to attain proper length, causing abduction at the wrist. Extra epiphyses may appear in the metacarpals and phalanges, and the second metacarpal is excessively long.

The pelvic bones appear underdeveloped with contraction and asymmetry of the pelvic canal. Fusion at the symphysis pubis may fail to occur. The sacrum and coccyx are often poorly formed; the latter is sometimes absent. The neck of the femur may be deformed to cause coxa vara. Abnormalities in the bones of the feet may be similar to those of the hands.

Poorly developed vertebrae with fusion defects of the spinous processes and laminae may cause lordosis, scoliosis or kyphosis.

There is marked disturbance in formation of the teeth. The deciduous teeth are usually normal though often delayed in eruption. Shedding of the deciduous teeth is usually delayed or does not occur so that eruption and growth of the permanent teeth are markedly impaired. Caries and premature periodontitis are excessive. Dentigerous cysts may develop.

The disturbance in dentition and difficulties in gait due to femoral neck deformity are the commonest causes of complaint. The failure of proper development of the clavicles causes little or no disability.

Rubin points out that the basis for this disturbance is the failure of the normal development of the midline junctions between bones. This might account for the open fontanelle, the wide metopic suture, the failure of fusion of the anterior mandibular and the neural arches and the proper development of the sacrum. Apparently the fibrous syndesmoses are involved. He relates the involvement of the clavicle on the basis that it is not preformed in cartilage like the cylindrical bones but is preceded by a fibrous condensation before the cartilage growth centers appear. Thus, if the condition were a disturbance in the formation of collagenous tissues related to bone development and if it were effective at the very outset of skeleton formation in embryonal life, the features of this disease might be explained.

CHONDROECTODERMAL DYSPLASIA (Ellis–van Creveld)

In 1940 Ellis and van Creveld[106] reported two patients who exhibited ecto-dermal dysplasia, chondrodysplasia, polydactylism and congenital cardiac anomalies and a third with the first three of these four features. Only a few reports have appeared subsequently,[107, 108] indicating that this condition is a rare syndrome.

The cardiac anomalies appear in approximately 60 per cent of cases and include interatrial and interventricular septal defects and large vessel transposition. These patients usually have cyanosis at birth and die shortly in congestive heart failure. The ectodermal dysplasia has included small, distorted and friable nails, defective dentition and, in two cases, alopecia. The upper lip is often short and bound down to the anterior portion of the gum. Chondrodysplasia was diagnosed because of dwarfing of the extremities, synostosis of the calvarium, failure of normal growth and deformity of the tubular bones. The distal segments of the limbs manifest greater shortening than do the proximal segments unlike achondroplasia in which the opposite is true. The hamate and capitate bones of the wrist are often fused. A defect in the lateral aspect of the proximal portion of the tibia causes genu

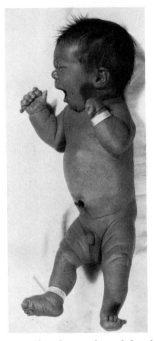

Figure 6–115   Chondroectodermal dysplasia (Ellis-van Creveld). There are flaring of the thorax, downward displacement of the liver and spleen, dwarfing of the extremities and polydactylism of both hands and both feet.

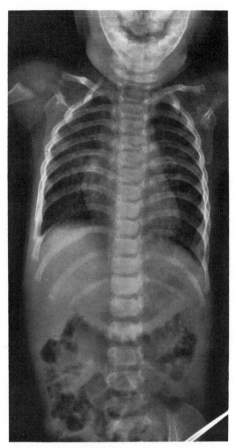

Figure 6-116 Chondroectodermal dysplasia. The thorax is narrow. There is cardiac enlargement and pulmonary vascular engorgement as a result of an intracardiac shunt. Teeth are present in the mandible, but none had erupted by the ninth month of life. The spine is normal. (Courtesy of Dr. J. W. Hope, Children's Hospital, Philadelphia.)

valgum. Polydactyly has been constant, appearing more often in the hands than in the feet. The patient lacking cardiac anomaly in the original series has been followed to adult life.[108] Except for her dwarfism and the short stubby deformity of her hands she is able to lead a normal life.

Microscopic sections were made in one case.[107] A decrease in the depth of the proliferating cartilage layer with too few and too short chondrocyte columns, absence of the provisional line of calcification and islands of cartilage cells within the metaphysis were reported. These changes are nonspecific and do not define the defect in physiology that causes this curious syndrome.

Hereditary and familial features have been lacking in most reported cases but the occurrence of three cases in the family cited previously is strong evidence for a familial incidence, and McKusick et al. in studying the Old Order Amish of Lancaster County, Pennsylvania, concluded that this dysplasia is autosomal recessive.

ASPHYXIATING THORACIC DYSTROPHY

In 1955 Jeune et al.[109] reported two infant siblings who died of respiratory distress associated with a small and relatively immobile thorax; hence the appellation. Such infants demonstrate, upon radiographic examination, very short ribs and variable degrees of shortening of the long tubular bones with peculiar notching of the metaphyses. The ilium in the young infant is short in its inferosuperior dimension with a broad acetabular roof in which there is apt to be a large V-shaped notch. The spine and skull are normal. A form of this dysplasia has been described in which the thoracic deformity is mild and the patients grow into childhood. Cone-shaped epiphyses in the hands are usually present. Intrinsic renal disease, interstitial fibrosis, may be encountered in this group of patients.[110]

The deformity of the pelvis is very similar to that observed in the young infant with chondroectodermal dysplasia. A relationship with this dysplasia, a part of a spectrum, has been suggested.[111]

OTHER AFFECTIONS ASSOCIATED WITH DWARFISM

There are a number of rather vague clinical entities and syndromes, less clearly definable than the conditions already described, that are emerging in the current literature. Two of these, thanatophoric dwarfism[112, 113] and metatrophic dwarfism[114, 115] have, until recently, been classified with achondroplasia. Some writers still feel that the former is but a severe, intrauterine form of achondroplasia and the latter a subtype in which the dwarfing factor involving the limbs is somehow corrected at birth.

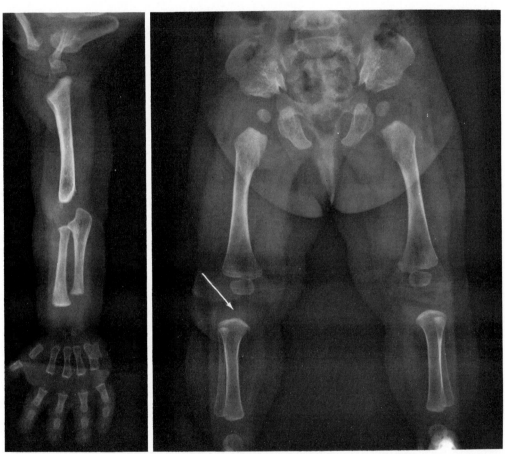

Figure 6–117 Chondroectodermal dysplasia. The bones of the extremities, particularly the distal ones, are short. A ridge is present in the proximal tibial epiphyseal line (arrow) and the center will appear adjacent to the medial slope. A rudimentary metacarpal is present. There is often fusion of several carpal centers. (Courtesy of Dr. J. W. Hope, Children's Hospital, Philadelphia.)

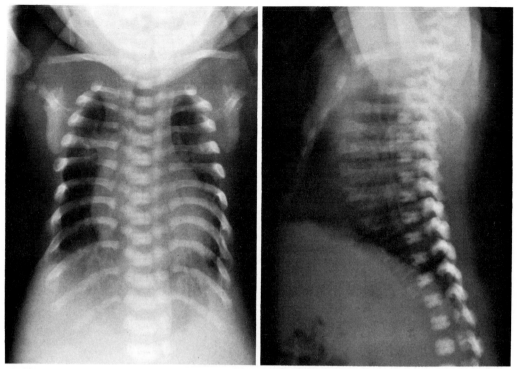

Figure 6–118 Asphyxiating thoracic dystrophy. The ribs are short so that the volume of the thorax is markedly reduced. The vertebrae are normal in appearance.

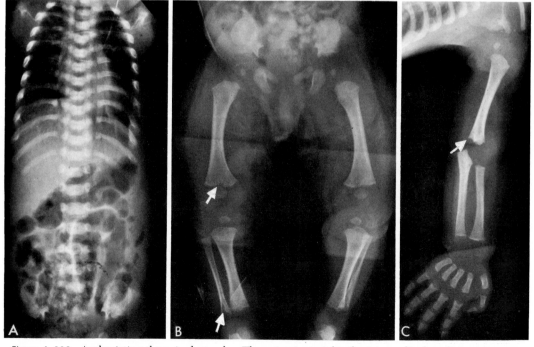

Figure 6–119 Asphyxiating thoracic dystrophy. The spine is straight; the interpediculate distances are normal (A). Notching of the acetabula associated with a flat and broad roof is evident. There are peculiar notches in the metaphyses of many of the long bones (A and B, arrows).

Other conditions in which the skeleton fails to grow normally are associated with multiple abnormalities in other systems and sometimes with premature aging as in progeria and Cockayne's syndrome,[116] the Hallerman-Streiff syndrome, Werner's syndrome, Seckel's dwarfism and bird-headed dwarfism.[117] Descriptions of these bizarre growth disturbances obviously belong elsewhere.

Finally the modern literature is replete with single or one-family case reports of an infinite variety of anomalies which may or may not involve the skeleton. Such exotic disturbances, e.g., familial osteo-dysplasia,[118] are admittedly fascinating but are of scarcely enough general importance to include in this text.

References

1. Fairbank, T.: Atlas of General Affections of the Skeleton. Edinburgh, E. & S. Livingstone Ltd., 1951.
2. Hunter, E.: Proc. R. Soc., 10:104, 1917.
3. Hurler, G.: Ztschr. F. Kinderich., 24:220, 1919.
4. Kressler, R. and Aegerter, E.: J. Pediatr., 12:579, 1938.
5. Reilly, W.: Am. J. Dis. Child., 62:489, 1941.
6. Brante, G.: Scand. J. Clin. Lab. Invest., 4:43, 1952.
7. Dorfman, A. and Lorincz, A.: Proc. Nat. Acad. Sci., 43:443, 1957.
8. Zellweger, H., Ponseti., I., Pedrini, V., Stamler, F. and von Noorden, G.: J. Pediatr., 59:549, 1961.
9. Pedrini, V., Lenuzzi, L. and Zambotti, V.: Proc. Soc. Exp. Biol. Med., 110:847, 1962.
10. Wallace, B., Kaplan, D., Adache, M., Schneck, L. and Volk, B.: Arch. Pathol., 82:462, 1966.
11. McKusick, V.: Heritable Disorders of Connective Tissue. Ed. 3. St. Louis, C. V. Mosby Co., 1966.
12. Morquio, L.: Arch. Med. Enf., 32:129, 1929.
13. Brailsford, J.: Am. J. Surg., 7:404, 1929.
14. Progress in Pediatric Radiology. Vol. 4. Intrinsic Diseases of Bones. Edited by H. ·J. Kaufmann. Basel, S. Karger, 1973.
15. Ellis, R., Sheldon, W. and Capon, N.: Quart. J. Med., 29:119, 1936.
16. Horrigan, D. and Baker, D.: Am. J. Roentgenol., 86:473, 1961.
17. Dawson, I.: J. Pathol. Bact., 67:587, 1954.
18. Wolfe, H., Blennerhasset, J., Young, G. and Cohen, R.: Am. J. Pathol., 45:1007, 1964.
19. Zellweger, H., Giaciai, L. and Fuzli, S.: Am. J. Dis. Child., 84:421, 1952.
20. Spillane, J.: J. Neurol. Neurosurg. Psychiatry, 15:246, 1952.
20a. Spranger, J. W., Langer, L. O. and Wiedemann, H. R.: Bone Dysplasias: An Atlas of Constitutional Disorders of Development. Philadelphia, W. B. Saunders Co., 1974.
21. Rubin, P. and Squire, L.: Am. J. Roentgenol., 82:217, 1959.
22. Caffey, J.: Am. J. Roentgenol., 80:458, 1958.
23. McKusick, V., Egeland, J. and Eldridge, R.: Bull. Johns Hopkins Hosp., 115:306, 1964.
24. McKusick, V., Eldridge, R., Hostetler, J., Ruangwit, U. and Egeland, J.: Bull. Johns Hopkins Hosp., 116:285, 1965.
25. Jansen, M.: Z. Orthop. Chir., 61:253, 1934.
26. Cameron, J., Young, W. and Sissons, H.: J. Bone Joint Surg., 36B:622, 1954.
27. Gram, P., Fleming, J., Frame, B. and Fine, G.: J. Bone Joint Surg., 41A:951, 1959.
28. Daeshner, C., Singleton, E., Hill, L. and Dodge, W.: Pediatrics, 57:844, 1960.
29. Schmid, F.: Mschr. Kinderheilk., 97:393, 1949.
30. Stickler, G., Maher, F., Hunt, J., Burke, E. and Rosevear, J.: Pediatrics, 29:996, 1962.
31. Miller, S. and Paul, L.: Radiology, 83:665, 1964.
32. Peterson, J.: J. Pediatr., 60:656, 1962.
33. Spahr, A. and Spahr-Hartmann, I.: Helv. Paediatr. Acta, 16:836, 1961.
34. Mahorner, H.: J. Pediatr., 10:1, 1937.
35. Ollier, M.: Bull. Soc. Chir. Lyon, 3:22, 1899.
36. Bean, W.: Arch. Intern. Med., 102:544, 1958.
37. Jaffe, H.: Arch. Pathol., 36:335, 1943.
38. Keith, A.: J. Anat., 54:101, 1919.
39. Jansen, M.: Association of Bone Growth, Robert Jones Birthday Volume. London, Oxford University Press, 1928.
40. Chang, C., Piatt, E., Thomas, K. and Watne, A.: Am. J. Roentgenol., 103:645, 1968.
41. Trevor, D.: J. Bone Joint Surg., 32B:204, 1950.
42. Fairbank, T.: J. Bone Joint Surg., 38B:237, 1956.
43. Keats, T.: Radiology, 68:538, 1957.
44. Lamy, M. and Maroteaux, P.: Presse Méd., 68:1977, 1960.
45. Taybi, H.: Radiology, 80:1, 1963.
46. Stover, C., Hayes, J. and Holt, J.: Am. J. Roentgenol., 89:914, 1963.
47. Wilson, D. W.: Arch. Dis. Child., 44:48, 1969.
48. Ford, N., Silverman, F. and Kozlowski, K.: Am. J. Roentgenol., 86:462, 1961.
49. Weinberg, H., Frankel, M., Mahin, M. and Vas, E.: J. Bone Joint Surg., 42B:313, 1960.
50. Freiberger, R.: Radiology, 70:379, 1958.
51. Yakovac, W.: Arch. Pathol., 57:62, 1954.
52. Rubin, P.: Dynamic Classification of Bone Dysplasias. Chicago, Year Book Medical Publishers, 1964.
53. Silverman, F.: Ann. Radiol., 4:833, 1961.
54. Scot, D. and Stiris, G.: Acta Med. Scand., 145:237, 1953.
55. Bergman, G. and Engfeldt, B.: Acta Pathol. Microbiol. Scand., 35:537, 1954.
56. Follis, R.: J. Pediatr., 41:713, 1952.
57. Follis, R.: Bull. Johns Hopkins Hosp., 93:225, 1953.
58. Weber, M.: Arch. Pathol., 9:984, 1930.
59. Engfeldt, B., Engstrom, A. and Zellerstrom, R.: J. Bone Joint Surg., 36B:654, 1954.
60. Karshner, R.: Am. J. Roentgenol., 16:405, 1926.
61. Zawisch, C.: Arch. Pathol., 43:55, 1947.
62. Pines, B. and Lederer, M.: Am. J. Pathol., 23:755, 1947.
63. Maroteaux, P. and Lamy, M.: J.A.M.A., 191:715, 1965.
64. Elmore, S., Nance, W., McGee, B., Montmollin, M. and Engel, E.: Am. J. Med. 40:273, 1966.

65. Grunebaum, M. and Landau, B.: Br. J. Radiol., 41:359, 1968.
66. Elmore, S.: J. Bone Joint Surg., 49A:153, 1967.
67. Pyle, E.: J. Bone Joint Surg., 29:874, 1931.
68. Jackson, W., Albright, F., Drewry, G., Hanelin, J. and Rubin, M.: A.M.A. Arch. Intern. Med., 94:871, 1954.
69. Mori, P. and Holt, J.: Radiology, 66:335, 1956.
70. Halliday, J.: Br. J. Surg., 37:52, 1949.
71. Camurati, M.: Chir. Arg. Mov., 6:662, 1922.
72. Engelmann, G.: Fortschr. Röntgenstr., 39:1101, 1929.
73. Sear, H.: Br. J. Radiol., 21:236, 1948.
74. Ribbing, S.: Acta Radiol., 31:522, 1949.
75. Lennon, E., Schechter, M. and Hornabrook, R.: J. Bone Joint Surg., 43B:273, 1961.
76. Cohen, J. and States, J.: Lab. Invest., 5:492, 1956.
77. Franklin, E. and Matheson, I.: Br. J. Radiol., 15:185, 1942.
78. Dillehunt, R. and Chainard, E.: J. Bone Joint Surg., 18:991, 1936.
79. Hurt, R.: J. Bone Joint Surg., 35B:89, 1953.
80. Hinsen, A.: Am. J. Surg., 45:566, 1939.
81. Martincic, N.: Br. J. Radiol., 25:612, 1952.
82. Schlumberger, H.: Milit. Surg., 99:504, 1946.
83. Freund, E. and Moffert, C.: Surg. Gynecol. Obstet., 62:541, 1936.
84. McCune, D. and Bruch, H.: Am. J. Dis. Child., 54:807, 1937.
85. Albright, F., Butler, A., Hampton, A., and Smith, P.: N. Engl. J. Med., 216:729, 1937.
86. Lichtenstein, L.: Am. J. Surg., 36:874, 1938.
87. Lichtenstein, L. and Jaffe, H.: Arch. Pathol., 33:777, 1942.
88. Thannhauser, S.: Medicine, 23:105, 1944.
89. Stauffer, H., Arbuckle, R. and Aegerter, E.: J. Bone Joint Surg., 23:323, 1941.
90. Aegerter, E.: Clin. Orthop., 19:19, 1961.
91. McIntosh, H., Miller, E., Gleason, W. and Goldner, J.: Am. J. Med., 32:393, 1962.
92. Aegerter, E. and Smith, L.: Am. J. Cancer, 31:212, 1937.
93. Holt, J. and Wright, E.: Radiology, 51:647, 1949.
94. Condow, V. and Allen, R.: Radiology, 76:444, 1961.
95. Caffey, J.: Pediatric X-ray Diagnosis. Ed. 5. Chicago, Year Book Medical Publishers, 1967, p. 1024.
96. Ducroquet, R.: Mém. Acad. Chir., 63:863, 1937.
97. Barber, C.: Surg. Gynecol. Obstet., 69:618, 1939.
98. Aegerter, E.: J. Bone Joint Surg., 32A:618, 1950.
99. Caffey, J.: Pediatric X-ray Diagnosis. Ed. 6. Chicago, Year Book Medical Publishers, 1972.
100. Langer, L.: Am. J. Roentgenol., 95:178, 1965.
101. Felman, A. H. and Kirkpatrick, J. A.: Radiology, 93:1037, 1969.
102. Whittaker, S. and Sheehan, J.: Lancet, 16:791, 1954.
103. Park, E. and Powers, G.: Am. J. Dis. Child., 20:235, 1920.
104. Kahn, A. and Fulmer, J.: N. Engl. J. Med., 252:379, 1955.
105. Soule, A.: J. Bone Joint Surg., 28:81, 1946.
106. Ellis, R. and van Creveld, S.: Arch. Dis. Child., 15:65, 1940.
107. Smith, H. and Hand, A.: Pediatrics, 21:298, 1958.
108. Caffey, J.: Am. J. Roentgenol., 68:875, 1952.
109. Jeune, M., Beraud, C. and Carron, R.: Arch. Franç. Pediatr., 12:344, 1955.
110. Roentgen Diagnosis of Diseases of the Bone. Vol. I. Ed. 2. Edited by J. Edeiken and P. J. Hodes. Baltimore, Williams and Wilkins, 1973.
110a. Langer, L. O.: The Clinical Delineation of Birth Defects. IV. Skeletal Dysplasias. Baltimore. Williams and Wilkins, 1969, p. 55.
111. Berdon, W. E. and Baker, D.: Pediatr. Clin. North Am., 13:1017, 1966.
112. Kaufman, R., Rimoin, D., McAlister, W. and Kissane, J.: Am. J. Dis. Child., 120:53, 1970.
113. Keats, T., Riddervold, H. and Michaelis, L.: Am. J. Roentgenol., 108:473, 1970.
114. Jenkins, P., Smith, M. and McKinnell, J.: Br. J. Radiol., 43:561, 1970.
115. La Rose, J. and Gay, B.: Am. J. Roentgenol., 106:156, 1969.
116. Fujimoto, W., Greene, M. and Sugmiller, J.: J. Pediatr., 75:881, 1969.
117. Fitch, N., Pinsky, L. and Lachance, R.: Am. J. Dis. Child., 120:260, 1970.
118. Anderson, L., Cook, A., Coccaro, P., Coro, E. and Bosma, J.: J.A.M.A., 220:1687, 1972.

Chapter 7

FUNCTIONAL DISTURBANCES OF THE RETICULOENDO- THELIAL SYSTEM

Many, perhaps all, of the skeletal dysplasias discussed in the previous chapter appear, at the time of this writing, to be caused by some abnormality in the formation of one or more components of collagen, chondroid or osteoid, usually either the collagen fiber or its mucopolysaccharide ground substance.

Appropriately, the next group of diseases to be discussed is the result of several types of disturbances in the metabolic routines of certain cell systems. The common denominator in these diseases is the manner in which the reticuloendothelial system reacts to the resulting metabolites which are abnormal in quantity or quality.

A dense fog of confusion has, from the outset, obscured our understanding of this most interesting group of diseases. They were originally described as separate entities under the general heading of "Reticuloendothelioses." They included Hand-Schüller-Christian disease, Niemann-Pick disease, Gaucher's disease, Tay-Sachs disease and later eosinophilic granuloma and Letterer-Siwe disease. For a while the Hunter-Hurler syndrome, then called lipochondrodystrophy, was included. The original concept suggested that these diseases resulted from a systemic disturbance in the metabolism of certain lipids. Eventually the Hunter-Hurler syndrome was removed because it was found that the offending substance within the histiocytes of this condition

was mucopolysaccharide rather than lipid in nature. Chemical analysis of the tissues of the other diseases allowed them to be grouped into three categories: those in which the dominant lipid involved is cholesterol (Hand-Schüller-Christian disease, Letterer-Siwe disease and eosinophilic granuloma), that in which a cerebroside is the offending agent (Gaucher's disease) and finally those in which the cells contain various phosphosphingosides (Niemann-Pick and Tay-Sachs diseases).

The next advance in our understanding of these curious processes was the report that Hand-Schüller-Christian disease, eosinophilic granuloma and Letterer-Siwe disease are only various manifestations of the same process.

As more cases became available for study in depth, it became apparent that these conditions were essentially idiopathic, abnormal proliferations of derivatives of the reticuloendothelial system. Lichenstein[1] coined the term "histiocytosis X" for the group in which cholesterol metabolism appears to be at fault. One might ask the significance of the "X" and because we do not know the answer we are prone to omit it.

Finally it has become apparent that we have been confusing two completely different processes, one metabolic and the other neoplastic, in the histiocytosis group. Both have been included under the heading of Letterer-Siwe disease, which was described as a universally fatal condition occurring in infants and young children. Then the same or a similar process was found to occur in older patients, and this was reported under several headings including "histiocytic medullary reticulosis."[2]

The fulminant, disseminated type of "metabolic" histiocytosis may be difficult or impossible to differentiate from neoplastic histiocytosis (or better, neoplastic reticulocytosis, since the neoplastic cell may be the reticulum or any one of its derivative cells) in the early stages. If the condition responds to antibiotic therapy, it is probably the non-neoplastic form of the disease.[3] Good results have been reported with cortisone[4] and with vinblastine sulfate.[5] Whether these cases were the neoplastic form is still uncertain. One of us had the opportunity of following a case of neoplastic reticulocytosis in a 22 year old male. His original, solitary lesion was considered to be eosinophilic granuloma. The lesion became multiple, and in the course of 18 months an eosinophilic leukemia developed and the patient died despite every conceivable type of therapy. We have also encountered a patient with Gaucher's disease who eventually died with multiple sarcomas, which appeared to be of reticulum origin. The histiocytoses may be classified as follows:

  I. Non-neoplastic or metabolic forms
    A. Subacute disseminated type
      Hand-Schüller-Christian disease
    B. Chronic focal type
      Eosinophilic granuloma
    C. Acute disseminated type
      Letterer-Siwe disease, childhood and adult
  II. Neoplastic forms
    A. A variety of sarcomatous and leukemic types involving a number of cell forms.

HAND-SCHÜLLER-CHRISTIAN DISEASE

Hand-Schüller-Christian disease, sometimes called lipoid granulomatosis, cholesterol reticuloendotheliosis or histiocytosis, is a condition in which multiple, microscopically characteristic, nonbacterial, focal granulomas develop first in relation to bones, in more severe cases extending to the extraosseous reticulum deposits and skin and, in some, invading the viscera. The cause is unknown, but a highly characteristic and peculiar part of the mechanism is the deposition of a variety of lipids, preponderantly cholesterol and its esters, within histiocytes.

Hand,[6] in 1893, was the first to report descriptions of the lesions as an entity. The etiology was presumed to be tuberculous though at the time he expressed doubt as to the correctness of this presumption. He later recognized it as a nontuberculous entity and published his opinion as such.[7] In 1915, Schüller reported three cases of the disease, and in 1919 Christian made his report[8] in which appeared the first description of the triad of exophthalmos, diabetes insipidus and multiple focal areas of deossification. Rowland[9], in 1928, recognized the condition as a disturbance in lipid metabolism with phagocytosis of excessive macromolecules of lipid by the reticuloendothelial system. It had previously been thought, because of the hypophyseal involvement in the reported cases, that the lesions were an expression of pituitary dysfunction. Rowland's report shifted opinion to a systemic disturbance of lipid metabolism and related the condition to Gaucher's disease and Niemann-Pick disease.

With the concept that the reticuloendothelial system played a secondary role in merely accumulating the lipids at fault, the disease was classified with the xanthomatoses. When Farber,[10] in 1941, directed attention to the similarity of the lesions of Hand-Schüller-Christian disease and those of eosinophilic granuloma, a condition that was presumed to be caused by an unknown infectious agent, opinion swung back again to approximately the original point of view.

Today, most will admit that the cause of Hand-Schüller-Christian disease is unknown. The lesions appear to result from the inability on the part of the reticuloendothelial components of certain regions to process several of the complex lipids, principally cholesterol. This inability may arise from a congenital enzymatic lack or from an alteration of metabolic capacity of the cells whose function is to handle these lipids. Or it might be caused by an outside agent, perhaps infectious in nature, such as a virus, though none has been isolated even though investigators have sought for it.

The former association with the hypercholesterolemic and hyperlipemic xanthomatoses seems to have dissolved with a better understanding of the physiology of these processes. The relationship to some of the other lipid reticuloendothelioses (Niemann-Pick and Tay-Sachs diseases) is uncertain because they often show hereditary features that are lacking in Hand-Schüller-Christian disease. It may be that an enzymatic deficiency is the basic difficulty in all these conditions, but the cause of this deficiency and the cells involved may be variable.

Hand-Schüller-Christian disease usually begins in infancy or early childhood. Less often it appears in adolescence and rarely it is first diagnosed during adult life. The earlier the onset, the more grave the prognosis is apt to be. Before x-ray therapy was generally used for this disease, cases beginning in childhood or earlier usually terminated fatally in from two to four years. With the benefit of proper therapy most patients now survive well into adult life. In some series there has been a preponderance of males; in other series this sex predilection has been lacking.

The commonest site of origin is the intraosseous reticulum and its derivatives. When manifestations are minimal, the skeleton is apt to be the only structure involved. In somewhat more florid cases the spleen, liver and lymph nodes may be the sites of granulomatous lesions, and the skin is often affected. In the cases that begin early in life and run a malignant course most of the tissues of the body are involved, including the lungs, brain, heart, kidneys, mucous membranes, tendon sheaths, fascia and serous surfaces. Rarely the disease may remain latent as a solitary lesion for a long period and then progress into typical multicentric Hand-Schüller-Christian disease. A few cases are reported to run a fairly classic course for several months and then to develop into a fulminant terminal phase, which is identical with that of Letterer-Siwe disease.

The fundamental lesion of Hand-Schüller-Christian disease is a focal granuloma that grows peripherally to agglomerate with other granulomas until a large irregular mass is formed. The blood supply to the normal tissue of the site is obstructed, normal structures degenerate and the granulomas replace them. Thus, the lesion compresses and pushes aside or destroys the normal tissue where it develops.

Actively hematopoietic marrow is most commonly involved and, therefore, flat bones are most frequently affected. Long bones are not spared, however, The affected areas may give rise to pain. In cylindrical bones, unlike most of the bone tumors, the lesion of Hand-Schüller-Christian disease may begin in any region. The metaphysis is no more frequently involved than is the mid-diaphysis. Bone supportive fibrous tissue is also frequently involved; the lesions may, therefore, begin in the periosteum or, when in the head, beneath the dura or the scalp tissues. They begin as miliary lesions, which enlarge and coalesce. Cancellous and cortical bone in their path melts away, leaving sharply delineated areas of deossification. This tissue is moderately firm, has a yellow or yellowish gray color and may show inconspicuous areas of hemorrhage or cystic degeneration in its active phase.

The bones of the head are most frequently involved (Fig. 7–1). The calvarium may become riddled with circular holes, which may be palpated through the scalp. Involvement of the base and the sella causes pituitary dysfunction in about one third of the cases. If the posterior pituitary lobe is affected there may be polydipsia and polyuria—diabetes insipidus. If the anterior lobe is involved there may be delayed somatic and sexual growth with infantilism, dwarfism, adiposogenital syndrome or Simmonds' disease. Compression on the base of the brain may result in hydrocephalus with symptoms of headache and vomiting. The jaw is frequently involved causing swelling of the gums and loosening of the teeth.

The spleen, liver and lymph nodes are not affected in the very mild cases and are never greatly involved. The reticulum of

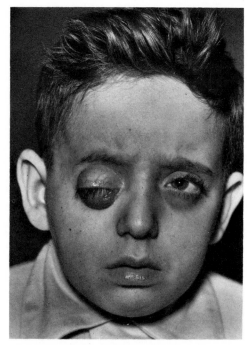

Figure 7–1 Hand-Schüller-Christian disease. Involvement of the bones of the orbit causes proptosis. This, plus pituitary dysfunction due to involvement of the sella, and x-ray rarefaction of other skull bones, constitutes a common and classic triad of the disease.

the marrow is frequently sufficiently invaded to cause an anemia.

The skin is involved in less than one third of the cases. The typical lesions are yellow nodules and plaques in the corium covered with a thin layer of epiderm. At times the latter ulcerates and chronic, ragged craters persist complicated by an indolent infection.

Hypercholesterolemia and hyperlipemia have been reported frequently, particularly in the earlier papers, but most authors now agree that alterations in the serum lipids are unusual and are probably not characteristic. Eosinophilia has been reported in a few cases, particularly since an association with eosinophilic granuloma has been stressed. The eosinophilic leukocyte count has never been very high and is probably of no significance. Mild fever and leukocytosis have been mentioned in a few instances.

Microscopy. The diagnosis of Hand-

For Roentgenographic Manifestations see page 214.

Schüller-Christian disease can be made with finality only by examination of involved tissue under the microscope. Even with this evidence it is frequently necessary to supplement the microscopic picture with clinical and roentgenographic evidence because the microscopy varies and in some stages is entirely nonspecific.

The typical lesion of Hand-Schüller-Christian disease suggests that the reticulum and its derivatives of a more or less circumscribed area have become unable to process certain lipid substances with which they have come in contact. It is a popular concept that these lipids are normally processed by these cells but that because of a fault in their metabolic activities the cells can now only absorb them into their cytoplasmic substance where, instead of being processed and passed on, the lipids accumulate and eventually cause cell death and rupture with a spilling of the lipids into the supportive tissues of the area. The hypothesis that the disease is a systemic fault in lipid metabolism resulting in the circulation of an excessive amount of this material, which is eventually picked up by the phagocytic reticulum elements, lacks support in that if this were the case and the reticulum were healthy, one might expect all units of the normal reticulum to be affected equally. Universal involvement is seen in only the most florid cases of histiocytosis.

For a proper concept of the microscopic features of the lesion of Hand-Schüller-Christian disease one must realize that the cells specifically involved are those of the reticulum and its derivatives, particularly the motile, phagocytic cells, and that the elements of this system have the capacity of morphologic and apparently functional interchange. Thus the lesion seems to undergo a series of changes throughout its life cycle, and the terminal phase is quite different in appearance from the early stage. It should be kept in mind also that cells other than the specifically affected reticulum elements are usually involved, so that the character of the lesion may vary depending upon the tissue site. Thus it is small wonder that the pathologist frequently misses the diagnosis unless he maintains a high level of suspicion for this rather rare disease or unless he has the benefit of the roentgenologic and clinical data when he examines his sections.

The exact sequence of events in the early stages of the lesions of Hand-Schüller-Christian disease is probably not known with certainty, though in all instances there appears to be a migration or proliferation of large macrophages, monocytes or histiocytes in the affected area. Before the other events of the cycle take place, large fields of these cells may closely simulate neoplasm, and one must guard against the temptation to diagnose the lesion as Ewing's tumor (Fig. 7–2). At some time during the early stages of the cycle there is an influx of eosinophilic leukocytes, lymphocytes, plasma cells and neutrophils, their numerical incidence being approximately in the order named. At times the inflammatory reaction is more apparent than is the histiocytic nature, and a diagnosis of nonspecific osteomyelitis may be made. In at least some lesions the eosinophilic leukocytes may completely dominate the picture, and unless the lesions are known to be multiple a diagnosis of eosinophilic granuloma is quite understandable. At some time in the course of the cycle, usually late, collections of lipids are noted within the cytoplasm of the histiocytes. At first the cytoplasm is granular, then vacuolated and finally swollen and foamy. Many of the nuclei appear to shrink and to become more pyknotic (Fig. 7–3). Tissue necrosis occurs and there is an admixture of detritus among the cell components. Eventually some of the histiocytes rupture and the lipid material collects in the intracellular spaces. In hematoxylin-eosin stained preparations one finds sharply pointed clefts in the tissue, the sites of crystals of cholesterol before they were dissolved in the processing fluids. A foreign body reaction is engendered by the presence of the lipids and multinucleated giant cells make their appearance. This is the cytologic picture that one usually thinks of as characteristic of Hand-Schüller-Christian disease (Fig. 7–4). The background is composed of histiocytes, many of them lipid-bearing, exudative inflammatory cells, particularly eosinophilic

leukocytes, necrosis, intercellular cholesterol crystals and giant cells. Soon the inflammatory reaction becomes less apparent and the exudative cells may disappear entirely. Collagenoblasts appear and gradually dominate the picture, probably as a transition of the histiocytes that were not too damaged by their lipid content. Eventually the lesion may be converted to a collagenized scar showing crystals of cholesterol and perhaps some foreign body reaction (Fig. 7–5).

The differentiation of Hand-Schüller-Christian disease and eosinophilic granuloma cannot be made on a cytologic basis alone. The majority of the solitary lesions occurring after the age of 10 years turn out to be the latter though occasionally even one of these cases may run a course with the development of multiple lesions that is much more like a mild Hand-Schüller-Christian disease.

The lesions of Letterer-Siwe disease are usually quite unlike those just described. The histiocytic aggregates are present and often an exudative inflammatory reaction occurs, but the lipid element is usually considerably less evident and sometimes cannot be found at all, leading to the term "nonlipid histiocytosis." The foreign body reaction usually does not appear.

There is usually very little attempt at regeneration of the destroyed bone in Hand-Schüller-Christian disease. This may possibly be accounted for on the basis of an interruption of the blood supply. If fracture occurs, there is apt to be callus formation with spicules of new bone and islands of cartilage. Then the picture may be exceedingly difficult to interpret.

Rarely, one may encounter cortical "expansion" over a large lesion of Hand-Schüller-Christian disease. In two such lesions we found accompanying aneurysmal bone cyst. The latter apparently may be superimposed on almost any type of bone injury and the cortical "expansion" is apparently the result of the aneurysmal bone cyst rather than the primary lesion.

Much of the lipid material that appears in the lesions of this disease can be stained with Sudan III or scharlach R. It is doubly refractile with polarized light, and analysis has shown it to consist largely of cholester-

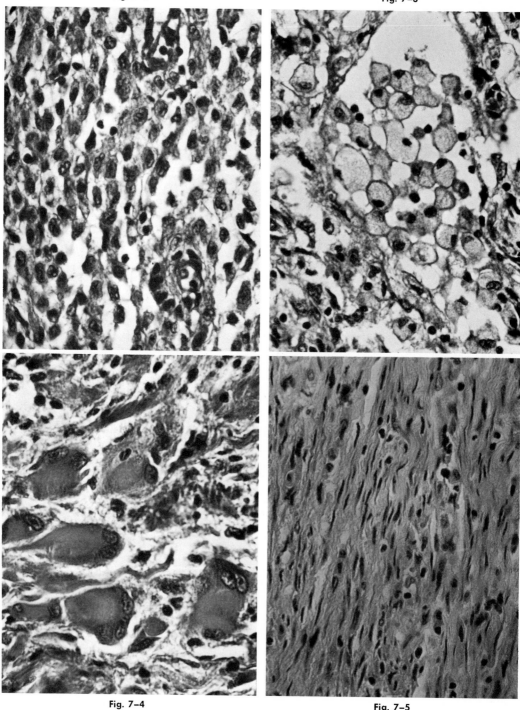

Fig. 7–2

Fig. 7–3

Fig. 7–4

Fig. 7–5

Figure 7–2 Hand-Schüller-Christian disease. The early lesion may consist largely of macrophages (histiocytes or epithelioid cells). The nuclei are large, pale and often have triangular or reniform outlines. Abnormal amounts of fat may be hard to demonstrate at this stage. The uniformity of the cells may suggest neoplasm. This type of lesion cannot be differentiated from eosinophilic granuloma. (× 450.)

Figure 7–3 Hand-Schüller-Christian disease. At some time (usually early) the macrophages begin to fill with lipid. The cytoplasm becomes swollen with pale granules or vacuoles. The nucleus shrinks and becomes pyknotic. (× 450.)

Figure 7–4 Hand-Schüller-Christian disease. Giant cells soon form and these with the other elements plus lymphocytes and eosinophilic cells constitute the characteristic picture of the disease. (× 450.)

Figure 7–5 Hand-Schüller-Christian disease. Following degeneration, the lesion is converted to collagenizing fibrous tissue which remains as the scar of the active lesion. (× 450.)

ol and cholesterol esters. However, it is almost certain that the lipids involved constitute a group in which, though cholesterol is most abundant, there are traces of a variety of other complex lipoid substances. This is another reason to suggest that the fault lies not in the systemic metabolism of a specific lipid but rather in a cellular defect involving a group of related chemical substances.

Prognosis. Approximately one half of the cases of Hand-Schüller-Christian disease have terminated fatally, though with proper roentgen therapy or prednisone many patients have survived over a period of years and as yet no one knows what the eventual prognosis will be. In the florid cases, beginning early in life, the outcome is dubious no matter what the therapy, though since a few cases of Letterer-Siwe disease have reportedly responded to antibiotic and other agents it is probable that this field has not been fully exploited as yet. Visceral involvement is a bad prognostic omen and if the infiltration is extensive, death is apt to occur within two years.

EOSINOPHILIC GRANULOMA

Eosinophilic granuloma of bone is a disease entity in which one or more focal areas of bone are destroyed by a granulomatous process of unknown etiology. The striking similarity of the microscopy of these lesions to those of Hand-Schüller-Christian disease has led most observers to consider the two conditions variants of the same process.

On January 13, 1940, Otani and Ehrlich[11] submitted for publication a paper entitled "Solitary Granuloma of Bone" and on January 19 of the same year Lichtenstein and Jaffe[12] submitted a paper entitled "Eosinophilic Granuloma of Bone" to the same journal. The first was published in July and the second in September of that year. These were the first papers in the American literature to report this common condition as a pathologic entity though both papers credit the Italian and German literature with earlier descriptions of the disease. In April, 1941, Farber,

Green and McDermott[13] read a paper before the American Association of Pathologists and Bacteriologists in which they stated that they believed that eosinophilic granuloma (using the name suggested by Lichtenstein and Jaffe), Hand-Schüller-Christian disease and Letterer-Siwe disease were all variants of the same process, and in 1942 they published a series of ten cases in support of this hypothesis.[14] Today, most observers subscribe to this opinion because enough data have been accumulated, both clinical and pathological, to corroborate the original observations.

Most cases of eosinophilic granuloma are seen in childhood, adolescence or early adult life and there is a considerable male predominance, when the reported cases are pooled. In almost half the cases there are two or more lesions. The most common site is in one or both frontal bones though lesions have been described in almost every bone of the skeleton. They rarely occur in the small bones of the hands and feet. When they involve the vertebrae they may cause vertebra plana.[15]

Extraosseous, soft tissue eosinophilic granulomas have been reported but when unassociated with bone lesions they constitute a vague group, the identity and significance of which is difficult to evaluate. Recently, multiple nodules within the lungs have been found accompanying typical bone lesions.[16] We have had the opportunity of examining material from one such case.

Eosinophilic granuloma usually causes some pain though as a rule it is not severe. When it occurs in the vicinity of a joint the symptoms may suggest the diagnosis of arthritis. Sometimes the onset is relatively sudden, which is hard to explain in terms of the underlying tissue alterations.

Unlike most of the true neoplasms of bone, eosinophilic granuloma has no predilection for any particular area within the bone, appearing within the diaphysis of long bones as often as within the metaphysis. The contiguous cortex melts away and the granuloma frequently extends out into the soft tissue. The surgeon may be surprised, having curetted an eosinophilic granuloma of one of the skull bones, to find that he has exposed the dura or even the brain. The lesion is usually small when discovered, often not more than a few millimeters in diameter, but it may become much larger. Occasionally very large, poorly delineated lesions are encountered. The curetted tissue is soft, nondescript red or mottled gray and rarely contains bone fragments. Its vascularity is not remarkable. Cultures of the tissue are sterile.

A few cases have manifested a moderately elevated eosinophilic leukocyte count in the peripheral blood, but this finding is so inconstant that it is of little diagnostic value.

Microscopy. The term "eosinophilic granuloma" is an admirably descriptive one for the majority of these lesions when examined through the microscope. The matrix usually consists of a reticulated mass of histiocytes infiltrated with eosinophilic leukocytes. The latter may be so numerous that they form solid masses occupying a large portion of the low power field, staining the area a deep brick red. The eosinophilic cells rarely may be filamented forms, but usually they are younger and often are eosinophilic myelocytes or more often bi-lobed structures. Charcot-Leyden crystals frequently have been reported within the cytoplasm. Ayres and Silliphant[17] found Charcot-Leyden crystals in 97 of 100 cases of eosinophilic granuloma. Because these crystals have been associated with allergic reactions, this pathogenesis has been suggested for eosinophilic granuloma. When these cells are numerous the diagnosis can hardly be missed (Fig. 7–6). At times, however, the eosinophilic cells may be scant or lacking. There may be a prevalence of lymphocytes, of plasma cells or even of neutrophilic granulocytes; all types may be represented, or there may be no leukocytes at all. Occasionally the lesion may consist entirely of masses of rather immature histiocytes (Fig. 7–7). Such lesions have led to the mistaken histologic diagnosis of myeloma in the past.

As the process matures, lipid material can be demonstrated within the cytoplasm of the phagocytic histiocytes (Fig. 7–7).

For Roentgenographic Manifestations see page 214.

Eventually this substance may become quite obvious even with routine hematoxylin-eosin stains though in the very early lesions it may be entirely lacking. Necrosis soon takes place and the histiocytes pick up nuclear fragments and debris. Apparently the lipid content of the macrophages becomes so great that they die and contribute this material to the detritus. Giant cells are formed (Fig. 7–8), probably by the agglomeration of histiocytes, and these too act as phagocytizing agents. The lipid accumulates in crystals to form slit-like, pointed clefts. Gradually the exudative inflammatory reaction subsides and fibroblasts begin to dominate the section. We assume that the lesion eventually becomes completely fibrosed. Much of the lipid material can be stained with scharlach R and it is seen to be doubly refractile when examined with polarized light. It has been identified as cholesterol and cholesterol esters.

When one examines a series of sections of eosinophilic granuloma of varying stages and compares the microscopy with that of Hand-Schüller-Christian disease, one is impressed with the similarity, within the broad range of the varying pictures of the two conditions. It is now generally believed that the former is a focal and often solitary manifestation of the latter. The clinical findings in a number of cases support this thesis.

Prognosis. Eosinophilic granuloma is usually considered an innocuous condition, completely cured by curettage, x-ray therapy or a variety of drugs. These lesions have been treated with cortisone and with various antimetabolic drugs with apparent success. In a few cases, however, the condition has progressed to a state that cannot be differentiated from Hand-Schüller-Christian disease. If the lesions are multiple, begin in early childhood and especially if there is accompanying visceral involvement, the prognosis should be guarded.

LETTERER-SIWE DISEASE

Letterer-Siwe disease, which has been called nonlipid reticuloendotheliosis, is a fulminant disturbance of the total body

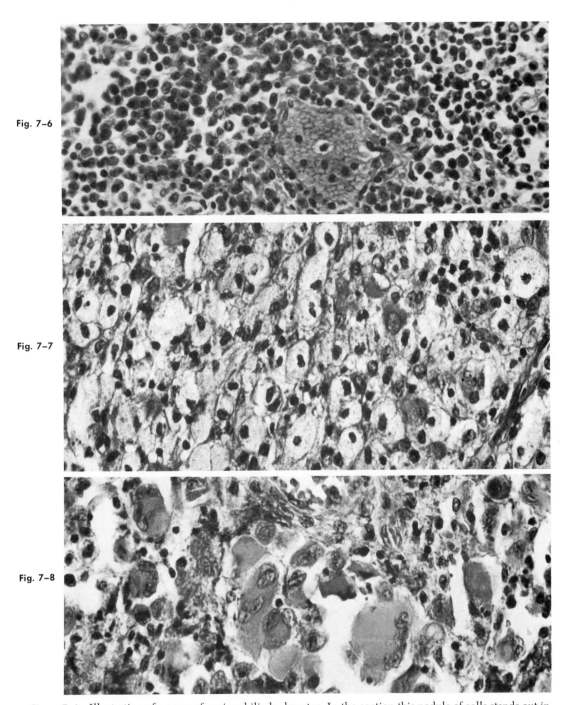

Fig. 7–6

Fig. 7–7

Fig. 7–8

Figure 7–6   Illustration of a mass of eosinophilic leukocytes. In the section this nodule of cells stands out in vivid contrast to the surrounding tissue but in the photograph it appears only as a rounded aggregate of cells the cytoplasm of which is darker. Some plasmacytes and neutrophils are intermixed with the eosinophils. Note that the nuclei of eosinophilic granulocytes are much less dramatically lobulated than those of neutrophilic leukocytes. (× 450.)

Figure 7–7   Macrophages have picked up large amounts of pale-staining lipid which swells the cytoplasm and causes the nuclei to become pyknotic. Some of the cells show evidence of bursting with escape of the lipid contents. (× 450.)

Figure 7–8   Eventually giant cells characterize the lesion. They probably arise as a result of the lipids which are spilled into the tissue. Exudative inflammatory cells are the result of degenerative changes. (× 450.)

reticulum apparatus with manifestations referable to the principal reticulum stations, the bone marrow, spleen, lymph nodes and liver and often the skin. It will be described only briefly here because it can be construed as orthopedic pathology only by virtue of its relation to Hand-Schüller-Christian disease and eosinophilic granuloma.

This condition as originally described by Letterer[18] and later by Siwe[19] is a disease of infants. The onset is usually quite sudden, often with symptoms of an acute infection. In the course of a blood analysis it is usually found that there is an anemia and a thrombocytopenia. If leukemia develops the condition should probably be diagnosed as neoplastic reticulocytosis. It becomes obvious that there is a disturbance in marrow function. The patient develops pallor and bleeding phenomena with petechial hemorrhages in the skin (Fig. 7–9) that become macular and finally confluent. Resistance to infection is lost. The spleen and liver become greatly en-

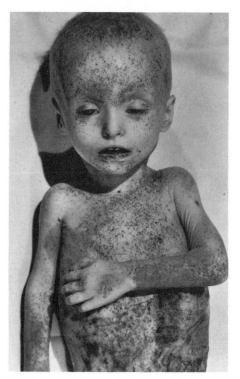

Figure 7–9 Letterer-Siwe disease. Replacement of bone marrow induces a myelophthisic anemia and bleeding phenomena. Petechial and macular hemorrhages are highly characteristic findings.

larged and lymphadenopathy of peripheral and deep nodes usually becomes prominent. Until relatively recently all cases terminated fatally, usually within one to three months. In 1940, Glanzman[20] suggested that Letterer-Siwe disease is a fulminant variety of Hand-Schüller-Christian disease, and in 1941 Farber et al.[21] expressed the belief that these two conditions and eosinophilic granuloma are all different manifestations of the same disease process. Since the last named is a granuloma and was thought at that time to be of probable infectious origin, massive doses of antibiotics were given in a few cases diagnosed as Letterer-Siwe disease with survival.

Today, the etiology of Letterer-Siwe disease remains unknown and the question of correct diagnosis must of necessity arise in any cases that survive. Most observers believed that the disturbance represents an incapacity of the reticulum apparatus to process certain lipids, of which cholesterol and its esters appear to predominate.

Microscopy. Knowledge of the cytologic aspects of Letterer-Siwe disease has come from needle aspiration biopsies of the bone marrow and spleen and from several thorough necropsy studies.[22]

The bone marrow is almost completely replaced by a proliferation of the reticulum and its derivatives (Fig. 7–10). This proliferation so packs the medullary regions that it may cause a diffuse demineralization and thinning of the cortex. At the ends of cylindrical bones where hematopoietic tissue predominates, the deossification may be so accentuated as to resemble tumor. The sections are composed largely of young histiocytes. In some cases lipid material was searched for and not found and this led to the term "nonlipid histiocytosis." In most instances, however, the lipid, though not as obvious as in Hand-Schüller-Christian disease, is quite apparent and its presence can be surmised even with hematoxylin-eosin technique.

The same type of cell dominates the sections of spleen, lymph nodes and liver (Figs. 7–11 and 7–12). In the first, large areas of necrosis and hemorrhage are apt to occur because of interference with the blood supply. There may be myeloid meta-

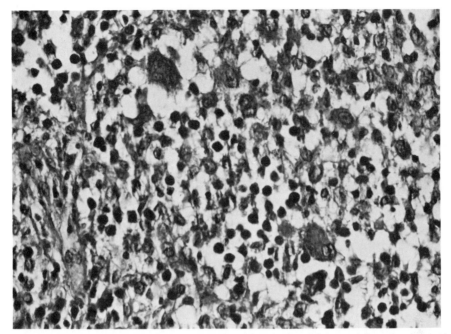

Figure 7–10 Letterer-Siwe disease. Marrow tissue has been replaced by a proliferation of reticulum. Note the large cells, some of them with multiple nuclei, and the lymphocytes which infiltrate the lesion. (× 450.)

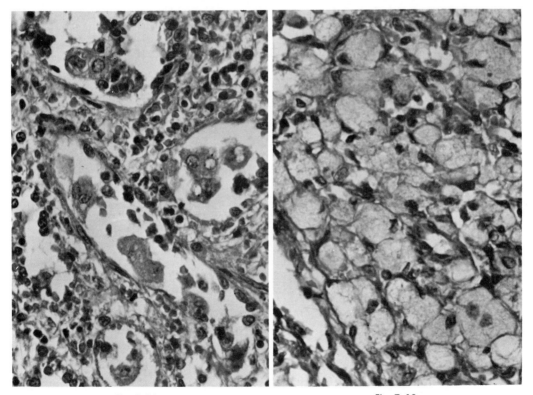

Fig. 7–11   Fig. 7–12

Figure 7–11 Letterer-Siwe disease. A section from the spleen reveals numerous lipid-filled macrophages within the sinusoids. (× 450.)

Figure 7–12 Letterer-Siwe disease. Section taken from a lymph node. The fibrous trabeculae are infiltrated with lipid-filled macrophages. (× 450.)

plasia, and occasional megakaryocytes occur. Unless the pathologist maintains a high index of suspicion for the lipid histiocytoses the sections may be misinterpreted as atypical leukemia. If the clinical aspects of the case are known the diagnosis should be apparent.

Prognosis. Typical Letterer-Siwe disease always occurs in infants, usually under 1 year of age. The originally reported cases all terminated fatally within a period of a few weeks or months. More recently some cases, treated with massive doses of antibiotics or cancerocidal chemotherapy or both, have survived. A few have developed a clinical picture like that of Hand-Schüller-Christian disease. It is still unproven that either of the agents

mentioned has been curative because doubt must always arise in the unautopsied case as to whether it was true Letterer-Siwe disease. If it can be shown that the antibiotics will cure a reasonable proportion of the cases, this would be strong evidence for an infectious agent as the cause of the three related cholesterol histiocytoses. On the other hand, if nitrogen mustard or another cancer chemotherapeutic agent can be shown to benefit Letterer-Siwe disease it would suggest that this particular type falls in the category of the neoplastic reticulocytoses. Since both diseases are dominantly characterized by a proliferation of histiocytes, therapeutic trial may be the only means of differentiating them in some instances.

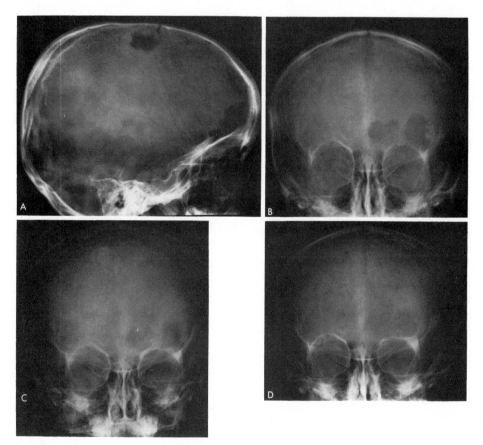

Figure 7–13 Multiple lesions of the cranial bones secondary to Hand-Schüller-Christian disease in a white male 5 years of age. Exophthalmos on the left was the presenting complaint. *A* and *B* represent the initial radiographs; *C*, a radiograph six months later and *D*, a radiogram exposed 12 months after the original examination. The initial lesions have sharply defined, although irregular, margins. Three large defects are evident, probably the result of confluence of multiple smaller ones. Healing, as shown in *C*, is manifest by an indistinctness of the borders of the lesions and a diminution in their size. In *D*, healing has progressed even further and the medial of the two defects is barely visible.

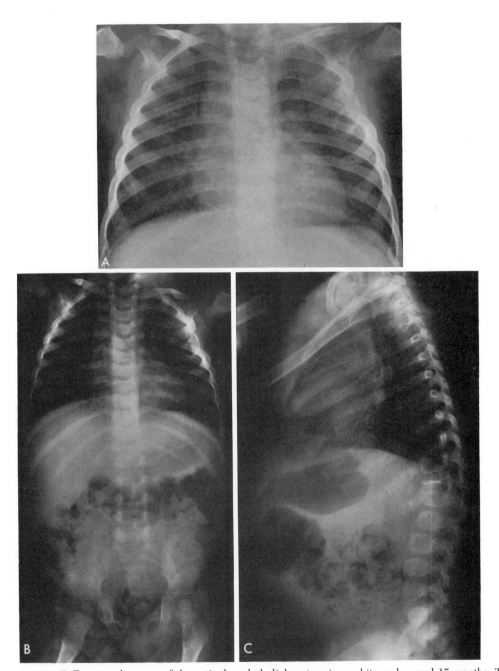

Figure 7–14 Diffuse involvement of the reticuloendothelial system in a white male, aged 15 months. The skin was involved as were numerous lymph nodes, the liver and spleen. The disease was fatal. The histologic findings were compatible with Letterer-Siwe disease, as were the clinical and radiographic manifestations. A illustrates miliary-like involvement of the lungs which may simulate tuberculosis. Such involvement may also be seen in Hand-Schüller-Christian disease and eosinophilic granuloma. B and C show deformity of the twelfth dorsal vertebra as well as lesions of the proximal left femur, the right pubic bone and the fourth left rib. The vertebral deformity may be seen as an isolated lesion and may be the only manifestation of an eosinophilic granuloma. The intervertebral disc above and below the involved vertebral body is of normal stature.

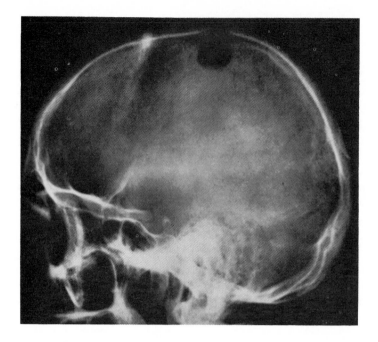

Figure 7-15 The solitary lesion of eosinophilic granuloma as it involved the skull of a 22 year old white male. A soft tissue mass was present over the defect in the parietal bone. The lesion is punched out but does present a sequestrum in its center. The latter is an unusual finding, but has been documented in the literature. There is no sclerosis about the round radiolucent defect.

Roentgenographic Manifestations of the Non-Neoplastic Histiocytoses. The radiographic manifestations of Hand-Schüller-Christian disease, eosinophilic granuloma and Letterer-Siwe disease will be considered together. The osseous lesions of all are secondary to granulomatous proliferation of the intraosseous reticulum and its derivatives, and radiographically have similar patterns. Radiographs may reveal hepatosplenomegaly and pulmonary infiltrates, which are the result of systemic reticulum involvement. The pulmonary involvement may present as miliary densities, as areas of linear infiltrate or result in diffuse cystic lesions.

A sharply defined radiolucent defect is the characteristic bony lesion. It is round or oval with no surrounding sclerosis and may be described as "punched out." The defect represents a granuloma that has destroyed bone and is of the density of soft tissue. There is no bony reaction to the destructive process except as the cortex of a cylindrical bone is destroyed and the periosteum elevated and stimulated to produce bone (Fig. 7-16). Flat bones are more frequently involved than are cylindrical bones.

Cranial bones are probably the most commonly affected, and often small lesions enlarge and coalesce to form a large irregular defect. Periosteal new bone is not a feature of the cranial lesions, and both inner and outer tables may be destroyed. Characteristically the lesion in the skull has a beveled edge so that the appearance is that of a hole within a hole.[24]

The area of destruction in a cylindrical bone initially involves the medullary canal in most instances. As it enlarges, the inner aspect of the cortex may be eroded and periosteal new bone may result if the erosion progresses. The lesion in this instance may mimic a malignant neoplasm of bone such as Ewing's tumor, although the new bone tends to be solid and not interrupted or spiculated. Periosteal new bone is evident too if a fracture occurs through a lesion. The epiphyseal centers may be involved.

When a vertebral body is affected, it loses stature. It may present as a thin dense plate. The intervertebral discs above and below maintain their normal width. Such an affected vertebra, when seen as an isolated lesion, should be considered as being due to one of the reticuloendothelioses until proved otherwise.

Healing of the osseous lesions starts at the periphery of the defect and proceeds centrally. The margins become indistinct, and gradually the lesion fills in with new bone. During the healing

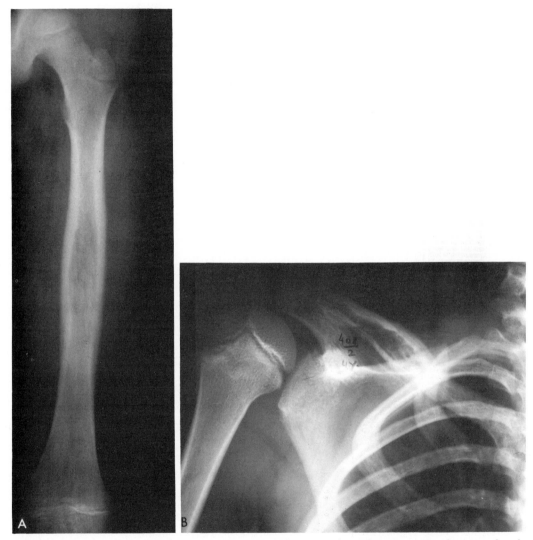

Figure 7-16 Eosinophilic granuloma. Two patients, each 4 years of age, demonstrate involvement of a tubular bone. In the femoral diaphysis (A) the medullary canal is wide and there is appositional new bone present that "expands" the shaft. The same phenomenon is present in the clavicle (B) but there are areas of more discrete endosteal destruction.

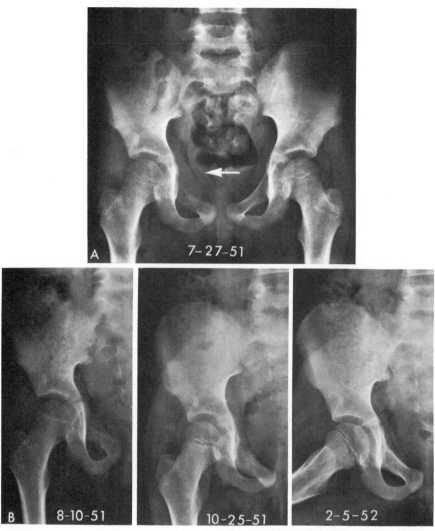

Figure 7–17 Eosinophilic granuloma. *A*, The initial examination reveals destruction of the right pubic bone associated with a soft tissue mass (arrow). *B*, Progress to healing is illustrated over the ensuing seven months.

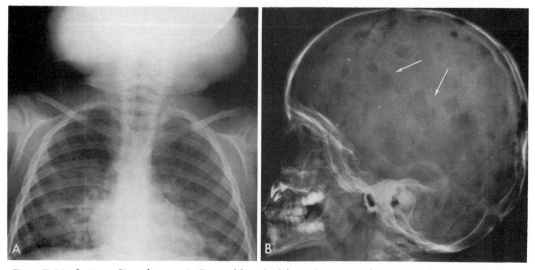

Figure 7–18 Letterer-Siwe disease. *A*, Cervical lymphadenopathy is present and the pulmonary infiltration is linear and patchy in contrast with the miliary densities illustrated in Figure 7–14 *A*. *B*, There are multiple lytic defects in the cranial bones; some are irregular in contour (arrows) reflecting confluence of smaller lesions.

phase, particularly if it is protracted, the margins become dense. There are no residual osseous manifestations in the majority of instances.

It must be recognized that the osseous defect is not an empty space but is occupied by a soft tissue mass. This mass of tissue causes secondary effects such as exophthalmos when bones of the orbit are involved. There may be increased intracranial pressure with widening of the cranial sutures. Mandibular involvement may destroy tooth sockets and be responsible for the extrusion of teeth. Mastoiditis may be suspected clinically when the temporal bone is involved.

THE NEOPLASTIC RETICULOCYTOSES

In the histiocytoses the organ affected is the reticuloendothelial system. The exact nature of the various types of this disease is poorly understood but the manifestations appear to relate to an inability of the reticulum, or a segment or area of reticulum, or one or more cell derivatives of reticulum (histiocytes) to process one or another lipid metabolite. The severity of the disease apparently depends upon the amount of the system involved. In the most grave of the three types, Letterer-Siwe disease, most or all of the reticulum system is involved; in Hand-Schüller-Christian disease multiple focal areas are affected, while in eosinophilic granuloma only one or at most a couple of sites are concerned.

Our understanding of the disease has been delayed because until recently we have confused cancer of the reticulum or its derivatives with these diseases, the histiocytoses.

This type of cancer is rare but it does occur in a variety of forms. It is most easily recognizable when it occurs as a leukemia of one of the reticulum cell derivatives, most commonly monocytic leukemia. But it may erupt as a fixed tissue sarcoma such as one we saw implanted on Gaucher's disease, or as in another case in our collection it may begin as a solitary lesion of eosinophilic granuloma and evolve into eosinophilic leukemia. A discussion of the neoplastic affections of the reticuloendothelial system does not belong in a text of orthopedic pathology. We mention them here only to emphasize that we occasionally must differentiate them from the histiocytoses.

GAUCHER'S DISEASE

Cerebroside reticulocytosis, usually called "Gaucher's disease," is a disturbance in which there is an excessive production of histiocytes, most of which become filled with a complex lipid, a cerebroside known as kerasin. Aggregates of these cells accumulate in the spleen, liver, bone marrow and skin. Symptoms are referable to enlargement of the spleen and liver, interference with marrow function and destruction of bone.

The disease was described in the French literature by Gaucher in 1882. Since then the condition has been extensively discussed by Pick[25] and others. It is stated that there are two forms, an infantile variety, which runs a fulminant course and is fatal within 18 months, and a more chronic form, the initial symptoms of which may appear at any period of life though usually before the age of 40. Clinically, the two types are completely different because in the infantile variety the brain is prominently involved and, therefore, the course is much like that of Niemann-Pick disease. Indeed, it is usually impossible, apparently, to distinguish the two except by chemical analysis of the involved tissues. Since in the fulminant, infantile types of lipid reticuloendothelioses a variety of complex lipids are usually involved, one might question whether, on the basis of the few analyses that have been done in these rare cases, a separate entity—acute, infantile Gaucher's disease—actually exists.

The usual form of the disease begins insidiously. The older literature states that Gaucher's disease usually begins during the first decade but more recent reports describe the onset of symptoms occurring quite equally scattered along the first half of the life span.[25] This discrepancy may arise from the possibility that incipient cases are frequently discovered today in the older age group by more efficient diagnostic tools, such as x-ray and liver and spleen puncture.

A familial and hereditary incidence is found in approximately one third of the cases. Though about half the cases are found among the Caucasian groups in the United States there appears to be a somewhat higher incidence in the Jewish race. The word "race" is used advisedly here because whether defined by geography, color or religion, interbreeding for centuries causes recessive features to recur with such frequency that they become characteristic of the group, thus establishing a distinct strain or race.

The most common site of involvement causing symptoms is the spleen, though if the bone marrow is carefully searched the characteristic tissue changes are found in possibly every case. The spleen may reveal a very moderate enlargement for many years. In most cases it eventually becomes huge and may fill practically the entire abdominal cavity. The small spleens are symptomless but, as they enlarge, they give rise to pain and a sense of dragging discomfort. These symptoms in themselves may necessitate splenectomy.

Enlargement of the liver in Gaucher's disease does not usually give rise to symptoms though in a few cases mildly altered liver function tests have been recorded.

Changes in the skin and conjunctivae are noted in a high percentage of cases if they are looked for. Irregular, poorly delineated, light tan areas appear in the skin of the exposed parts. It is uncertain what causes this pigmentation though it is assumed that the color is due to excessive lipochrome pigment within the reticulum elements of the corium. Brownish tan pingueculae may appear in the sclerae. These lesions have led some authors to classify Gaucher's disease with the idiopathic xanthomatoses, unjustifiably because the offending lipid of the xanthoma is cholesterol.

Symptoms of bone marrow involvement are usual though they may not appear until the disease is well advanced. These findings arise from a marrow depression due to replacement of hematopoietic tissue. All three elements are involved. The anemia is of the hypochromic type and is usually not more than moderately severe. The fall in erythrocyte count is usually accompanied by a leukopenia. A thrombocytopenia may be suspected in a high percentage of patients who complain of ecchymoses on mild trauma. The blood picture is apt to return toward normal, at least for a considerable period, following splenectomy. The lymph nodes are usually not prominently involved until the late stages of the disease and then often only the deep nodes become enlarged.

The changes in the skeleton are usually found by a roentgenographic skeletal survey, done only after the diagnosis is suspected because of an enlarged spleen or a depressed marrow function. Since it is the marrow reticulum that is involved, any bone bearing hematopoietic tissue may be affected; thus, depending upon the age, any or nearly all bones may show the lesions. A particularly high incidence has been reported in the femurs, vertebrae, ribs, sternum and flat bones of the pelvis. It is said that the cylindrical bones of the lower extremity are involved more often than are those of the arms. Masses of lipid-bearing marcophages may pack the intramedullary spaces causing erosion of the cortices from the inside. Since the process is very slow, appositional bone is laid down on the outer cortical surfaces of the involved areas and thus an "expansile" lesion is produced at the ends of long, cylindrical bones, particularly at the lower ends of the femurs. The process does not involve cartilage so that the epiphyses are spared except by extension from nearby centers of hematopoiesis. When this occurs there may be collapse of the head like that of epiphyseal ischemic necrosis (Perthes' disease). Gaucher's disease must always be considered when idiopathic ischemic necrosis of the femoral head is encountered in the adult. This may lead to symptoms of arthritis and severe disability. The cortices may be so extensively eroded and weakened that pathologic fractures result. Compression fractures of the vertebrae are relatively common in the advanced stage of the disease. Fractures of the ribs and long bones of the extremities are also reported (Fig. 7–21).

The focal lesions develop so slowly that, like enchondromas, they usually do not cause bone pain. Occasionally pain is the presenting symptom but it is probable that in these cases there has been infraction or the joint is affected.

The blood chemistry reveals no alterations of diagnostic significance.

Several analyses have been done of the lipid material that appears to be the offending agent in Gaucher's disease. All are in accord that the lipid in greatest abundance is a cerebroside, i.e., a lipid-linked carbohydrate with nitrogen. Here agreement ends. The carbohydrate of normal kerasin is galactose. Some chemists have isolated galactose, others glucose, and still others a combination of both. Phospholipids and cholesterol in smaller amounts have also been found. It has been suggested that there may be two types of Gaucher's disease, one with a cerebroside containing galactose and the other with glucose. Since, as yet, there is no evidence that the clinical course is influenced by the chemistry of the lipid at fault, it is probably wiser to accept the concept that Gaucher's disease is a disturbance resulting in the inability of the reticulum and its motile derivatives to process certain carbohydrate-linked lipids. Because a variety of cerebrosides are found, along with other lipids, in an acute process of infancy, a disease that is quite different clinically from Gaucher's disease, this does not necessarily make it belong to this group.

The involved cerebroside is apparently phagocytized by the motile derivatives of the reticulum, most prominently the histiocytes. The material accumulates within these cells because of an inherited deficiency of glucose cerebrosidase.[26] The source of this lipid is probably degraded blood cell membranes. Since the molecules of glucose cerebroside cannot be broken down further they collect, distending the cell and converting it to a useless component of the lesion. In masses these cells interfere with the presence and function of vital tissues.

Gross Pathology. The spleen may enlarge to a huge mass weighing as much as 5000 grams. The consistency usually remains about normal or somewhat softened. The capsular surface of the large spleens usually shows areas of necrosis or hyalinized scars of healed necrotic portions. Throughout the parenchyma one usually finds mottled areas of pale yellow or gray, often intermixed with areas of necrosis and hemorrhage. The latter resemble irregular infarcts.

The enlarged liver may or may not reveal the aggregates of lipid material to the naked eye. Small pale areas against a red background may be identified in the bone marrow. These may coalesce to form large patches and streaks of obviously abnormal tissue.

Roentgenographic Manifestations. When abnormal reticulum cells accumulate in marrow the osseous lesions of bone destruction may become evident radiographically. The proliferation of Gaucher cells may involve the marrow cavity of one or more bones either in a

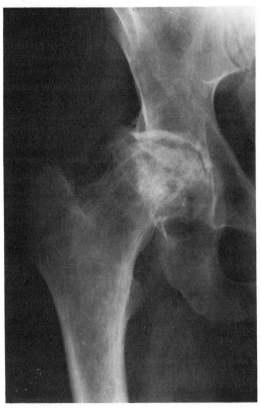

Figure 7-19 Gaucher's disease involving bone. Involvement of the femoral head in this male adult has resulted in destruction with deformity that may be confused with osteoarthritis. In the child, involvement of the femoral capital epiphysis mimics ischemic necrosis (Fig. 7-21). Note the radiolucent areas with irregular sclerosis about them.

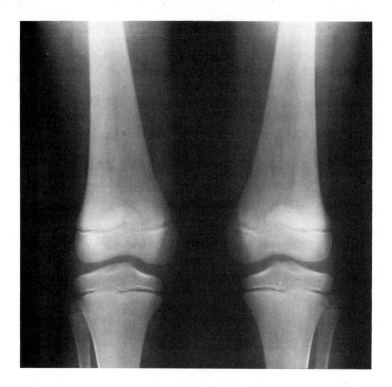

Figure 7-20 Gaucher's disease in a young girl as manifest by wide distal femurs, thin trabeculae and narrow cortices.

diffuse or localized manner. In either instance the lesions are predominantly radiolucent, although some observers believe that sclerosis about the lesions is common, the result of the formation of new bone. Any bone may be affected, but involvement of cranial bones and bones of the hands and feet is rare.

Diffuse involvement of the marrow cavity results in a wide medullary canal, a thin cortex and sparse trabeculae. Femoral involvement is usually of this type and expansion of the distal diaphysis is common (Erlenmeyer flask deformity). Localized radiolucent defects, sometimes cyst-like, may occur in any portion of a bone and pathologic fracture of weight-bearing bones so involved, particularly the femurs and vertebrae, is not uncommon. In those instances in which the disease is of long duration, periosteal new bone may be present as well as medullary sclerosis and evidence of infarction of bone. Epiphyseal destruction causes growth disturbance.

In the infant with Gaucher's disease visceral changes are more prominent than are osseous ones. Hepatomegaly and particularly splenomegaly are seen as well

as pulmonary infiltration. The patient with the infantile form of the disease lies in hyperextension.

The radiographic manifestations of Gaucher's disease may, therefore, present great variability, depending on the extent of osseous involvement, the speed with which the process progresses and the effects of bone destruction.

Microscopy. The diagnosis of Gaucher's disease may be made by aspiration biopsy of the bone marrow, the spleen or the liver. A careful search of the smears from the marrow may be necessary but usually the pathognomonic cells are found.

These cells are motile reticulum derivatives. They are often huge, measuring up to 75 microns. The substance of the cytoplasm is pale with the hematoxylin-eosin technique. It may have a crackle-glaze or crushed tissue paper appearance. These have been called "foam cells." The appearance is due to the presence of the kerasin that has accumulated within the cytoplasm that with electron microscopy is seen in long twisted strands. The nucleus is somewhat smaller and more heavily stained than that of the normal macrophage or histiocyte. This pyknosis is

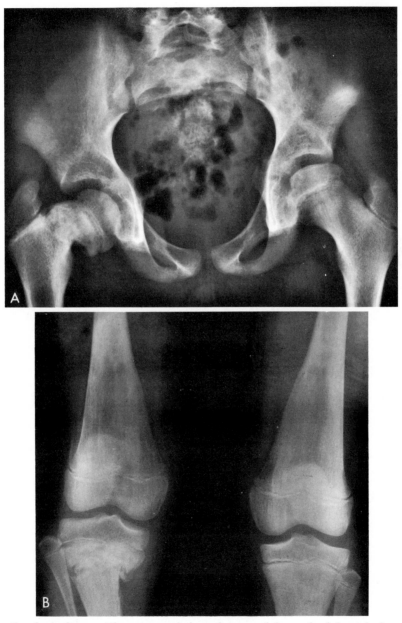

Figure 7–21 Gaucher's disease. There is a pathologic fracture of the neck of the right femur (A) and the proximal end of the right tibia (B). The left femoral capital epiphyseal center is opaque, and flat as a result of epiphyseal ischemic necrosis. The distal femurs are wide and their cortices thin. Sclerosis within the medullary canal of the femoral diaphysis is present.

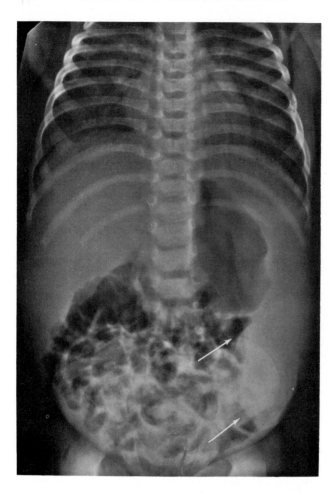

Figure 7–22 Gaucher's disease in a young infant. Hepatic and splenic (arrows) enlargement and pulmonary infiltration are present.

probably due to the altered intracellular metabolism. The nuclei may be multiple.

The foam cells may occur singly though they are usually found in aggregates, which may coalesce into huge sheets. In this event their appearance is monotonously similar. In the spleen they are found in the spongiosa between and often compressing the follicles (Fig. 7–23). In the liver they infiltrate the portal areas, and in the intramedullary regions they replace the marrow (Fig. 7–24).

Prognosis. The prognosis of the chronic form of Gaucher's disease is less grave than any of the other types of idiopathic lipid reticulocytosis with the exception of eosinophilic granuloma or some cases of xanthomatosis. The earlier the symptoms appear the more extensive the disease is apt to be, and the patient may succumb after a period of years because of the interference with marrow function. Splenectomy should alleviate these symptoms. It has been said that splenectomy increases the rate of bone involvement. When the reports of many cases are reviewed this does not appear to be true. Most patients, properly treated, lead a comfortable and uncurtailed life.

We have seen one patient in whom, after a number of years of Gaucher's disease, a sarcoma apparently of reticulum cell origin (Fig. 7–25) arose in the involved areas and rapidly metastasized, killing the patient. This event must be exceedingly rare because no account of a similar behavior can be found in the published reports.

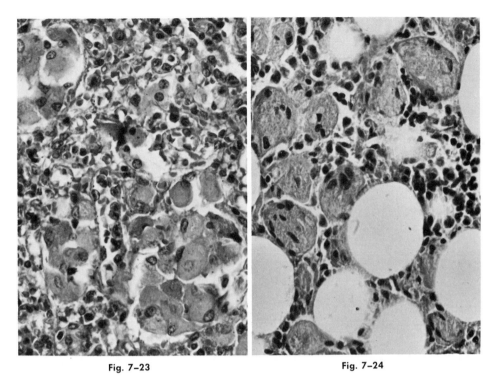

Fig. 7–23   **Fig. 7–24**

Figure 7–23 In the spleen one may find the sinusoids filled with lipid-containing macrophages (Gaucher's cells). This accumulation causes splenomegaly. (× 450.)

Figure 7–24 Large lipid-filled macrophages can be identified between the normal fat cells (the circular clear spaces) in the bone marrow. (× 450.)

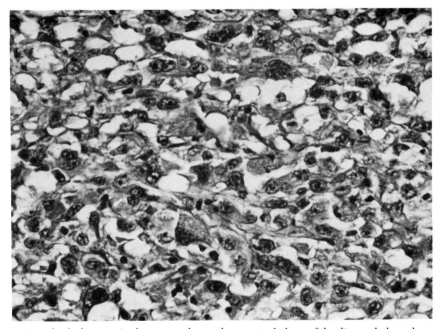

Figure 7–25 Gaucher's disease. In this unusual case the terminal phase of the disease behaved as a reticulum cell sarcoma. The section is composed of tumor reticulum cells. (× 450.)

NIEMANN-PICK DISEASE

Niemann-Pick disease is a disturbance in which abnormal quantities of the phospholipids and cholesterol are deposited in most of the mesenchymally derived tissues of the body and some of epithelial derivation. A brief account is given here only because the marrow is involved and because of the relation of this disease to the other lipid reticulocytoses.

The condition is rare. Members of the Jewish race are affected in about half the cases. Parental consanguinity has been noted in several of the cases in Gentiles. The disease practically always occurs in infants of less than 18 months of age though three cases of a very similar nature have been reported in adults. The disease is probably always fatal, usually within a year of onset.

The reticulum of the spleen, liver and lymph nodes is most dramatically involved, though deposits of lipid-bearing macrophages have been found in most other tissues. The cause of the disease is unknown though there is a strong familial incidence. Several siblings may be affected and in some series the adult blood relatives have shown nonsymptomatic enlargement of the spleen and liver.

Both fixed and motile phagocytic cells become engorged with a variety of lipids of which sphingomyelin predominates. These deposits of phosphosphingosides cause the remarkable enlargement of all the normal reticulum stations and typical cells have been found in the circulating blood. Marrow involvement eventually causes a hypochromic anemia. The serum neutral fat, cholesterol and phospholipid levels may be elevated.

Niemann-Pick disease is frequently associated with amaurotic familial idiocy (Tay-Sachs disease). It was originally thought that the cerebral involvement was merely an extension of the generalized process but analysis of the brains of some cases has shown a predominance of lecithin rather than sphingomyelin in the nerve tissue. When the brain is involved the cherry red macula and mental deterioration are to be expected. It is probable that the difference in the predominating phospholipid in the systemic tissues and the brain is due to native metabolic variation in the cells involved because it seems highly unlikely that two such rare entities would occur in the same patient if their mechanisms were distinctly different.

Abnormal pigmentation has been noted at the normal sites of lipochrome pigment, and a brownish discoloration has been described in the skin of the extensor surfaces of the joints.

The cells that store the involved lipid become swollen to many times their normal size, ranging from 20 to 60 microns. The material is seen within the cytoplasm with the Lorrain Smith and Weigert techniques, and by routine methods the cells have a foamy appearance. The striations that characterize the foam cells of Gaucher's disease are not seen and the Niemann-Pick cells are more finely vacuolated.

The reticulum of the bone marrow is probably always involved and the diagnosis may be corroborated by marrow aspiration. Since the disease is of relatively short duration, the bone itself may not be affected. In some cases a diffuse deossification has been noted and in at least one reported case there was said to be delay in the development of the ossification centers.

FAMILIAL NEUROVISCERAL LIPIDOSIS

In 1964 Landing and co-workers[29] reported eight cases of what appears to be a specific clinicopathologic entity in infants with radiologic features very similar to the Hunter-Hurler syndrome, marrow and hematologic characteristics suggesting Niemann-Pick disease, and failure of mental development and cherry red spots in the retina, which caused it to be classified with Tay-Sachs disease. Indeed, it had been reported previously under various titles, such as "pseudo-Hurler disease," "Hurler-variant" and "Tay-Sachs disease with visceral involvement."

Many types of cells throughout the body, including the blood leukocytes and monocytes, the marrow histiocytes, the ganglion cells of the brain, the parenchymal cells of the liver and the endothelial lining cells

Fig. 7-26

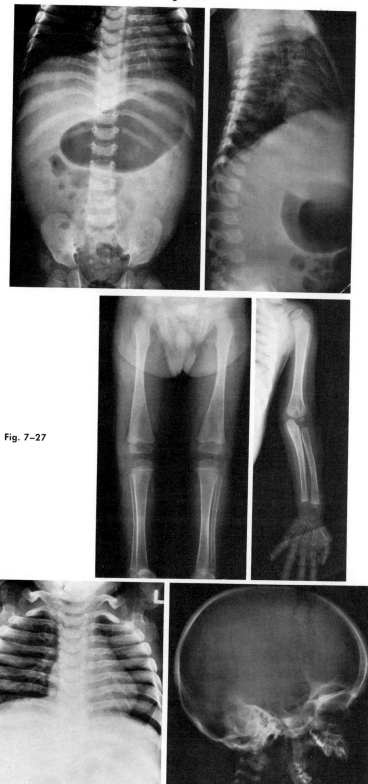

Fig. 7-27

Fig. 7-28   **Fig. 7-29**

Figures 7-26 to 7-29 Neurovisceral lipidosis. There are many features suggestive of Hurler's disease. The bodies of the twelfth thoracic and the first three lumbar vertebrae have an inferoanterior beak. The long bones are of normal length, but their cortices are thin and there is failure of modeling (Figs. 7-26 and 7-27). The ribs and clavicles are broad (Fig. 7-28). The cranial vault is enlarged, the sella is elongated and the articular condyle of the mandible is flat (Fig. 7-29).

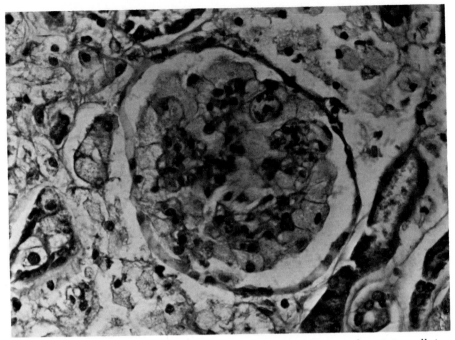

Figure 7-30   Neurovisceral lipidosis. Section of a glomerulus. A ring of large, pale-staining cells is seen about the periphery of the glomerular tuft. These cells contain the glycolipid that characterizes the disease. In severe cases the material may be seen within the lining cells of both Bowman's capsule and the tubule.

of the glomerular capillaries of the kidneys, contain intracytoplasmic granules and "vacuoles" of a chemical substance that has been identified as a soluble acidic lipid consistent with a ganglioside. All patients were dead by the twenty-first month, usually of chronic respiratory infection though one succumbed of myocardial arrhythmia due presumably to infiltration of the heart muscle with histiocytes laden with the sugar-linked lipid.

The radiologic features in the skeleton are very similar to those of Hurler's syndrome but probably occur earlier and run a more florid course. It has been suggested that probably many of the severe infantile cases of "Hurler's disease" with early death were, in truth, cases of neurovisceral lipidosis.

Mental involvement is profound, there is failure of development of motor function, the peripheral leukocytes contain Reilly granules, there is massive enlargement of the liver and spleen and a constant and pathognomonic feature is the presence of large quantities of the offending substance in the glomerular tufts, which may cause eventual kidney failure. Involve-

ment of bone marrow causes an anemia. The condition is familial.

Knowledge to date suggests that the pathogenesis of this condition is similar to that of the mucopolysaccharidoses, i.e., genetic depletion or alteration in enzymatic constitution resulting in abnormal metabolism of a ganglioside. It is at last becoming apparent that a number of the entities now grouped with the skeletal dysplasias or the reticuloendotheliosis have a common denominator in this type of pathogenesis, the variant being the chemical protagonist. Eventually we may find our classifications considerably simplified as, one after another, the skeletal alterations are explained on the basis of a metabolic defect in the osteoid-forming cells. For example, there is evidence to suggest that this disease is one of a group of abnormalities which have been characterized as mucolipidoses. The storage material affects the same cells as are involved in the mucopolysaccharidoses, hence the similarity in clinical and radiological findings. Thus neurovisceral lipidosis is classified as GM_1 gangliosidosis, type I. Mucolipidosis II, inclusion cell

(I-cell) disease, is a condition with similar findings in which inclusions are found in cultured skin fibroblasts and in which the lipid content of I-cells is increased but in which no specific lipid is stored.[30] Roentgen findings early in life are usually quite severe.

References

HAND-SCHÜLLER-CHRISTIAN DISEASE

1. Lichtenstein, L.: J. Bone Joint Surg., 46A:76, 1964.
2. Greenberg, E., Cohen, D., Pease, G. and Kyle, R.: Proc. Mayo Clin., 37:271, 1962.
3. Bierman, H.: J.A.M.A., 196:368, 1966.
4. Cox, P.: Gt. Ormond Str. J., 10:104, 1955–1956.
5. Siegel, J. and Cottman, C.: J.A.M.A., 197:123, 1966.
6. Hand, A.: Trans. Phila. Pathol. Soc., 16:1891–1893.
7. Hand, A.: Penn. Med. J., 9:520, 1905–1906.
8. Christian, H.: Contributions to Medical and Biological Research. New York. Paul B. Hoeber, vol. 1:390, 1919.
9. Rowland, R.: Arch. Intern. Med., 42:611, 1928.
10. Farber, S.: Am. J. Pathol., 17:625, 1941.

EOSINOPHILIC GRANULOMA

11. Otani, S. and Ehrlich, J.: Am. J. Pathol., 16:479, 1940.
12. Lichtenstein, L. and Jaffe, H.: Am. J. Pathol., 16:595, 1940.

13. Farber, S., Green, W. and McDermott, L.: Am. J. Pathol., 17:625, 1941.
14. Green, W., Farber, S. and McDermott, L.: J. Bone Joint Surg., 24:499, 1942.
15. Compere, E., Johnson, W. and Coventry, B.: J. Bone Joint Surg., 36A:969, 1954.
16. Childers, J., Middleton, J. and Schneider, M.: Ann. Intern. Med., 42:1287, 1955.
17. Ayres, W. and Silliphant, W.: Am. J. Clin. Pathol., 30:323, 1958.

LETTERER-SIWE DISEASE

18. Letterer, E.: Frankfurt. Z. Pathol., 30:377, 1924.
19. Siwe, S.: Z. Kinderheilkd., 55:212, 1933.
20. Glanzman, E.: Ann. Paediatr., 155:1, 1940.
21. Farber, S., Green, W. and McDermott, L.: Am. J. Pathol., 17:625, 1941.
22. Levinsky, W.: Arch. Pathol., 48:462, 1949.
23. Arcomano, J., Barnett, J. and Wunderlich, H.: Am. J. Roentgenol., 85:663, 1961.
24. Mosely, J. E.: Bone Changes in Hematologic Disorders. New York, Grune & Stratton, 1963.

GAUCHER'S DISEASE

25. Pick, L.: Med. Klin., 18:1408, 1922.
26. Lee, R.: Bull. Pathol. 234, July–August, 1969.
27. Medford, A. and Bayrd, E.: Ann. Intern Med., 40:481, 1954.
28. Levin, B.: Am. J. Roentgenol., 85:685, 1961.

FAMILIAL NEUROVISCERAL LIPIDOSIS

29. Landing, B., Silverman, F., Craig, J., Jacoby, M., Lahey, M. and Chadwich, D.: Am. J. Dis. Child., 108:503, 1964.
30. Progress in Pediatric Radiology. Intrinsic Diseases of Bones. Vol. 4. Kaufmann, H. J. (ed.). Basel, S. Karger, 1973.

SECTION THREE

DISTURBANCES IN THE NORMALLY FORMED SKELETON

Chapter 8

THE REPAIR OF FRACTURES

An understanding of fracture healing is a prerequisite of successful fracture treatment. It is regrettable that the physiology of the commonest of bone ailments cannot yet be completely described. We know a good deal about the formation of new bone and somewhat less about the lysis of dead bone, but the accounts of the chronologic order of the several stages in bone healing and the stimuli that direct their order find little agreement among authors who have written on the subject. The detailed examination of the entire pathologic structure at multiple intervals over the healing course in the experimental animal demands techniques that are unavailable to most. Such studies in man are obviously impossible and so much of our knowledge consists of fragments derived from animal experimentation pieced together with what fortuitous biopsies of human bone the surgeon has contributed. The danger of application of findings observed in the experimental animal to human physiology need not be emphasized here, but it is hardly out of place to remark that the processes of bone healing in the cat and in the dog are little more alike than their temperaments and are probably quite as different from the process as it occurs in the human.

Several modern writers[1] regard the hematoma consequent to fracture as an inactive by-product of no importance, an incidental occurrence that affects callus formation neither positively nor negatively. This opinion is apparently derived by observation of fracture healing in the animal. One should not contradict such opinions without carrying out the same experiments, but the experienced pathologist finds it

hard to believe that the hematoma of fracture can be so innocently innocuous when elsewhere in the body the hematoma plays such a very important role in the response to trauma. Moreover, the meager bits of tissue that we have been able to retrieve from human fractures of various ages strongly suggest that the hematoma does organize and that from the collagenous tissue that is thus provoked come important elements that eventually constitute the callus.

Some writers state that all or most of the bone tissue of callus is produced by the osteoblasts of the viable cambium and the endosteal lining cells.[2] Thus the callus is said to develop by the formation of two collars, one about the end of each fragment, which grow toward each other and eventually unite to form a bridge over the hiatus produced by the fracture. Examination of sections of fracture material leaves little doubt that these cells do produce bone and perhaps the preponderant part of the callus, but the ability of collagenoblasts to change into osteoblasts and chondroblasts in the callus medium is equally striking, and the bone and cartilage therefrom appear to be very important components of the healing process. Since healthy osteoid is mineralized and therefore becomes opaque to x-rays within a matter of hours to days after formation, if the collar or bridge hypothesis were correct one should be able to follow the progress of the advancing margins as these collars approach each other by a series of correctly timed roentgenograms. But such roentgenograms do not support this theory. Instead one perceives the full-blown callus as soon as its

Fig. 8–1

Fig. 8–2

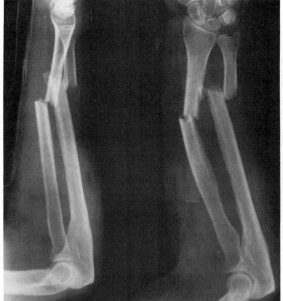

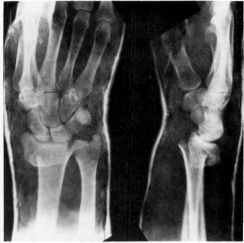

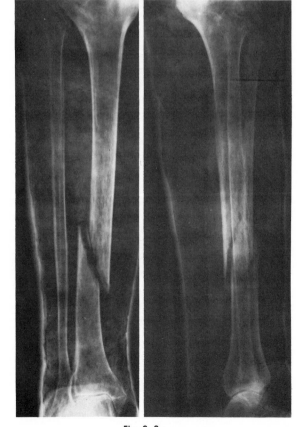

Figure 8–1 Transverse fracture of both bones of the forearm. A fracture line is radiolucent by virtue of discontinuity in the bone. Deformity is best described as the distal fragment relates to the proximal fragment.

Figure 8–2 Colles' fracture (distal radius and ulnar styloid).

Figure 8–3 Comminuted, oblique fracture of the tibia. The comminuted fragment lies adjacent to the medial aspect of the end of the proximal fragment.

Fig. 8–3

opacity is greater than the surrounding soft tissue, and though it increases in x-ray density as it collects osteoid and mineral, this density is diffuse rather than polar concentrations that eventually merge.

There has been a tendency recently to minimize the proclivity of collagenoblasts to form bone and cartilage by metaplasia. The experienced general pathologist who examines tissues from all parts of the body is not surprised to find this phenomenon in the most unexpected places. It has long been known that the presence of periosteum is not necessary for the formation of bone. If one causes a fracture in the experimental animal, strips the periosteum well back from the fracture ends, and ensheaths and connects the bare bone with a plastic cylinder, the hiatus is soon bridged by a rod of bone, which forms from granulation that has grown into the plastic sheath. More often than not, fragments of newly formed bone are found in the vicinity of abnormal calcium deposits in mesenchy-

mal tissues. It is as though the presence of calcium salts induces a change in collagen so that it now accepts mineral just as does osteoid. Whether the influence is upon the collagenoblasts or on their intercellular product is not known, or indeed, whether the mineral is the initiating agent or merely a by-product of some unknown force that induces both metaplasia and calcification.

The entire subject of cell induction[3] is fascinating but it seems unnecessary to imagine some mysterious agent passed from one cell to another to comprehend fibro-osseous metaplasia. The collagen of connective tissue, the chondroid of cartilage and the osteoid of bone are all remarkably similar substances despite the obvious differences in their physical properties. They are elaborated in the presence of three types of cells, the collagenoblast, the chondroblast and the osteoblast, all of which arise from a common stem cell, the fibroblast. The factors that induce the fibroblast to differentiate into one of these three

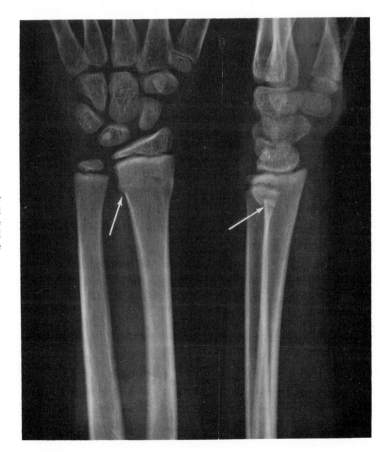

Figure 8–4 An impacted or "buckle" fracture of the distal end of the radius (arrows). Most of the deformity involves the dorsal cortex. This is a common fracture of childhood.

types are unknown but they are related to environmental circumstance and probably involve pH, the amount of blood supply, motion, the presence of mineral salts, stress and perhaps other factors as yet unsuggested. A specific humoral substance may be the dominant agent but as yet none has been isolated, and explanations based on its presence sometimes sound like the older theories concerned with the Galenic humors.

The repair of fractures is like the reparative processes elsewhere in mesenchymal tissue except that the end product is bone rather than collagenous scar. The differences between unmineralized osteoid and collagen are largely physical and can probably be accounted for on the basis of the type of bonding of the three polypeptide chains of which bone collagen fibers are constructed. It is our contention that the osteoblast forms osteoid because of its metabolic resources. If we knew more about its metabolic habits we probably would find that it can produce chondroid or collagen with equal facility. It is probable that under normal circumstances the osteoblast elaborates osteoid only in the presence of preexisting bone or cartilage. In fracture healing this method of osteoid production predominates but probably does not account for all new bone formation.

Bone fracture heals by the production of a callus. This callus tends to immobilize the bone fragments. When immobilization is achieved, stress trajectories are established and further bone production is directed by the principle of the attainment of the greatest strength with the least mass. Bone production takes time. The greater the amount of callus necessary to reestablish continuity of the fragments, the longer will be the healing time. Thus the principles of fracture treatment are obvious. Reduction should bring the ends as close together as possible in the nearest approximation of normal alignment in order that

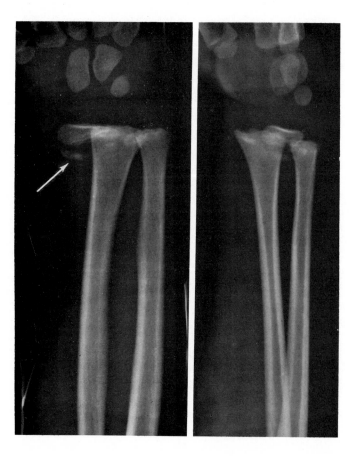

Figure 8–5 A fracture through the epiphyseal line with displacement of the distal radial epiphysis. A fragment of the dorsal cortex and metaphysis (arrow) accompanies the displaced epiphysis.

the smallest possible callus may suffice. Immobilization should be designed to control motion to a degree that prevents any disturbance in the rigid callus structure. In most instances immobilization should be as complete as possible. Muscle tension and movement of the part as a whole should provide sufficient stress to stimulate osteoblastic action. Finally, the multiple factors in callus and normal bone production should be kept constantly in mind with every effort to provide these factors when they are deficient. Splints, casts, plates, pins and nails as well as traction appliances should be used where necessary with the least interference to blood supply. Adequate caloric intake with sufficient ascorbic acid and vitamin D should be maintained. If endocrine deficiencies are apparent, especially estrogen, they should be corrected. Under optimal conditions, 1 to 3 centimeters of large cylindrical bone tissue should be formed within a year.

If bone production is deficient and the healing process delayed substantially beyond a year, especially in the areas in which there is repeated motion, a pseudarthrosis is likely to be formed. The organism is slow in bridging with rigid bone an area in which motion is constant. Instead the callus remains fibrous and pliable. Eventually a bursa-like sac develops in the region and its walls may undergo cartilaginous metaplasia. This is a marvelous imitation of a joint with articular plates covering the bone ends, an illustration of the adaptability of tissues to new environmental conditions.

The factors that cause non-union and delayed union may be exceedingly complex and difficult to determine. A discussion of these factors and of the mechanics of fracture treatment is not pertinent to the subject matter of this text. These subjects belong to the experienced orthopedist and none other should try to explain them.

We attempted to establish the sequence of events that constitute fracture healing. With the kind assistance of Dr. Stewart Lewis, material was collected from the Medical Examiner's Office over a period of two years. To the extent that practicability would allow us, whole sections were made of a series of fractured bones and arranged in chronologic sequence ranging from six

hours to 116 days. This material was supplemented by surgical specimens to fill in the time sequences and by a series of fractures in dogs. It is obvious that one must be cautious in interpreting this material literally because, ideally, comparisons of fractures at various times in the healing process should be made on the same bone, in patients of the same age and sex who maintained about the same amount of activity while on a constant diet. The amount of bone destruction, hemorrhage and displacement would also have to be taken into consideration. Since control of these factors is obviously impossible in the human, one can only draw broad conclusions from such investigation, but at least this is better than applying the results of animal experimentation directly to the human process.

When fracture of a bone occurs, the soft tissues on either side of it are lacerated. The periosteum is usually torn and the vascular channels of the parosteal and endosteal soft tissues are opened. Arterial blood flows out into the tissues to produce a hematoma. The continuity of the small channels within bone that carry nutrient material to the lacunar osteocytes is interrupted and these cells die. Thus the edges of the fragments, back as far as the junction of collateral channels, consist of dead bone. The hematoma forms within and outside the cortical walls. Within a matter of hours a network of fibrin is precipitated, first at the edges and then into the center of the clot. Soon collagenoblasts penetrate the hematoma from the labile mesenchymal tissues surrounding the injured area. As these climb through the network of fibrin strands the torn capillaries send endothelial buds after them, and soon the hematoma is organized and gradually becomes converted to a mass of granulation (Fig. 8–6). The hyperemia thus induced probably plays a role in the lysis of the ragged fragments of dead bone that constitute the fracture edges, surcharging the intercellular fluids with mineral salts. As the inflammatory reaction subsides the pH probably is altered.[4]

During this time the viable osteoblasts begin to produce osteoid, and new fibroblasts within and without the cortex mature into osteoblasts (Fig. 8–7) and chondro-

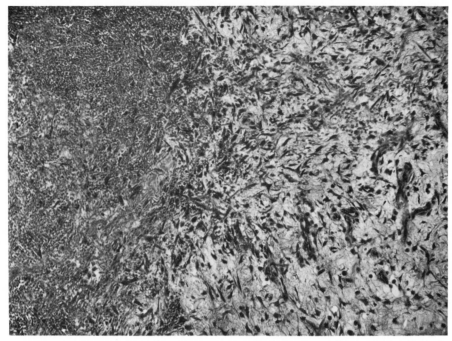

Figure 8–6   The central portion of the hematoma is seen at the left and granulation at the right. At the junction of the two zones fibroblasts and capillary buds are entering the former, thus converting it to the latter. ($\times$ 180.)

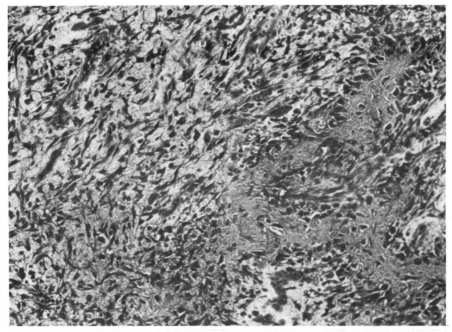

Figure 8–7   A spicule of recently formed fiberbone (on the right) ensheathed with osteoblasts is found in a mass of granulation which was probably formed from hematoma. Thus the hematoma enters indirectly into the formation of bone. ($\times$ 180.)

blasts (Fig. 8–8). As the collagenoblasts lay down collagen the recently formed vascular channels are squeezed out of existence and the blood supply is consequently diminished. Osteoid is laid down wherever a nidus of solid tissue will serve as a base: on fragments of old bone (Fig. 8–9) and on islands of newly formed cartilage (Fig. 8–10). Mineralization follows soon after osteoid production. Throughout the area one can find small masses of cartilage surrounded by fiberbone, osteochondroid (Fig. 8–11). The osteoid at the periphery appears to merge into the cartilaginous centers, and some observers have interpreted this as the direct transition of cartilage into bone. A more plausible explanation to us is that fibroblasts first mature into chondroblasts and produce chondroid. As the lesion ages, fibroblasts become osteoblasts, which continue the laying down of intercellular substance that eventually becomes recognizable as osteoid. When a large cartilage island persists, usually at the periphery of the lesion, the chondroblasts mature and columnate just as in the enchondral plate, and a line of provisional calcification is laid down. At this point the irregular cartilage edge takes on the appearance of an epiphyseal line, producing a scaffolding of mineralized chondroid for the deposition of osteoid. This manner of enchondral bone formation is apparently neither necessary nor exceedingly common, judging from the number of times it turns up in sections made of callus tissue.

Why cartilage is produced in some areas and bone in others remains a mystery to us. Some authors have proposed the theory that cartilage thrives in ischemic areas that are too barren for osteoid to survive. If variation in oxygen tension is the reason, the theory is hard to support on morphologic grounds because these areas are scrambled in a patternless array.

The metaplasia of fibroblasts into bone and cartilage-forming elements is by no means the whole explanation for callus formation. When the cambium is torn from the compacta one can see the diligent production of new bone between the periosteum and old cortex (Fig. 8–12). A solid mass of bone also replaces the marrow tissue, forming a plug or core that merges through the cortical hiatus with the out-side callus (Fig. 8–13). Thus the shaft of a cylindrical bone is braced both within and without. All of this cellular activity constitutes a composite, the callus. This again is an illustration of the ability of the organism to adapt itself by cellular activity and metaplasia to the circumstances of a new environment.

The bone of the callus consists largely of fiberbone that must be replaced with adult bone if it is to withstand the stress of normal function. Trajectories of stress determine the shifting of bone without diminishing mass and thereby strength. New adult bone is being laid down on one side of a piece of fiberbone while the other side is undergoing lysis (Fig. 4–24). Thus strong adult bone moves into the areas in which strength is needed, and the weaker fiberbone disappears. The organism is able to straighten the angulations of malposition even though side-to-side rather than end-to-end approximation resulted from the reduction (Fig. 8–14). As adult bone is exchanged for fiberbone the need for bulk is diminished and, therefore, the callus is reduced in size. If the fragments are perfectly aligned, the need for extracortical callus disappears and it melts away, leaving a perfectly smooth cortex. Since stress is borne through the cylindrical cortex, the medullary core of callus is no longer needed and it undergoes lysis, allowing a reestablishment of communication between the medullary cavities of the two fragments (Fig. 8–15). Should infection complicate an open fracture the normal sequence of healing events is disturbed, as one might expect it would be. The callus is prevented from performing its normal function, and an imperfect result is inevitable (Fig. 8–16).

To summarize the process in chronologic sequence, one finds proliferation of the cambium cells of the disturbed periosteum at the end of the second day post fracture. By the sixth day one can find traces of osteoid being laid down by these cells on the preexisting cortex. It seems that the cambium can produce osteoid directly only in the presence of preexisting bone but this it does immediately, forming the first new bone found in the healing process. Thus it would appear that fractures in which the periosteum is not devitalized begin callus

(Text continued on page 241.)

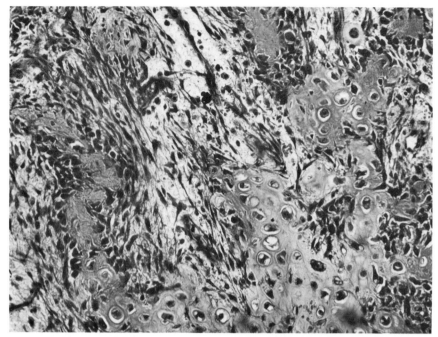

Figure 8-8 An island of young cartilage cells is surrounded by granulation. These cells appear to have been derived from the fibroblasts of granulation about the periphery of the cartilaginous island. Osteoblasts are laying down fiberbone. This combination of central cartilage and peripheral bone in a field of granulation is seen wherever callus is formed. The material has been called osteochondroid. (× 180.)

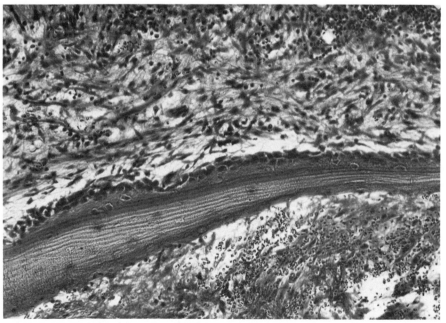

Figure 8-9 A spicule of normal adult bone which survived the lytic process following fracture. It acts as a nidus for the apposition of new bone. Along its upper surface a layer of osteoblasts can be seen laying down a seam of new osteoid. (× 180.)

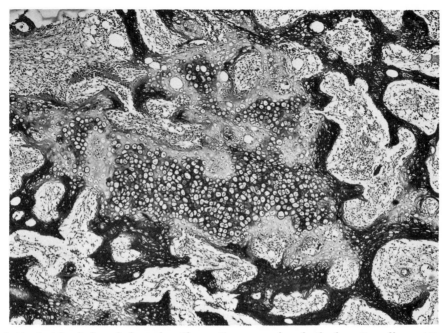

Figure 8–10   An island of newly formed cartilage acting as a nucleus for the formation of bone at its periphery. There is apparently a normal progression: hematoma to granulation to fibrosis to cartilage to bone. (× 40.)

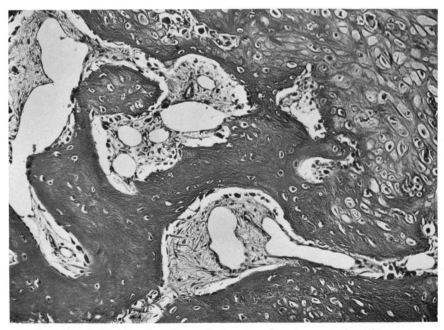

Figure 8–11   Osteochondroid. The edge of a cartilaginous nucleus is seen in the right upper corner. About it new bone is being formed. (× 180.)

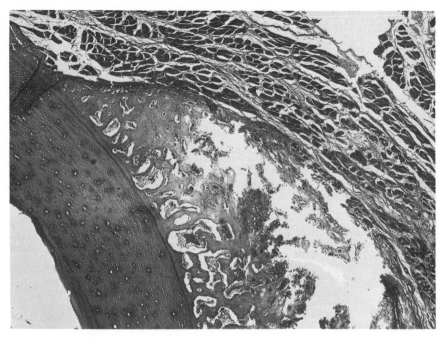

Figure 8-12   A segment of the cortex of a cylindrical bone is shown in the left lower portion. The muscle and periosteum in the right upper half of the picture have been detached by the fracture. The cambium has laid down a thick layer of new bone between the periosteum and the external cortical surface. (× 28.)

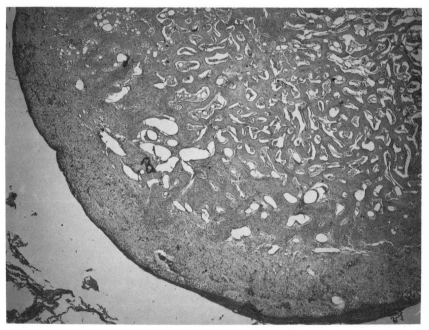

Figure 8-13   A segment of the cortex of a fractured bone. The medullary tissues have been replaced by a solid core or plug of callus that is annealed to the inner cortical surface. (× 16.)

ments probably create multiple foci of osteochondroid formation and thereby an increase in the size of the callus.

While these events are taking place outside the bone about the fracture site, a more complex mechanism takes place within. The hematoma begins to organize about its periphery immediately, and within six hours one can find fibroblasts penetrating the outer zone of the clot. Within three days budding capillaries are apparent and there is obvious collagen production. Thus the hematoma is gradually converted from the periphery inward, the center of a large hematoma remaining liquid for as long as 42 days and probably

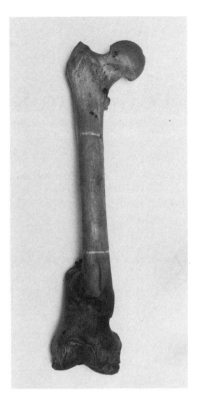

Figure 8–14 A femur with old fracture through the lower third and side-to-side approximation. Callus annealed the two fragments allowing full weight-bearing although with considerable shortening.

formation earlier than do those in which there is widespread periosteal destruction. This also emphasizes the virtue in utilizing the native periosteum in bone grafting.

At the hiatus where no cortical bone exists there is no direct osteoid formation by the cambium cells. Instead, the more primitive capacity of the periosteum to form cartilage is relied upon. Thus at each fracture edge, merging with the new subperiosteal appositional bone, which incidentally is always laid down in heavy spicules running vertical to the cortical surface, there is a ring of cartilage extending around the bone and defining the fracture line. This begins to appear at about the eleventh day after fracture. The presence of this ring is important because it is the nidus from which the extracortical callus will form. Movement of the fracture edges and disturbance of this ring probably inhibit firm callus formation. Breaking up of the ring and dissemination of the frag-

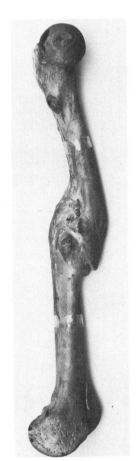
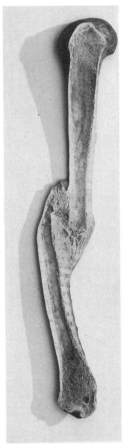

Figure 8–15 The outer surface and the cut surface of a femur with old fracture and healing. Note how the callus persists along the trajectory lines but has disappeared within the medullary areas of the two fragments. Because there was side-to-side rather than end-to-end apposition the continuity of the medullary spaces of the two fragments was never reestablished.

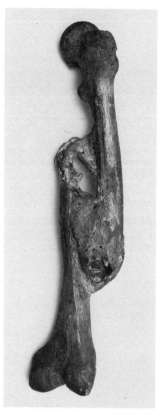

Figure 8-16 Osteomyelitis complicated this fracture so that repair was inhibited and the callus developed numerous sinuses.

longer. As early as the ninth day one can find metaplasia of the fibroblasts to chondroblasts. Isolated foci of cartilage merge with each other forming a zone of cartilaginous nidi across each fracture end and merging with the ring about the periphery. After the extracortical and intracortical cartilage aggregates have formed, a situation is established that is identical with that of the primary ossification center in embryonic bone growth. By the sixteenth day there is conversion to osteoid production, and at the end of 30 days a good endosteal osteochondroid callus has been formed. In one specimen 116 days old the hematoma had been entirely converted to a callus of osteochondroid with a collagen center (Fig. 8–17).

It should be noted that the timing given in this account is approximate and more often than not deduced by observation of a single specimen. There may be considerable variation depending upon the varied circumstances of the fracture and postfracture treatment. But these observations suggest several important principles of fracture healing.

1. Early and complete stabilization is important for rapid, solid callus formation.

2. Viable periosteum produces the first new bone of the callus. It should be utilized to provide the first natural scaffolding for future callus production.

3. Though the periosteum is important for early bone formation, new bone is produced in its complete absence. Since osteoid can be formed apparently only in the presence of cartilage or bone, the bulk of the callus depends upon fibroblastic proliferation, fibrocartilaginous metaplasia and then chondro-osseous metaplasia.

4. Though there is probably considerable variation in time sequence, subperiosteal appositional bone begins to form in about six days, hematoma cartilage in about nine days and metaplasia to primitive osteoid in about sixteen days.

Organized tissues, like organized societies, respond in an astonishing manner to emergencies. Callus may form in response to a fracture in a bone that was poorly constructed in the beginning—osteogenesis imperfecta—or normally constructed but unable to maintain itself—fibrous dysplasia and pseudarthrosis. One might reason that the newly formed bone in these instances is the product of the osteoblasts that are recently formed from the emergency fibroblasts or capillary endothelial cells. It is said that muscle cells undergo atrophy to supply to the emergency tissues the building blocks with which to construct callus. It is of interest that the bone formed under such circumstances is not durable. After the emergency is past, this bone responds in the same manner as the original bone of the fragments.

AVULSION OF THE ANTERIOR INFERIOR ILIAC SPINE

This lesion is not uncommon in rapidly growing teenage boys, particularly those who subject this area to unusual strain during competitive racing events. Sometimes the onset is insidious and the patient

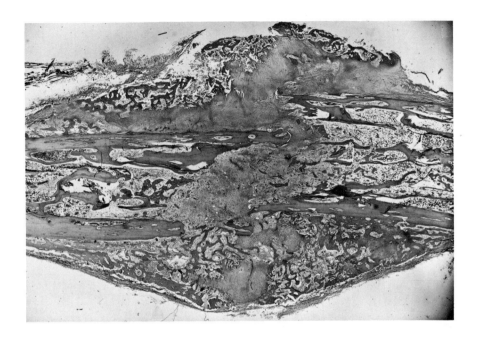

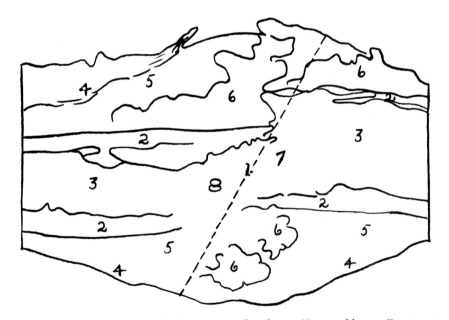

Figure 8–17 Low magnification through fracture site of a rib in a 60 year old man. Fracture was approximately four months old. 1, Fracture line. 2, Original cortex. 3, Original cancellous bone. 4, Elevated periosteum. 5, Subperiosteal new bone. 6, Subperiosteal chondroid. 7. Center of old hematoma. 8, Intracortical chondroid.

is unaware of the initial strain. Recurrent pain over a period of weeks is usually caused by running. The lesion is often misdiagnosed by radiologist and pathologist alike. The callus forming in response to the avulsion may be interpreted as tumor in both roentgenograms and tissue sections.

THE BATTERED CHILD

Inflicted trauma during infancy is frequently responsible for skeletal abnormalities. The lesions are unique to this age group because of the nature of the skeleton. It is growing rapidly, the periosteum is quite vascular and but loosely applied. The infant may be subjected to stresses not readily applicable to the older child such as shaking and hyperextension of joints, e.g., the knees and elbows. A history of trauma cannot always be obtained, and there may be a paucity of signs and symptoms. Thus the lesions are often discovered incidentally at the time of a roentgenographic examination for a seemingly unrelated illness. Subdural hematoma is often an associated abnormality.[5]

Radiographically, the lesions tend to be multiple, often asymmetric, and to be superimposed on bones of normal density and architecture. When there have been multiple episodes of trauma, fractures in various stages of healing are seen. There is apt to be elevation of the diaphyseal periosteum of the long bones by hemorrhage manifested by the appearance of subperi-

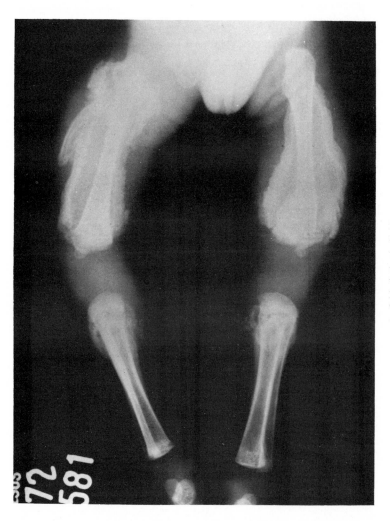

Figure 8–18 Trauma has resulted in massive subperiosteal hemorrhage manifest at this time by exuberant periosteal new bone. There is displacement of the distal femoral epiphyses and there are fractures across the proximal tibial metaphysis on each side. (Courtesy of Dr. A. Amoedo, Rio de Janeiro, Brazil)

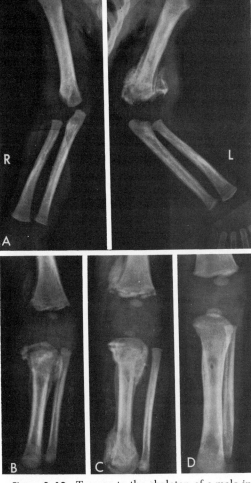

Figure 8–19 Trauma to the skeleton of a male infant 4 months of age. The lesion involving the left elbow (A) was noted on an x-ray of the chest and this finding prompted a skeletal survey. Both legs were involved. The left leg is shown at the time of the initial study (B) and as healing progressed, two weeks later (C), and four months later (D). Bilateral subdural hematomas were also present.

osteal new bone which may be exuberant. Fragmentation of the metaphysis and zone of provisional calcification is common and is frequently most evident at the elbows, knees and ankles, possibly related to hyperextension of these joints. There may be epiphyseal displacement and gross fractures of the diaphyses.[5, 6]

The differential diagnosis includes scurvy, congenital syphilis, infantile cortical hyperostosis and even neoplasm. Trauma is not manifest by a radiolucent zone adjacent to the zone of provisional calcifica-

tion or by osteopenia, as in scurvy. Areas of destruction do not appear in the metaphysis, in contrast to syphilis. Infantile cortical hyperostosis is not associated with fractures of the metaphyses. Skeletal involvement is spotty, not generalized as in metabolic bone disease. Note that the distal ends of the radius and the ulna are intact and that the distal end of the humerus, an area of relatively slow growth, is involved in the patient illustrated in Fig. 8–19. Recognition of the nature of the skeletal alterations is essential to the well-being of the infant or child, as the mortality rate is said to approximate 4 to 5 per cent and the morbidity, 40 per cent.

INSENSITIVITY TO PAIN

Congenital absence of sensation of pain may be divided into two categories: congenital indifference to pain in which no other sensory abnormalities and no detectable anatomic or physiological defects are present; and congenital sensory neuropathy in which there are detectable abnormalities of sensation (Table 8–1).[7]

Radiographically, one may see evidence of either infection or trauma. Patients with purulent arthritis may have a full range of motion during the acute phase of infection when a joint is obviously distended by pus. Old trauma may be manifest by deformity that is frequently metaphyseal in location and characterized by cupping and disturbances in growth. There may be periosteal reaction or myositis ossificans as well. Sclerosis and healing fractures in the absence of osteopenia may be expected. Self-mutilation is often associated with loss of soft tissue, and even bone, e.g., the finger tips and distal phalanges. As in unsuspected trauma encountered in infants, there may be fractures in various stages of healing.

PATHOLOGIC FRACTURE

A pathologic fracture is one that occurs through a bone that has been weakened by an underlying disease process. Generally, such fractures are transverse in nature and upon roentgenographic examination the area of abnormality is usually evident.

TABLE 8–1 COMPARISON OF CONGENITAL AND HEREDITARY CAUSES OF INSENSITIVITY TO PAIN*

Parameter	Congenital Indifference	Congenital Sensory Neuropathy	Hereditary Sensory Radicular Neuropathy	Familial Dysautonomia	Familial Sensory Neuropathy with Anhidrosis
Intelligence	Normal	Dull to normal	Normal	Dull to normal	Defective
Heredity	None D-trisomy mosaicism	Mostly sporadic; occ. dominant	Dominant	Recessive	Recessive
Age at onset	Birth	Birth	Late childhood	Birth	Birth
Distribution of sensory loss	Universal	Incomplete	Predominantly distal extremities	Incomplete	? Incomplete
Temperature perception	Normal	Absent	Absent	Reduced	Reduced
Touch perception	Normal	Lost	Lost	Present	Present
Axon reflex	Normal	None	None	None†	None
Physiologic pain reactions	Present	None	None	None‡	None
Sensory nervous system anatomy	Normal	No myelinated fibers or dermal nerve networks	No myelinated fibers	Absence of fungiform papillae and taste buds on tongue	Absence of Lissauer's tract and small dorsal root axon; myelinated fibers and dermal nerve networks present

*From Pinsky, L. and DiGeorge, A. M.: J. Pediatr., 68:1, 1966.
†Axon reflex is restored during intravenous infusion of mecholyl.
‡No response to cold pressor test.

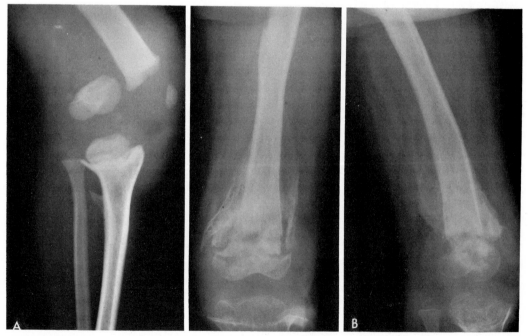

Figure 8–20 Congenital familial sensory neuropathy with anhidrosis. This white male 5 years of age presented with a swollen knee of two weeks' duration. There is obvious soft tissue swelling and a fracture through the distal femoral epiphyseal line (A). The patient damaged his cast and walked before healing occurred with the resultant destruction and sclerosis as seen in B.

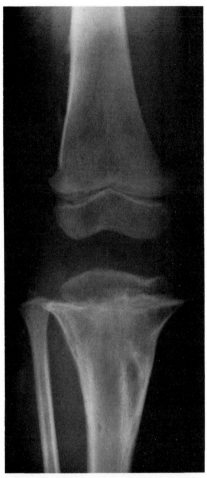

Pathologic fractures are commonly associated with metastatic malignancy and may be the first manifestation of metastases.

In other instances, the underlying disease may be congenital or developmental in nature, such as a simple cyst, the lesions of fibrous dysplasia, enchondromatosis or Paget's disease. Fractures may be associated with osteomalacia, osteoporosis and hyperparathyroidism. A pathologic fracture may occur through a bone that has been weakened by a primary malignancy of bone and, uncommonly, before the tumor is apparent radiographically.

Depending on the nature of the lesion through which the fracture has occurred, healing either proceeds in a normal manner or is delayed.

STRESS FRACTURE

A stress fracture is one that occurs through an otherwise normal bone that is subjected to repeated episodes of stress, less severe than that necessary to produce an acute fracture. Such fractures are encountered in athletes, particularly the teen-aged athlete, and in people participating in strenuous activities to which they are not acclimated.[8] The bones most commonly involved are the metatarsal, calcaneus,

Figure 8–21 Insensitivity to pain. There is evidence of old trauma to the tibia with deformity.

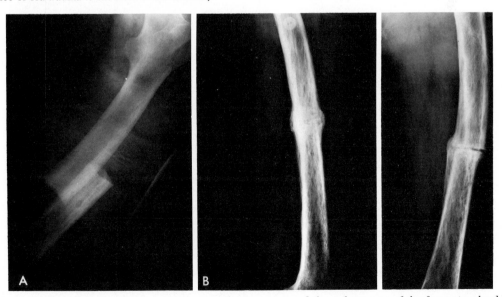

Figure 8–22 Pathologic fracture. A transverse fracture occurred through an area of the femur involved by Paget's disease (A). Later studies reveal healing reaction about the site of the fracture (B).

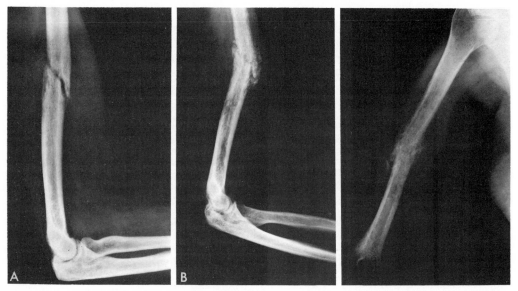

Figure 8–23 Pathologic fracture. The fracture has occurred through an area of destruction secondary to metastatic carcinoma of the breast (A). Healing reaction did appear about the site of the fracture (B).

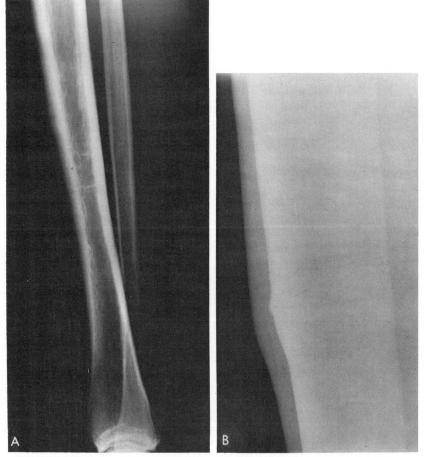

Figure 8–24 Stress fracture. The fracture line is barely visible in the anterior cortex of the tibia (A). There is local soft tissue swelling and periosteal reaction (B).

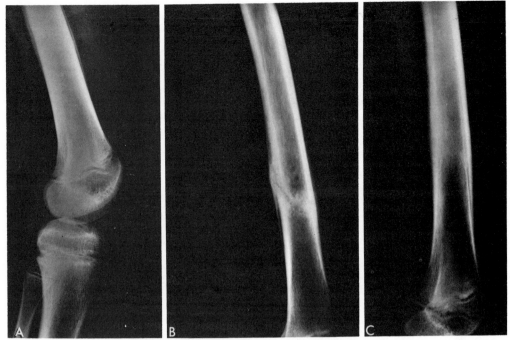

Figure 8–25 Stress fracture. The initial examination of the femur revealed only periosteal thickening around the distal epiphysis (*A*). One month later the fracture line was clearly visible (*B*). Healing occurred as manifest by thickening of the cortex and disappearance of the fracture line (*C*).

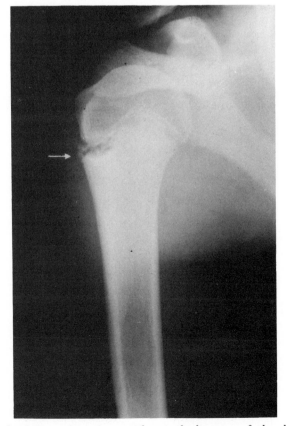

Figure 8–26 Metaphyseal infractions (arrow) are evident in the humerus of a baseball pitcher, age 12 years.

the proximal diaphysis of the tibia, the distal diaphysis of the femur, the femoral neck and the pubic rami.[9]

The fractures may involve medullary bone or the cortex or both and are manifest clinically by pain and local tenderness.

Radiographically, one may see only an area of periosteal new bone formation or a thickened area of cortex. This reaction may closely mimic a malignant tumor of bone. Differential diagnosis is facilitated by the obvious presence of a fracture line. If, however, the lucent fracture is not seen on conventional exposures, laminography or multiple projections should be employed. The fracture line may not become apparent until the part is put at rest and healing is established. If the medullary portion of bone is primarily involved, the fracture is manifest by a zone of sclerosis. Metaphyseal infractions may occur in children as a result of relatively continuous trauma, e.g., the humerus in those who are baseball pitchers.[11] The appearance may suggest the destructive foci associated with infection (Fig. 8–26).

References

1. Ham, A. and Harris, W.: In Bourne, G., Ed.: Biochemistry and Physiology of Bone. New York, Academic Press, Inc., 1956, p. 475.
2. McLean, F. and Urist, M.: Bone. Chicago, University of Chicago Press, 1955, p. 139.
3. Spemann, H.: Embryonic Development and Induction. New Haven, Yale University Press, 1938.
4. Schram, W. and Fosdick, L.: J. Oral Surg., 1:191, 1943.
5. Caffey, J.: Pediatric X-Ray Diagnosis. Ed. 6. Chicago, Year Book Publishers, 1972.
6. Bakwin, H.: J. Pediatr., 49:7, 1956.
7. Pinsky, L. and DiGeorge, A.: J. Pediatr., 68:1, 1966.
8. Kroening, P. and Shelton, M.: Am. J. Roentgenol., 89:1281, 1964.
9. Blickenstaff, L. and Morris, J.: J. Bone Joint Surg., 48A:1031, 1966.
10. Winklemann, R., Lambert, E. and Hayles, A.: Arch. Dermatol., 85:323, 1962.
11. Torg, J. S.: Am. Fam. Physician, 6:71, 1972.
12. Caffey, J.: Am. J. Roentgenol., 108:451, 1970.

Chapter 9

INFECTIOUS DISEASES OF BONE

SUPPURATIVE OSTEOMYELITIS
  Acute
  Chronic
  Focal (Brodie's abscess)
  Salmonella osteomyelitis
NONSUPPURATIVE OSTEOMYELITIS
  Tuberculosis
  Osteomyelitis caused by other acid-fast bacilli
  Syphilis
  Brucellar osteomyelitis
  Fungus infections of bone
  Virus osteomyelitis
  Boeck's sarcoid
  Sclerosing osteitis of Garré
  Congenital rubella syndrome

SUPPURATIVE OSTEOMYELITIS

ACUTE AND CHRONIC SUPPURATIVE OSTEOMYELITIS

Bone is no less vulnerable to the ravages of animate, biologic agents than are soft tissues. Because, under normal circumstances, bone is never exposed to the external environment, these agents must reach their site of colonization by the blood or lymphatic stream, usually the former, except in compound fracture or iatrogenic infection due to surgical manipulation. It is probable that transient episodes of asymptomatic bacteremia are common. Because the organism is usually nonpathogenic or of very low virulence or because the host resistance is high, these agents are killed before they have the opportunity of establishing growth and tissue damage. If the host resistance is low or the resistance of a focal area has been impaired, a virulent organism may find a situation suitable to its reproduction and a site of infection becomes established. Suppurative osteomyelitis has a high incidence in the debilitated and in bone regions that have suffered trauma. It is probable that minor trauma causes a minute hemorrhage that lowers the resistance of a focus. If there happens to be a bacteremia and the organisms are carried to this exact area, they are able to multiply because bactericidal factors are inhibited.

Bone that suffers from the lowered oxygen tension of sickle cell disease is prone to develop one or more foci of osteomyelitis.[1] It is peculiar that in these instances

251

organisms of the *Salmonella* group have been most often reported. These infections are more apt to involve the shaft than the metaphyseal region and children appear to develop this type of osteomyelitis more often than adults.

In perhaps a third of the cases of ordinary suppurative osteomyelitis a primary focus of infection can be found. Furuncles, subcutaneous abscesses and paronychiae are the usual sources of the organisms that contaminate the blood. Visceral or serosal pus collections may supply the infectious agent and produce the debility that predisposes to secondary bone involvement. Other diseases, such as lobar pneumonia and typhoid fever, may be responsible for the bone focus during the stage of systemic infection.

The *Staphylococcus aureus* accounts for the great majority, perhaps as many as 90 per cent, of cases of suppurative osteomyelitis. A member of the streptococcus group is involved in about half of the remainder and a small percentage are caused by *Escherichia coli*, *Salmonella typhi* and *Neisseria gonorrhoeae*.

Suppurative osteomyelitis occurs most often in children under 12 years though it may occur, of course, at any age in situations conducive to its development. It is from two to four times more common in boys than girls, the reason usually offered to explain this preponderance being the greater occurrence of trauma in the former. The disease usually affects the large cylindrical bones of the extremities, with the femur, the tibia, the humerus and the radius being involved in the order named.

Suppurative osteomyelitis may involve any part of any bone but the great majority of the primary foci are found in the metaphyses and usually at the end of most rapid growth. Thus the knee region, lower end of the femur and upper end of the tibia are most commonly involved, just as with tumors. This predilection is difficult to explain though there apparently is an association with areas having the richest blood supply. In adults the shaft may be affected as often as the metaphysis.

The onset is usually sudden though occasionally it is insidious. Pain which is usually deep and often intense, ushers in the bone involvement. Tenderness is focal and usually exquisite. Soon there is swelling of the soft tissues over the area of bone involved and heat and redness appear. The systemic signs and symptoms are those of infection wherever it occurs. There are fever, malaise and anorexia, a sharp rise in the leukocyte count and a marked shortening of the sedimentation time.

The infection probably always starts in the soft medullary tissues. In the early stages there is hyperemia, change in capillary permeability and edema. Granulocytic leukocytes soon infiltrate the area in most types of infection. These are destroyed by the bacteria or their products and liberate a proteolytic enzyme. Tissue necrosis ensues and the bacteria, the lytic products of necrosis, the pus cells and debris are mingled to form a focus of suppuration.

The fate of this lesion now depends upon many factors including, of course, the virulence of the organism and the resistance of the host. But much also depends upon the portion of the bone involved and the integrity of the blood supply to the area.

In the metaphyseal area the compacta is very thin and the infection finds ready ac-

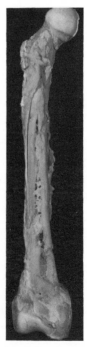

Figure 9–1 Suppurative osteomyelitis. The infection has extended through the length of the shaft. A "troughing" operation was done for drainage.

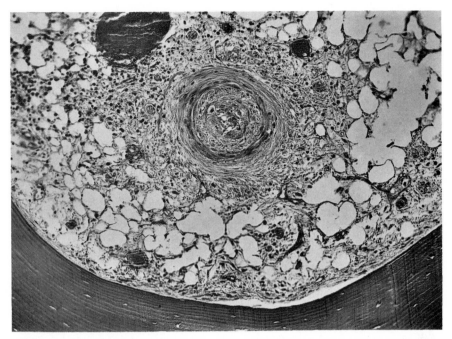

Figure 9–2 Osteomyelitis. Cross section through a small cylindrical bone. Portion of compacta at bottom. The fatty marrow shows an infiltration with inflammatory cells. A medullary vessel is completely thrombosed. The alteration of blood supply, decreased by thrombosis and increased by granulation, produces the characteristic x-ray changes of the disease. (× 109.)

cess to the subperiosteal tissue of this region. It pushes up the periosteum and travels along the external cortical surface. Spread in this fashion may be quite rapid in growing bone in which the periosteum is only loosely attached. Advancing along the venous and lymphatic channels of the spongiosa, the infection permeates the cancellous metaphysis (Fig. 9–1) and works its way toward the mid-diaphysis. Thus the cortical cylinder becomes bathed in pus on both sides.

The initial hyperemia results in bone absorption that may be sufficient to register on the roentgenograms within one week. The inflammatory reaction causes thrombosis of vessels producing irregular areas of bone ischemia (Fig. 9–2). As the infection is controlled or contained there is production of excess osteoid, which becomes mineralized, revealed as irregular areas of increased density on the roentgenogram. As the infection travels along the tortuous channels of the spongiosa and through the haversian canals, granulation is formed in the wake of the advancing acute process. With the increased blood supply carried by

the numerous budding capillaries of the granulation there again is lysis of bone. The haversian canals are increased in diameter causing the compacta to become porous.

Vascular thrombosis induces varying degrees of ischemia. In cases in which the blood supply is decreased below normal but is still sufficient to maintain the life of the bone tissue, the osteoblasts respond by laying down excessive amounts of osteoid. In cases in which nutrients are diminished beyond the point of viability, the osteocytes die and after a few days appear as pyknotic masses or disappear entirely, leaving the lacunae empty. Now the bone is dead and as such it is inert. Until the circulation is reestablished it remains exactly as it was at the time of cell death. What happens to this piece of dead bone depends greatly upon its size. If it is small, fingers of granulation from the contiguous living tissue bring in a fresh blood supply that causes its lysis. Eventually, it is completely removed and replaced first by granulation, then by fiberbone and eventually by mature, lamellated bone. If it is a large piece, the granulation extends into its substance as far as its vessels will support it. The periphery of the dead bone becomes canalized and eventually lysed and surrounded by a zone of granulation. The central residuum remains as a static mass. This piece of bone is known as a sequestrum (Fig. 9–3). The sequestrum remains intact until it is revascularized or surgically removed.

The sequestrum may be composed of a mass of cancellous bone, an area of compacta or a combination of the two. It varies in size from a minute fragment to the entire shaft. In cancellous bone it is identical with a bone infarct except that it is complicated by infection. If the process is in spongiosa the surrounding zone of granulation collagenizes, calcifies and then is converted into a shell of living bone that encapsulates the dead fragment. If the sequestrum is composed of compacta, a surrounding shell is produced by the overlying periosteum. In either case this ensheathing layer of bone is called an involucrum. The involucrum may be intact or incomplete depending upon the stage of the incar-

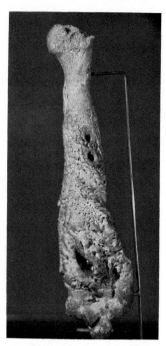

Figure 9–4 Suppurative osteomyelitis. Infection has traveled the full length of the shaft and penetrated the cortex at numerous points to produce sinuses.

cerated infection. Usually it is punctured with numerous channels through which pus may escape from inside. The nature of the lesion now tends to wall off pockets of infection that may lie dormant for long periods and then undergo exacerbations of activity. Thus chronic sinuses are formed (Fig. 9–4) that eventually reach the surface and drain. They suppurate until the infection becomes static and then the channels are plugged with granulation and remain closed until the pressure of the pus within builds up to the point of reopening the sinuses or establishing new ones. Thus the process may continue over a period of many years or until the bone becomes so riddled and useless that amputation is imperative. In a small percentage the sinus tract opening onto the skin becomes lined by stratified squamous epithelium growing down from the surface. Constant inflammation of these lining cells may induce cancerous change. The resulting neoplasm behaves in all respects like an ordinary squamous cell carcinoma (Fig. 9–5).

A fatal chronic granulomatous disease of childhood has been described recently.[2]

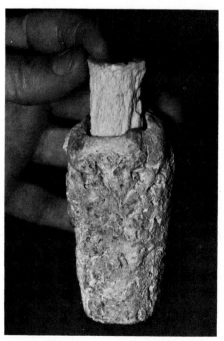

Figure 9–3 Suppurative osteomyelitis. There are two separate cylinders of bone. The inside cylinder (the sequestrum) represents the residuum of the original bone. The outside cylinder (the involucrum) represents new bone laid down by the elevated periosteum. The inner cylinder is separate from the outer and can be removed intact.

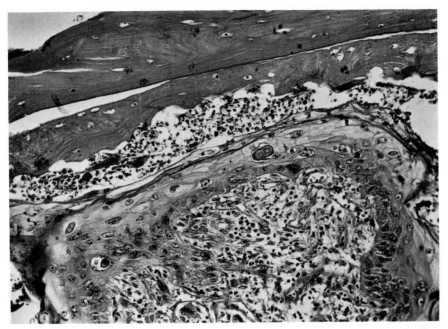

Figure 9–5   Chronic suppurative osteomyelitis. The squamous cell carcinoma seen in the lower half of the picture arose in a chronic sinus and penetrated into the bone. (× 117.)

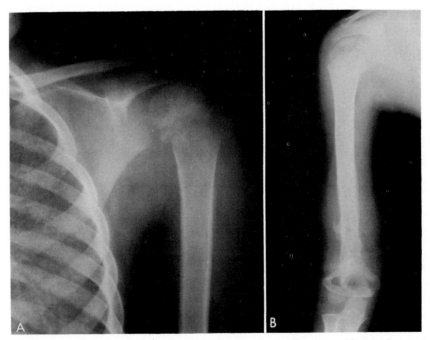

Figure 9–6   Chronic granulomatous disease, male, 5 years of age. There is evidence of acute infection involving the proximal metaphysis of the left humerus (A). Chronic osteomyelitis is present in the distal end of the right humerus characterized by periôsteal new bone, deformity and destructive foci (B).

Osteomyelitis is a frequent component of this disease. It is a sex-linked disease of boys, the defective gene being carried by the mother. Polymorphonuclear leukocytes from these patients with chronic granulomatous disease of childhood have a defective bactericidal capacity for certain bacterial species. The cells have normal phagocytic function, serum antibody response and skin sensitivity tests but the organisms remain viable within the cells (Fig. 9–6).

Roentgenographic Manifestations. The roentgenographic manifestations of suppurative osteomyelitis are related to the destruction of bone, to the formation of new bone as a reaction to infection and to the presence of devitalized bone. Radiographic examination reveals no abnormalities of bone early in the course of the process and changes are not apparent until there is macroscopic evidence of bone destruction or of new bone formation, usually seven to ten days after the onset of infection. The early administration of antibacterial agents further modifies the radiographic manifestations, so that with mild infections there may be no radiographic

evidence of the disease or with more severe infection there may be a marked delay in the radiographic manifestations of the process. Because osseous changes are dependent upon destruction of bone or new bone formation, the first evidence of an underlying osteomyelitis may be the presence of soft tissue swelling adjacent to the affected bone as manifest by displacement of the overlying lucent planes of fat. With progression, edema obliterates these fatty deposits. Associated with further deep soft tissue swelling, the muscle mass may become larger and more opaque. In some instances there will be extension to the more superficial soft tissues which results in irregular opacity of the subcutaneous fat (Fig. 9–7).[2a]

In the untreated case, small irregular areas of radiolucency are evident in the spongiosa, usually in the metaphyseal end of the bone. These represent areas in which trabeculae have been resorbed as a result of local hyperemia and necrosis. The spread of infection through the cortex causes elevation of the periosteum with resultant production of a thin, visible layer

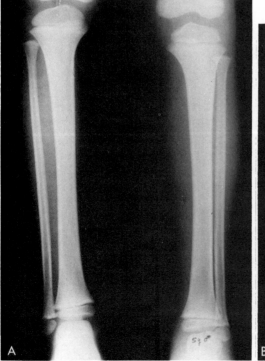 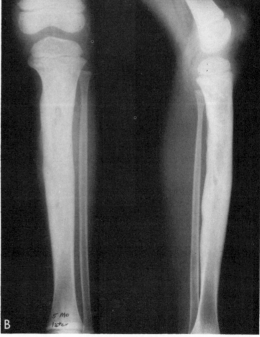

Figure 9–7 Osteomyelitis, left tibia. The initial examination (A) reveals deep and superficial soft tissue swelling along the tibia. Five months later (B) chronic osteomyelitis is obvious.

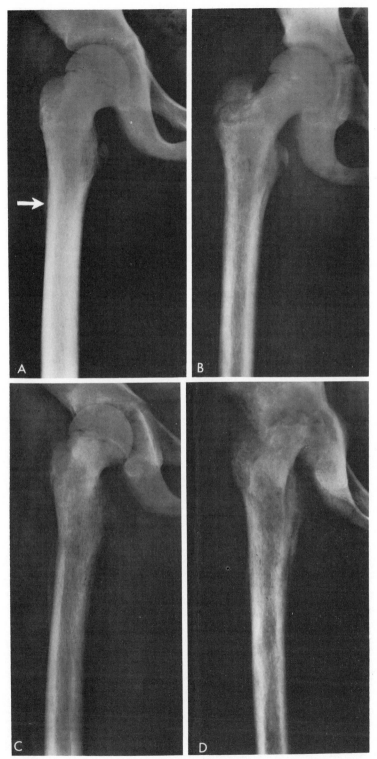

Figure 9–8 Suppurative osteomyelitis. The initial radiograph (A) shows only minimal periosteal reaction along the lateral aspect of the proximal femur (arrow). Ten days later (B) periosteal reaction is more marked and small irregular radiolucent areas are evident within the cortex and spongiosa. The joint is narrowed. Two months later (C) further bone destruction and narrowing of the joint are evident. Eight months after the onset (D) there is gross destruction of the joint and the proximal femur and more new bone about the femur.

of bone. The appearance of new bone produced by the periosteum parallels the appearance of the destructive foci.[3] The configuration of this new bone is variable and depends in large degree on the severity of the infection (Figs. 9–8 and 9–9). Extension of infection through the tissues of the medullary canal results in the extension of osseous destruction and the presence of more and larger areas of radiolucency.

Thrombosis of vessels by the inflammatory process causes ischemia and death of bone. Spicules of devitalized bone appear quite opaque in contrast to the surrounding granulation tissue and demineralized bone. This is accentuated by the fact that the dead bone cannot respond to hyperemia as does the surrounding living bone. These spicules of dead bone (sequestra), which may be cortical or medullary in location, vary in size, are usually smooth in outline and are surrounded by a radiolucent area of granulation tissue, which in turn is surrounded by an area of reactive living bone (involucrum). Multiple openings are pres-

ent in large involucra and it is through these cloaca that drainage of debris occurs, often to the skin surface.

Infection may penetrate the epiphyseal line and cause disturbances of growth (Fig. 9–11). If the joint is involved, rapid destruction of the articular cartilage follows initial distention of the joint. This is followed by narrowing of the joint and ankylosis. Involvement of a joint is not uncommon in cases in which the affected metaphysis is within the capsule of the joint such as the hip.

After the initial roentgenographic manifestations of osteomyelitis appear, roentgenographic examination is invaluable in delineating the extent and chronicity of involvement and the presence or occurrence of subsequent disturbances in growth.

Microscopy. The microscopic appearance of suppurative osteomyelitis depends upon the stage of the process at which the tissue is taken. In the early stage the section is dominated by fields of polymorpho-

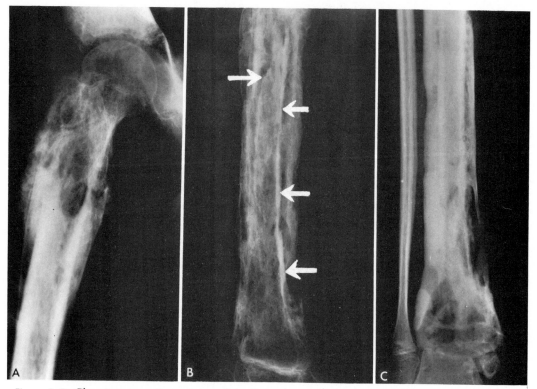

Figure 9–9 Chronic suppurative osteomyelitis. Examples of chronic suppurative osteomyelitis are illustrated. In *B* the original cortex (arrows) is a sequestrum, opaque and smooth in outline. A large involucrum surrounds it, in which there are multiple cloaca. The ankle joint has been destroyed (*C*).

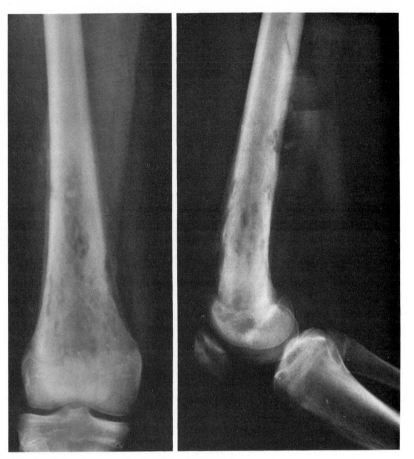

Figure 9–10 Suppurative osteomyelitis. The roentgen appearance is like that of a malignant tumor of bone. Compatible with infection are the sequestra, the rough and irregular periosteal new bone and the absence of a soft tissue mass.

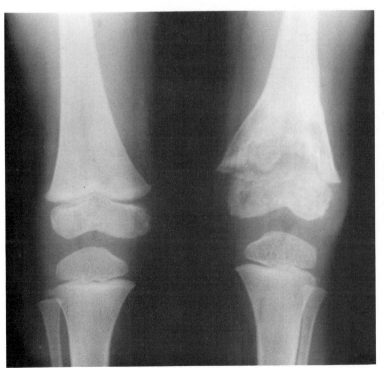

Figure 9–11 The metaphysis is distorted as a result of infection that interfered with the normal processes of longitudinal growth in the epiphyseal plate.

259

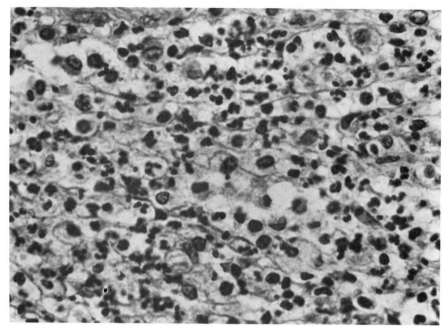

Figure 9–12   Suppurative osteomyelitis. There is necrosis with a rich infiltrate with exudative inflammatory cells. Note the numerous polymorphonuclear leukocytes. (× 534.)

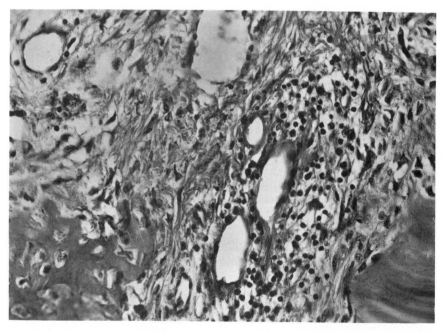

Figure 9–13   Suppurative osteomyelitis. There is a piece of new bone in the lower left corner and of old bone in the lower right corner. Between the two there is fibrosis with a perivascular infiltration with lymphocytes. (× 247.)

nuclear leukocytes, living and dead with areas of liquefaction necrosis and cell detritus (Fig. 9–12). Later the exudate is composed largely of lymphocytes, macrophages and plasma cells. Eventually a fibrotic marrow becomes the predominating feature and it may be necessary to search through numerous fields to find exudative cells (Fig. 9–13). Spicules of quite normal appearing bone may be found in which the lacunae are empty. If no lacunar osteocytes can be demonstrated in entire fields, the bone is quite probably dead. The compacta often shows enlargement of the haversian canals. Some of these are empty, others are filled with granulation and still others have collagenized connective tissue. Regeneration of new bone is found in areas in which the infection has been controlled and the debris removed by macrophage activity. The novice may have difficulty in differentiating exudate in cancellous bone from normal marrow. This mistake is not as ridiculous as it may sound because the components of an exudate, polymorphonuclear granulocytes, plasma cells, lymphocytes and red cells, may all be found in normal bone marrow. But marrow always has a distinctive fat cell pattern—large, circular, clear spaces evenly distributed throughout the cell aggregates. Exudate never contains these evenly dispersed fat cells.

Long continued infection in the subepiphyseal region, though it rarely violates the enchondral plate, may inhibit enchondral bone growth so that a long bone may fail to achieve normal stature. In some instances the excessive blood supply to the growth area consequent to nearby infection may speed growth so that the cylindrical bone becomes longer than its opposite member. Longstanding suppurative disease of medullary tissues predisposes to secondary amyloidosis, most often occurring in the spleen, kidneys and liver. The mechanisms of amyloid formation are not well understood but apparently the function of the globulin-forming tissues is perverted, so that instead of producing specific antibody gamma globulin they produce an abnormal globulin, which is somehow incorporated into the chemical constituency of amyloid.

BRODIE'S ABSCESS

In certain cases a suppurative osteomyelitis may be established but the host may be able to confine the infection to cancellous tissue and its spread to the subperiosteal region does not occur. Instead, the central area of suppuration and necrosis becomes incarcerated by a wall of granulation, which collagenizes to form a fibrous capsule. Thus a focal abscess of bone develops and becomes static. The offending organisms are killed and the pus is usually found to be sterile. Because auto-drainage is impossible the abscess remains until surgical intervention.

Brodie's abscess represents an aborted acute suppurative osteomyelitis. Early symptoms of the latter may disappear entirely or there may remain a focal area of bone pain and tenderness. In cases that have yielded positive bacterial culture the same organisms have been found as in cases of diffuse suppurative osteomyelitis. It is probable that the mechanisms of development are the same.

SALMONELLA OSTEOMYELITIS

The *Salmonella* group may produce suppurative osteomyelitis though this disease is very much less common than that caused by staphylococci. Chronic osteomyelitis as a complication of typhoid fever has been recognized since medical antiquity. More recently bone infections following paratyphoid fever and other salmonella septicemias have been reported.

In the past decade several accounts[4] of Salmonella osteomyelitis have appeared. These infections are most often encountered in patients with sickle cell anemia. The reason for the association of the two conditions is not clear. It has been suggested that the anemia plus the autosplenectomy that frequently accompanies it may lower the resistance to the Salmonella organisms. It has also been suggested that the minute infarctions of the intestinal wall induced by the poor oxygen-carrying capacity of the erythrocytes promote the diffusion of the organisms. Recently it has been shown that patients with sickle cell anemia and those with hemoglobin S-C

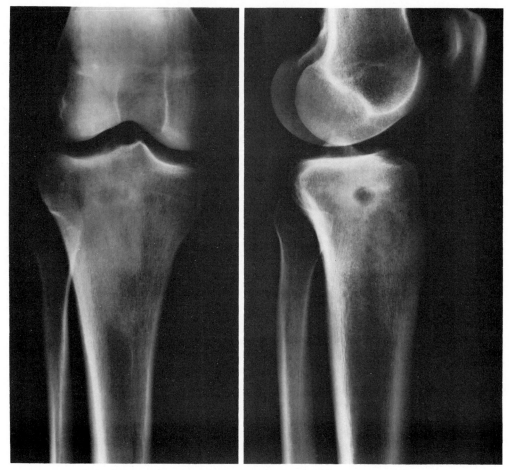

Figure 9–14 Brodie's abscess. A localized area of osteomyelitis is present in the proximal tibia. There is a well defined, radiolucent lesion surrounded by opaque reactive bone. Culture of the material obtained from the lesion at surgery revealed *Staphylococcus aureus*.

disease have a high incidence of multiple infarction of bone. In most cases these infarcts are aseptic. It appears probable that these areas of aseptic necrosis provide the locus minoris resistentiae, which allows the Salmonella organisms to flourish and that the disease can occur only in patients whose red cells contain hemoglobin S or hemoglobin C and who develop a salmonella septicemia.

The condition occurs more commonly in children than adults though any age may be affected. The foci of infection are usually multiple, apparently conforming to the multiple areas of infarction. The disease is much more serious than ordinary staphylococcal osteomyelitis because the

several foci of infection plus the sickle cell anemia may lead to a fatal terminus.

Salmonella osteomyelitis should be suspected in patients with a hemolytic anemia, a high reticulocyte count, erythroid hyperplasia of the marrow, splenomegaly or, of course, frank sickling of red cells. Salmonella osteomyelitis has not as yet been reported in hemoglobin S-C disease.

Radiographically, salmonella osteomyelitis in patients with sickle cell anemia usually involves more than one bone. Characteristically there are multiple destructive lesions throughout the diaphysis, extensive periosteal new bone formation and irregular sclerosis (Fig. 9–15). This

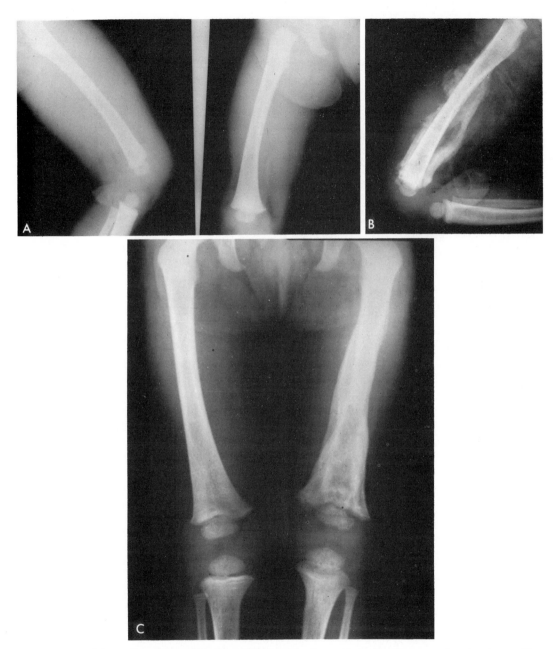

Figure 9–15   Salmonella osteomyelitis. The initial examination at 8 months of age reveals extensive swelling of the deep soft tissues of the thigh (A). Three weeks later there is abundant periosteal new bone present (B). Four months after the onset (C) remodeling is incomplete and there is disturbance of growth at the distal end of the femur. (Courtesy of Dr. M. Haskin, Hahnemann Hospital, Philadelphia.)

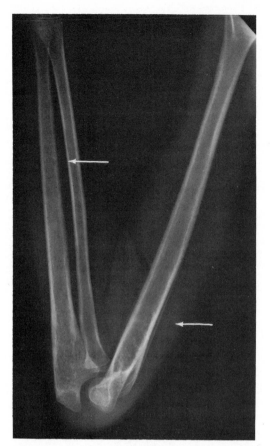

Figure 9–16 Salmonella osteomyelitis. The humerus and ulna are surrounded by a cloak of periosteal new bone (arrows). Minute radiolucent areas of destruction are evident in the cortex and medullary canal of the ulna. This patient had sickle cell anemia.

degree of involvement may be due to the wide haversian canals associated with sickle cell anemia and hence easy spread of the infection through the cortex as well as the medullary canal (Fig. 9–16).

Prognosis. Suppurative osteomyelitis is no longer the dreaded disease of the past. Antibiotic therapy has completely changed the mortality and the morbidity. Treated early and efficiently the infection may be expected to yield with the same consistency as like processes in soft tissues. The principal difficulty is in making a firm diagnosis before extensive bone destruction has occurred. Because clinically and radiologically the differential diagnosis often includes Ewing's tumor, a biopsy and culture should be resorted to if necessary. Recently numerous cases have appeared that seem to be attenuated infections caused by the antibiotic used. These may run a smoldering course, which makes diagnosis exceedingly difficult because the cultures may be consistently negative. Usually the biopsy showing a fibrotic marrow with scattered aggregates of lymphocytes and plasma cells supplies the last piece of information necessary for accurate diagnosis. Cultures should always be made in all cases that might appear even remotely to be infectious in origin. This rule is all too frequently forgotten or ignored by surgeons.

Rarely a nonpathogenic organism or one of extremely low virulence gains access to bone. A very low-grade infection is established that may progress so slowly that osteomyelitis is not suspected. Such lesions are sometimes seen in the vertebrae months or even longer after a spinal puncture, and it is assumed that the organism has been introduced by a nonsterile needle. The very best bacteriologic work may be required to culture the organism and some cases have been shown to continue for years before the cause is determined.

NONSUPPURATIVE OSTEOMYELITIS

TUBERCULOSIS OF BONE

Tuberculous osteomyelitis used to be one of the most important problems of orthopedic practice. With but rare exception it is secondary to a tuberculous infection elsewhere in the body, usually in the lungs. With the advent of a much more ef-

ficacious therapy of this disease both the incidence and morbidity have decreased.

Tuberculous osteomyelitis may occur at any age but the great preponderance of cases affect the prepubertal child. The vertebral bodies are the most common sites of involvement, after this the upper end of the femur and the ends of cylindrical bones near large joints. In most instances there is a related tuberculous arthritis and it is impossible to state whether the infection begins within the joint or the cancellous tissue of the metaphysis. A good review of the tuberculous infection of joints and bones in adults seen at the Mayo Clinic has been published by Kelly and Karlson.[4] The close physiologic relationship between the subchondral cancellous tissue of the metaphysis and the soft tissues that constitute the joint has been pointed out in several instances. In rheumatoid arthritis, if biopsy material is taken from the metaphysis contiguous to the affected joint, an exudative reaction similar to that of the soft tissues is found. A like condition pertains in villonodular synovitis. Apparently the lymphatic channels of the joint capsule serve as the pathways by which processes in one area gain access to the other. It is not remarkable that tuberculosis often involves both sites. It is remarkable that tumors and suppurative arthritis so rarely do the same.

The pathology of tuberculous osteomyelitis may be classified for the sake of discussion into four groups: (1) tuberculosis of the spine, (2) combined tuberculous arthritis and osteomyelitis, (3) tuberculosis of the shaft and (4) tuberculoid reactions in bone.

Tuberculosis of the spine is almost invariably a combination of tuberculous arthritis and osteomyelitis. Since the paper describing this disease by Percivall Pott in 1779, the condition is widely known as Pott's disease. The organisms reach either the joint tissues or the spongiosa of the vertebral body through the blood. They usually spread from an involved area to a healthy site beneath the anterior longitudinal ligaments but they may advance directly by necrosis from one vertebral body to the next. At times a normal body or joint may intervene between two foci of infection.

The infection develops slowly, spreading from the joint synovia to destroy the discs and from the cancellous tissue of a vertebral body to the supportive compacta. Lysis of cartilage and necrosis of bone occur. The trunk is shortened by collapse of the vertebrae and discs and by interference at the growth centers.

With destruction of the discs and bodies, severe distortion of the normal spinal curves and alignment occur. The lower thoracic and lumbar regions are the usual sites of involvement. The anterior portion of the vertebral body is commonly most severely involved and necrosis at this site produces a kyphotic angulation, a kyphosis (Fig. 9–17). The normal anteroposterior curves must increase to compensate for this angulation. Muscle spasm and weakness are early symptoms; later there is deformity, pressure upon spinal nerves and spread of the infection to the soft tissue to produce "cold abscesses."

The latter are slowly developing, necrotizing abscesses that result from tuberculous channels that emerge from the bone or joint. They dissect along fascial planes and come to the surface in the paraspinal region or dissect along the sheath of the psoas muscle to appear in the inguinal region or on the medial aspect of the thigh. They may rupture spontaneously to cause a chronic sinus. They may produce large, fluctuant, subcutaneous masses that persist for a long period. If

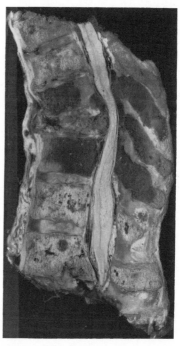

Figure 9–17   Tuberculous osteomyelitis. A sagittal section of a portion of the vertebral column. Two vertebrae are involved and have collapsed, causing kyphotic angulation with compression of the spinal cord.

they remain uncontaminated by pyogenic organisms, the whole process may be the site of an extensive precipitation of calcium salts. Sinuses may rupture through the dura and drain into the spinal canal. A tuberculous meningitis usually follows with a high mortality. Angulation and distortion of the vertebral column may cause pressure on the cord but actually this complication occurs less commonly than one might expect. The infection usually stimulates a considerable growth of granulation and this tissue may sufficiently narrow the canal to produce symptoms of a transverse myelitis.

Tuberculous infections in cylindrical bones are usually found in the metaphyses and there is almost always an infection in the corresponding joint. Thus the disease is a combined arthritis and osteomyelitis. The regions of the hip and knee are the most commonly involved. The joints are destroyed by a replacement of the synovial lining with tuberculous granulation. The articular cartilages undergo lysis, particularly about their peripheries. A tuberculous abscess develops within the metaphysis and sinuses develop and open onto the surface. Sequestration is less common than in suppurative osteomyelitis. A well established infection rarely heals without considerable bone and joint destruction. If large amounts of cancellous tissue are involved over a long period, secondary amyloidosis of the liver, kidney and spleen may develop.

Tuberculous infection of the shaft without joint involvement is much less commonly encountered. It heals more readily and extensive bone destruction is unusual. We have seen only one instance of multiple tuberculous infection of the metacarpals, a condition that earlier writers called spina ventosa. Infection of the entire shaft of one or more of the short cylindrical bones occurs with expansion of the shafts by subperiosteal apposition of bone.

When the joint tissues are involved in a tuberculous infection, the contiguous end of a long bone often reveals evidence of deossification that is out of proportion to the disuse atrophy one might expect. Surgical investigation at this site reveals a disappearance of cancellous bone tissue, thinning of the compacta and replacement with what grossly appears to be tuberculous granulation without actual necrosis or abscess formation. The process is apt to be sterile to culture and the pathologist is unable to find the granulomas that characterize the disease. This occurs often enough to have impressed earlier writers with the difficulty of demonstrating the microscopy of tuberculosis in these cases. In pulmonary tuberculosis the patient may develop what is known as an "id" reaction in the skin. This is a sensitivity response in the skin to a remote infection. Without laboring the matter, it has occurred to us that some bone lesions that are sterile and fail to reveal granulomas on biopsy may be a similar type of reaction within the bone to an infection in a nearby joint. This may account for some of the cases of "tuberculosis sica" of the earlier writers.

Roentgenographic Manifestations. The roentgenographic manifestations of tuberculosis of bone are those of slowly progressive bone destruction, which is usually associated with a minimum of bone reaction and little or no formation of sequestra. Radiolucency may be a prominent radiographic feature, as well as involvement of the related joint. In cases in which a joint is affected, the destruction of articular cartilage is much slower than is the case with suppurative infections because proteolytic enzymes are not present in the exudate. Joint involvement is manifested by widening of the joint followed by destruction of the subchondral cortex, particularly where the joint surfaces are not opposed. Later, narrowing of the joint occurs but this might require six months or more.[3] Tuberculosis of a joint in a child is often associated with enlargement of participating epiphyses presumably related to hyperemia of long standing.

Involvement of the spine is characterized by destruction of one or more intervertebral discs and apposition of the adjacent vertebral bodies, accompanied by destruction of one or more vertebral bodies (Fig. 9–18). The destruction is especially apt to occur anteriorly with resultant formation of a gibbus. A soft tissue swelling is usually evident around the area and a soft tissue mass of varying size is commonly associated; this mass, which is often pear-shaped and which may calcify, represents a cold

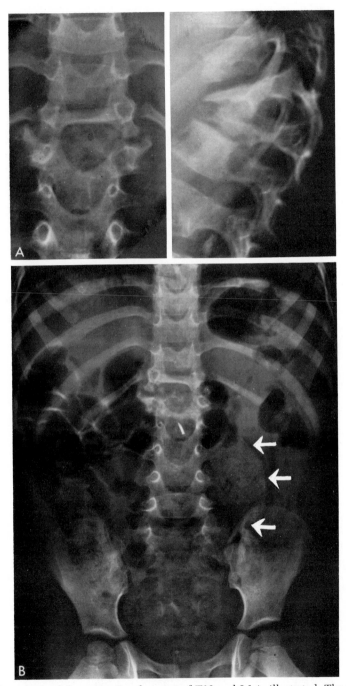

Figure 9–18   Tuberculosis of the spine. Involvement of T12 and L1 is illustrated. The intervertebral discs are narrowed and the affected vertebrae have lost stature, resulting in a gibbus. A cold abscess (arrows, *B*) is evident; speckled calcification is present in the abscess.

abscess. At times, the disease spares the intervertebral disc but produces destructive lesions in the vertebral body, the pedicles or lamina that do not result in collapse of vertebral bodies and deformity.

In the long bones there is usually severe radiolucency of the involved area. The response of the surrounding bone is often minimal so that destruction in the spongiosa may not be surrounded by reactive bone and there is little or no periosteal reaction. Occasionally, the areas of destruction are disseminated and cystic in nature. Diaphyseal lesions may be associated with considerable destruction and periosteal new bone formation, e.g., the phalanges. In some instances, however, the process may resemble pyogenic osteomyelitis and a definitive diagnosis of tuberculosis is usually not possible radiographically.

Because of the chronicity of the disease, atrophy of surrounding soft tissues is apt to occur.

The Microscopy of Tuberculosis. Tuberculous infection, whether it be in lung, bone or anywhere else in the body, characteristically manifests itself as a granulomatous inflammation.

The very earliest evidence of tissue damage by the tubercle bacillus is a focal area of necrosis with an aggregate of polymorphonuclear leukocytes, but within a very short time the epithelioid cell becomes dominant. The term "epithelioid cell" is used here to avoid a term that would more exactly designate the origin of these cells. They resemble macrophages or histiocytes and are phagocytic with nuclei characteristic of the "endothelial" elements of the reticulum. They appear to arise from the young collagenoblasts at the periphery of the lesion. It is probable that the latter may become motile and phagocytic if the infection is severe enough to call forth this response. In this instance the margins of the lesion advance, epithelioid cells are

(*Text continued on page 272.*)

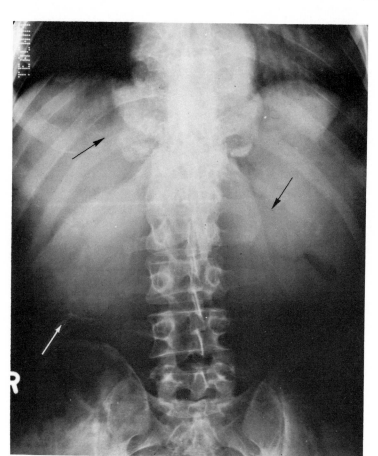

Figure 9–19 Tuberculosis of the spine, male, 35 years of age. There is considerable bone destruction involving the lower dorsal segments of the spine. Paraspinal masses with calcification are present (arrows).

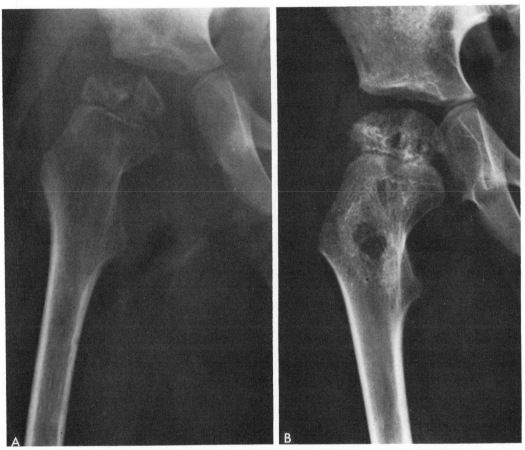

Figure 9–20 Tuberculosis. *A* shows displacement of the proximal femur from the acetabulum as a manifestation of joint involvement. Destructive lesions in the femoral capital epiphyseal center are present and marked osteopenia is apparent. One year later (*B*) destructive lesions in the femur are present but there is little bone reaction. The joint in this instance did not suffer permanent damage.

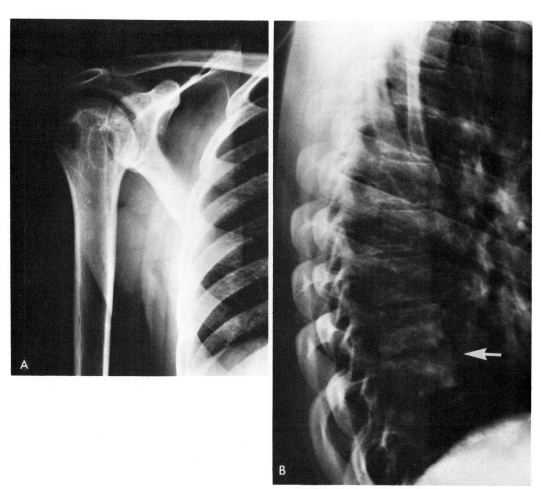

Figure 9–21   Tuberculosis. The initial examination of the shoulder was obtained because of pain and revealed lucent defects surrounded by a thin sclerotic margin (A). Biopsy resulted in the diagnosis of tuberculosis. Two months later, a lesion of the spine became apparent (B).

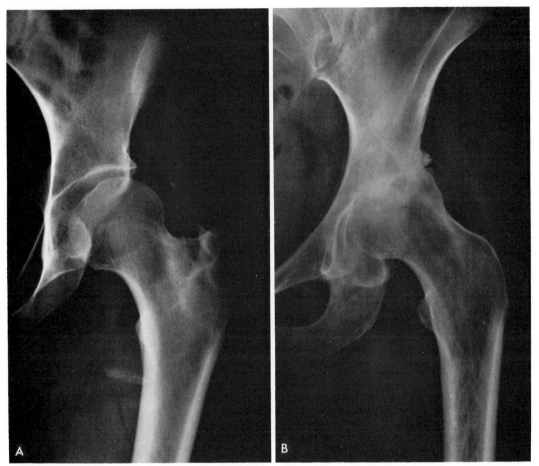

Figure 9–22 Tuberculosis. The initial involvement of the greater trochanter was associated with a large soft tissue mass with calcifications (*A*). The greater trochanter was resected. Overt destruction of the hip joint ensued over the following months (*B*).

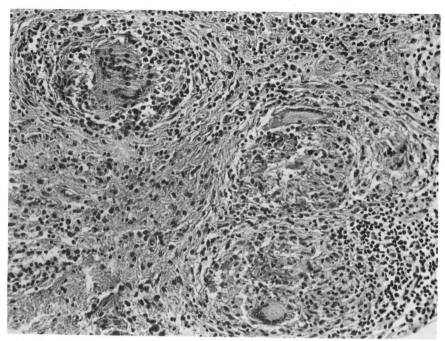

Figure 9-23 Three tubercles are seen. The ones in the upper left and lower right each contain a giant cell in the central area. About this there is an epithelioid cell reaction, lymphocytic infiltration and a peripheral zone of fibrosis. (× 186.)

formed and in turn form giant cells and perish in the necrotizing reaction at the vortex of the struggle. As the offending organisms are mastered, the peripheral collagenoblasts remain fixed and lay down collagen to wall off the quiescent process. Lymphocytes infiltrate the margins. The result is a fairly well delineated lesion that is called a granuloma (Fig. 9-23).

The term "granuloma" should not be confused with granulation. The former is a specific reticuloendothelial tissue reaction to a specific type of irritant. The latter is a nonspecific repair phenomenon found in any tissue and called forth by any injurious agent. Most fungi cause a granulomatous response. Some bacteria, the tubercle bacillus, for example, a few viruses, a few parasites and some chemical substances, especially the lipids and waxes, produce this granulomatous reaction. One cannot, with absolute assurance, name the specific agent on the evidence found in a tissue section. The granuloma (tubercle) of tuberculosis and that of Boeck's sarcoid often cannot be distinguished. If an acid-fast tissue stain is done and characteristic organisms found (less than 50 per cent of

granulomatous reactions in bone are positive for organisms), it is probable that these organisms are pathogenic and the cause of the reaction. Even then it may be necessary to do definitive culture work to be sure that the acid-fast organisms found in the tissue are pathogenic tubercle bacilli.

OSTEOMYELITIS CAUSED BY OTHER ACID-FAST BACILLI

In the past two decades several cases of infection by acid-fast microbacteria that are different from the tubercle and leprosy bacilli have been reported. These have produced focal and systemic infections, some of which have been fatal. The organisms resemble human leprosy and avian tubercle bacilli but they are not pathogenic for guinea pigs, they are resistant to antibiotics, the tuberculin skin test is negative and they usually grow on culture media to form orange or yellow colonies. They have been called chromogenic bacteria or the yellow tubercle bacillus. They produce lesions that are indistinguishable from that caused by mammalian tuberculosis.

More recently an acid-fast bacilliform microorganism that is not a mycobacterium has been isolated. Because it grows with branching it more closely resembles *Nocardia*. It causes intracellular parasitism and the lesions characteristically reveal numerous large foam cells similar to those seen in Gaucher's disease. This organism has been called *Nocardia intracellularis*.

In 1958, van der Hoeven et al.[6] reported a case of fatal multiple focus osteomyelitis from the island of Curaçao. They isolated an organism that grew with branching and produced tuberculomas with large numbers of foam cells (Fig. 9–24) containing the acid-fast bacteria. The patient had a high leukocyte count, fever, enlargement of lymph nodes, spleen and liver, inversion of the albumin-globulin ratio, elevated alkaline phosphatase level and a negative skin tuberculin reaction. The destructive lesions in the bones were similar or identical to those of tuberculosis (Fig. 9–25).

We have had the opportunity, by courtesy of Drs. Yakavac and Hope, of seeing material from a case studied at Children's Hospital, Philadelphia, which very closely resembles the previously described lesion.

Infections of bone by these exotic organisms are unquestionably unusual but they probably account for at least some of the cases of "atypical" tuberculous osteomyelitis. When these cases present unusual features, produce negative skin tests and do not respond to treatment, careful bacteriologic work-up may uncover a nontuberculous acid-fast organism as the cause.

SYPHILIS OF BONE

The *Treponema pallidum* infects bone just as it does the soft tissue of the body. It may be acquired in utero (congenital syphilis) from an infected mother or in postnatal life by contact (acquired syphilis). The modern treatment of syphilis by antibiotic therapy in its early stages has greatly lessened the incidence of acquired bone syphilis, and effective therapy plus compulsory premarital and prenatal serologic examinations has made congenital syphilis something of a rarity in enlightened communities.

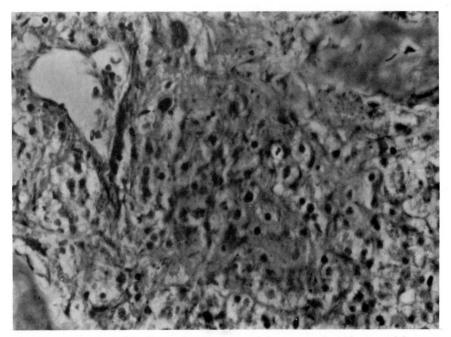

Figure 9–24 "Atypical tuberculosis" osteomyelitis caused by a nontuberculous, acid-fast organism that characteristically produces large numbers of foam cells in a granulomatous lesion.

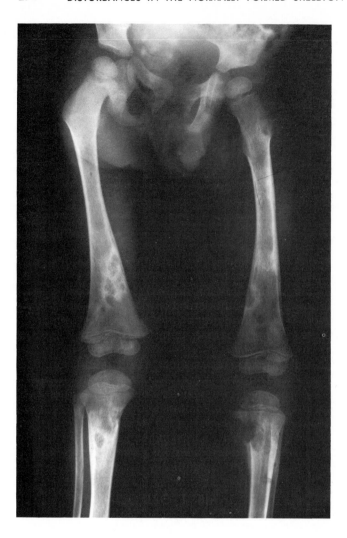

Figure 9–25 Roentgenogram of the lower extremities in the case illustrated in Figure 9–24. The lesions are sharply defined; some are associated with surrounding sclerosis and periosteal reaction. (Courtesy of Dr. J. W. Hope, Philadelphia.)

Acquired Bone Syphilis

The spirochete is carried to the site of infection by the blood. Bone syphilis occurs late and is usually classified as a tertiary form of the disease. In some instances subperiosteal lesions may be noted along with the skin manifestations of secondary lues. It should be remembered that systemic syphilis is a blood-borne infection and the walls of the arterioles are the primary sites of involvement. A luetic osteomyelitis of cancellous tissue is seen in the metaphysis. In most cases the periosteum is involved first, and without treatment the infection may spread to the cortex and even through the cortex to the medullary tissues. Both long and flat bones may be involved,

predominantly the large bones of the lower leg and the bones of the skull. Alteration of the blood supply secondary to involvement of arterioles induces both necrotizing and proliferative reactions in the tissues involved.

The necrotizing reaction may be circumscribed and surrounded by a zone of collagenized connective tissue. The central portion of the lesion undergoes a characteristic degenerative process that transforms it into a moderately firm, gray, amorphous mass. This lesion is called a gumma. More often the reaction merges imperceptibly into the surrounding tissues producing a type of granulation in which there are areas of necrosis, fibrosis and exudative cell reaction. The exudate is composed

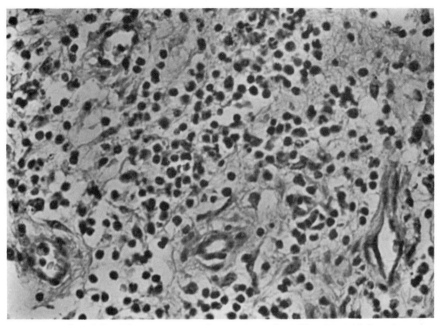

Figure 9–26   Acquired syphilis. The section reveals a perivascular infiltration with lymphocytes and plasma cells.

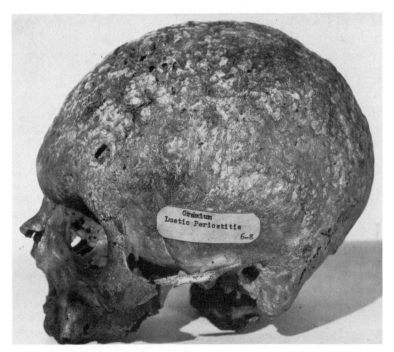

Figure 9–27   Acquired syphilis. A skull showing the roughened outer surface due to the apposition of bone by a periosteum, the site of luetic infection.

largely of lymphocytes and plasma cells. The microscopist encountering any chronic inflammatory lesion of bone composed of granulation with large numbers of plasmacytes (Fig. 9–26), particularly if the latter have a perivascular arrangement, should always think of syphilis, though in most instances the diagnosis eventually turns out to be something else.

The proliferative reaction is interesting because very few infections provoke the formation of an excessive amount of the tissue involved. New bone may be apposed to both the inner and outer cortical surfaces. Thus a thickening of the bone and sometimes narrowing of the medullary area are achieved. Because syphilis is, in reality, a disease of the walls of small and large arterial channels, reducing the blood carrying lumina and thereby causing ischemia, and because lowered oxygen tension apparently increases osteoid formation, excess bone production is seen in this disease. The subperiosteal new bone formation is quite irregular so that the cortical surface becomes roughened by numerous irregular craters and jagged linear depressions (Fig. 9–27). The interstices are filled with syphilitic granulation.

Congenital Syphilis

The spirochete characteristically attacks the metaphyseal areas in skeletal syphilis of the unborn. Any or all cylindrical bones may be involved. The normal metaphyseal tissues are replaced by syphilitic granulation. The infection prevents the emergence of the osteoblasts from the capillary lining of the fibroblast pool and consequently osteoid production is inhibited or prevented. Because the epiphyseal cartilage is avascular the organisms are unable to gain access to this region and, therefore, the chondroid scaffolding is usually produced. However, because a regular pattern depends upon the invasion of the foot of each column of chondrocytes by a tongue of granulation, and because the latter is replaced by infected granulation, the chondroid masses are irregularly shaped and dispersed. Because the mineralizing mechanism is unaffected, these cartilage masses become densely infiltrated with opaque

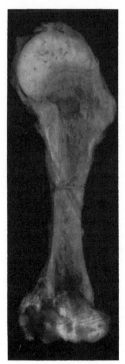

Figure 9–28   The femur of a syphilitic newborn cut in sagittal section. At the upper end the white line represents the juxta-epiphyseal zone of granulation caused by the infection.

calcium salts. Thus a broad, dense "epiphyseal line," which is often quite irregular in contour (Fig. 9–28), appears on the roentgenograms. Because osteoid production is inhibited, a paucity of cancellous bone in the subchondral area produces a zone of abnormal translucency. This lack of spongiosa causes the area to be weakened and fractures through this site are common. The epiphysis may be displaced or more often crushed down into the defective ends of the shaft.

Sections through this region disclose a replacement of normal tissues with infected granulation (Fig. 9–29), an absence of or poor osteoid production and a scrambled pattern of irregular masses of densely mineralized chondroid. The spirochete can often be demonstrated in florid cases if the proper silver staining technique is employed.

The periosteal reaction is like that of acquired syphilis. A proliferative reaction most often predominates. Because this reaction is slowly progressive and most active after birth, it is usually not noted until

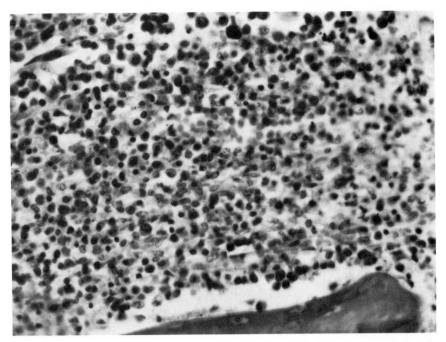

Figure 9-29   Congenital syphilis. A higher magnification of a section from the area shown in Figure 9–28. The normal tissues are replaced by infected granulation in which the plasmocyte predominates. (× 450.)

early childhood. The tibia is most often affected and the subperiosteal apposition of bone to the anterior cortical surface produces a forward bowing and sharpening of the anterior margin, the saber shin of congenital syphilis (Fig. 9–30).

BRUCELLAR OSTEOMYELITIS

Chronic osteomyelitis due to *Brucella* infection is not uncommon among farmers, meat packers and those who drink unpasteurized milk. The age group is older than that affected by the more common suppurative osteomyelitis, the great majority in a series reported by Kelly et al.[7] being over 30 years. A variety of the *Brucella* species may be involved including *abortus, melitensis* and *suis*. The patient usually has symptoms of systemic brucellosis with fever, weight loss, mild leukocytosis and decreased sedimentation time. The vertebrae are most commonly involved, then the large cylindrical bones of the extremities and finally the flat bones of the trunk. There are pain and tenderness at the site of involvement. Joints and bursae may be involved independently or in combination

with bone infection. The organisms may be cultured from the tissues in about half the cases, rarely from the blood. In the late stages there is positive serum agglutination

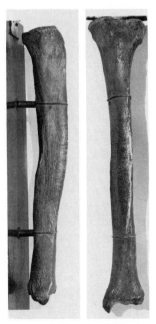

Figure 9-30   The "saber shin" of congenital syphilis. The anterior bowing is illustrated on the left. The prominent, sharp margin is seen on the right.

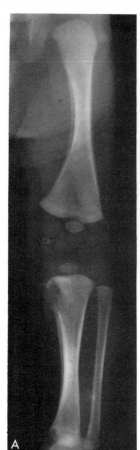

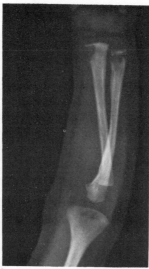

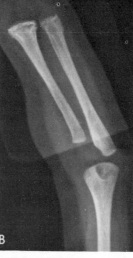

Figure 9–31 Congenital syphilis. *A*, There are radiolucent defects adjacent to the zones of provisional calcification and periosteal new bone around the diaphysis. The defect in the proximal tibia is symmetrical (Wimberger's sign). *B*, Reexamination of the forearm three weeks later reveals evidence of healing of the metaphyseal lesions.

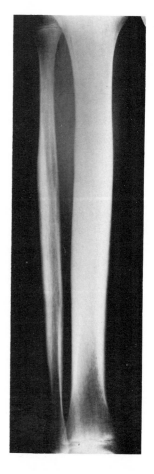

Figure 9–32 Late congenital syphilis of bone. Periosteal reaction about the tibia and fibula is marked. There is endosteal thickening of the cortex of the tibia with encroachment on the medullary canal.

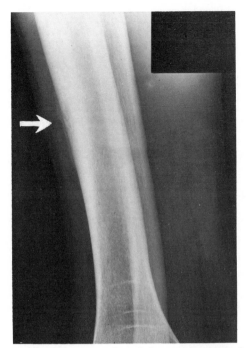

Figure 9–33 Acquired syphilis. A destructive lesion in the tibia is associated with the formation of periosteal new bone (arrow), which is irregular in outline and thickness.

and titers of 1 to 800 and above are significant. Roentgenographic findings are those of suppurative osteomyelitis with bone destruction and periosteal thickening.

Brucellar osteomyelitis is more difficult to treat than is ordinary suppurative osteomyelitis. It usually responds to tetracycline combined with streptomycin therapy, but recurrence is not uncommon and superimposed staphylococcus infection is apt to occur late in the course of the process.

FUNGUS INFECTIONS

A number of fungi may establish growth within bony tissue. These diseases are referred to as mycotic osteomyelitis. Actually they make up a very small percentage of bone infections. The four fungi most often reported in skeletal infections are *Actinomyces bovis* producing actinomycosis, *Coccidioides immitis* causing coccidioidomycosis, *Blastomyces dermatiditis*, blastomycosis, and *Sporotrichum schenckii*, sporotrichosis.[8, 9, 10] All of these fungi affect soft tissues more often than

bone and the latter is usually invaded by extension of the primary infection. Coccidioidomycosis is an exception in that bone is sometimes involved as part of a generalized infection due to hematogenous dissemination of the organism.

Actinomycosis usually involves the soft tissues of the head and neck and may spread to the mandible, to the lungs involving the ribs or dorsal vertebrae, or to the appendiceal region and extend to the pelvic bones. If the organisms gain access to bone they form multiple abscesses that are connected by sinuses. The ray fungus has a powerful lytic action on all tissues and the sinuses are formed by liquefaction necrosis with a wall of granulomatous inflammatory tissue. Colonies of the fungi removed in the pus may appear as amorphous yellow granules, which are referred to as sulfur granules. Actinomycosis is a chronic type of infection and when it involves bone it is difficult to eradicate. Surgical measures have been used in the past but recently antibiotic therapy in infections of soft tissues has been so successful that a trial of this type of therapy is warranted.

Coccidioidal infections are usually contracted in the southwest part of the United States, most often in the region of the San Joaquin Valley. When the infection spreads to involve bone there are usually multiple foci and the prognosis is grave. The granulomatous reaction is much like that of tuberculosis and can be differentiated only by finding the fungus forms in the sections.

VIRUS OSTEOMYELITIS

Bone infections of viral origin are so rare that insufficient material is available for adequate and conclusive descriptions of the process. Most accounts are of cases that have complicated smallpox. We have seen one instance of this condition (by courtesy of Dr. McNair-Scott) accompanying severe vaccinia. The patient eventually recovered following. massive soft tissue necrosis and multiple areas of bone destruction. The x-ray appearance, except for its multiplicity, could not be distinguished from that of ordinary staphylococcal osteomyelitis.

Recently a considerable amount of cir-

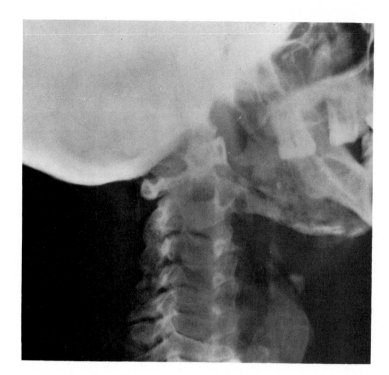

Figure 9–34 Actinomycosis of the mandible in a white female, 55 years of age. The involved portion of the mandible is irregularly thickened and contains lucent areas surrounded by extensive sclerosis. (Courtesy of Dr. George T. Wohl.)

Figure 9–35 Blastomycosis. The lesion in the fibula is purely osteolytic with a minimum of periosteal new bone formation. Reaction to this infection is not apt to occur for months after the onset of the disease. (Courtesy of Dr. George T. Wohl.)

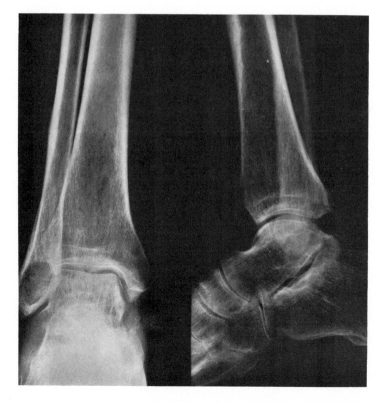

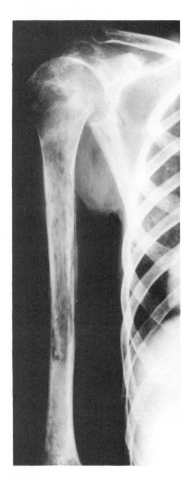

Figure 9–36 Blastomycosis. In the humerus the destruction of bone is diffuse but there is minimal sclerosis and periosteal new bone. (Courtesy of Dr. R. Perreira, Campinas, Brazil.)

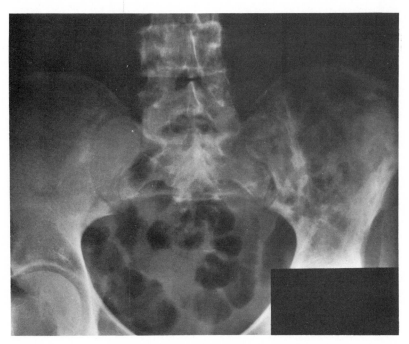

Figure 9–37 Torulosis. The extensive involvement of the left ilium is characterized by osteolytic lesions with minimal reactive new bone formation. (Courtesy of Dr. George T. Wohl.)

cumstantial evidence has been collected to indict a virus as the cause of infantile, cortical hyperostosis. Though cultures for virus and bacteria have been consistently negative it has been pointed out that the early stages are quite characteristic of an infectious inflammatory reaction.

BOECK'S SARCOID IN BONE

Boeck's sarcoid is a peculiar, granulomatous inflammatory reaction that is usually seen in the lymph nodes, spleen, lungs and liver. A combined involvement of the eyes and parotid glands has been called uveoparotid fever. Involvement of several soft tissue sites is usual and bone lesions, rarely seen independently, are usually a part of a systemic infection.

The cause of Boeck's sarcoid is unknown. For many years it was widely believed to be a manifestation of a benign type of hematogenous tuberculosis. However, the mycobacterium tuberculosis cannot be isolated from proven sarcoid lesions, the tuberculin skin test is negative in uncomplicated Boeck's sarcoid, tuberculous involvement to the extent of a multiple sarcoid dissemination has a much higher mortality than the latter, and a specific skin reaction, the Nickerson-Kveim test, can be obtained in sarcoidosis. Boeck's sarcoid and tuberculosis have frequently been reported in the same patients, but it must be added that sarcoidosis, a relatively benign disease, often is found associated with several other conditions.

Because Boeck's sarcoid is endemic in regions of large pine forests and because pine pollen has been shown to produce granulomas in the experimental animal, it has been suggested that this condition is a hypersensitivity reaction to this substance.

Almost no tissue is invulnerable to this disease but the deposits of reticuloendothelial tissue appear to be the favorite media for the etiologic agent. Even with massive involvement of large amounts of tissue the ultimate prognosis is relatively good, though occasionally infection of the lungs, liver, spleen and kidneys may cause death. The marrow tissue of bones is involved in perhaps 10 per cent of cases.

The skeletal parts most commonly af-fected are the small bones of the hands and feet, particularly the metacarpals, metatarsals and phalanges. The large bones are much less frequently involved.

Sometimes the disease is symptomless but often the patient complains of malaise and has fever. The diagnosis may be exceedingly difficult to make and can be substantiated only by biopsy. If an enlarged superficial node can be found it should be sampled. Roentgenograms of the mediastinum may disclose bilateral lymph node enlargement, which is highly suggestive. The lung fields are sometimes characteristic, having the appearance of hematogenous miliary tuberculosis except that the multiple opacities are often coarser. Needle aspiration of the liver should be done[11] and the sarcoid lesions may be obtained in a surprisingly large number of cases. We had the opportunity of studying the liver aspiration biopsies of 21 cases of sarcoidosis that were initially thought to be tuberculous. Positive material was obtained in 16 of these. Biopsy of the skin lesions may be diagnostic.

Analysis of the serum proteins, calcium, phosphorous and alkaline phosphatase levels should always be done. The globulin level is frequently elevated, usually with a reversal of the albumin-globulin ratio. The serum phosphorus level is usually not disturbed but it may be a little high. Most characteristic is the elevation in the levels of calcium and phosphatase. The former has been investigated[12] and it is thought that, though there is bone involvement, the calcium levels are out of proportion to the amount of deossification. It is postulated that the patient with sarcoidosis metabolizes a substance that is, or has an action like, vitamin D. These patients are sometimes sensitive to vitamin D therapy and, moreover, if the fecal calcium is bound by a phytate so that it cannot be absorbed, the serum calcium level falls. The elevated serum alkaline phosphatase level may be due as much to the involvement of the liver as of bone.

Because of the elevated serum calcium and alkaline phosphatase levels, the differential diagnosis between Boeck's sarcoidosis and hyperparathyroidism may be exceedingly difficult, particularly if impaired kidney function due to nephrocalcinosis has occurred. If kidney function is normal the serum phosphorus level should be low in hyperparathyroidism. In a case referred to one of us, a diagnosis of parathyroid adenoma had been made and the surgeons were instructed to search for a parathyroid adenoma. In the course of the operation a parathyroid gland showing "primary" clear cell hyperplasia was removed, and next to it a small lymph node showing unmistakable granulomas of Boeck's sarcoid. This poses an interesting question concerning the cause of the hypercalcemia in these patients.

Actually the high serum calcium level may be one of the most troublesome features of the disease because it leads to metastatic calcification of soft tissues, particularly of the kidneys. Nephrocalcinosis and urinary tract stones may cause the symptoms that bring the patient to see his physician. Snapper[13] emphasizes the frequency of lesions in the skin over the involved bone site.

Roentgenographic Manifestations. The osseous lesions of Boeck's sarcoid most frequently involve the phalanges of the hands and feet. The granulomatous process in the marrow cavity destroys bone but causes no bone reaction or periosteal new bone formation. Radiographically, the lesions usually present as small focal areas of radiolucency or the process may be diffuse within the involved bone to cause destruction of smaller trabeculae and irregular erosion of the cortex, resulting in a coarse reticular trabecular pattern. Uncommonly, the skeletal lesions are sclerotic in nature, perhaps to the extent that osteoblastic metastases are suspected (Fig. 9–40).[14] A combination of localized areas of radiolucency and the reticular pattern is most apt to be seen.

Microscopy. The lesions of Boeck's

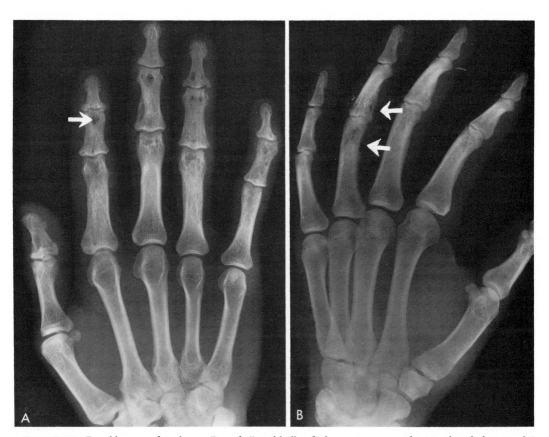

Figure 9–38 Boeck's sarcoid in bone. Round, "cystlike" radiolucencies are evident in the phalanges of A (arrow). A reticular pattern of destruction is evident in the phalanges of B (arrows).

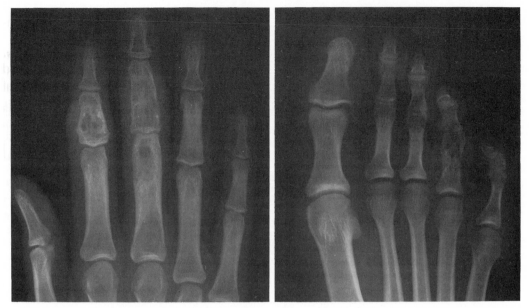

Figure 9–39   Boeck's sarcoid. There are extensive lesions in the phalanges of the hand and foot; some are confluent as in the middle phalanx of the third digit of the hand.

sarcoid are found in the interspicular marrow tissue. The microscopic appearance of the lesion depends upon its age. It begins as a minute area of necrosis measuring less than a millimeter in diameter. At first there is little cellular reaction but soon there is an infiltration of macrophages, epithelioid cells. Often the center of the lesion is occupied by a small mass of acellular, pink-staining material that has the appearance of amyloid but does not take the amyloid stain. It is probably what Teilum calls para-amyloid. Giant cells are frequently seen among the epithelioid cells. They may contain cytoplasmic condensations, which if stellate and pink-staining are called asteroid bodies and if blue and laminated are called Schaumann bodies. It was once thought that these structures were pathognomonic of the disease but they have since been demonstrated in giant cells of a variety of granuloma types. There is a tendency for the granulomas to merge (Fig. 9–41) but their peripheral outlines usually remain discernible because of the reserve cells, which develop into collagenoblasts and lay down collagen. As the lesions age the latter cells become more prominent until they eventually replace the epithelioid cells. Necrosis does occur

but it is usually not as prominent as that in the tuberculoid granuloma and it is rarely if ever caseous. There is usually a sprinkling of lymphocytes about the periphery of the lesion. The granuloma of Boeck's sarcoid cannot be differentiated from those of a host of other diseases, but if granulomas are found with typical clinical and laboratory findings and roentgenograms the diagnosis can usually be established with a fair degree of certainty.

SCLEROSING OSTEITIS (GARRE)

In 1893, Garré described a type of osteomyelitis as a low-grade, chronic, diffuse inflammatory reaction that caused thickening and increased density in cortical and cancellous bone. Several reports stress the lack of suppurative exudate, the increase in bone mass, sometimes with fibrous replacement of the interspicular tissues, and the usual inability to culture organisms from the lesion. The process is said to involve the shafts of long bones particularly, causing a fusiform thickening. Mild to moderate bone pain, especially at night, is said to be the chief and sometimes only symptom.

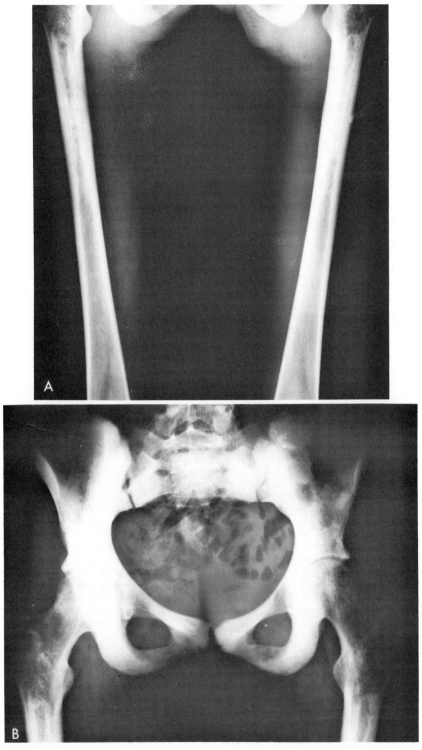

Figure 9–40 Boeck's sarcoid. Osteosclerotic alterations of the femurs and the bones of the pelvis are marked. (Courtesy of Dr. A. Bonakdarpour, Temple University Hospital, Philadelphia.)

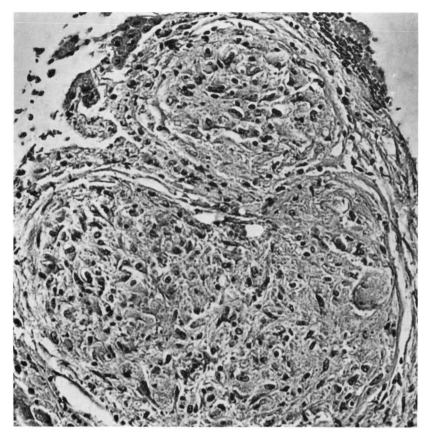

Figure 9–41   Three granulomas of Boeck's sarcoid. The top lesion is quite discrete. All are composed of an epithelioid cell reaction surrounded by a fibrous collar. (× 267.)

Other writers, unable to identify a causative agent for the condition, have suggested that the lesion may be caused by an interference with the blood supply. They point out that if the normal oxygen tension in bone is reduced but still adequate for bone viability, organic osteoid is laid down and soon becomes mineralized. They suggest that the increase in bone mass produces tension that could cause pain. They fortify their argument by stating that surgical incision or drilling frequently relieves the pain. This presumably is brought about by the formation of granulation and thereby an increase in the blood supply to the area.

Many orthopedists today believe that if the lesion that appears on clinical and roentgenographic evidence to be sclerosing osteitis is carefully studied it will be found to be one of a variety of other conditions. They suggest that there is no entity as Garré described. Because the roentgenographic findings might be produced by a number of sclerosing conditions and because the microscopic structure is certainly far from pathognomonic, there is no way of proving whether the entity exists. It is certain that the diagnosis is much less frequently made today than it was in the past in many large clinics.

CONGENITAL RUBELLA SYNDROME

It has been documented that infection of the pregnant female by the virus of rubella during the first trimester of pregnancy carries the risk of damage to the newborn infant. In general, the abnormalities that result fall into several broad categories: (1) generalized disease with retardation of growth, hepatosplenomegaly, thrombocytopenia and central nervous system disease, (2) abnormalities of the skeleton as noted radiographically, 3) abnormalities of the eye characterized by cataracts and glaucoma and (4) congenital cardiac disease.

It has been possible to obtain positive cultures of the rubella virus in a large percentage of affected infants, most often from throat swabs. Continuous excretion of virus over a period of months after birth has been documented as well.

Radiographically, the most striking manifestations of the rubella syndrome are noted in the long bones. The bones at the knee tend to be most involved. There are longitudinal streaks of alternating sclerosis and lucency in the metaphyses, often associated with irregular density and contour of the zone of provisional calcification (Fig. 9–43). At times a broad, transverse band of metaphyseal lucency is seen, alone or in association with the previously mentioned manifestations. The lesions tend to disappear over a period of two to three months; unusual thickness of the zone of provisional calcification may persist, however.

Histologically, there would seem to be a defect in the formation of bone, particularly in the deposition and mineralization of osteoid. Adjacent to the line of ossification, one sees poorly calcified cartilage and

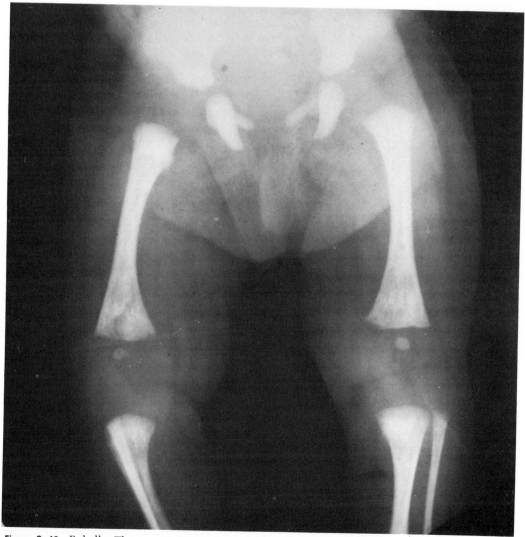

Figure 9–42 Rubella. The roentgen examination of the lower extremities of a newborn infant reveals the zone of provisional calcification to be irregular in contour. Within the metaphysis and extending into the diaphysis there are alternating lucent and sclerotic streaks. The midportion of the diaphyses is spared.

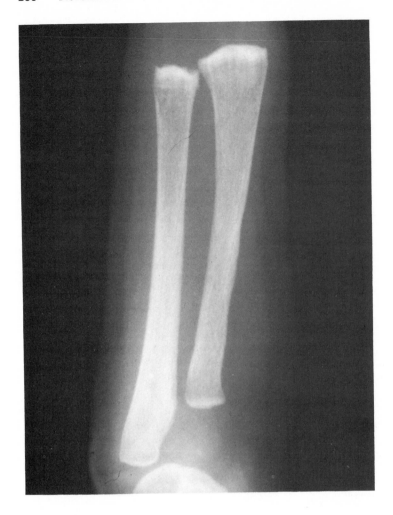

Figure 9–43 Rubella, male, 7 months of age. There are longitudinal streaks of density and lucency within the metaphysis and diaphysis of the distal radius and ulna. The zone of provisional calcification is quite thick and dense.

poorly formed osteoid. Individual trabeculae have a central core of hyaline cartilage surrounded by islands of osteoid. Fragments of cartilage persist and extend into the diaphysis.[9]

The nature of the osseous alterations is not completely understood. The absence of evidence of inflammatory reaction in the bone would suggest that the alterations reflect a metabolic and nutritional disturbance; a viral inflammatory process cannot be positively excluded.

References

1. Hughes, J. G. and Carroll, D. S.: Pediatrics, *19*: 184, 1957.
2. Quie, P. G., Kaplan, E. L., Page, A. R. et al.: N. Engl. J. Med., *278*:976, 1968.
2a. Capitanio, M. A. and Kirkpatrick, J. A.: Am. J. Roentgenol., *108*:488, 1970.
3. Steinbach, H. L.: Seminars in Roentgenol., *1*:337, 1966.
4. Kelly, P. and Karlson, A.: Mayo Clin. Proc., *44*:73, 1969.
5. de Torregrosa, M. V., Dapena, R. B., Hernandez, H. and Ortiz, A.: J.A.M.A., *174*:354, 1960.
6. van der Hoeven, L. H., Rutten, F. J. and van der Sar, A.: Am. J. Clin. Path., *29*:433, 1958.
7. Kelley, P. J., Martin, W. J., Schirger, A. and Weed, L. A.: J.A.M.A., *174*:347, 1960.
8. Reeves, R. J. and Pedersen, R.: Radiology, *62*:55, 1954.
9. Rudolph, A. J., Singleton, E. B., Rosenberg, H. S., Singer, D. B. and Phillips, C. A.: Am. J. Dis. Child., *110*:428, 1965.
10. Gehweiler, J. P., Capp, M. P. and Chick, E. W.: Radiology, *108*:497, 1970.
11. Shay, H., Berk, J. E., Sones, M., Aegerter, E., Weston, J. K. and Adams, A. B.: Gastroenterology, *19*:441, 1951.
12. Henneman, P. H., Dempsey, E. F. and Albright, F.: J. Clin. Invest., *35*:1229, 1956.
13. Snapper, I.: Bone Diseases in Medical Practice. New York, Grune and Stratton, 1957.
14. Bonakdarpour, A., Levy, W. and Aegerter, E.E.: Am. J. Roentgenol., *113*:646, 1971.
15. Rosen, R. S. and Jacobson, G.: Seminars in Roentgenol., *1*:370, 1966.

Chapter 10

CIRCULATORY DISTURBANCES

BONE INFARCT

Sudden and complete obstruction of the arterial blood supply to bone results in death of the tissue supplied — an infarct — in much the same manner that infarction occurs in such soft tissues as the heart, spleen and kidney. In the diaphysis, cancellous tissue is involved and the overlying cortex spared so that there is no change in the external aspect of the bone. Because the periosteum is not involved, the infarct is without symptoms. In cases in which the infarction involves the epiphysis, the support for the articular cartilage may be destroyed and then the condition is known as epiphyseal ischemic necrosis, aseptic necrosis, epiphyseal osteochondritis or, in childhood, Perthes' disease or coxa plana. For these reasons, bone infarct was quite neglected until Kahlstrom, Phemister and Burton[1] published their paper in 1939. The condition had been recognized in 1878 when Bert described the lesion in patients who had worked in environments with high atmospheric pressure. A few subsequent reports appeared, emphasizing the arthritic aspect and describing roentgenographic features.

Because all of the early reported cases were associated with increased atmospheric pressure, the condition has long been known as caisson disease. Kahlstrom and Phemister[2] reported the disease in a patient in 1946 who denied ever doing caisson work and numerous other cases are now known. They contend that bone infarct occurs as often in noncaisson workers as in those who are exposed to high pressure. They state that if a high index of suspicion is maintained the diagnosis will be made much more frequently. Such is certainly the experience of any radiologist who remains alert for the condition.

The history of caisson disease should cause one to explore the possibility of bone infarct as a part of the complex of multiple infarction of soft tissues. The caisson worker is exposed to atmospheric pressures of 25 to 50 pounds. As the worker is compressed, gas is absorbed by the blood. Fat has a greater affinity for nitrogen than does the blood, estimated at about fivefold. Tissues composed largely of lipids, the omentum and mesentery, the subcutaneous tissue and the marrow of long bones, absorb large quantities of nitrogen under conditions of compression. As the worker is decompressed, this nitrogen is released into the blood but the lungs are unable to clear it as fast as it is released, so that it accumulates in minute bubbles, which may coalesce to form pockets of intravascular nitrogen. This unabsorbed nitrogen causes gas embolism in the vicinity in which the gas is released.

In the skin and subcutaneous tissue there are usually flushing, areas of lividity and pruritus. Bleeding occurs from the mucosa of the gastrointestinal, respiratory and urinary tracts. Cramplike pains may occur in the abdomen because of multiple small infarcts of the viscera. If enough small bubbles are delivered to the lungs there may be dyspnea. Infarcts occurring in the spinal cord and brain may cause a variety of signs including visual disturbance, tinnitus, hypesthesias, motor paralysis and even collapse and death. Most of the symptoms occur while decompression is being accomplished or within three hours but in a few cases they have appeared as late as 23 hours after decompression.[3]

It is probable that bone infarcts occur in the majority of these cases, but because there are no immediate symptoms they are missed. The long bones are involved almost exclusively, the upper end of the femur most commonly and then the lower femur, upper tibia and upper humerus. These areas are doubtless most vulnerable because of their proximity to fat stores and because they are supplied by long arteries with few collaterals. Cancellous tissue is involved, whereas the overlying cortex escapes. The infarct may occur at any point in the bone, but the incidence is highest at the bone ends. The lesion varies in size from a few millimeters in diameter to involvement of the entire half of the shaft. If the infarct is restricted to the diaphysis, symptoms may never develop and the area is noted only when roentgenograms are made for other reasons. In cases in which the epiphysis is involved, the supportive columns of the articular plate eventually give way, resulting in unevenness or actual collapse of the latter. Symptoms of arthritis usually develop within six months to a year.

When an area of bone tissue is deprived of its arterial blood supply it dies. The soft, fatty marrow undergoes coagulation and liquefaction necrosis. In the bone spicules the osteocytes die and leave their lacunae empty. As long as there is no circulation through the area, it must remain more or less intact, as dead tissue. But at the margins of the infarct, at the point at which it adjoins healthy tissue, there is circulation and here phagocytes enter to clean up the debris and dead bone can be absorbed. Vessels sprouting from the healthy area surround the infarct with a capsule of granulation tissue. Fingers of the latter insert themselves as far into the dead tissue as its vasculature will support it. It is probable that small infarcts are completely absorbed and replaced by new and healthy cancellous tissue. In larger lesions, the aging granulation collagenizes before it completes its task and soon the vessels are choked off by shrinking scar tissue. The fibrous capsule calcifies, perhaps because of the abundance of calcium salts in the area or possibly because of its chemical make-up. The calcified collagen frequently goes on to ossification. Thus, the area of dead bone and marrow is surrounded and isolated by a layer of dense fibrous scar (Fig. 10–1), of calcified collagen, of new bone or, as in most cases, of a combination of these tissues. The encapsulated infarct may be suspended in cancellous tissue or it may abut against the cortical wall. Here it remains indefinitely, usually unsuspected unless some unrelated event leads to roentgenographic or surgical investigation in later life. Osteoporosis, disuse atrophy or degenerative disease in a nearby joint may cause symptoms that lead to x-ray investigation. When these areas turn up on a roentgenogram they introduce a serious diagnostic problem. Though the radiologist may surmise their true nature, if there is no history of caisson exposure the diagnosis can be confirmed only by biopsy.

Infarcts in the epiphysis usually run an entirely different course. Here, failure of the support of the articular plate leads to impairment of the weight-bearing surface and degenerative joint disease sets in. Pain, deformity, disability and even ankylosis may occur. The gross appearance of the infarct is altered by the motion and pressure of usage and eventually even large amounts of dead tissue may be converted to granulation and then to new bone. But by this time the normal anatomy is so distorted that function may be impossible without surgical repair.

It is certain that the nutrient vessels of bone uncommonly are closed by agents other than the nitrogen emboli of caisson disease. There appears to be no reason why thrombosis and thrombus embolism cannot occur in vessels of bone just as they occur in those of soft tissue. The incidence of this accident, like that of idiopathic hemorrhage, is probably much greater than we have heretofore suspected.

A rapid and massive necrosis of bone and joint tissues is occasionally encountered in patients taking cortisone compounds either systemically or locally injected. The mechanisms are not well understood and perhaps are not the same for bone and for the cartilage of joints. The massive and tragic necrosis of the spine and less often other bones is thought to be

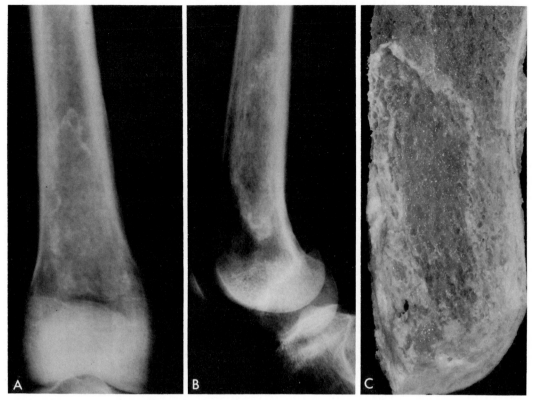

Figure 10–1 *A*, Anteroposterior and *B*, lateral projections of the lower end of the femur; *C*, a sagittal section through the bone. This area is on the site of a large infarct, which in *C* is outlined by a sclerotic margin of hard, white, mineralized collagen.

an ischemic necrosis by Fisher et al.,[4] who reported a case of fat embolism in the head of a femur. Moran[5] established a relationship between systemically administered corticoids and elevated serum lipids, fatty liver and fat emboli in rabbits. Hill[6] reported a death due to multiple fat embolism in viscera, and Jones and Engelman[7] suggest the relationship of ischemic necrosis in femoral heads of alcoholics due to fat emboli. Fatty livers may be found in both types of patients.

Microscopy. Sections taken from the center of a well established bone infarct show spicules of dead bone with empty lacunae (Fig. 10–3). The intervening marrow has been converted to an amorphous mass of tissue debris. There are areas of liquefaction necrosis surrounded by irregular patches of fibrous collagen in which may be embedded crystals of cholesterol. With the routine hematoxylin and eosin technique these appear as fusiform clefts with sharply pointed ends. Coarse granules

of deep blue calcium salts are scattered about and there is usually evidence of old hemorrhage with finer hemosiderin particles. In some areas there is coagulation necrosis and a retaining of the architecture of masses of fat cells. Elsewhere, the sections take a washed-out bluish stain indicating the partial splitting of neutral fats.

About the periphery of this region one should find fields of mature fibrous tissue (Fig. 10–4), and often this is so densely infiltrated with mineral that it may require decalcification for sectioning (Fig. 10–5). There is usually some bone formation about the periphery where circulation has been reestablished.

Prognosis. Bone infarcts in the diaphysis have been known to exist for years without giving any symptoms. Their chief importance is the diagnostic problem they introduce when turned up as an incidental finding. Infarcts in the epiphysis (epiphyseal ischemic necrosis, aseptic necrosis) cause severe arthritis and crippling. It may

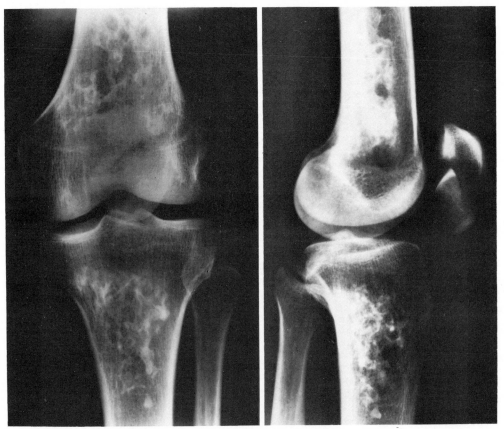

Figure 10–2   Bone infarct. The spongiosa of the distal femur and the proximal tibia is involved. The cortex is spared. Irregular opacities within the marrow cavity are evident, a reflection of calcified or ossified collagen about and within the infarcted areas. The radiolucent areas are the residua of areas of necrosis.

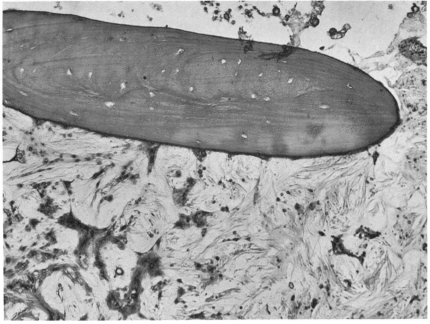

Figure 10–3   A spicule of dead bone lying in a mass of necrotic medullary soft tissue. The osteocytes have disappeared from the lacunae. Surrounding the bone is an oily mass of necrotic tissue containing only a few fibroblasts. ($\times$ 180.)

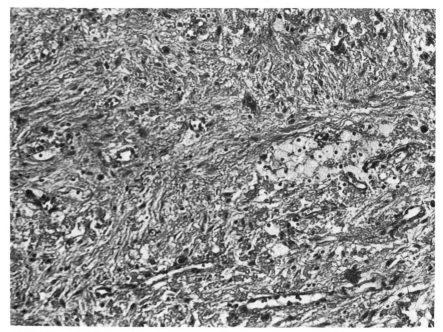

Figure 10–4 Section taken from the periphery of an infarct showing a fibroblastic proliferation. An aggregate of lipid-bearing histiocytes appears at right center field. (× 180.)

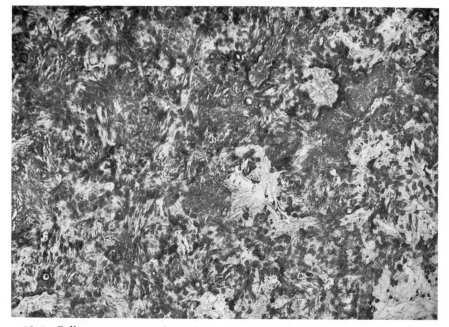

Figure 10–5 Collagenous margin of an infarct with massive deposition of mineral salts. (× 180.)

be necessary to reconstruct an articular surface and its support to reestablish function.

EPIPHYSEAL ISCHEMIC NECROSIS

By this term we refer to the condition that is variously called osteochondritis deformans juvenilis, the osteochondroses, epiphyseal osteochondritis or epiphyseal aseptic necrosis. When the process involves the capital epiphysis of the femur it is usually called Perthes' disease or Legg-Calvé-Perthes disease or simply coxa plana. When it involves the secondary or less frequently the primary epiphyses of other bones, it is often designated by an eponym such as Osgood-Schlatter disease (tibial tubercle), Köhler's disease (tarsal navicular and sometimes the patella), Freiberg's disease (second metatarsal head), Scheuermann's disease (vertebral bodies), Panner's disease (capitellum of the humerus), Thiemann's disease (proximal phalanges) and others, depending upon the site. Harvard Ellman recently has described an ischemic necrosis of the radial head in youngsters who produce a valgus overload in pitching a baseball. Today most orthopedists agree that the pathogenesis of these lesions is the same and that the benumbing array of eponyms should be discarded for the sake of clarity and common sense.

The process is essentially a degeneration and eventual replacement of the osseous nucleus of an epiphysis, almost certainly the result of an interference with its blood supply. In a sense, it is an infarct of the bony epiphysis, which then collapses under pressure and causes distortion of the surrounding healthy tissues that it is supposed to support. To use the term "osteochondritis" is to imply that inflammation is an important factor, which in most cases it certainly is not. Although there is a very convincing array of data to support the ischemia hypothesis, the offending vessels have not yet been conclusively demonstrated. In addition, because a few cases have yielded positive bacterial culture, the name "aseptic necrosis" is untenable. Jones and Sakovich[8] injected lipiodol into rabbits and found that over the course of

hours the fat droplets accumulated in the epiphyseal arterial capillaries. They concluded that many cases of Perthes' disease are caused by multiple microinfarcts secondary to fat embolism.

Most types of the disease occur more commonly in males in a ratio of about four to one. Because the more important types occur in the unclosed epiphysis of a growing bone it is usually seen in the younger age groups, most often children, with some of the less common types appearing in adolescents and adults. The primary epiphyses are apt to be involved at an earlier age than the secondary. Thus, the primary epiphysis of the tarsal navicular is usually affected between the ages of 4 and 6 years, whereas the secondary epiphyses of the vertebral bodies show involvement during adolescence. In certain types in which the vessel damage is probably caused by repeated trauma, the head of the second metatarsal and the carpal lunate reveal the characteristic changes, in most cases, in adult life. The most important type of epiphyseal aseptic necrosis occurs in the superior epiphysis of the femur in children between 3 and 12 years old.

The cause of epiphyseal ischemic necrosis has been the subject of polemic debate since Osgood and Schlatter each wrote their separate papers on the condition in 1903. It might be entertaining to review the various theories, their authors and the authors' supportive arguments, but such a review would probably do little to enhance one's understanding of the disease. It will suffice to list the more popular theories, such as chronic repeated trauma, congenital and hereditary factors, infection, embolism and endocrine disturbances. It is probable that most of these causes have played a role in the vasculature and blood supply of the affected epiphyses in the past, but the resultant ischemia is the common denominator of all the lesions. All the acceptable, well documented facts support this hypothesis. In brief, the vessels may rarely be closed by emboli (supported by cases in which embolism occurs in other soft tissue vessels), the vessels may be torn or thrombosed by trauma (ischemic necrosis has occurred in those cases of trauma in which all vessels were involved), and the lesion has yielded indubitably positive cultures in a very few cases. A dysgenesis of the superior femoral epiphysis that has much the same appearance as epiphyseal ischemic necrosis occurs in cretinism. Caffey has reported his painstaking study of 30 cases[9] and made several observations which support the hypothesis that degenerative changes are initiated by fracture followed by the to-be-expected ischemic necrosis. He suggests that the name be changed to "chronic stress injury" and if his observations are as valid as they appear at this writing it is certainly a sensible suggestion. In any event a careful reading of his paper is mandatory for anyone wishing to understand this interesting and important condition.

The failure of true coxa plana to occur after puberty is probably due to the change in vasculature that is incident to epiphyseal ossification. The excessive incidence of this lesion in boys conceivably may be due to their propensity for traumatizing activity. Though papers[10] still appear, associating epiphyseal ischemic necrosis with hypothyroidism, there is little beyond the slender substance of which they are composed to convince one that hypothyroidism, per se, is a cause of this condition. The congenital and hereditary hypotheses probably stem from the similarities of lesions in such conditions as Morquio's and Hurler's disease that have been mistaken for epiphyseal ischemic necrosis.

Pain in the region of the tibial tubercle during adolescence is an exceedingly common occurrence. Radiographs often have shown variations that have been interpreted as epiphyseal ischemic necrosis, Osgood-Schlatter disease. Today it is recognized that most of these changes are nothing more than variations of the normal growth pattern. Some writers do not recognize the existence of the entity ischemic necrosis of the tibial tubercle but most agree that the bona fide lesion is one of tibial tubercle avulsion.

Another debatable lesion occurs in the medial proximal epiphysis of the tibia resulting in an idiopathic type of lateral bowing of that bone. This condition is called osteochondrosis deformans tibia, tibia vara or Blount's disease. It has been widely ascribed to ischemic necrosis in the proximal medial epiphysis, but because it

is frequently bilateral, many writers contend that it is a congenital growth defect (multiple epiphyseal dysplasia, see p. 137).

The most important member of the epiphyseal ischemic necrosis group from the standpoint of both incidence and morbidity is the process in the capital epiphysis of the femur, commonly called coxa plana or Perthes' disease. Because the morbid physiology of the various members of the group is the same, only the clinical and radiologic aspects differing with the various sites, a detailed discussion of coxa plana will serve to illustrate the process in general.

Before discussing ischemic necrosis of the superior femoral epiphysis, an understanding of the vasculature of the head and neck of the femur is essential.[11] The epiphysis is almost completely supplied by two arteries: the lateral epiphyseal artery arises from the medial femoral circumflex and is the dominant source of blood for the epiphysis; the medial epiphyseal artery is a continuation of the artery that courses through the ligamentum teres, which in turn arises from the acetabular branch of the obturator. These vessels anastomose with each other and send branches toward the articular cartilage. These branches form single large capillaries that supply the zone immediately beneath the articular plate. To date no vascular channels have been demonstrated within the substance of the articular cartilage. The metaphysis of the femoral neck is supplied by two groups of vessels. The inferior metaphyseal arteries supply the greater portion of fresh blood and the superior metaphyseal arteries, from two to five in number, supply the lesser portion.

Until ossification of the enchondral plate, there is little communication between these two sets of vessels. Following closure of the epiphyseal line, anastomosing branches between the epiphyseal and metaphyseal groups have been demonstrated. Neither group is intimately associated with the main nutrient artery of the femoral shaft.

Until 1910, ischemic necrosis of the superior femoral epiphysis was confused with other diseases of the hip joint, principally tuberculosis. In that year, there appeared three separately authored papers in the American,[12] French[13] and German[14] literature distinguishing the condition as an entity. Though Perthes originally suggested the ischemic nature of the condition, the realization that it is an example of a process that may affect any epiphysis was not general until many years later.

Coxa plana is a relatively common orthopedic disease. It affects males more often than females in a proportion of about four to one. The peak age incidence is about 6 years though it may occur between the ages of 3 and 12. It probably never starts, at least in its typical form, after 12 years though the regenerative stage may progress well into adolescence. It is bilateral in perhaps 10 per cent of cases. It is rarely seen in the Negro.

The symptoms may be insidious in onset or sudden, the latter frequently associated with trauma. Pain of varying degrees of severity, limp and limitation of motion are usually the presenting complaints. The pain frequently starts in the knee region and may persist here for weeks or even months, obscuring the actual source. The pain may be referred to the inner thigh or the groin following the distribution of the obturator nerve. It is usually worsened by activity and relieved by rest. Motion is often limited, particularly on internal rotation and in flexion and abduction. There may be anterior and posterior tenderness. Eventually the pain disappears spontaneously and motion is restored. If a limp persists it is due to mechanical factors rather than pain. At this time one may note minimal atrophy of the thigh muscles and eventually slight shortening (growth failure) of the involved extremity. Having run its course, the disease may leave a crippled hip, the patient adjusting his activity to the amount and type of joint impairment. In later adult life, degenerative joint disease (osteoarthritis) often sets in because of the altered stress trajectories and weight-bearing surfaces.

Ischemic necrosis of the capital femoral epiphysis runs its morbid course in two to six years. The process is usually divided into three active phases and a fourth or healed period of static altered joint and bone structure.

The first stage lasts two weeks to two months. Because weeks or even months elapse before the changes in bone consequent to deprivation of its blood supply become obvious, the changes of the first period are those that appear in the soft tissue. There is swelling and a low-grade inflammatory reaction in the joint synovia and capsule. Caffey believes that fracture through or into the epiphyseal osseous nucleus can be demonstrated early in the lesion if proper x-ray technique[9] is used. Eventually fibrosis with thickening intervenes.

During the second phase the predominant feature is a necrotizing process within the osseous nucleus and underlying enchondral plate. The articular plate derives almost all of its nourishment from the joint fluid, and though there is edema and congestion of the soft tissues of the joint incident to the epiphyseal ischemia, the articular cartilage usually survives intact until its osseous support collapses. Then surface irregularities, flattening and spreading occur. The osseous nucleus dies in part (according to Caffey, the anterior, superior, lateral quadrant), or in toto. Vessels are apparently torn or thrombosed. Because the enchondral plate derives its blood supply from the same vessels, it too usually softens. Enchondral growth is inhibited or stops completely. The second phase, that of necrosis, persists for 6 to 18 months or somewhat longer. Because the osseous nucleus is small and is supplied by more than one vessel, it is rare that the entire epiphyseal blood supply is lost. Thus, though the bone and contiguous cartilage die, granulation can still generate from the persisting mesenchymal cells. Deltas of new arterioles and capillaries bring in sufficient blood to partially demineralize the bone and weaken its supportive strength. It collapses and becomes condensed owing to stress pressures. It may fragment or give the appearance of fragmentation because of the inroads of granulation.

In the third phase the predominant feature is the replacement of dead tissue by new bone and cartilage. Its duration varies from a year to several years depending upon the size of the area affected, the availability of a new supply of vessels and the extent of the distortion that occurs in the second phase. If the original epiphyseal vessels are completely lost, the area must await granulation to penetrate from the metaphysis and during this period the lesion appears to be static. Eventually the debris of the dead bone, cartilage and marrow is removed and replaced by new bone, or by densely collagenized fibrous tissue. The flattened head, the shortened and thickened neck and the corresponding modeling changes that occur in the acetabulum remain as the residuum, sometimes referred to as the fourth phase.

Roentgenographic Manifestations. The radiographic manifestations of epiphyseal ischemic necrosis parallel the alterations in anatomy and physiology. These are the same no matter which epiphyseal center is involved, so that a discussion of the process as it involves the femoral capital epiphysis applies to other epiphyses. The radiographic recognition of this process as it involves the hip is important because of the desirability of early treatment.

During the first stage of the disease there may be only meager radiographic changes, consisting of bulging of the joint capsule, as a result of synovial thickening and fluid within the joint. The capsule may be visualized by virtue of more radiolucent fat contiguous to it. At this time, slight lateral displacement of the proximal femur in relation to the acetabulum may be appreciated. The earliest osseous manifestation may be the visualization of a lucent crescent[15, 16] that parallels the subchondral surface of the femoral epiphysis, usually anterolaterally (Fig. 10–6). This, it has been postulated, represents a fracture. Later the femoral capital epiphyseal center appears more opaque than is normal, particularly in the absence of weight-bearing. This probably does not represent a real increase in mineral content, but rather reflects demineralization of the surrounding bony structures as a result of disuse secondary to pain or immobilization by hyperemia coupled with persistent mineralization of the epiphyseal center. The latter cannot demineralize because its blood supply is lost. The radiolucent epiphyseal line widens and becomes irregular, often showing localized radiolucencies that may involve a large portion of the metaphysis and persist into the third stage of the process (Fig. 10–8). The epiphyseal line undergoes such

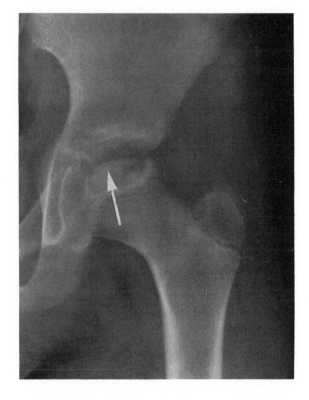

Figure 10–6 Epiphyseal ischemic necrosis. A subchondral lucent defect is visible (arrow). This defect may be seen before any other osseous alteration; in this patient, fragmentation of the epiphyseal center has begun.

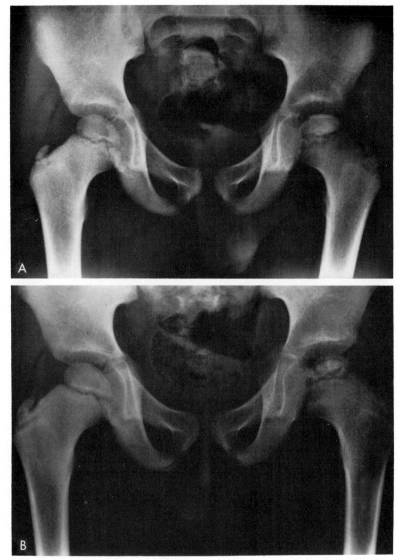

Figure 10–7   Epiphyseal ischemic necrosis. In the latter portion of the first stage (A) the opacity of the left femoral capital epiphysis is evident. The surrounding bony structures are demineralized, which accentuates this opacity. The joint space is widened, the metaphysis is broad and more radiolucent than is normal and the femoral neck is deformed. One year later (B) fragmentation is evident and dead bone (opaque) may be seen. The joint space is wide. This radiograph presents the second stage of the process.

alterations because its blood supply is absent; it is supplied by the same vessels that nourish the epiphysis.

The second stage is characterized by opacity, fragmentation and flattening of the epiphyseal center. These changes reflect the invasion of the necrotic epiphyseal center by granulation tissue and the effects of stress on this weakened structure. The increase in opacity of the epiphyseal cen-

ter now is probably real and reflects the collapse of the center and apposition of its fragments.

In the third or healing stage, new bone is formed and the outline of the epiphyseal center again becomes regular and intact. Often the process appears to be completely healed on radiographs made in the antero-posterior projection, but when the hip is examined in the lateral projection radiolucent areas in the anterior aspect of the epiphyseal center may be evident and are the last to heal (Fig. 10–9).

In addition to the changes in the epiphyseal center itself, alterations occur in the metaphysis as a result of which the femoral neck becomes broad and short. The acetabulum must adapt itself to the flat, broad femoral head. Thus, the fourth stage is represented by a short, broad femoral neck that is often angled anteriorly more than is normal, a flat, broad head and an enlarged acetabulum that corresponds roughly in shape to the femoral head. The fourth stage is represented by the final deformity of the hip joint (Fig. 10–10).

Pathologic Morphology. Pathologists have had little opportunity of studying the lesion as a whole because the disease is not fatal and rarely has the orthopedist resorted to resection of the entire head and neck as a means of therapy. Because modern treatment with reasonably early diagnosis is entirely conservative and without surgery, adequate material, even fragments, has

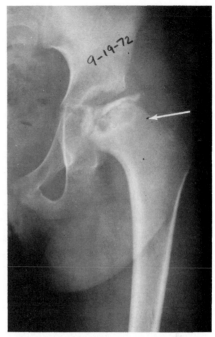

Figure 10–8 Large lucent defects are evident in the metaphysis (arrow); the margins are sclerotic. The epiphyseal center is flat and dense.

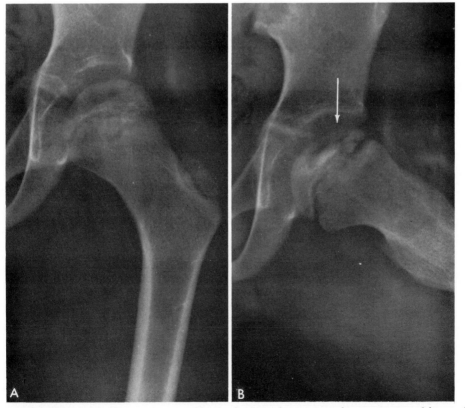

Figure 10–9 Epiphyseal ischemic necrosis in the third stage. There is partial reconstitution of the epiphyseal center, which, however, is flat. The anterior aspect of the center that is least healed is best seen in the lateral projection (arrow, *B*).

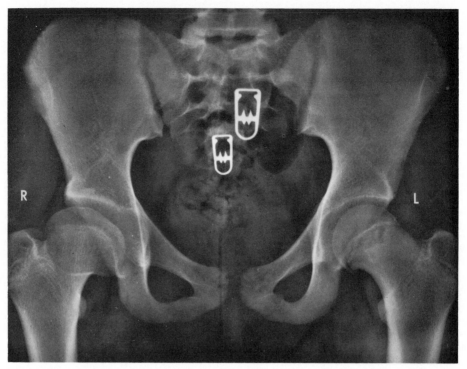

Figure 10-10   The fourth stage of epiphyseal ischemic necrosis is evident on the right. The left femur shows the early changes of epiphyseolysis.

rarely been available for conclusive studies. Our information has been picked bit by bit from a number of sources. When this is fitted together and correlated with the clinical and roentgenographic details, the lesion emerges as an area of epiphyseal bone that has been deprived of a blood supply adequate for continued life and health.

Gall and Bennett[17] had the opportunity of doing an autopsy study on a patient with coxa plana who died of secondary parathyroid hyperplasia and kidney failure. The head of the femur was flattened and though the articular surface was widened and irregular it was still intact. The osseous nucleus was necrotic, compressed and fragmented. There was evidence of old hemorrhage, cystic degeneration and replacement fibrosis. The enchondral plate was softened and distorted, the epiphyseal line irregular and, in the central portion, completely replaced by fibrous granulation growing in from the metaphysis.

The paper of Zemansky[18] gives one of the most complete descriptions of the microscopy. The cytologic findings depend upon the phase in which the lesion is sec-

tioned. In the first phase, the bone and cartilage are intact though one may note changes in or death of the osteocytes. The vessels are dilated and filled with static blood. Degenerative changes soon become apparent in the marrow. The contiguous soft tissues reflect the altered physiology of the vascular accident. The synovial membranes and capsule are thickened by congestion and edema (Fig. 10-11). The dilated vessels may be circled by small aggregates of lymphocytes. If the stasis persists long enough, a fibroblastic action eventually takes place. In the second phase one finds irregular fragments of well preserved dead bone interspersed with areas of necrotic bone that is undergoing lysis. Between and around the fragments is granulation. The cartilage of the enchondral plate may show enlargement of its lacunae and distortion of the cellular pattern. The soft interspicular tissue is converted to an amorphous mass of extravasated red cells, degenerating fat and marrow cell debris (Fig. 10-12). Shadow cells may be discernible, such as those that appear in soft tissue infarcts. Osteoclasts are in evidence

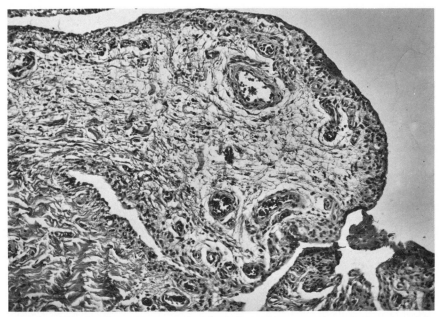

Figure 10–11 Epiphyseal ischemic necrosis (Perthes' disease). Section through the synovial lining of the joint. A villous process is pictured. It is thickened by edema and a mild inflammatory process. (× 180.)

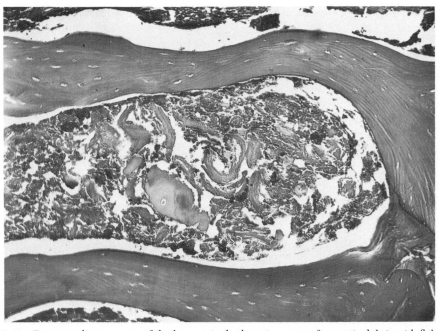

Figure 10–12 Between the two arms of the bone spicule there is a mass of necrotic debris with flakes of bone and soft tissue intermixed.

and there may be occasional giant cells. Masses of tissue with a microscopic resemblance to "giant cell tumor" have been described. Such an extravagant giant cell reaction has never occurred in our material and it is rarely noted in the literature.

During the third phase there is a gradual lysis of dead bone and cartilage by newly formed granulation. The rate of granulation formation is dependent upon the extent to which a healthy vascular bed has been retained around the necrotic nucleus. If all the blood supply to the epiphysis has been obliterated, the necrotic center may have to wait until granulation grows up from the metaphysis before a sufficient blood and macrophage supply can accomplish lysis. Irregular masses of cartilage and bone may be found. It is difficult to be certain whether these are newly formed as a part of the repair process or the residuum of areas whose blood supply was less severely jeopardized than the necrotic fragments. In some cases the destroyed area is eventually replaced by a densely collagenized mass that extends from the undersurface of the remaining articular cartilage and merges with the fibrous tissue of the metaphyseal medullary area. In some cases this area is converted to bone and then resembles a closed, albeit deformed, epiphysis.

Prognosis.   The course and ultimate deformity of coxa plana depend upon the age of onset, the number of vessels occluded and, thereby, the size of the epiphyseal infarct and finally the amount of usage to which the injured member is put. In general, the damage is apt to be greater in the younger age group, from 3 to 6 years. Most orthopedists agree that some motion in the healing stage acts as a stimulus to new bone growth. The stress must be so calculated that it will encourage and not distort the newly formed epiphyseal structures. Sometimes surgery is necessary to remove large areas of dead tissue that might never resolve or to reshape a deformed articular plate or femoral neck that would handicap normal motion when healing is at last achieved.

OSTEOCHONDRITIS DISSECANS

Osteochondritis dissecans is essentially a type of epiphyseal ischemic necrosis in which only a peripheral segment of the bony epiphysis is involved. Because in the unclosed epiphysis of childhood its blood supply and that of the metaphysis is almost entirely separate, usually the entire bony nucleus or a considerable portion is involved when the epiphyseal vessels are affected because there is insufficient collateral circulation from the metaphysis. This results in epiphyseal ischemic necrosis. Consequently, though osteochondritis dissecans can occur at any age its most frequent incidence is shortly after epiphyseal closure, in late adolescence and young adult life.

A fragment of the peripheral osseous epiphysis underlying the articular cartilage undergoes ischemic necrosis. A plane of cleavage separates the dead fragment from the surrounding healthy bone and eventually it may loosen and fall out into the joint space taking along the layer of healthy cartilage that covers it. The cartilage remains viable because it derives its nutrition from the synovial fluid, until the trauma incident to its dislodgement may cause it to degenerate.

Loose joint bodies associated with an epiphyseal defect were probably first described by Alexander Monro[19] and later in 1870 by Sir James Paget,[20] but König[21] described the lesion as an entity in 1888 and gave it the name by which it is known today.

Osteochondritis dissecans is a rather common orthopedic condition. Lavener[22] found 33 cases in 891 roentgenograms of the knee region. This is probably somewhat higher than the general incidence because his material was from military service personnel and the disease is more frequent in active young adult males. In most series the peak incidence occurs between the ages of 15 and 25 and one frequently finds the statement that it is rarely seen in children. However, Green and Banks[23] were able to collect 27 cases in patients under 15 years of age. In reviewing the literature they were able to find reports of only 9 cases in children.

The disease has about the same male predominance as epiphyseal ischemic necrosis, i.e., four to one, though in at least one series the ratio was as high as thirteen to one. In perhaps 10 per cent of cases two or more lesions are found. Multi-

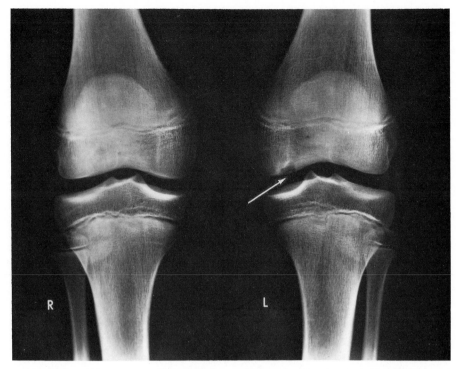

Figure 10–13 Osteochondritis dissecans. A radiolucent defect is evident in the left medial femoral condyle (arrow). A tiny fragment of bone is present within the defect.

ple lesions have a tendency to be symmetrical. Osteochondritis dissecans is sometimes associated with one or more lesions of epiphyseal ischemic necrosis.

Osteochondritis dissecans may be symptomless and found incidentally on roentgenograms made for other reasons. More often it causes mild to moderately severe pain in the affected joint. The onset may be sudden or insidious. There is usually some limitation of extreme motion and moderate disability. Eventually, there may be muscle weakness and some disuse atrophy. In a few cases the fragment of bone and cartilage that has become loose in the joint has caused locking. In some instances there is swelling and joint effusion. There may be tenderness.

The process usually runs its course over a period of months. The defect caused by the separation of the bone and cartilage fragment becomes filled with fibrous scar and the continuity of the articular surface is reestablished though an indentation often remains. If the fragment does not interfere with normal joint motion the patient may become symptomless after a year or more. This is particularly true of cases occurring in children. In adults, pain and disability are apt to persist until surgical intervention.

Ischemic necrosis of a segment of the bony arch that supports the articular cartilage has occurred in most of the weight-supporting bones of the skeleton, but in about 85 per cent of the cases the medial condyle of the femur is involved. No completely satisfactory explanation of this incidence has been offered. Other sites occasionally encountered are the femoral head, the elbow (capitellum), the distal humerus, the head of the humerus and the superior aspect of the astragalus. Involvement of other regions is a rarity. In the commonest site, the medial femoral condyle, an area of bone necrosis appears on its lateral border, extending to the margin of the intercondylar fossa adjacent to the posterior cruciate ligament. A circumscribed segment of the arch of bone that supports the articular cartilage dies and then proceeds to necrosis. Pressure causes it to collapse so that a depressed area occurs in the overlying articular plate. Just as in an infarct of soft tissue, a zone of hemorrhage occurs about the dead fragment and soon a capsule of granulation tissue is formed.

This granulation, bringing with it an increased blood supply, nibbles away the surface of the infarcted dead fragment until a line of separation is established. The lesion now is essentially a sequestrum. The disc of cartilage that overlies the dead fragment usually survives because it does not depend upon the epiphyseal vessels for its nourishment, though as its support gives way it becomes indented to mark the trouble spot beneath. As a sequestrum, the lesion may persist indefinitely in this state. Sometimes the lysis of the surface of the dead fragment is so extensive that it is completely separated from the surrounding bone, though often the densely collagenized fibrous tissue arising from the granulation may bind it in place. If the loosening process predominates without much scar formation the piece may drop out, taking with it the overlying disc of living cartilage. A vascularized pedicle may persist and tie the loose fragment to its original bed, or the diseased bone tissue and its associated cartilage may be freed to become a loose joint body.

Morbid Anatomy. The ischemic area of bone is first demarcated by an area of congestion and then a zone of hemorrhage (Fig. 10–14). If sectioned at this time, the bone of the central nidus is seen to be dead or dying; that is, the lamellae remain intact but the osteocytes within the lacunae are lacking or show degenerative change. Next, granulation begins to creep in from the surrounding healthy vessels and soon the hemorrhagic area becomes organized and the dead bone melts away along the advancing granulation surface. Tongues of granulation insinuate themselves along the haversian canals and interspicular spaces bringing sufficient fresh blood and phagocytes to cause bone necrosis. The fate of the lesion now depends upon the degree to which a new vasculature may be supplied. If it is minimal the granulation matures and the crater in the bony epiphysis becomes lined with dense fibrous tissue. If it is more adequate the fragment becomes loosened and eventually detached.

The behavior of the affected cartilage is

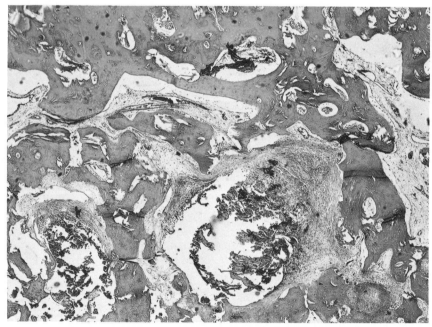

Figure 10–14   Osteochondritis dissecans. Two small areas of hemorrhage are surrounded by zones of fibrosis in the bone contiguous to the articular plate. (× 15.)

interesting. Abnormal pressure incident to its lack of support or change in position may cause it to degenerate. If it escapes this fate it may survive even though the fragment becomes completely detached. In this circumstance it usually proliferates to form a complete capsule about the necrotic bone nidus and thus the loose body may become spheroid and actually increase in size.

It cannot be said that the cause of osteochondritis dissecans is known, because the obstructed or interrupted vessels have not actually been demonstrated. The theory of trauma has always been emphasized, and a history of trauma, either acute or chronic, can be obtained in approximately 50 per cent of the cases. It is possible that acute trauma may cause avulsion of an epiphyseal fragment in a few cases in certain sites. However, the most frequently involved areas, such as the medial femoral condyle, are so well protected from acute trauma that it is difficult to accept this as a cause even in cases in which it appears in the history. Chronic trauma undoubtedly plays a role but its mechanism is almost surely through a thrombosing action upon the vessels. The mechanism of osteochondritis dissecans is almost certainly an ischemic necrosis. Chronic trauma may cause the ischemia by thrombosing the vessels and acute trauma may be the trigger mechanism that dislodges the diseased fragment. It is possible that infection may occasionally cause thrombosis and rarely an embolus may occlude the precise vessel that supplies the area. It is probable, however, that the common sites and the prevalent age incidence are the result of factors conditioned by the development of the normal vasculature pattern. It seems likely that an area on the lateral aspect of the medial femoral condyle is involved in about 85 per cent of the cases because this area normally has a narrow margin of vascular reserve after the epiphysis is ossified.

HYPERTROPHIC OSTEOARTHROPATHY

Generalized hypertrophic osteoarthropathy (pulmonary or secondary hypertrophic osteoarthropathy) is a syndrome, a triad consisting of clubbing of the fingers and toes, periosteal bone formation of the shafts of the cylindrical bones of the extremities, and a type of degenerative joint disease. It is almost always associated with visceral disease, usually situated within the thorax. There is a rarer congenital form of clubbing, unaccompanied by periosteal thickening and joint disease, that appears to be a separate entity.

Clubbing of the digits was described in ancient times but the syndrome as a triad and its accompanying pulmonary lesions were not described until the last decade of the last century when Marie and Bamberger independently reported the condition. A recent review by Gall, Bennett and Bauer[24] adequately summarizes what is known about the disease and describes the morphologic changes in seven cases.

Pulmonary neoplasm or longstanding suppurative disease of the lung—bronchiectasis, abscess, empyema or tuberculosis—is usually found to be a precursor of hypertrophic osteoarthropathy. Heart disease, usually of congenital type, was noted frequently in the early reports and, therefore, the term "pulmonary osteoarthropathy" was adopted to incorporate the chest pathology. Later it was discovered that primary pulmonary cancer, metastatic tumors to the lung and even benign lesions of the mediastinum and pleura, such as lymphadenopathy and fibromas, were occasionally associated. At length it was realized that diseases with sites and pathogenesis as widely diversified as those of syphilis, cirrhosis, osteosarcoma, chronic alcoholism and pyelonephritis apparently may cause the condition; therefore, the "pulmonary" portion of the title must be omitted for the sake of accuracy.

The syndrome is much more common in males than females, and though it may occur at any period during adult life it is relatively frequent before the age of 40. During the early phase the complex is usually first manifested by a widening of the ends of the fingers and toes. As this widening progresses the nails curve in both directions, growing down over the ends of the digits to accentuate the typical clubbed appearance. Though clubbing usually occurs first, pain over the shafts of the extremities may lead to an x-ray examination that reveals periosteal thickening in the distal thirds of the diaphyses of the bones of the forearms and legs and the shafts of the phalanges. Stiffness and joint pains are somewhat less common and often later in onset. The pain and periosteal thickening usually spread proximally to involve the remainder of the affected bones and progress to the shaft of the femur and humerus. The symptom complex waxes and wanes with exacerbations and remissions of the primary disease and in a few cases has disappeared when the latter has been cured. Some patients note a worsening of their symptoms during periods of warm and humid weather. Edema of the extremities may be a troublesome complication.

The pathogenesis of hypertrophic osteoarthropathy is unknown though it has been a target for explanation for over a half century. At first it was thought that the suppurative disease within the chest elaborated a toxin that caused the peripheral changes. When cases were discovered without accompanying infection it was proposed that the poor blood supply and stasis in the extremities resulting from cardiac inadequacy caused a proliferative fibrosis at the periphery. Then came the disturbing experimental work of Mendlowitz and Leslie[25] who produced hypertrophic osteoarthropathy in dogs by increasing the peripheral blood flow, and the measurements of Mendlowitz[26] in 35 cases of clubbing (of a variety of causes, excepting the congenital type) in which there was increased arterial pressure and blood flow in the affected digit in all cases with the exception of those with the complete symptom triad of hypertrophic osteoarthropathy. They concluded that secondary clubbing is always caused by an increase in arterial pressure and blood flow in the clubbed member, and that in some cases following clubbing the mean brachial and mean digital pressures equalize so that the digital pressures now appear normal, but the tissue alterations progress to the periosteum and joints and thus produce the triad of hypertrophic osteoarthropathy. If the Mendlowitz hy-

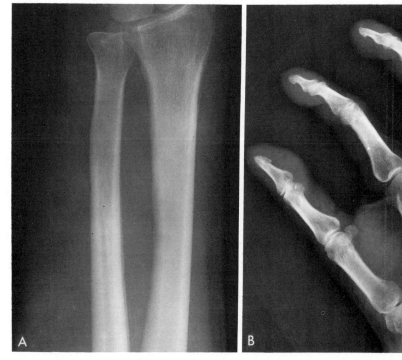

Figure 10–15 Hypertrophic osteoarthropathy. Cortical thickening and periosteal new bone is evident in *A*. There is an increase in soft tissue about the distal phalanges, clubbing, without underlying bony alteration (*B*).

pothesis applies, there is still to be explained why the heterogeneous variety of visceral diseases causes increased peripheral blood flow and indeed why this increased pressure and flow cause the characteristic changes. We must wait for further work before the pathogenesis of hypertrophic osteoarthropathy is clarified.

Roentgenographic Manifestations. The roentgenographic manifestations of hypertrophic osteoarthropathy reflect the changes in the periosteum and cortex that are visible microscopically. Periosteal new bone is laid down about the diaphyses of tubular bones. Early, this new bone may present a smooth outer surface, but later becomes rough and irregular. When the changes are severe, the periosteal new bone may blend with and thicken the cortex but a radiolucent line may be apparent between this new cambial bone and the underlying cortex. This line represents the fibrous matrix in which the new bone is first formed and in which actual bone marrow appears between the new bone and the cortex. In some areas, perpendicular spicules of bone may be visualized passing through the marrow from cortex to the new cambial bone. Radiographs may reveal the increase in soft tissue about the terminal phalanges of the digits.

Microscopy. Sections made through the clubbed portion of the digit are disappointing. The bulbous enlargement shows little more than hyperemia, edema and a mild infiltration with lymphocytes and plasma cells. The periosteum of the terminal phalanx is usually normal; sometimes the bone is actually atrophic. It appears that the soft tissue enlargement is the result of a purely circulatory disturbance.

The periosteum of the large cylindrical bones, and to a lesser extent the metacarpals and metatarsals and at times the proximal phalanges, shows an interesting alteration. The cambium lays down spicules of bone between it and the cortical surface. At first, the spicules are perpendicular to the cortical surface, unattached to it and embedded in a loose fibrous matrix. As the layer of new bone widens, however, it becomes annealed to the cortex, the spicules become incor-

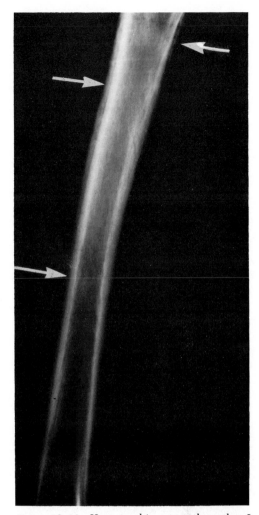

Figure 10–16 Hypertrophic osteoarthropathy. Irregular, shaggy periosteal new bone is evident about the femur (arrows). The patient, 48 years of age, had pulmonary tuberculosis.

porated in lamellae that run parallel to the cortical lamellae and marrow tissue appears. Thus, though the medullary region remains constant the cortex is thickened to as much as twice its normal width. The new bone is quite normal in structure.

The articular structures develop changes that are quite similar to those of osteoarthritis. The changes apparently begin in the synovia with vascular sclerosis and a resultant fibrosis that produces changes like those of a mild villonodular synovitis. The capsule becomes thickened by fibroblastic proliferation. Focal areas of degeneration appear in the articular cartilage and eventually cause roughening and narrowing. A few advanced cases have developed a pannus of granulation like that of rheumatoid arthritis, which eventually destroys the cartilage and leads to ankylosis.

Prognosis. Simple clubbing of the digits is a common complication of a wide variety of visceral diseases, most of which involve the lung, pleura or mediastinum. Today, bronchogenic cancer and pleural neoplasms are probably the commonest exciting factors. Some cases of clubbing progress to involve the periosteum of the extremities and the joints, these elements being necessary for the diagnosis of hypertrophic osteoarthropathy. In a few instances the disease has been so severe that practically all bones, including those of the spine and skull, were involved. Complete disappearance of the osteoarthropic signs and symptoms has occurred in cases in which the primary disease was completely alleviated. In many cases the osteoarthropathy has appeared as a forerunner of demonstrable evidence of metastatic disease in the lungs. The ultimate outcome depends upon the underlying visceral disease. Because many cases are caused by malignant tumor the prognosis should be guarded until the condition has been thoroughly studied.

NON-OSTEOGENIC FIBROMA

Non-osteogenic fibroma is a rather common degenerative and proliferative lesion of the medullary and cortical tissues of bone. It occurs most commonly near the ends of the diaphyses of the large long bones, particularly of the lower extremities. It has a predilection for the bones of late childhood, adolescence and early adult life, the great majority of cases occurring between the ages of 5 and 15 years. It is frequently multiple. This lesion has been and in some quarters still is called xanthoma or xanthofibroma, and because of the failure of many to recognize it as an entity it is widely confused with solitary cyst, giant cell tumor, fibrous dysplasia, lipid histiocytosis, chronic osteomyelitis, bone infarct and subperiosteal cortical defect. Despite its common incidence there is surprisingly little written on the subject and most of the older literature is so hopelessly vague and inaccurate because of the lack of a clear concept that it is scarcely worth the reading.

Non-osteogenic fibroma, though badly named, is a definite entity, and with the now available knowledge of its clinical, radiologic and microscopic features the diagnosis rarely should be missed.

Jaffe and Lichtenstein[27] were the first to realize that this lesion has a highly characteristic behavior and appearance, which enables one to disentangle it from the unusually large number of similar conditions that masked its recognition as a separate process until 1942. They gave it the name "non-osteogenic fibroma," believing it to be a benign fibrous neoplasm of bone lacking the ability to form osteoid. One wonders why they did not call it simply "fibroma of bone" but because an entity—ossifying fibroma—had already been described, it is possible that they thought the prefixed "non-osteogenic" was warranted to distinguish it. Actually, knowledge of the process that has been garnered since their original paper makes it quite certain that the lesion is entirely non-neoplastic in nature so the term "fibroma" is an unfortunate one, because it has thrown it into the classification of bone tumors in which it almost certainly does not belong. If one accepts the definition of neoplasm, as most oncologists are beginning to, as a hyperplasia of cells that progresses until therapeutic intervention or death of the host, non-osteogenic fibroma cannot be a true neoplasm, even a benign one, because the natural course of the lesion is one of healing, albeit several years are required.

One may justifiably question the grouping of non-osteogenic fibroma with the circulatory disturbances of bone, though Hatcher[28] and some others have apparently reached that conclusion. It is so placed in this monograph to stress the important (from a therapeutic standpoint) point that it is not a neoplasm. Because we freely admit that we do not know its morbid physiology there is no absolutely correct category for its inclusion and we place it here because it is like some other lesions of the group.

Approximately 50 per cent of the lesions diagnosed as non-osteogenic fibroma have given no symptoms and are discovered incidentally in skeletal roentgenograms made for other diseases. For this reason the true incidence of the condition is unknown and difficult to surmise. It is probable that every busy radiologist sees at least a half dozen of these cases each year. Of the cases that show symptoms, the history of trauma can often be obtained just as in a large proportion of all bone diseases. Because the mechanism of the lesion is unknown it cannot be stated whether trauma plays a causative role. Pain is the common complaint and it may be of weeks' or even months' duration, suggesting that it usually is not severe. Because the lesion is usually near the end of the diaphysis of a long bone the pain is often interpreted as a type of arthritis. Occasionally enlargement of a bone, particularly if it be a slender bone such as the fibula or the ulna, may be the presenting sign.

Most non-osteogenic fibromas occur during adolescence and the last half of the first decade. Older patients are not entirely spared, however, and in our material a classic lesion developed in the proximal femur of a 32 year old woman. Until recently it was thought that non-osteogenic fibroma occurred only in the large cylindrical bones of the extremities, but it is now known that they occasionally develop in flat bones. We have made the diagnosis in a lesion of the ilium near the sacrum. Two or more areas may appear in the same bone or in different bones. It is often bilateral.

In its classic form the lesion appears near the end of the shaft a centimeter or more from the unclosed epiphyseal line. Over a period of weeks and months it gradually enlarges, attaining an average size of 3 to 5 cm. In its fully developed state it gives one the impression that it is composed of several confluent areas of deossification, the whole having a bosselated outer "surface." It involves both

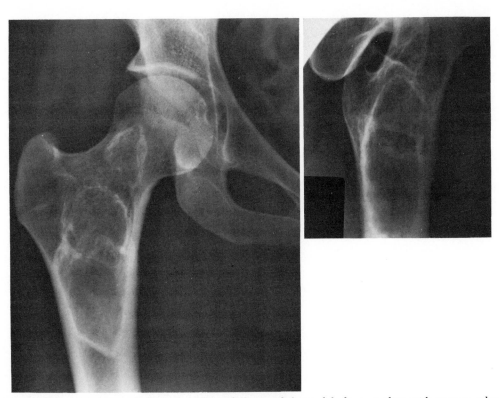

Figure 10–17 Non-osteogenic fibroma. The radiolucent defect is lobular in outline with opaque, sclerotic borders. It is sharply limited. There is erosion of the inner aspect of the cortex.

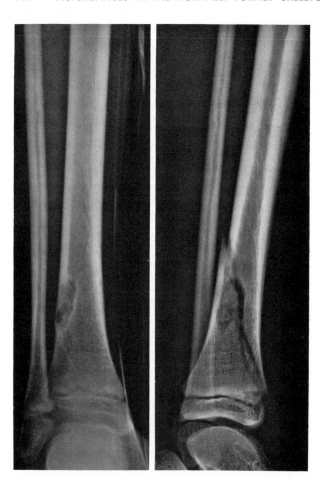

Figure 10–18 Non-osteogenic fibroma. There is a fracture through the tibia in the region of the lesion.

cancellous and compact bone and appears to begin just deep to the cortical laminae and destroys bone tissue in both directions. It progresses slowly so that the periosteum is enabled to lay down a thin shell of bone over its exterior surface producing cortical expansion, and the cancellous tissue at the inner margin undergoes sclerosis. Eventually, the lesion may extend across the entire diameter of the bone and then it becomes sealed off from the normal medullary tissues above and below by a margin of sclerotic bone and laterally it is covered by a fusiform bulging shell of cortex. If the lesion is followed long enough it will be seen to "drift" toward the mid-diaphysis as enchondral growth pushes the epiphysis away from it. Eventually, it may come to lie well down in the shaft but usually does not extend beyond the midpoint. In a few cases that have been observed throughout the entire life of the lesion, new bone grows in from the periphery and eventually obliterates the area. The time from the date of diagnosis to that of complete healing in these few cases has been recorded as two to five years. A curetted lesion may appear to heal only to recur later further toward the mid-diaphysis, at a point corresponding to the original site in the younger bone.

The average lesion produces such a characteristic radiograph that there is no difficulty whatsoever in making the diagnosis. But occasionally these lesions are huge, crossing the entire diameter of the shaft and extending longitudinally to involve a considerable proportion of the diaphysis. They often must be biopsied in order to rule out less innocuous conditions.

Occasionally infractions of the cortical shell or, as in one of our cases, complete fracture may occur. Then the surrounding normal tissues are stimulated to produce callus and the clinical radiologic and microscopic picture becomes more complex. Pain appears or becomes more severe, the delineating margin changes and unless the biopsy material is chosen from the right area the usual microscopy is replaced by irregular masses of young bone and cartilage in a fibrous matrix, i.e., callus.

We have encountered a few cases in which there is aneurysmal bone cyst. In such cases the lesion appears to explode. It increases in size rapidly, often perforates the cortex and extends into the soft tissues. Fractures are common and pain usual.

Microscopy. Non-osteogenic fibroma is essentially an area of cancellous and overlying cortical deossification and replacement by fibroblastic proliferation. It is uncertain whether a true ischemic degenerative process precedes the fibrous hyperplasia or whether a primary and uncontrolled fibrous hyperplasia causes the bone erosion to accommodate its bulk. The expansion of the cortex over many of these lesions suggests the latter explanation. The cause for the fibrous tissue overgrowth is quite unknown. The history of trauma is not constant enough to account for even the majority of the lesions. The results of bacterial culture have been too inconsistent to be impressive. The fact that the process goes on to normal healing appears to exclude a neoplastic nature.

Focal ischemia due to vascular occlusion by trauma or embolism has been suggested as the initiating agent. If the cortical expansion could be accommodated to this reasoning, the other features might conceivably align themselves on a hypothetical basis. It is true that the microscopy of non-osteogenic fibroma is quite different from that of the lesion that we have come to accept as infarct. But the nidus of dead bone in the latter, with its surrounding zone of fibrous and bone sclerosis, is probably the residuum of an infarcted area that was too large for the ingrowing granulation to resolve completely. If the area of tissue death were small enough to be completely deossified by the granulation growing in from the surrounding normal tissues, it is possible that this process might initiate the fibrosis and other microscopic features that characterize non-osteogenic fibroma. Against

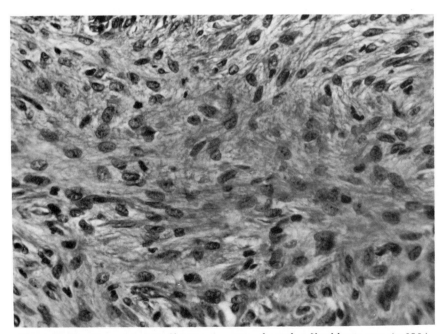

Figure 10–19 Non-osteogenic fibroma. A section through a fibroblastic area. ($\times$ 396.)

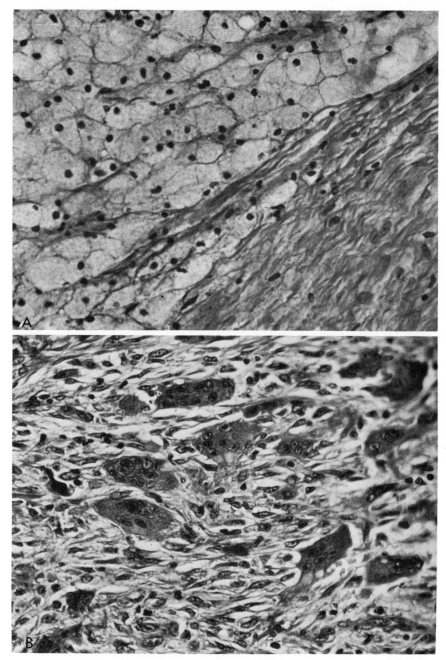

Figure 10–20 *A,* An aggregate of xanthoid cells in the left upper half of the picture. (× 396.) *B,* Giant cells are frequently scattered through the matrix. (× 396.)

this rather fanciful hypothesis is the occasional finding of infarcts no larger than the ordinary non-osteogenic fibroma, and the fact that one is not happy about accrediting the ischemia mechanism as a cause for the progressive enlargement of the lesion and the overlying cortical expansion.

All the microscopic features are consistent with a healed infarct of bone. There is a matrix of rather loosely arranged spindled cells that one has every reason to suppose are collagenoblasts and more adult collagenocytes. They are characteristically arranged in rather vague whorls and less prominent trabeculae (Fig. 10–19). Collagen production is lacking in most areas but at times small fields of collagen may appear. There is no osteoid production. Lesions with osteoid production and an identical collagenoblastic matrix are usually called osteoblastomas. In most lesions at least a few xanthoid cells, large, pale polyhedral cells with abundant, finely granular cytoplasm can be found (Fig. 10–20A). Often these cells are arranged in aggregates or cell islands and occasionally they dominate the microscopic field. These cells are macrophages, or phagocytizing fibroblasts if a distinction can be made, that have taken up lipid material, largely cholesterol. Higher magnification discloses the presence of coarse pigment granules within the more spindled elements. A Prussian blue reaction identifies this material as hemosiderin, further evidence suggesting origin in an infarct. Scattered through most fields one finds giant cells (Fig. 10–20 B). The nuclei are morphologically identical to those of the fibroblasts and they probably represent either a failure of complete division or a tendency of these elements to agglomerate. One gets the impression that these giant cells are

somewhat smaller and more spindled than those usually found in the reaction to bone injury. The periphery of the lesion is usually quite sharply delineated and surrounded by a layer of sclerotic bone (Fig. 10–21).

Differential Diagnosis. SOLITARY CYST. The surgeon should be able to differentiate these two lesions inasmuch as non-osteogenic fibroma is probably never cystic.

FIBROUS DYSPLASIA. The diagnosis cannot be made without the presence of at least some bone spicules. Non-osteogenic fibroma by definition cannot produce bone.

LIPID HISTIOCYTOSIS. Hand-Schüller-Christian disease is a disturbance of the reticulum and its derivatives. Epithelioid cells are prominent and there is usually an eosinophilic infiltration or the presence of other exudative inflammatory cells in response to the presence of the lipid.

CHRONIC OSTEOMYELITIS. The diagnosis of infectious inflammation is exceedingly risky without the presence of at least some inflammatory exudate.

BONE INFARCT. All of the microscopic features of non-osteogenic fibroma might be accounted for on the basis of ischemic

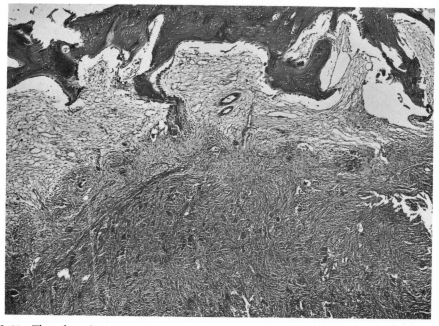

Figure 10–21   The edge of a typical non-osteogenic fibroma. It is surrounded by a thinned layer of cortical bone. (× 34.)

necrosis in which complete resolution of dead bone has been accomplished. Because our concept of bone infarct at present includes a nidus of dead bone with surrounding tissue reaction, the lesions are not compatible as we now understand them.

SUBPERIOSTEAL CORTICAL DEFECT. This lesion erodes cortical bone from without. Actually, the mechanism and microscopy are probably identical though there appears to be less evidence of a whorled pattern and the presence of pigment granules and a greater tendency to form chondroid. Giant and xanthoid cells may appear, usually more prominently than in the subcortical variety.

Prognosis. From the evidence currently available, one should expect a non-osteogenic fibroma to disappear in two to five years from the time it is diagnosed. If it is unusually large, and thereby jeopardizes the strength of the bone, or if infraction causes pain, the most conservative surgical management may be necessary. Diagnostic biopsy is unnecessary except in atypical cases or those that are complicated by other bone disease. It is the opinion of some that fibrosarcoma may be derived from a preceding non-osteogenic fibroma. We have not encountered a case in which this was evident.

A new name should be devised to designate more accurately the correct character of the lesion. Fibroma is a bad designation if the condition is not a true neoplasm. The name "xanthoma" should be abandoned because not all of the lesions contain xanthoid cells, at least not at the outset, and this name implies that a disturbance in lipid metabolism is a major etiologic factor. Perhaps both non-osteogenic fibroma and subperiosteal cortical defect should be included in the common term "fibrous defect of bone."

SUBPERIOSTEAL CORTICAL DEFECT

Subperiosteal cortical defect is a symptomless rarefaction of cortical bone. To date it has been described only in cylindrical bones and almost exclusively in the large, long bones of the extremities. Though it has been discovered in the skeletons of adults, these lesions appear to represent the persisting residuum of processes that began much earlier. Most subperiosteal cortical defects develop between the ages of 22 months and 8 years and they rarely, if ever, develop after the age of 15 years. There is a preponderance in males, rated in some series as high as two to one.

The condition is common. Caffey[29] estimates that it probably occurs in some bone at some time in 20 per cent of all male skeletons and 10 per cent of all female skeletons. It is commonly multiple, sometimes two or more lesions occurring in the same bone, more often a single affected area appearing in each of two or more bones. It may be bilateral and it is sometimes symmetrical.

Despite the considerable incidence of cortical defect, the combined clinical, radiologic and pathologic aspects have not been studied in a sufficient number of cases to insure a thorough and correct concept. Because it is symptomless, it is usually considered of minor importance. When diagnosed by the radiologist it is usually not followed and rarely biopsied. Consequently our factual knowledge at this time depends upon one aspect or another but in no large series has a thorough study of all features, including the microscopy, been reported.

Actually, subperiosteal cortical defect is important. Its nature should be understood by all those dealing with bone disease lest it be overdiagnosed and overtreated. In at least one series a needless amputation has been forthrightly reported. Because this is a common lesion it frequently accompanies more serious bone conditions. Should it accompany a correctly diagnosed malignant tumor, how easy it would be to presume it to be a metastasis and thereby alter therapy.

Kimmelstiel and Rapp were the first to report[30] a series of cases in which the concept of the lesion is one that is limited to the cortex. Later, Caffey[29] reported the clinical and radiologic aspects of a much larger series and applied the name, "cortical defect." We have prefixed "subperiosteal" to denote the pathology more exactly and to separate it from other cortical lesions of a variety of causes. In the earlier report of Ponseti and Friedman[31] one cannot be sure that the condition is an entity or that it is confined to the cortex. In the series reported by Sontag and Pyle,[32] cases of what is now known as non-osteogenic fibroma are included with subperiosteal cortical defect. Caffey fails to take cognizance of this in spite of the appearance in the report of such statements as "All of them are situated in the metaphysis or adjacent shaft where they are usually eccentrically placed. The defect often abuts on the cortex or occupies a portion of it," and "In the process of tubulation of the metaphysis the defect may eventually occupy a part of the cortex bone." Also in the illustration of the roentgenogram of case four of Sontag and Pyle, there is shown a lesion of the fibula that in both the anteroposterior and lateral projections extends completely across the diameter of the bone and causes a fusiform expansion of the cortex. Obviously they are describing at least some cases of non-osteogenic fibroma and any conclusions drawn from the report may not be applied to subperiosteal cortical defect.

Subperiosteal cortical defect begins most often on the external surface of the medial and posterior cortical walls of the lower end of the femur in children between the ages of 3 and 6 years. The second commonest site is the upper end of the tibia where it occurs in the anterior as well as the posterior wall. It is less frequently encountered in the upper end of the humerus and probably occurs occasionally at the ends of all the long bones of the extremities. It always begins near or perhaps at an epiphyseal line. It enlarges slowly from a spheroid area of demineralization to an ovoid lesion, the greatest diameter in the long axis of the host bone. It grows slowly, requiring months and sometimes years to reach its maximal size. It usually attains a greatest diameter of 3 to 4 cm. and probably never reaches the size of the larger non-osteogenic fibromas. As it grows it may change shape and relative position. Some of the lesions have been seen to drift toward the mid-diaphysis as the growing epiphysis pushes away from it. Others maintain their relative position to the epiphyseal line indicating that they progress in the direction of bone growth

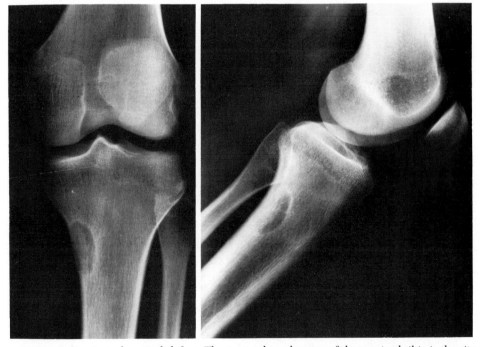

Figure 10–22 Subperiosteal cortical defect. The posterolateral cortex of the proximal tibia is the site of the lesion. The radiolucent defect is surrounded by a sharply defined opaque border. Incidentally, this lesion was observed to heal over a period of months.

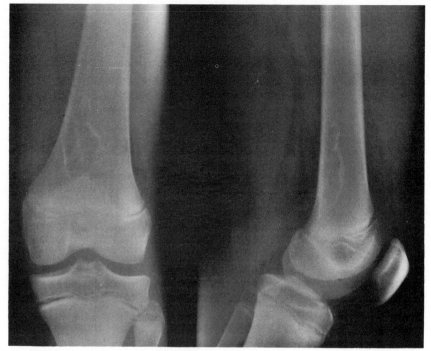

Figure 10–23 Subperiosteal cortical defect. The lesion is located in the posteromedial aspect of the femur. This portion of the femur is an area of rapid growth and is the most frequent site of the cortical defect.

and heal in the older portion, thus keeping pace with the normally growing bone. They may heal in a matter of months or persist for a decade or longer but one may expect complete disappearance in two to five years in most cases.

Certainly the majority of these defects are symptomless. In cases in which pain is a feature, one cannot be sure that it is not due to the trauma that often calls attention to the lesion. Because the involved area is never very large, it rarely leads to fracture.

In cases that have been adequately studied the defect always begins in the cortical surface directly contiguous to the overlying periosteum. As it enlarges it apparently erodes the bone, producing a dishlike crater. In a few instances a thin subperiosteal shell of bone has roofed the lesion, apparently the product of the related cambium, but there is no evidence to show that the lesion begins within the cortex. As the defect expands, the space is filled with a growth of collagenous tissue from the periosteum. No one knows whether the process of deossification is

primary and the collagenous proliferation an attempt at healing or whether there is an uncontrolled periosteal collagenous proliferation that erodes bone. There has been a tendency to accept the latter explanation without much justification.

Microscopy. It is almost impossible to obtain a clear concept of the microscopic appearance of subperiosteal cortical defect from the published reports. In the largest series, that of Caffey, no biopsies were taken and the source of the photomicrographs submitted by Jaffe is not absolutely clear. In the series reported by Sontag and Pyle, both non-osteogenic fibroma and subperiosteal cortical defect are included so that one cannot be sure which lesion they are describing. Kimmelstiel and Rapp describe the microscopy of their four cases and include several photomicrographs that are quite different in appearance from those illustrating Caffey's paper. Our very limited material most closely resembles the descriptions of Kimmelstiel and Rapp.

In our sections the process appears to be a proliferation of collagenous cells

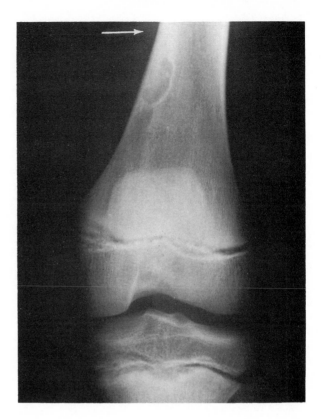

Figure 10–24 Subperiosteal cortical defect. Healing in this male, 13 years of age, has commenced and is manifest by sclerosis at the superior aspect of the lesion (arrow).

from the periosteum, which fills the defect produced by a bone erosion (Fig. 10–25). The appearance of the cells is reminiscent of those that compose the normal fibrous periosteum. Multinucleated giant cells similar to those found in non-osteogenic fibroma are present but xanthoid cells, though present, are usually less in evidence. There are some foci of hemosiderin granules. The chief distinction between the two lesions, if an over-all distinction can be made, is the presence of chondroid and some intercellular substance resembling osteoid in the subperiosteal cortical defect. The presence of the intercellular products of chondroblasts and osteoblasts, if examination of a large number of cases shows them to be consistently present, is of major importance. Numerous studies of non-osteogenic fibroma have shown chondroid and osteoid to be consistently absent. Little more can be said about the microscopy of this common lesion until a sufficient number of biopsies have been taken to answer our numerous questions.

One can no more than conjecture the pathogenesis of subperiosteal cortical defect. Caffey considers the evidence for trauma and proposes the possibility that muscle pull at points of tendon attachment may initiate the process. After reviewing the evidence for this hypothesis he reminds us that the defects occasionally occur in areas in which there are no tendon attachments, that they may be symmetrically bilateral, that two symmetrical lesions may appear and heal synchronously and that a defect may drift away from the point of its origin. These data suggest that the lesion is a variant in normal bone growth.

One is tempted to consider the probability that non-osteogenic fibroma and subperiosteal cortical defect are the same process, the one developing on the inner surface of the cortex and the other on the outer. There may be some criticism for considering cortical defects under the category of vascular disturbances in bone. This would be quite justifiable but the reasons for placing non-osteogenic fibroma in this category have been given and the two lesions should be considered together, at least for the present.

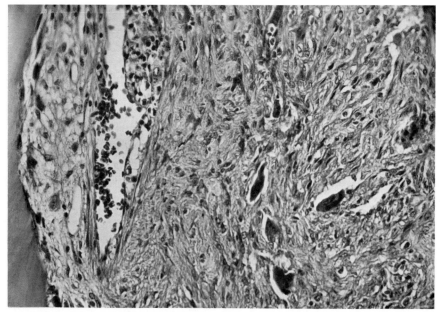

Figure 10–25   Subperiosteal cortical defect. A dishlike erosion is made in the bone seen at the left margin. A fibroblastic reaction with giant cells and xanthoid cells is found between the bone and periosteum. (× 396.)

THE CHRONIC HEMOLYTIC ANEMIAS

The osseous alterations associated with the chronic hemolytic anemias reflect an abnormality common to all, hyperplasia of the bone marrow. This latter is the result of the production of abnormal erythrocytes followed by their premature destruction by the reticuloendothelial system. Skeletal abnormalities are most marked in Cooley's anemia, less common in sickle cell anemia and uncommon in spherocytic anemia. In the latter two, the only recognizable alterations may be in the cranial bones.

Hyperplasia of the bone marrow results in an increase in the diameter of the medullary cavity, thinning of the cortex and at times an increase in the diameter of the bone. The trabecular pattern is distorted relative to the severity of the process. In some instances all of the trabeculae are sparse and diminished in size; in others, the smaller trabeculae are absent so that the larger ones stand out in sharp relief. This latter appearance is accentuated by thinning of the overlying cortex. The entire skeleton may be involved, but the changes tend to be most marked in the metacarpals and the long bones.

The bones of the skull may be thickened, particularly the frontal and parietal bones owing to an increase in width of the diploë. Spicules of bone form in the diploë to lie perpendicular to the inner table. The outer table becomes indistinct. When the process is severe there is bony encroachment on the paranasal sinuses and enlargement of the zygomas, maxilla and mandible. The cranial changes tend to be most severe in Cooley's anemia, but in general the severity of this alteration need not parallel the alteration of the remainder of the skeleton.

In sickle cell disease the osseous changes are often absent during childhood. Irregular areas of sclerosis may be seen in the spongiosa of long bones as a result of infarctions and these may occur in epiphyses and be so extensive as to mimic idiopathic epiphyseal ischemic necrosis (Legg-Calvé-Perthes disease). In the adult, epiphyseal necrosis is characterized by sclerosis, deformity, lucent defects that represent areas of bone resorption and narrowing of the cartilage of the joint. Biconcave deformities of the vertebral bodies are sometimes evident, particularly in the adult, and are often characterized by relatively perpendicular margins (Fig. 10–29).

(*Text continued on page 324.*)

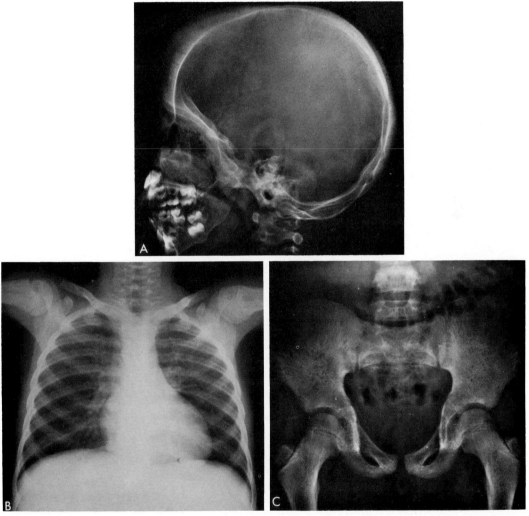

Figure 10–26   Cooley's anemia. The diploë of the frontal bone is wide, the outer table is indistinct and there are radiating spicules within the diploë that are perpendicular to the inner table (A). The ribs are radiolucent, their medullary cavity is wide and their trabeculae are sparse (B). The coarse trabecular pattern of the pelvic bones is evident (C).

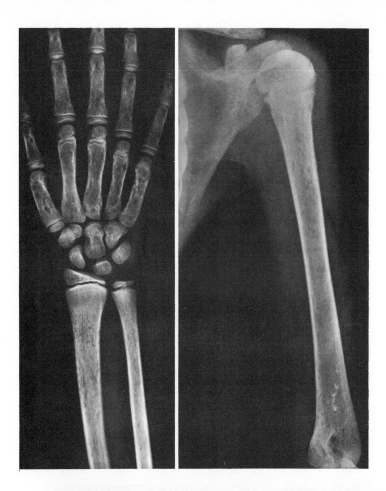

Figure 10–27 Cooley's anemia. The widened medullary cavity and distorted trabecular pattern are evident.

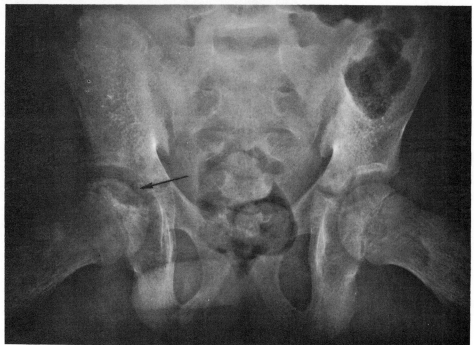

Figure 10–28 Sickle cell anemia. The trabecular pattern of the pelvic bones is coarse. An area of ischemic necrosis is present in the right femoral capital epiphyseal center (arrow).

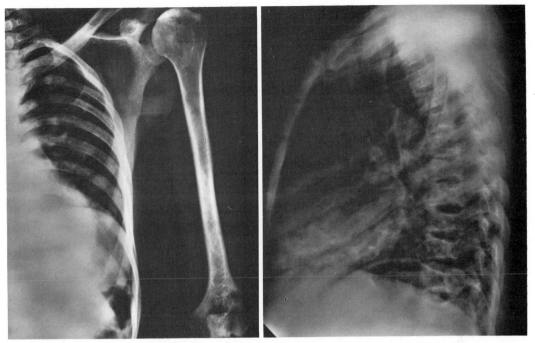

Figure 10–29 Sickle cell anemia in a black male, 24 years of age. Irregular areas of sclerosis are evident in the head of the humerus and the trabeculae in the diaphysis are sparse. There are biconcave deformities of the vertebral bodies; some of the concavities have almost vertical margins, particularly posteriorly.

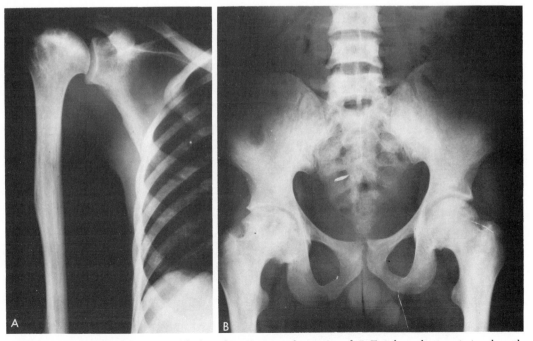

Figure 10–30 Sickle cell anemia, black male, 25 years of age. *A* and *B*, Epiphyseal necrosis involves the proximal end of each femur and the proximal end of the humerus. Sclerosis and subchondral lucencies are apparent as well as deformity, particularly of the right femoral head.

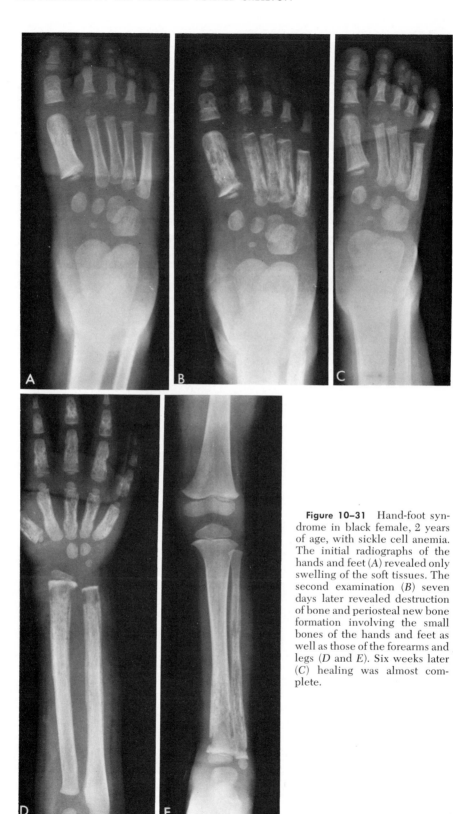

Figure 10–31 Hand-foot syndrome in black female, 2 years of age, with sickle cell anemia. The initial radiographs of the hands and feet (A) revealed only swelling of the soft tissues. The second examination (B) seven days later revealed destruction of bone and periosteal new bone formation involving the small bones of the hands and feet as well as those of the forearms and legs (D and E). Six weeks later (C) healing was almost complete.

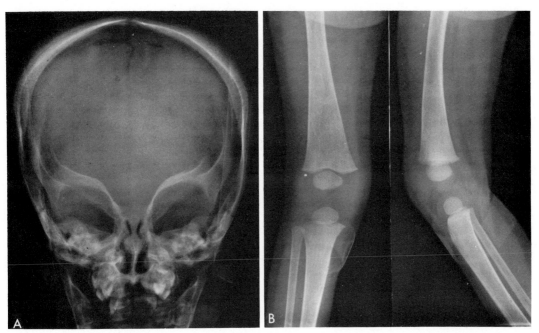

Figure 10–32   Iron deficiency anemia. There is thickening of the frontal bones as is seen in the hemolytic anemias. Mild but definite alterations in the trabecular pattern and the shape of the bones of the knee are evident.

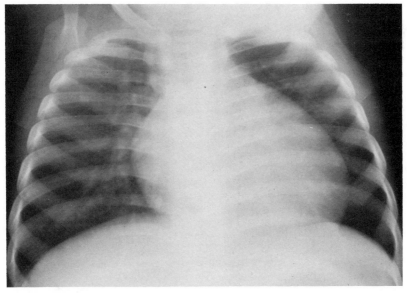

Figure 10–33   Iron deficiency anemia. Cardiac enlargement is evident. It is common in patients in whom the anemia is marked.

There is a curious manifestation of sickle cell anemia, usually in children under the age of 2 years, that has acquired the name of hand-foot syndrome. Multiple infarctions occur in the small bones of the hands and feet. There is swelling of the soft tissues of the area, heat, pain and tenderness. Fever is common and the temperature may rise to 103°F. X-ray changes are lacking until about the seventh to fourteenth day, then lesions can be noted in the tarsals and metatarsals, carpals and metacarpals and less frequently in the phalanges (Fig. 10–31).[33] In the majority no complicating infection can be demonstrated. When infection is present it is usually of the salmonella type.

Iron deficiency anemia is not a hemolytic anemia but it is associated with hyperplasia of the bone marrow. Changes in the cranial bones identical with those of the hemolytic anemias have been reported.[34] The long bones are said to be normal but one of our cases did show mild widening of the femurs and a coarse trabecular pattern (Figs. 10–32 and 10–33).

POST-HEMATOMA CYSTS

The concept of simple, solitary or so-called unicameral bone cysts has been well established for several decades. Though the pathogenesis is still unknown, they apparently always originate in the metaphysis of a cylindrical bone of the growing skeleton. They are smoothly ovoid in shape and appear to "drift" toward the mid-diaphysis as normal bone growth proceeds beyond them. They contain fluid that is bloody, amber or clear, apparently depending upon their age, and the wall of condensed cancellous bone is lined by a layer of collagenous tissue containing hemosiderin and usually a few giant cells and some lipid-laden histiocytes. There is much about the appearance and behavior of this lesion to suggest that it was caused by an extravasation of blood into the metaphysis of a young, growing bone,[36] but we lack factual evidence for this hypothesis. Hemophiliacs occasionally bleed into cancellous bone tissue and produce lesions that are called pseudo-

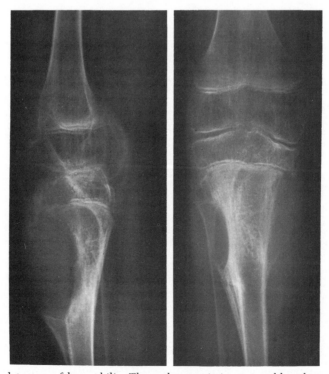

Figure 10–34 Pseudotumors of hemophilia. The pathogenesis is presumably a hematoma. What happens thereafter is unknown because biopsy studies have not been done. We suggest that the hematoma may organize to bring an excessive amount of blood to the area, thus causing bone lysis. The large size and the rapidity of development suggest the possibility of aneurysmal bone cyst development.

tumors of hemophilia (Fig. 10–34). Little is known of the pathology of these lesions because biopsy is contraindicated for obvious reasons. For many years we have known that subperiosteal hematomas stimulate appositional new bone formation by the periosteum (Fig. 10–35). These are most often seen in children with neurotropic diseases or spina bifida. In adults they occur in various types of paralysis. In the growing skeleton the new bone may be incorporated into a remodeled shaft.

Occasionally one encounters cysts of the same radiographic, gross and microscopic features as the typical simple solitary cyst but the clinical features are so different that one is loath to include them in the same category. They usually appear in bones that are mature and in areas other than the metaphysis.

This difference was emphasized to us some years ago on finding such a cyst in the shaft of a rib of a 36 year old male. The involved portion of the rib was completely resected and we had the opportunity of studying the lesion in toto (Fig. 10–36). The rib cortex was expanded, partially lined by recently formed bone inside of which was a fibrous sheath containing the residua of old hemorrhage surrounding a fluid-filled cavity. There was a history of trauma at this site three months earlier. We have since seen 16 more such cases, all in ribs, usually in young adult males. About half have given a history of trauma two to five months before diagnosis.

The radiograph reveals a localized segment of rib with cortical expansion (Fig. 10–37). One may search the American literature in vain for accounts of post-hematoma bone cyst. Apparently no such entity is recognized by American orthopedists and pathologists. In 1952 Hans Cottier[37] surveyed the German literature in which this entity has been recognized for many years. He was able to produce reasonably similar cysts in rabbit bones by injection of partially hemolyzed, acidified blood.

One is strongly tempted to ascribe these lesions to preceding hematomas that have organized, formed a fibrous capsule and then have undergone lysis. If such could be established, this hypothesis could be extended to explain the pathogenesis of other atypical simple cysts that occur in the mature skeleton. We have collected several of these with well documented histories of trauma. In a few cases they have been removed en bloc so that we were able to section the entire lesion (Fig. 10–38). The microscopy is precisely the same as that of ordinary solitary cyst of growing bone and of the rib cysts in adults. They usually occur in the ossified epiphysis of long bones; occasionally they occur in flat bones. We have included illustrations of two cases, one in the proximal tibia of a middle-aged stonemason (Fig. 10–39) and the second in the distal

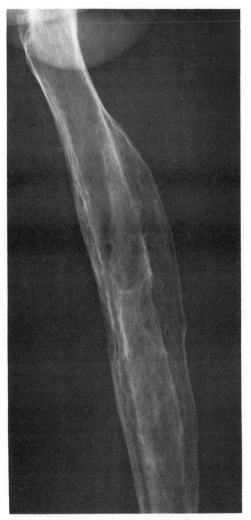

Figure 10–35 Massive subperiosteal hematoma in a 17 year old paraplegic. The periosteum has been dissected up and has formed a shell of bone over the entrapped blood.

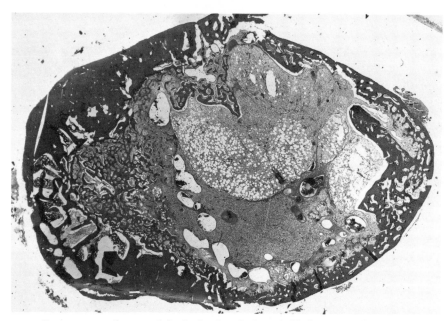

Figure 10–36 Cross section of a cyst of the body of a rib. It probably began as a hematoma within the cancellous tissue. Bleeding may be spontaneous or post-traumatic. (× 8.)

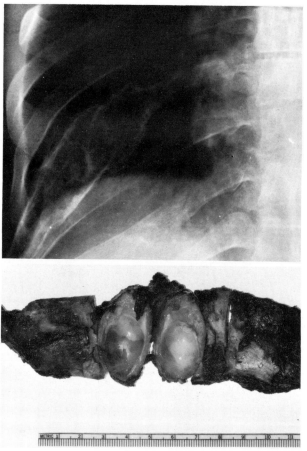

Figure 10–37 Above, a radiograph of a post-hematoma rib cyst. There is a fusiform cortical expansion about a collagenous walled space. Below, the lesion has been resected, cut in half and opened to show the cyst.

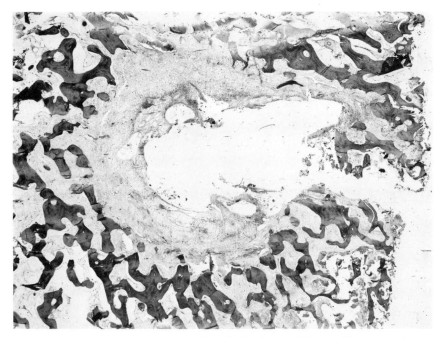

Figure 10–38 Post-hematoma cyst in the femoral head of a 58 year old male. There was a history of trauma, which is probably significant. (× 10.)

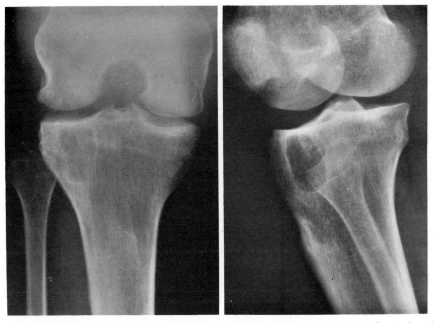

Figure 10–39 Post-hematoma cyst in the epiphysis of a 50 year old stonemason. Radiographs of one year earlier showed no evidence of lesion. (Courtesy of Dr. James Hardy.)

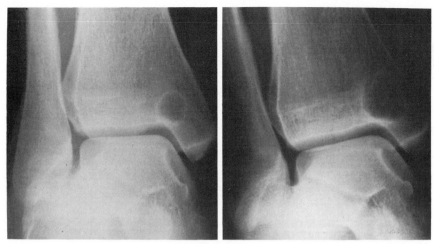

Figure 10–40 Post-hematoma cyst in the distal epiphysis of a mature tibia, which has enlarged over a two year period. There was a history of trauma.

tibial epiphysis, which was followed over a two year period (Fig. 10–40). In both it was shown that the lesion arose in the ossified epiphysis.

FOCAL OSTEOLYSIS

Several instances of focal or localized lysis of bone have been reported.[38] An area of radiolucency may appear in a soli-

tary bone, in contiguous bones or the bones about a major joint, e.g., the wrist. The area of involvement may increase in size until a major portion or entire bone is affected, e.g., phantom bones, disappearing clavicle. The process is asymptomatic until it causes function loss and deformity. There appear to be three types.[39] The most common, now usually called massive osteolysis or Gorham's disease,[40] is usually unifocal and has no hereditary or

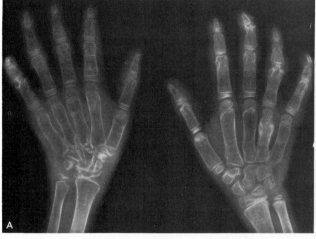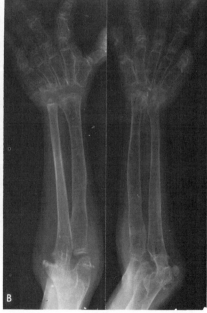

Figure 10–41 Hereditary multicentric osteolysis without nephropathy. Over a period of three years the bones of the extremities became osteopenic and loss of the carpus was noted at 7 years of age. Subchondral destruction in some of the interphalangeal joints occurred (A). A sibling, 10 years of age, demonstrates marked alterations at the wrist, the carpal bones are absent and the wrist has lost stature (B).

22. Lavener, G.: Am. J. Roentgenol., 57:56, 1947.
23. Green, W. T. and Banks, H. H.: J. Bone Joint Surg., 35A:26, 1953.

HYPERTROPHIC OSTEOARTHROPATHY

24. Gall, E. A., Bennett, G. A. and Bauer, W.: Am. J. Pathol., 27:349, 1951.
25. Mendlowitz, M. and Leslie, A.: Am. J. Pathol., 17:458, 1941.
26. Mendlowitz, M.: J. Clin. Invest., 20:113, 1941.

NON-OSTEOGENIC FIBROMA

27. Jaffe, H. L. and Lichtenstein, L.: Am. J. Pathol., 18:205, 1942.
28. Hatcher, C. H.: Ann. Surg., 122:1016, 1945.

SUBPERIOSTEAL CORTICAL DEFECT

29. Caffey, J.: Adv. Pediatr., 7:13, 1955.
30. Kimmelstiel, P. and Rapp, I.: Bull. Hosp. Joint Dis., 12:286, 1951.
31. Ponseti, I. V. and Friedman, B.: J. Bone Joint Surg., 31A:582, 1949.
32. Sontag, L. W. and Pyle, S. I.: Am. J. Roentgenol., 46:185, 1941.

CHRONIC HEMOLYTIC ANEMIAS

33. Moseley, J. E.: Bone Changes in Hematologic Disorders. New York, Grune & Stratton, 1963.
34. Caffey, J.: Pediatric X-Ray Diagnosis. Ed. 5. Chicago, Year Book Publishers, Inc., 1966.
35. Burko, H., Mellins, H. Z. and Watson, J.: Am. J. Roentgenol., 86:447, 1961.

POST-HEMATOMA CYST

36. Cohen, J.: J. Bone Joint Surg., 42A:609, 1960.
37. Cottier, H.: Schweiz. Z. Allg. Path., 15:46, 1952.

FOCAL OSTEOLYSIS

38. Torg, J. and Steel, H.: J. Bone Joint Surg., 51A:1649, 1969.
39. Torg, J. and Steel, H.: J. Bone Joint Surg., 50A:1629, 1968.
40. Gorham, L. and Stoub, A.: J. Bone Joint Surg., 37A:985, 1955.
41. Shurtleff, D., Sparkes, R., Clawson, D., Guntheroth, W. and Mottet, N.: J.A.M.A., 188:363, 1964.
42. Torg, J. S., DiGeorge, A. M., Kirkpatrick, J. A. and Trujillo, M. M.: J. Pediatr., 75:243, 1969.

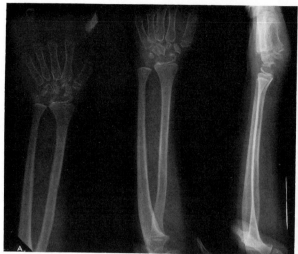
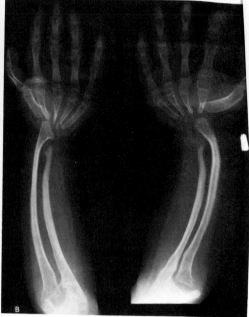

Figure 10–42 Essential osteolysis with nephropathy (female). At 4 years of age the carpal bones are present but irregular in outline (*A*). At 10 years of age the carpal bones have resorbed; the wrist has become narrow; and the proximal end of the metacarpals, especially two, three and four, and the distal ulna have been resorbed as well (*B*). Similar alterations are present at the elbow. (Courtesy of Dr. J. Torg.)

familial features. It is caused by the growth of a hemangioma or, less frequently, lymphangioma within the bone. Since these growths are hamartomas rather than true neoplasms, the invasion and destruction may be extensive but there is never metastasis to cause death of the patient. A second type is called essential osteolysis with nephropathy. This is a rare disease[39] in which there is a progressive and ultimately complete resorption of the carpus and tarsus and partial resorption of adjacent tubular bones. The mechanism is unknown; vascular hamartomas have not been demonstrated. The bone loss is accompanied by a renal disease that eventuates in hypertension, azotemia and death in early adult life. Still a third type, or perhaps a subtype of the above[41] has been called idiopathic hereditary osteolysis with dominant transmission. Familial involvement and absence of renal disease characterize this type. Again the mechanism is unknown.

References

BONE INFARCT

1. Kahlstrom, S. C., Phemister, D. B. and Burton, C. C.: Surg. Gynecol. Obstet., 68:120, 1939.

2. Kahlstrom, S. C. and Phemister, D. B.: Am. J. Pathol., 22:947, 1946.
3. Coley, B. L. and Moore, M.: Ann. Surg., 111: 1065, 1940.
4. Fisher, D., Bickel, W. and Holley, K.: Mayo Clin. Proc., 44:252, 1969.
5. Moran, T.: Arch. Pathol., 73:300, 1962.
6. Hill, R.: N. Engl. J. Med., 265:318, 1961.
7. Jones, J. and Engelman, E.: Arthritis Rheum., 10:287, 1967.
8. Jones, J. and Sakovich, L.: J. Bone Joint Surg., 48A:149, 1966.

EPIPHYSEAL ISCHEMIC NECROSIS

9. Caffey, J.: Am. J. Roentgenol. 103:620, 1968.
10. Emerick, R. W., Corrigan, K. E., Joistad, A. H. and Holly, L. E.: Clin. Orthop., 4:160, 1954.
11. Trueta, J. and Harrison, M. H. M.: J. Bone Joint Surg., 35B:442, 1953.
12. Legg, A. T.: Boston Med. Surg. J., 162:202, 1910.
13. Calvé, J.: Rév. Chir., 42:54, 1910.
14. Perthes, G.: Dtsch. Z. Chir., 107:111, 1910.
15. Caffey, J.: Pediatric X-Ray Diagnosis. Ed. 5. Chicago, Year Book Publishers, Inc., 1966.
16. Norman, A. and Bullough, P.: Bull. Hosp. Joint Dis., 24:99, 1963.
17. Gall, E. A. and Bennett, G. A.: Arch. Pathol., 33:866, 1942.
18. Zemansky, A. P.: Am. J. Surg., 4:169, 1928.

OSTEOCHONDRITIS DISSECANS

19. Monro, A., Quoted by Phemister, D. B.: J. Bone Joint Surg., 61:278, 1924.
20. Paget, J.: St. Bartholomew's Hosp. Reports, 6:1, 1870.
21. König, F.: Dtsch. Z. Chir., 27:90, 1888.

Chapter 11

METABOLIC DISEASES
OF BONE

Most writers concerned with the metabolic diseases of bone agree that this category denotes a generalized reduction in bone mass due to subnormal osteoid production, subnormal osteoid mineralization or excessive rate of deossification. This is about all they do agree upon and the definitions and explanations of the pathogenesis of the so-called metabolic diseases are almost as numerous as the authors who write them. An important cause of some of the confusion and seemingly contradictory evidence for explaining the pathogenesis of these conditions is semantic, a failure to define carefully the language used. Thus, when the internist uses the term "osteoporosis" to denote a clinical entity resulting from a number of pathogenic mechanisms, the orthopedist uses it to mean an area of weakness in bone, the radiologist uses it in describing a localized region of abnormal radiolucency and the pathologist defines it as a subnormal rate of osteoid production, it is small wonder that none of them understands what the others are talking about. Also there has been a tendency in the past decade for certain writers to attack the accepted principles by which we have explained the metabolic processes in bone without offering acceptable explanations to replace them, a type of intellectual vandalism that creates more chaos than comprehension.

It seems self-evident that any generalized reduction in bone mass must be due to one of the mechanisms previously enumerated. To repeat, a normal osteoid balance must depend upon a normal rate of osteoid elaboration, normal rate of mineralization and normal rate of physiologic bone lysis. A change in any one of these rates without adjustment of the others results in an imbalance. Because the various diseases characterized by increase in bone mass or density (Paget's disease, osteopetrosis, diaphyseal sclerosis) are not included in the metabolic diseases of bone we may confine our remarks to the conditions in which we find a deficit of normal osteoid tissue, i.e., a negative osteoid balance.

The factors that maintain the normal osteoid balance are complex and poorly understood. There can be no doubt that one of the most important agents, perhaps the only agent, causing osteoblasts to elaborate osteoid is stress. Estrogen and androgen appear to be necessary for this activity but they may act not upon the osteoblasts that produce osteoid but upon the osteoclasts that destroy it, or better perhaps, upon parathormone, which appears to stimulate osteoclastic activity. Conceivably, parathormone and the steroid "sex" hormones may act as reciprocal influences governing the balancing activity of osteoblasts and osteoclasts in the elaboration and lysis of osteoid. It has become apparent recently that parathormone and thyrocalcitonin play a similar role in the mineralization of osteoid. If factors other than parathyroid influence regulate the rate of bone lysis, they are at present unknown. Bone maintenance is highly sensitive to slight shifts in pH values of the serum toward the acid side but this is probably through the mechanism of the resultant lowered serum calcium level, which stimulates parathyroid secretion. We are only now beginning to appreciate the influence of thyrocalcitonin on the flow of mineral ions from bone and we are still uncertain of the exact role of vitamin D in relation to this activity.

We may simplify the discussion of the metabolic diseases if we carefully define the terms we use. For more than a century the term "osteoporosis" has been used to denote a clinical entity usually encountered in the latter trimester of life in which a reduction in bone mass is brought about by a combination of dietary, hormonal and limited activity factors. It would be futile to attempt to designate this entity by any other name. But in the name of scientific accuracy we may use specific terms to indicate the conditions that result when only one of these factors is the important pathogenetic agent. Thus we might use the term "osteopenia" to designate the condition that manifests a reduced bone mass due to a decrease in the rate of osteoid synthesis to a level inadequate to compensate normal bone lysis. The term "osteomalacia" (rickets when the process occurs in the growing skeleton) has always been satisfactory in designating an inability to normally mineralize osteoid. The term "osteolysis" might be used to indicate the condition in which the reduced bone mass is secondary to an increase in bone destruction by osteoclastic means regardless of what stimulates the proliferation and activity of these cells. Thus decreased bone mass secondary to gonadal hypogenesis or surgical castration should be called osteopenia, that due to renal rickets of either type, osteomalacia and that due to hyperparathyroidism, osteolysis. Only the clinical entity which may be idiopathic or caused by a combination of the above factors should be called osteoporosis.

DISEASES DUE TO INADEQUATE OSTEOID SYNTHESIS (OSTEOPENIA)

The mechanism of osteoid elaboration appears to be very complex. Collagen is apparently synthesized within the cytoplasm of the osteoblast and extruded as short rods onto the cell surface. These rods are joined to form fibers outside the cell to provide the intercellular matrix. Certain amino acids and vitamin C appear to be necessary for collagen synthesis. A deficiency in these elements might be called deficiency or dietary osteopenia. If the amino acids are used up in the synthesis of sugars—glyconeogenesis, which probably occurs in diabetes mellitus and Cushing's disease—or if the catabolic destruction is greater than the supply, as in thyrotoxicosis, we might designate these types of osteopenia as endocrine. In post-traumatic osteopenia, causalgia or Sudeck's disease the cause may lie in a disturbance in neurocirculatory regulation. Stress must certainly be the most important factor in causing the metaphyseal capillary endothelial cells or the cells of the primitive mesenchymal pool to change into osteoblasts and finally it is becoming increasingly apparent that cells may inherit a deficient or defective set of enzymes. There may be a congenital disability of these cells to differentiate into osteoblasts, a condition we recognize as osteogenesis imperfecta. Thus we may set up a classification of osteopenia into five groups:

Dietary
Endocrine
    Cushing's disease
    Hyperthyroidism
Disuse atrophy or stress deficiency
Post-traumatic
Congenital

Dietary Osteopenia

Elderly patients may shun the difficult-to-masticate meats, which would provide them with an adequate amino acid intake, because of dental problems. Vegetarians and dietary eccentrics may find themselves in like trouble but the most common cause of protein deficiency osteopenia is an inability to absorb these materials because of a defective gut wall or digestive enzyme secretory system. Such difficulties are encountered in malabsorption syndromes or chronic inflammatory disease of extensive segments of the digestive tract, regional enteritis or ulcerative colitis.

SCURVY

Scurvy is the result of (1) an inability on the part of the finer ramifications of the vascular tree to hold blood and (2) an inability to manufacture adequate normal intercellular collagen and organic bone matrix. One is strongly tempted to link the two inabilities as a part of the same mechanism, and it has been hypothesized that the capillary extravasations are due to a failure in the production of a normal cement substance, supposedly of the same chemical order as collagen and osteoid, which binds the vascular lining endothelial cells and makes the vessel walls impervious. Factual proof of such cement substance and its lack in scurvy is still undemonstrated, though all recent studies do show a lack of osteoblastic activity with failure of osteoid production and some data suggest a similar inactivity of fibroblasts in stimulating collagen production. Because osteoblasts in the metaphyseal area are probably derived from capillary endothelial lining cells the defect in scurvy may possibly be related to the cells rather than their intercellular product, or possibly an inability to elaborate normal collagen fibrils may cause a weak or fenestrated capillary wall.

The disease is caused by a deficiency in vitamin C. This substance was isolated by Szent-Györgyi in 1928 and is known to be levo-hexuronic acid, now called ascorbic acid.

The history of scurvy is a long and romantic one since in the past it was a disease of peoples who because of distant travel or siege were forced to accommodate their dietary intake to stored supplies. Because adequate quantities of ascorbic acid are found only in fresh dairy products, fruit and vegetables and because in its raw state the vitamin cannot be adequately stored, adult scurvy played an important role in the history of exploration, war and frontier life. Accounts of the condition that is now recognizable as scurvy were recorded during the thirteenth century crusades by de Joinville and later by others. Lind proved in his unique experiments on 12 sailors that the disease was caused by a deficiency of a factor that resides in citrus fruits, and so reported in 1753 in his "Treatise of the Scurvy."

Until the latter nineteenth century, though adult scurvy was adequately diagnosed and treated, the incidence and importance of infantile scurvy was unappreciated largely because it is symptomatically different (the disturbances in bone growth obviously can be manifested only in younger patients) and because of the prevalence and similarity of rickets, with which it was confused, in the same age group. In 1883 Sir Thomas Barlow[1] separated infantile scurvy from rickets and since that time the condition frequently has been called "Barlow's disease." Other important contributions were made by Hess,[2] who in 1917 called attention to and stressed the importance of latent infantile scurvy, and by Szent-Györgyi who isolated ascorbic acid in 1928.

In the world of today, there is practically no incidence of full-blown adult scurvy except in those who are accidentally deprived of fresh food and medical supplies. Recently, however, there have been reports[3] of latent adult scurvy brought on by a too casual consideration of dietary requirements in a harassed business population. The symptoms of fully developed scurvy in the adult are due largely to hemorrhages in soft tissue and to a lesser extent in bone and subperiosteal tissues. The gums are especially involved. They become greatly enlarged, soft, spongy, edmatous and discolored. They bleed upon pressure. Macular hemorrhages appear in the various mucous membranes and eventually in the skin. Hemorrhages into the joint spaces cause arthralgia and those in the muscles and beneath the periosteum make movement painful and eventually impossible. An anemia develops and finally there may be frank hemorrhage from the mucosa of the gastrointestinal tract and even the conjunctivae. If ascorbic acid is not soon introduced into the diet, death may result from a variety of infections that the body is unable to resist.

Latent scurvy may be suspected in

adults who complain of weakness, weight loss, poor appetite, diarrhea, bleeding from the gums, hypermenorrhea and a hemorrhagic perifollicular skin rash. An anemia that is resistant to therapy with iron, vitamin B_{12} and folic acid yields to ascorbic acid. This is a nutritional type of anemia that may be due to the limitation of conversion of pteroylglutamic acid to the citrovorum factor.[4] The diagnosis is made by finding a positive tourniquet test and a blood ascorbic acid level of less than 0.8 mg. per 100 ml.

In modern medical practice the term scurvy usually refers to infantile scurvy unless otherwise designated. The condition almost always develops between the sixth and eighteenth months. It is rarely seen after the second year. The onset is insidious with a loss of appetite, listlessness and a failure of normal weight gain. The gums become swollen and ecchymotic, and hemorrhages appear in the oral mucous membranes and at the growing ends of the bones. There is little clinical evidence of the latter until the metaphyseal cortex is penetrated and blood extravasates under the periosteum. Then exquisite tenderness becomes a prominent symptom. Listlessness and laxness of the muscle tone may be noted. A swelling of the ends of the long bones occurs and the costochondral junctions become prominent. If the condition is allowed to continue there is a retardation of growth. Hematuria may occur and the capillary resistance test is found to be positive. Laboratory examination reveals subnormal levels of serum alkaline phosphatase and ascorbic acid.

Roentgenographic Manifestations. The radiographic manifestations of infantile scurvy are a reflection of osteopenia and hemorrhagic phenomena. Alterations are first apparent and are most marked in areas in which the growth of bone is most rapid, e.g., the wrists, knees and costochondral junctions. Because there is a dissociation of chondroblastic and osteoblastic activity, the changes are first manifested at the growing ends of the bones but there is little evidence of disturbance in longitudinal growth of the long bones. The zone of provisional calcification is normally formed. An increase in the opacity and the width of the zone of provisional calcification occurs as a result of failure of resorption of the calcified cartilaginous matrix. An inability to synthesize osteoid plus the extravasation of blood into the area result in a deficiency of new trabeculae of bone in the metaphysis, and hence a radiolucent band is found adjacent to the zone of provisional calcification, the so-called scorbutic zone. This band may be first evident at the periphery of the metaphysis and present as a notch, the corner sign.

Epiphyseal centers are altered in the same way as is the metaphysis. The zone of provisional calcification around the centers becomes thicker than normal and, combined with the thin, sparse trabeculae of the center, results in a radiographic appearance described as "ringing of the epiphyses"

The trabeculae of bone become small as a result of continued resorption of bone combined with defective formation of new bone. Many of the finer trabeculae completely disappear. Thus the bone of the spongiosa offers little contrast to the soft tissues of the marrow cavity and the medullary cavity therefore appears almost uniformly opacified, the so-called "ground glass" appearance. The cortex becomes thin as a consequence of bone resorption and deficient periosteal new bone production.

The opacity of the zones of provisional calcification does not connote strength, but rather these areas are brittle and multiple impaction fractures occur within these zones. These are evident radiographically as irregularity of the zone of provisional calcification. The metaphyseal area, weakened as a consequence of hemorrhage, deficient production of osteoid (trabeculae) and persistence of unutilized calcified cartilaginous matrix and cells, is readily separated from the adjoining diaphysis. Such fractures through this zone superficially suggest epiphyseal separations, but are really subepiphyseal; hence, healing occurs without deformity. They are responsible for lateral spurring at the end of the shaft.

Subperiosteal hemorrhage may be recognized at times only as a vague, irregular shadow of the density of soft tissue ad-

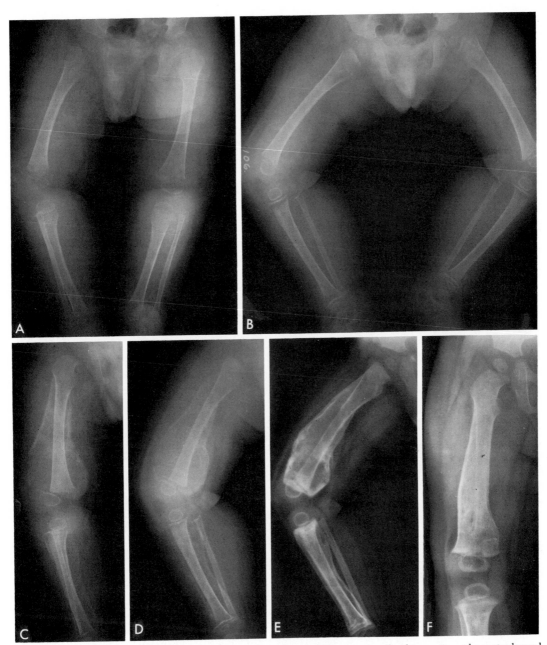

Figure 11-1 Infantile scurvy. The uniform opacity of the medullary cavity, the thin cortices, the metaphyseal rarefaction and the opacity of the zone of provisional calcification around the epiphyseal centers and at the ends of the shafts are illustrated in A and B. A vague soft tissue shadow is evident around the distal diaphysis of the right femur. Anteroposterior (C) and lateral (D) projections of the right femur made 10 days later and after the initiation of therapy demonstrate anterolateral displacement of the distal femoral epiphyseal center and zone of provisional calcification and calcification in subperiosteal hematoma. Such calcification is also evident about the right tibia. E and F are radiographs of the same area seven weeks and six months later, respectively. These demonstrate progressive calcification of the subperiosteal hematoma and remodeling of the femur.

jacent to the shaft. When healing begins, calcification in the subperiosteal hematomas is seen and is probably one of the earlier signs of healing.

That the radiolucency of the skeleton associated with scurvy may in part be the result of disuse is probable. In any event, the radiographic alterations in infantile scurvy can be correlated with the histopathology.

Microscopy. Scurvy is essentially a matter of blood extravasation from the capillaries and a failure of osteoid and collagen production. Examination of the vasculature of scorbutic tissues fails to reveal the cause of the multiple hemorrhages that occur, especially into the mesenchymal tissues. Because an intercellular cement substance between the endothelial lining cells has not been seen by all who have looked for it, the explanation involving its deficiency must be regarded as hypothetical. Adequate studies of the endothelial cells themselves and of the subendothelial wall have not been done. It is possible that a failure in the maintenance of the vascular collagen supportive substance may be at fault in this aspect of the disease or that there is a defect in endothelial cell metaplasia to osteoblasts which form the collagen fibers of osteoid.

In respect to the skeletal system, the hemorrhages occur in the metaphyses, in the central portions of the epiphyses and beneath the periosteum, particularly at the ends of the cylindrical bones. In the metaphysis the extravasations interfere with normal bone growth and hematopoiesis. About the vessels in the center of the epiphysis they delay the appearance of the osseous nucleus. In the juxtacortical region they lift the periosteum in a collar about the metaphysis, and gradually dissect it toward the midshaft until the periosteum may become virtually detached from the diaphysis, except at the point at which it merges with the perichondrium. The latter is never raised from the cartilaginous epiphysis.

Ascorbic acid is apparently not required for the normal growth and maturation of chondroblasts and the formation of chondroid. But it is necessary for the production of osteoid. Thus, in scurvy there is the rare dissociation of chondroblastic and osteoblastic activity. This same dissociation is seen in osteogenesis imperfecta and other types of osteopenia, loss

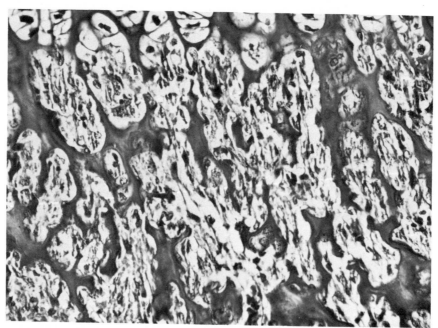

Figure 11–2   Scurvy. The epiphyseal line is seen along the upper border of the picture. The scaffolding of chondroid has been laid down in good order and is now mineralized. No osteoid seams appear around the hyalin bars because there is an inability to produce osteoid. ($\times$ 396.)

of skeletal mass caused by a negative osteoid balance due to an inability to form osteoid. Combined with the failure of osteoid production, there is a deficient growth in the metaphyseal granulation. These two factors appear to cause most of the disturbance in the regions of enchondral bone formation.

The chondroblasts of the epiphyseal plate reproduce normally and align themselves in columns. Intercolumnar chondroid bars are formed and a line of provisional calcification appears because there is no disturbance in mineral supply or deposition. At this point the normal process is interrupted. There is inadequate penetration of the bases of the cartilage cell columns by the fingers of granulation (Fig. 11–2) and thus, as in rickets, the mature cartilage cells are not utilized and so persist and are pushed downward into the metaphysis. This creates a widened zone of chondroid, which mineralizes and causes the white line of Fraenkel seen on the roentgenograms.

In the complete scorbutic state osteoblasts do not emerge from capillary endothelial lining cells or the multipotent cell mass. Follis has noted that osteoblasts that can be identified lose the basophilic quality of their cytoplasm. By special staining methods he concludes that this is due to a loss of ribose nucleic acid. There is also a disappearance of intracytoplasmic phosphatase and cytochrome oxidase activity. It is quite possible that cells so disabled are incapable of maturing as osteoblasts and of producing organic bone matrix. If osteoblasts actually contribute a cell-synthesized substance to osteoid, this would seem to be a tenable hypothesis. It is noteworthy that electron microscopic studies of scorbutic osteoid show an alteration in the number and quality of the collagen fibers. Because these fibers in both osteoid and fibrous collagen have been shown to consist largely of protein, this fault may be linked to the altered enzymatic activity of the cells concerned. It remains to be shown that ascorbic acid is an essential building block for this particular metabolic activity.

The persistence of unutilized cartilage cells, the lack of osteoid production and the hemorrhage into the metaphysis all contribute to a weakening of or, rather, a failure of development of a strong, stress-bearing metaphyseal area. Infractions occur in the regional cortices and it is quite usual to find fractures through the entire region with displacement of the epiphysis and its epiphyseal line. It is notable, however, that with realignment and proper antiscorbutic therapy, enchondral bone formation may proceed without permanent scarring.

The failure in production of organic matrix precludes the deposition of mineral salts in this region. This accounts for the zone of subnormal x-ray density that lies shaftward from the widened line of provisional calcification. The central area of the bony epiphyseal nucleus is translucent and its periphery, the widened zone of provisional calcification, is denser than normal. This presents the roentgenographic picture that has been called "ringed epiphysis."

Extravasations of blood within tissues normally induce fibrosis. In scurvy there is an inability to produce normally collagenized fibrous tissue. The hematopoietic marrow of the metaphyseal area is replaced by a primitive type of connective tissue, sometimes called areolar connective tissue, with very little or no intercellular collagen. The extent of this marrow replacement is probably not sufficient to cause the anemia that is seen in scurvy. This appears to be a nutritional type, which results from a metabolic defect similar to that which causes an inability to form normal osteoid and collagen. The collagen-forming defect likewise may be reflected in the diminished tensile strength of tendons and fascia that is reported.

Roentgenologists long ago emphasized the curious diffuse loss of density that occurs throughout the skeleton. It is difficult to explain this phenomenon without involving the principle of disuse atrophy. It is quite true that pain greatly limits activity, and pediatricians frequently mention listlessness and refusal to move the extremities as early signs of the disease. It is quite probable that this is at least an important factor in the etiology of this finding.

Prognosis. Scurvy is a preventable disease and one that is readily amenable to dietary adjustment. Moreover, massive doses of vitamin C do not produce toxicity. Unless the fully developed ascorbic state has persisted for a very long time all signs of its presence are erased by adequate therapy. Even the evidence of retarded growth may eventually disappear.

Endocrine Osteopenia

It has long been known that estrogen, androgen or a combination of the two is necessary for normal osteoblastic activity. The estrogen level begins to fall soon after menopause and within 5 to 15 years may reach a level at which it is incapable of supporting this function. The decrease in androgen and estrogen due to adrenal cortical atrophy of senility is usually considerably later; thus the onset of osteopenia in males is usually in an older age group.

The mechanism by which the sex hormones affect osteoid synthesis is unknown. Some recently acquired evidence indicates that in postmenopausal osteopenia the rate of osteogenesis appears to be normal but the rate of osteolysis is increased. This suggests that the hormones' action is not directly on the osteoblasts as originally supposed, but that they neutralize parathormone, thus inhibiting osteoclastic activity.

The osteopenia of Cushing's syndrome is poorly understood largely because the pathogenesis of the latter has never been satisfactorily explained. Most cases show adrenal cortical adenomas, adrenal cortical hyperplasia or adenocarcinomas of the adrenal cortex. Because the osteopenia of Cushing's syndrome, as well as many other features of the disease, can be induced by the administration of cortisone, which is one of the sugar-active hormones, it is assumed that excessive amounts of this steroid cause accelerated glyconeogenesis at the expense of the proteins that

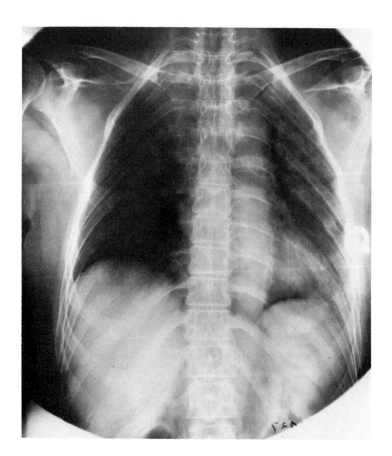

Figure 11–3 Cushing's syndrome. The bones are more lucent than normal; the cortices of the vertebral bodies are sharply defined.

are needed by the osteoblasts to form organic matrix.

The osteopenia of thyrotoxicosis and diabetes mellitus may be due to an over-utilization of proteins, in the first as an attempt to balance the increased rate of catabolism and in the second because of its conversion into much needed glycogen. Scurvy is a specific type of osteopenia. The hemorrhagic factor combined with the inability to form organic matrix makes it a specific entity so that it is never called osteopenia.

Stress Deficiency Osteopenia (Disuse Atrophy)

The osteopenia of disuse is important and interesting. It is well known that without the stress stimulus, the osteoblasts refuse to lay down osteoid. The transitory quality of bone, its continuous dissolution and replacement, is necessary to keep the bone fit for the functional stresses that it must bear. As stress trajectories change old laminae dissolve and are replaced by new ones arranged in the new stress lines. If there is no stress, the laminae are not re-formed and the bone mass decreases to the status of osteopenia. A disuse osteopenia can be noted after only a few weeks of absolute bed rest. If a limb is immobilized in plaster the osteopenia is more dramatic. As the bone undergoes lysis the minerals are released into the blood. The serum calcium and phosphorus rise,[26] presumably because there is insufficient osteoid production to recapture the bone salts, and calcium is spilled into the urine. Urinary calcium excretion may be sufficient to make it necessary to take precautionary measures against nephrocalcinosis and kidney and bladder calculi.

Post-Traumatic Osteopenia

Post-traumatic osteopenia, sometimes called causalgia or Sudeck's disease, is a curious phenomenon. Following an injury that may be insignificant there is pain, sometimes referred, often swelling and eventually a dramatic decrease in bone substance (Fig. 11–4). In many instances the osteopenia appears to be due to an in-

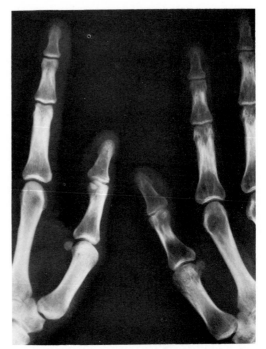

Figure 11–4 Causalgia. Deossification of the meta-carpals and phalanges of the thumb and index and middle fingers is shown on the right. Normal mineral content is seen on the left. Osteopenia occurred following a minor injury in the forearm.

creased blood supply caused by neurogenic insult. In other instances the mechanism is not as obvious and the disuse secondary to pain may play a role.

Congenital Osteopenia (Osteogenesis Imperfecta)

This condition is sometimes called osteopsathyrosis. It is essentially an inability to produce osteoid as rapidly as it is lysed. Most authors believe this inability resides in a subnormal production, though some have attempted to prove that there is excessive lysis. Morphologic studies suggest that an insufficient number of primitive fibroblasts or of endothelial cells, whichever is the source of osteoblasts, differentiate into osteoid-forming cells. Because the disturbance is due to an inadequate organic matrix (osteoid) production, either absolute or relative, it is a congenital, hereditary and familial form of osteopenia, i.e., a skeletal dysplasia, and as such is discussed more fully in Chapter 6.

The condition has been diagnosed on the basis of roentgenograms taken in utero and it is often obvious in the newborn or young child, or it may take a latent form in which there is undue fragility of the skeleton resulting in fractures with minor trauma throughout a life of normal duration.

Because the osteoblast rather than the cartilaginous elements are involved, there is an inadequacy of both cancellous and compact bone. The cartilaginous epiphyses form normally and there is an attempt to maintain normal stature growth rate. In severe cases this rate cannot be maintained and there is dwarfing, though much of the latter is due to repeated fractures with shortening. Though length growth may be normal, subperiosteal osteoid formation is never adequate to give the bone normal strength. Thus the limb bones appear long and gracile with thin cortices and scant spongiosa.

A paradoxical feature of osteogenesis imperfecta is the ability in many cases to form hyperplastic callus. In general, fractures in osteogenesis imperfecta heal, though sometimes slowly, but in many instances there is a remarkable proliferation of callus tissues, which may extend considerable distances from the fracture site. Callus proliferation may be so florid that the roentgenogram is misinterpreted as malignant neoplasm. If biopsy is done the microscopist encounters great masses of very active primitive bone formation, and he too may be misled into the diagnosis of osteosarcoma. In a case studied by us there was an unusual amount of hemorrhage about the fracture site, which may have acted as the stimulus for callus formation. Cases of dentinogenesis imperfecta have a tendency to excessive bleeding from ruptured vessels. In another case, in a child of 19 months, we suspected the diagnosis of dentinogenesis imperfecta because the mandible enlarged to many times its normal size with wildly proliferating tissue resembling callus.

The microscopic sections of bone from a case of osteogenesis imperfecta may reveal poor lamellar organization with a lack of haversian systems, but in most instances the bone appears to be normal in quality though deficient in quantity. The epiphyseal centers show nothing of pathognomonic significance.

Cases of osteogenesis imperfecta may become less severe after skeletal maturation. In our experience this has been more obvious in males than females. In one instance a patient who had suffered numerous fractures during childhood and adolescence ceased to be troubled after skeletal maturation and at middle age fell from a third story window incurring not a single fracture. Roentgenograms of the skeleton of his son at the age of 19, who had also had numerous fractures during childhood, showed normal cortical width and apparent strength. It has been our opinion that in moderate cases of osteogenesis imperfecta fractures are suffered during youth because bone production is too slow to keep up with the demands of growth, but after maturation bone production can establish a balance with the needs of maintenance. If this is true in the male but not in the female, inability to produce normal quantities of osteoid may be associated with steroid hormone activity. Because this is certainly true in the case of postmenopausal osteopenia, this aspect of the disease should be investigated.

DISEASES DUE TO INADEQUATE OSTEOID MINERALIZATION (OSTEOMALACIA)

Under this heading we have grouped a variety of skeletal diseases in which the production of osteoid apparently is normal or near normal but in which mineralization of this osteoid is defective. In all but hypophosphatasia the fault lies in an inadequate amount of available calcium or phosphorus, or both, in the fluid that permeates the inorganic matrix. This deficiency is brought about in a number of ways that can be summarized as inadequate dietary intake, defective absorption through the gut wall or a failure of the kidneys to conserve the mineral supply. In the osteomalacia of multiple pregnancies the deficit of mineral is due to an increased need to meet the demand for fetal skeleton and lactation. In hypophosphatasia the mineral supplies are normal but apparently the formed osteoid does not accept it.

The common denominator in all these conditions is a lack of rigidity in the areas affected, in the immature skeleton at sites of growth and in mature bones at points of stress where turnover (physiologic lysis plus replacement) is most rapid. Defective replacement becomes apparent first at these sites because of the greater demand for new bone production. Failure of mineralization and consequent inability to resist stress because of lack of rigidity result in a similarity in symptoms and in the radiographic evidence of the disease. It is logical, therefore, at least from the clinical viewpoint, to group these conditions together. A classification of the various entities, each of which will be discussed separately in the following paragraphs, can thus be constructed.

DISTURBANCES OF OSTEOID
MINERALIZATION

1. Rickets — usually due to inadequate vitamin D intake and synthesis in the growing skeleton.

2. The osteomalacias — may be due to inadequate mineral or vitamin D intake or absorption, excess mineral demand or renal loss in the mature skeleton.

3. Renal osteodystrophy (renal rickets) a calcium deficiency state — due to glomerular and tubular renal disease or possibly a disability to metabolize vitamin D_3 to 1,25-dihydroxycholecalciferol which is necessary for calcium transport across the gut wall.

4. Hypophosphatemic (vitamin D refractory rickets) — a phosphorus deficiency state due to inability of renal tubules to conserve phosphate.

5. Hypophosphatasia — due to inability of newly formed osteoid to mineralize.

All of these conditions are, in a sense, rickets when they occur in growing bone and osteomalacia when they are found in the mature skeleton. Because the pathogenesis of each is different in some degree from that of the others, each must be discussed separately.

Rickets

Rickets is a disturbance in the formation of bone in the growing skeleton caused by a failure of deposition of bone salts within the organic matrix of cartilage and bone. This failure is the consequence of an inadequate supply of calcium or phosphorus ions or both in the fluid that perfuses the matrix tissue. The inadequacy is due to a deficiency in the dietary intake or to a failure of adequate absorption through the gut wall. In an attempt to maintain a normal serum calcium level, salts may be withdrawn from the portions of bone that were mineralized before the onset of the disease with resultant softening of the previously normal skeleton. The ability to produce chondroid and osteoid organic matrix is retained. The effects of the disturbance are manifested in the growing skeleton and, therefore, do not pertain to bones after their secondary ossification centers have closed, though the distortions resulting from defective enchondral bone mineralization and secondary bone softening may persist for the life of the parts involved.

The earliest reports of a condition that can be indubitably identified as rickets come from England in the seventeenth century. It is almost certain that rickets must have existed among the ancients, but it may not have been common or severe enough to arouse general concern. Because most rickets results from insufficient vitamin D to maintain normal calcium absorption and because vitamin D is synthesized in vivo by the action of sunlight on the cholesterol supplies of the skin, it may be presumed that the geography of civilization played an important role in the incidence of the disease. The regions around the Mediterranean owe a considerable part of their enviable climatic reputation to the quantity and quality of their sunshine. England and especially Scotland are not as fortunate in this respect. There, where fog and industrial smoke filter out most of the sunlight, and where cold and the niceties of civilization necessitate a covering of the body surfaces, there may be too little naturally synthesized vitamin D to prevent the condition.

Since the work of Mellanby[5] and Park[6] the civilized world has learned that it is possible to prevent rickets even among its poorer populations. In lieu of sunshine, fish liver oils and the more accurately controlled synthetic preparations supply the necessary vitamin D. Both calcium and phosphorus are fairly ubiquitous minerals in most populations because of their high content in milk and dairy products. Consequently, the incidence of symptomatic rickets has diminished in most areas until now it is difficult to obtain adequate material for teaching purposes. Only in unenlightened areas, starvation populations and races and cults with dietary eccentricities does the fully advanced disease occur in numbers.

Most rickets today is caused by an inadequate intake of vitamin D in infancy and early childhood. Dietary calcium, normal in amount, is excreted in the feces because of failure of absorption. It is quite unusual for the infant diet to be deficient in either calcium or phosphorus because milk is a rich source of both. Rarely severe fibrocystic disease of the pancreas and more often idiopathic steatorrhea (celiac disease), because of the disturbance in fat metabolism at the intestinal level, may interfere with calcium absorption. This result is probably due largely to incomplete vitamin D utilization because it is a fat-soluble vitamin. The presence of excessive fatty acids, which may combine with calcium to form non-absorbable soaps, and the resultant diarrhea, which does not allow sufficient time for mineral absorption, may play some part in the diminished absorption of calcium. It is probable that all three mechanisms combine in this type of rickets.

Because active rickets is manifested only in the growing skeleton, its most obvious expression is seen in the period of most active growth, between 6 months and 3 years, though its effect may be encountered earlier and the less florid late rickets may manifest itself in the prepubertal years.

In infancy, the brain is the most rapidly growing organ of the body and the bones that surround it must keep pace. The enlargement of the cerebral cavity is accomplished by the intramembranous apposition of osteoid along the flat-bone edges within the fibrous sutures. The molding is the result of osteolysis of the inner table in areas that result in a flattening of the curve and apposition on the outer table to maintain thickness. Because

in rickets osteoid production is not impaired and osteolysis continues until the bone surface is covered with a more resistant but unmineralized and, therefore, soft osteoid, the calvarium enlarges, but it is thin and more pliable, the outer contours expressing more intimately the shape of the brain. When to this conformation there is added the external osteoid apposition in areas of normal bone growth together with the lag in anteroposterior growth at the base, the frontal areas become prominent and boxlike. This frontal bossing and thinning are called craniotabes.

The softening of the normally mineralized vertebral bodies allows the intervertebral discs to expand and the stress of weight-bearing results in further compression so that the spine becomes twisted and bent. The lumbar spine and sacrum telescope into the softened pelvis, which must bear the weight of the trunk, head and upper extremities. The acetabular roofs are pushed upward and inward to further narrow the pelvic outlet. The resultant pelvic deformity making parturition impossible, is one of the most serious consequences of the disease. The loss of rigidity of the weight-bearing long bones of the lower extremities leads to a characteristic bowing. If the progress of the disease is arrested before skeletal deformity due to softening is too far advanced, remodeling in the normal stress lines during uncomplicated skeletal growth erases much of the distortion. But, if the effects of rickets are severe and if the disease is active even though slowed throughout childhood and adolescence, the abnormalities harden into permanent deformities.

In the areas of enchondral bone growth the inadequate mineral supply interferes with bone formation and conformation. Length growth is inhibited so that the bones fail to achieve normal stature. If there is an inadequate supply of mineral salts the band of provisional calcification in the epiphyseal plate cannot form. This interferes with cartilage cell maturation and utilization. The bars that make up the mineralized lattice of the metaphysis are not produced. Consequently, there is no scaffolding for the deposition of osteoid. Moreover, the tufts of metaphyseal granulation are not properly guided in their invasion of cartilage. The result is that their course is erratic and masses of cartilage cells that should have been used in the process of provisional calcification are isolated and overtaken by the advancing frontier of bone formation until they eventually come to lie deep within the metaphysis. The osteoblasts provoke osteoid formation as they are intended, but there is no preformed pattern to guide this process. Because the unmineralized osteoid remains flaccid, there can be no modeling due to normal stress stimuli. The useless osteoid piles up about islands of still viable cartilage cells and eventually fills the entire metaphyseal region.

It appears that mineralization of the layer of chondroid matrix that supports the columns of mature chondrocytes, the line of provisional calcification, plays an important curbing function in cartilage cell proliferation. In rickets the formation of a provisional line of calcification cannot occur and the columnated cartilage cells behave as though a restraining influence had been removed. They proliferate and persist until large, irregular masses of cartilage widen the epiphyseal line and extend into the metaphysis, there to mingle with the patches of osteoid in an irregular, patternless aggregate.

The normal flaring of the diaphyseal ends cannot be reduced by the modeling process, perhaps because of a lack of rigidity or because of the abnormal deposits of cartilage and osteoid. Consequently, the ends of long bones reveal the graduated widening that has been so aptly called "trumpeting." This metaphyseal widening produces the enlarged joints that are so characteristically seen at the wrists, knees and ankles. It also produces a bulbous enlargement of the costochondral junctions and when marked this results in the "rachitic rosary." Sometimes this row of subcutaneous bumps fails to appear on the external thoracic surface, but is quite apparent on the pleural side of the plastron (Fig. 11–5). The negative intrathoracic pressure, which sucks the sternum inward while the ribs are being raised in inhalation expansion, may produce a deep, midline furrow down the anterior part of the chest. The pull of the diaphragm along its line of attachment creates a second, coronal furrow with flaring of the lower thoracic margins called "Harrison's groove." These various deformities of the chest may persist throughout adult life and stamp the owner as a victim of rickets in his early childhood.

One would expect the serum calcium level to be below normal in the actively rachitic patient, because the disturbance here is in the dietary supply or more often the failure of absorption. As long as the parathyroid function remains intact, the inadequate extrinsic supply of calcium is compensated by the stored calcium in

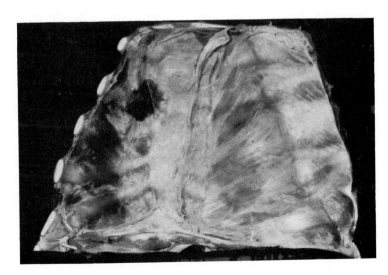

Figure 11–5 Rickets in a child. Plastron removed at autopsy. Internal surface. Along the right side of the specimen one notes the prominent nodules at the costochondral junctions. This is the cause of the "rachitic rosary," which is often seen on the external surface.

the skeleton. Thus the serum level is usually on the low side of normal even though the bones must be demineralized to maintain it. Examination of the parathyroid glands is said to reveal a moderate secondary hyperplasia. The low calcium levels stimulate the parathyroid glands to excessive secretion and their hormone affects the distal convoluted tubules of the kidney to inhibit reabsorption of the phosphorus that has passed the glomerular filters. Consequently, the serum phosphorus level is usually low. The sacrifice of the normally mineralized bone to this end causes excessive activity of the osteoblasts in an attempt to keep abreast of the eroding skeleton and, therefore, the alkaline phosphatase in the serum is apt to rise.

Roentgenographic Manifestations. Rickets or osteomalacia involving growing bone is manifested radiographically by alterations secondary to a deficiency of mineral salts associated with alterations in the maturation and proliferation of cartilage. The relationship of the radiographic changes to the altered physiology is best illustrated in the long bones. Although generalized osseous alterations occur, the first and most apparent are at the sites at which the growth of bone is most rapid, e.g., the wrists, knees and costochondral junctions.

The earliest radiographic sign is haziness of the zone of provisional calcification, which is soon followed by disappearance of this zone. This reflects the failure of deposition of mineral salts within the organic matrix of the degenerated cartilage cells. Failure of degeneration of the cells of the epiphyseal cartilage results in irregularities in the metaphysis and in the

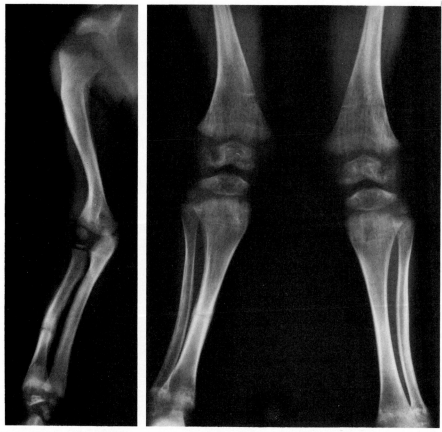

Figure 11–6 . Rickets. The alterations are extensive. The metaphyses are wide; the zone of provisional calcification is absent and the metaphyseal trabecular pattern is coarse. Lucent streaks are evident in the cortices. A pseudofracture (Looser zone) of the right tibia and the radius is evident. The osseous alterations are less marked at the elbow where growth of bone is slower than at the shoulder, wrist and knee.

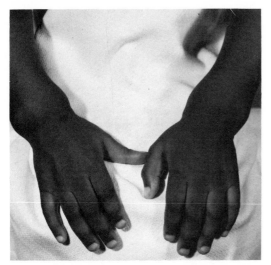

Figure 11-7 Rickets. Enlargement of the wrists is evident, a result of overgrowth of cartilage.

generation of cartilage cells results in an actual increase in the width of radiolucent cartilaginous matrix interposed between the epiphyseal center and the metaphysis, and on radiographs this zone is further increased in width as a result of failure of calcification of cartilaginous matrix as well as of osteoid tissue. Because the failure of degeneration is not complete along the line of ossification, but occurs in a patchy, irregular manner, any osteoid that is deposited is laid down along this irregular line of ossification in the metaphyseal zone. Attempts at ossification of the irregularly deposited osteoid enhance the irregularity of the metaphyseal region, resulting in a radiographic appearance that has been compared to the bristles of a paint brush. Cupping of the ends of the bones probably results from mechanical factors acting upon the soft, nonmineralized osteoid tissue at the metaphysis, which in addition resists modeling.

epiphyseal center; the changes in the latter site are less apparent, however, because the growth of bone is very slow in the epiphyseal center as compared with the metaphyseal zone. Failure of de-

In the shaft, resorption of bone continues, possibly at a faster rate than is normal as a consequence of increased parathyroid

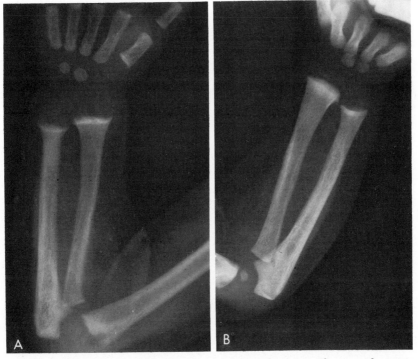

Figure 11-8 Rickets. A illustrates the early changes of rickets at the wrists. The zone of provisional calcification is hazy and irregular. Mild widening of the ends of the bones is evident. The cortex is not well defined and the trabecular pattern is coarse. After two months of therapy (B), the cortex is more dense as are the zones of provisional calcification. The epiphyseal center at the distal end of the radius has appeared.

activity due to a low serum calcium level. The smaller trabeculae may be completely lysed so that radiopacity is that of the soft tissue marrow. The larger trabeculae appear prominent and are often arranged longitudinally. The cortex is deceptively thick. It is made up of poorly ossified osteoid and radiolucent streaks may be seen within it. This undermineralization of the cortex contributes to the ease with which the larger trabeculae are seen radiographically and hence to the coarse trabecular pattern. In the infant, apparent widening of the cranial sutures is the result of the failure of mineralization at these sites of bone growth.

Greenstick fractures are common and the soft osteoid predisposes to bowing. Sharply defined, focal areas of decreased density may be seen traversing the shaft of the long bones. The origin of these "umbauzonen" or Looser zones has never been completely understood but their radiolucency is related to the fibrous tissue and osteoid present at these sites.

When healing of the rachitic process begins, the zone of provisional calcification appears at the site it would normally occupy if there had been no interference with mineralization. Later, the radiolucent metaphysis fills in with new bone. At this time, concavity of the ends of the bones may be most marked. The epiphyseal centers are reconstituted hemispherically since the base of the center grows at a slower rate than the periphery (Fig. 11–9). Epiphyseal centers that were delayed in their ossification appear, suggesting falsely a rapid increase in the bone age.

Microscopy. The most characteristic microscopic picture is obtained by making a longitudinal section through the epiphyseal and metaphyseal areas of a long bone in the rachitic infant. The cartilage cells and their chondroid matrix deeply situated in the epiphyseal chondral plate are normal in morphology and pattern. Maturation begins on schedule, but the cells, having obtained their normal component of glycogen and enzymatic potentialities, are not used; therefore they persist while new cells are added at the top of the column. Depending upon the degree of calcium and/or phosphorus paucity, there is usually some attempt at mineralization of the chondroid in contact with the mature cells, but a continuous line of provisional calcification is not

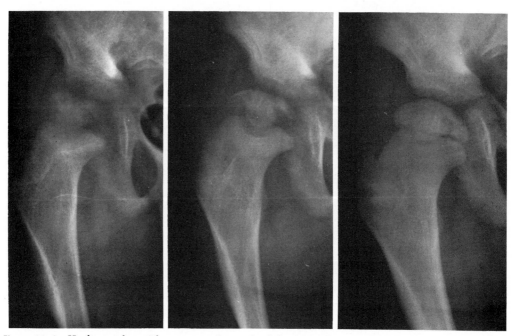

Figure 11–9   Healing rickets. The pattern of growth of the femoral epiphyseal center is illustrated by the pattern of healing of the rickets. The epiphyseal center is reconstituted in a hemispherical fashion about its base.

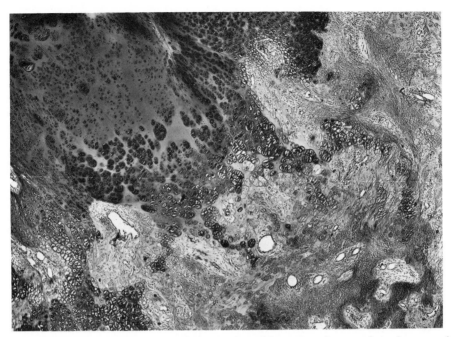

Figure 11–10   Rickets. Section taken through the epiphyseal line. Note the irregularity because of a lack of rigidity due to a failure of deposition of calcium salts. Stress probably causes the deformity. (× 28.)

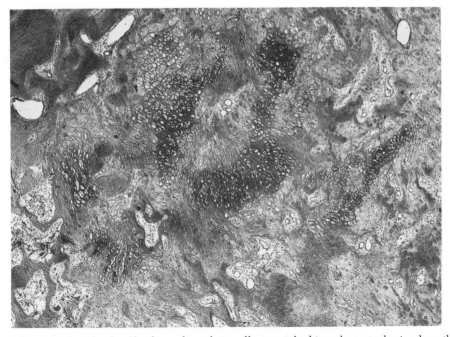

Figure 11–11   Rickets. Islands of hyalin and cartilage cells are pushed into the metaphysis where they serve as nuclei for the deposition of osteoid. The latter remains unossified because of a lack of mineral salts. (× 30.)

formed (Fig. 11–10). The persistence of unused chondrocytes, which are pushed farther and farther into the metaphysis, creates the impression that the fingers of vascularized granulation invade farther than normal into the chondral plate. The failure of the appearance of the calcified chondroid bars allows this granulation to progress along unguided routes so that the normal vertical pattern is destroyed and islands of cartilage cells drift into the metaphysis. The islands as well as fragments of imperfectly mineralized, primitive bone serve as foundations for the apposition of newly formed osteoid (Fig. 11–11). The latter also remains uncalcified so that there can be no alignment of lamellae and therefore no haversian system formation.

In the full-blown state of rickets, there is no condition that exactly duplicates this picture with the possible exception of metaphyseal dysostosis. Several of the congenital disturbances of enchondral growth result in poor columnation, scaffolding formation and spicule production, but there is never an excessive cartilage cell persistence plus abnormal amounts of osteoid without mineral deposition.

Prognosis. The addition of an adequate amount of vitamin D to the diet is usually all that is required to halt the progress of the disease. In the rare instances in which this is not effective, the diet should be critically examined and the bowel habits and stools analyzed. In the case that obstinately persists, the fault will almost surely be found to be in the function of the kidney. These cases have been called renal osteodystrophy if both glomeruli and tubules are involved or hypophosphatemic–vitamin D refractory rickets if the fault lies in phosphate conservation of the tubules.

Osteomalacia

Osteomalacia is a disease of mature bone occurring in adult life after the epiphyseal ossification centers have closed. The pathogenesis of this disease, an inadequate amount of calcium or phosphorus or both for mineralization of the osteoid that is formed to replace bone lost by normal catabolic lysis, is the same as that of rickets, which can occur only in growing bone. The symptomatic differences in the two conditions are due only to the difference in response of the growing and the mature skeleton in a state of chronic deficiency of calcium or phosphorus or both.

In children, the cause of the disease is almost always a lack of vitamin D in the diet or too little sunlight to synthesize the natural body sources. In adults, the causes are numerous, including deficiencies of calcium, phosphorus or vitamin D in the diet, disturbances in absorption of calcium or vitamin D and excessive serum phosphorus loss from the kidneys. Because full-blown osteomalacia is rare and its causes multiple, the nature of the disease has been poorly understood until relatively recently.

It was not until 1891 that osteomalacia and osteitis fibrosa cystica (parathyroid adenoma) were clearly separated by von Recklinghausen, but he, clinging to the ideas of Virchow, attributed the loss of rigidity of the skeleton to a solvent action of acid in the blood. Cohnheim, in 1889, had a more accurate concept of the disease, but it was not until the publication of McCrudden[7] in 1910 that the mechanism of osteomalacia was accredited to a deficiency of the mineral salts because of either an impoverished supply or an excessive loss.

Even today there is general confusion among clinicians regarding the two conditions, osteomalacia and osteopenia (osteopenic osteoporosis). Osteomalacia is a disease of mineralization; there is no interference with organic matrix formation. Osteopenia is a disease of organic matrix formation; mineralization mechanisms would be normal if sufficient matrix could be produced. Both terms have been in the past, and still are, used loosely to mean a softening of the mature skeleton. Such usage is inexact and leads to confusion. Actually, osteomalacia in the older age groups may eventually lead to a combined and superimposed disuse osteopenia because of pain and deformity. Adding to the leaching action of the former is the inhibition of the matrix formation of the latter. Combined the two diseases produce the most generalized and the most grotesque of the skeletal destruction diseases (Fig. 11–12).

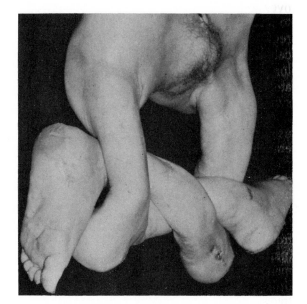

Figure 11-12 Combined osteoporosis and osteomalacia. A postmenopausal woman lived for a prolonged period on a starvation diet. Many factors played a role in the deossification and failure of osteoid maintenance, chief of which were inadequate intake of proteins, vitamins C and A and minerals.

The causes of the inadequate mineral supplies for skeletal maintenance are numerous. Dietary deficiencies of calcium and phosphorus cause osteomalacia but are so rare in most civilized populations that the disease practically does not occur from this cause. In remote areas, in which the simplest dairy products that abound in these minerals are unavailable, the disease is common.

Vitamin D lack is a much more common etiologic factor, particularly among politically oppressed groups who are forced to live on inadequate rations and are denied sunlight. Deprivation of the actinic rays because of social practices is reported to cause osteomalacia among women of India and the Orient. More common are the fat absorption disturbances that result from chronic disease of the bowel and pancreas. Chronic steatorrhea, sprue, fibrosing pancreatic disease, disturbances in the biliary duct system or even extensive and longstanding ulcerative colitis may result in conditions that inhibit the absorption of the fat-soluble vitamin D. The accompanying excess of fatty acids, which may form insoluble soaps with the available calcium, and the concomitant diarrhea, which moves the intestinal contents too fast for efficient absorption, may all add to the difficulties in the transport of adequate calcium and phosphorus from the bowel lumen to the blood.

A rather rare type of osteomalacia among women of the lower social strata is known as puerperal or multiple pregnancy osteomalacia. In young women who bear several children in rapid succession and nurse them between confinements, the calcium and phosphorus demand necessitated by the growing fetus and the milk supply for the infant may actually outpace the dietary supply. The skeletal stores are utilized and osteomalacia is the result.

Full-blown osteomalacia rarely occurs in the Western Hemisphere. Latent or early symptomatic osteomalacia, Milkman's syndrome, is seen occasionally in every active orthopedic clinic. These patients complain of pain, and if a roentgenogram is made early a focal area of demineralization in the cortex is found. These are more often seen in the diaphyses of large cylindrical bones but flat bones, particularly of the pelvis, may also be involved. According to Steinbach, the commonest site of occurrence of these pseudofractures, and the site most commonly missed, is the medial border of the scapula. The inferior ramus of the pubis is another common site in his material. He believes that these ribbon areas of deossification are produced by the pulsation of contiguous arterial channels, either normal or heterotopic. We have been unable to find evidence of such arteries in our small series of cases.

If periodic roentgenograms are taken over a span of weeks the focal area is seen to extend slowly across the bone in an irregular ribbon of translucency. These are called Looser zones. They were described long before their significance was appreciated. They are usually multiple, often symmetrical. They have the appearance of fractures without loss of alignment and usually there is no history of trauma. Several such cases were reported in the latter part of the last century and the first three decades of this century under a variety of headings. In 1934, Milkman[8] reported a case that he had studied thoroughly. He believed it to be a distinct entity, different from osteomalacia, osteitis fibrosa cystica (parathyroid adenoma) and osteitis deformans (Paget's disease). He called it "multiple, spontaneous idiopathic symmetrical fractures," and since this report the condition has been known as "Milkman's syndrome."

In 1946, Albright and co-workers[9] reported six cases of this condition with carefully controlled mineral balance studies. They concluded that the disease was caused by a chronic, low grade calcium deficiency due to renal tubule dysfunction and classified it as early, symptomatic osteomalacia. Their report has been amply corroborated by numerous workers since and Milkman's syndrome is now considered to be a mild type of osteomalacia. Albright et al. believed that a specific inability resided within the lining cells of the distal convoluted tubules of the kidneys to form an adequate amount of ammonia for urine secretion. There was a resultant withdrawal of the basic ions of the blood, especially calcium, to satisfy this need. The profligate use of calcium in this fashion necessitated a spending of the bone stores, producing symptomatic demineralization.

It is now generally conceded that most cases of Milkman's syndrome are instances of one or another of the types of hypophosphatemic–vitamin D refractory rickets that have survived the latent form of the disease in childhood or adolescence, or cases in which a similar dysfunction of the kidney tubules has been induced by plasma cell myeloma,[10] by metal poisoning including copper (Wilson's disease), lead, uranium and cadmium, in glycogen storage disease and in Lysol poisoning.[11] It is assumed that, in rare instances of plasma cell myeloma, the Bence Jones protein is reabsorbed by the lining cells of the proximal portion of the proximal convoluted tubules and inhibits the reabsorption of phosphates from the glomerular filter or increases the secretion of phosphates by these cells. Whichever mechanism applies, a lowering of the serum phosphorus (hypophosphatemia) with phosphaturia results and there is insufficient available mineral to supply the new osteoid of bone maintenance. Areas of weakness appear at points of stress and the lack of calcium salts at this site gives the roentgenographic appearance of a fracture. Alignment is maintained by the osteoid, which is strong but not rigid.

In this type of osteomalacia, Milkman's syndrome, there are pseudofractures, hypophosphatemia with hyperphosphaturia and slightly elevated alkaline phosphatase level. There may be massive aminoaciduria with a normal plasma amino acid level and glycosuria. There may be albuminuria, alkaline urine, mild systemic acidosis, hypokalemia and hypouricemia. Glomerular function is usually, though not in all types, normal.

As the disease progresses from Milkman's syndrome into florid osteomalacia the fractures increase in number and severity. Eventually, malalignment takes place and then it is noted that the entire skeleton is beginning to show deossification. Why certain focal areas (the regions of partial and finally complete fracture) are selected in early involvement is unknown. The Looser zones are usually, though not always, found at points of stress. Even in stress areas it is difficult to understand why a circumscribed portion of the bone undergoes demineralization and replacement with fibrous tissue while the adjoining region remains relatively normal.

As the skeleton softens, weight-bearing inflicts greater deformity. The long bones, particularly those of the lower extremities which must support the trunk, bend and twist. The pelvis becomes flattened laterally causing the pubic bones to protrude anteriorly. The vertebral column wilts like

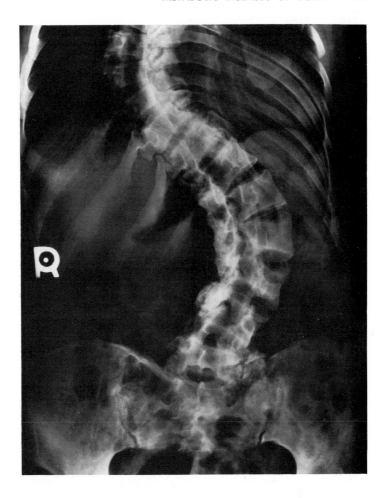

Figure 11–13 Severe osteomalacia. The vertebral column has suffered deossification until it can no longer bear the normal stresses to which it is exposed.

a warm candle (Fig. 11–13). Eventually, the directions of stress are so altered that the articular cartilage surfaces no longer serve their normal purpose and degenerative change induces a traumatic osteoarthritis. Pain from arthritis and fracture and disability due to deformity completely inactivate the patient. Then, disuse osteopenia sets in and the progress of the disease is hastened to a state of helplessness and eventual death.

Roentgenographic Manifestations. The roentgenographic manifestations of osteomalacia may be difficult to differentiate from those of osteopenia or osteoporosis, because in all three the skeletal structures are more radiolucent than is normal. Early in the course of osteomalacia only a coarse trabecular pattern associated with focal areas of radiolucency (Looser zones) may be evident or the skeleton may appear normal. The cortices then become less opaque and thinner. Deformities of the long bones, pelvis and spine follow as a result of softening of the bones. In the final stages, osteopenia as a result of disuse complicates the picture so that severe and marked radiolucency of the skeletal structures is evident (Fig. 11–15).

The coarse trabecular pattern is a consequence of inadequate mineralization of secondary trabeculae; the larger primary trabeculae are well seen in contrast with the unossified osteoid and soft tissues of the marrow. Radiolucent streaks in the cortex, representing unossified osteoid, precede thinning of this compact bone. In contrast with the brittle bones of osteopenia and osteoporosis, the unossified osteoid in osteomalacia permits deformities such as extensive bowing and bending.

Looser zones are radiolucent by virtue of their composition of osteoid and fibrous

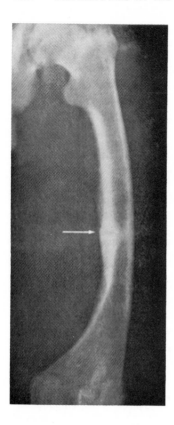

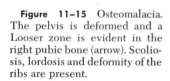

Figure 11–14 Osteomalacia. The femur is more radiolucent than is normal and the trabecular pattern is coarse. Bowing is evident and there is a Looser zone in the mid-diaphysis (arrow).

Figure 11–15 Osteomalacia. The pelvis is deformed and a Looser zone is evident in the right pubic bone (arrow). Scoliosis, lordosis and deformity of the ribs are present.

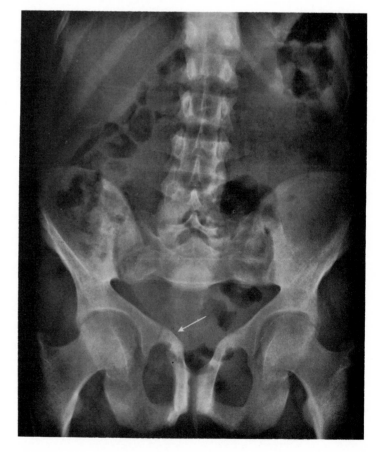

tissue. They often occur early in the course of the disease before the generalized skeletal manifestations of osteomalacia are apparent radiographically. These focal areas of radiolucency may be seen in other diseases, e.g., Paget's disease and fibrous dysplasia, but when evident in bones that appear otherwise normal radiographically, they strongly suggest the presence of osteomalacia. The pubic bones, the medial aspect of the neck and diaphysis of the femur, the axillary border of the scapula and the bones of the forearms are common sites of this lesion.

Microscopy. Sections made through areas of osteomalacia have much the appearance of rickets without the participation of cartilage. Sections through the Looser zones have shown a transverse stratum of bone destruction with replacement by a rather loose feltwork of fibrous and osteoid tissue. Mineral salts are completely lacking. As the disease advances the entire skeleton melts away. At the ends of the long bones the spicules of the spongiosa become thinner and thinner. Wide seams of osteoid are laid down to ensheath them and the interstices are filled with collagenizing fibrous tissue (Fig.

11–16). Osteoblasts and osteoclasts are abundant. There is less hemorrhage than in osteitis fibrosa cystica (parathyroid adenoma) and, therefore, giant cells are not so prevalent. The cortices become more and more attenuated by enlargement of the haversian canals until they come to resemble spongiosa. There is less osteoid proliferation in these areas except at the sites of infraction and frank fractures. Here the disarray of osteoid masses reminds one of callus formation.

Prognosis. The bone lesions of osteomalacia are much more insidious in their development than those of parathyroid adenoma. An early distinction between the two processes is important because of the completely different therapy. The cause of the bone softening must be ascertained. Dietary deficiencies are easy to supplant. Intestinal disease may require replacement or even surgical treatment. The method of alleviation of multiple pregnancy osteomalacia is obvious. Cases of Milkman's syndrome due to renal tubular insufficiency are usually treated by making available an alkaline salt to substitute the calcium ions being used, massive doses of vitamin D to stimulate tubular phosphate

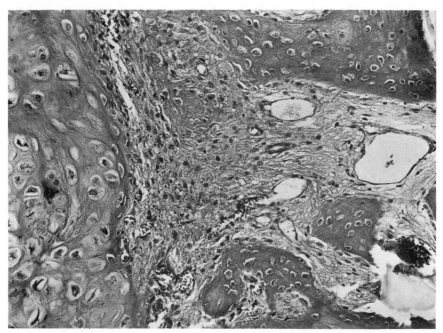

Figure 11–16 Osteomalacia. Cartilage and osteoid are normally produced but the latter is not mineralized to produce normal rigidity. The section reveals scrambled islands of cartilage between which there are masses of unmineralized osteoid. (× 150.)

reabsorption and a high calcium and phosphorus diet. Results depend largely upon the cause and available means to eradicate it. Most cases diagnosed early respond completely but in some the nature of the disturbance in physiology that causes the process may be so obscure that treatment is never very successful.

Renal Osteodystrophy (Renal Rickets or Secondary Parathyroid Hyperplasia)

The term "renal rickets" by which this disease has been known for so many years is no longer appropriate because it is now known that rachitic changes in the skeleton are produced by a number of types of kidney dysfunction, and moreover an important component of the bone manifestations is due to excessive parathyroid activity. Secondary hyperparathyroidism is a somewhat better term but inadequate because it does not include the important renal pathogenesis. It has become necessary to invent a new term that refers specifically to that disease of the skeleton that is secondary to dysfunction of the entire kidney, both glomeruli and tubules, with an overlay of hyperparathyroidism. Fraser[12] has suggested the name "pannephritic osteodystrophy," which appears to us to be the most suitable, but since in most clinics the condition is being called "renal osteodystrophy" this is the one that will be used here.

Renal osteodystrophy is the result of a chronic disease of the kidneys. It is widely believed that a dissipation of the serum calcium and an elevation of phosphorus, the former resulting in a stimulation of parathyroid hyperactivity, constitutes the pathogenesis of this disease. Recently it has been shown that healthy kidneys may be essential to reduce vitamin D_3 to 1,25-dihydroxycholecalciferol, the metabolite necessary for calcium ion transport from gut to blood stream. Whichever explanation pertains, the low serum calcium level makes it impossible to mineralize newly formed osteoid of growing bone, and the presumable excess of parathormone causes deossification of bone that has been normally mineralized. The result in rela-

tion to the skeleton is that of a combination of rickets and hyperparathyroidism.

The association of renal and skeletal disease was first called to the attention of the profession by Lucas in 1883.[13] During the next 30 years numerous such cases were reported, but it was not until the physiology of the parathyroid glands was carefully mapped that our present concept of the skeletal disturbance on the basis of parathyroid hyperplasia was presented. Even today, all the steps in the complex mechanisms of the disease have not acquired the security of factual proof, but from analysis of experimental data and of the morbid physiology of other types of renal disease and of parathyroid adenoma we are able to assume much that has hitherto been complete mystery.

The type of parathyroid hyperplasia known as "renal osteodystrophy" is by definition a disease of growing bone and, therefore, occurs only in children. Its counterpart in the mature skeleton is frequently called "renal osteomalacia" and, in a sense, differs from the childhood form just as vitamin D deficiency rickets differs from other types of osteomalacia.

The disease is almost always seen in childhood. The earlier it occurs, the more profound the bone changes are apt to be. Skeletal changes are rarely manifest sooner than two years after kidney insufficiency has become apparent. The background is usually a congenital disturbance in kidney development. Polycystic disease or hypogenesis is common, or there may be alteration in the pressure of the calyces because of congenital ureteral stricture or valves of the urethra. The congenital malformation is usually overlaid by a chronic pyelonephritis so that there is a gradual but progressive limitation of renal efficiency. Thus, a chronic uremic state is induced. It is unusual for renal osteodystrophy to be caused by a pure glomerulonephritis though this may be a cause of renal osteomalacia.

The signs of impaired kidney function are usually present if sought. Albuminuria and polyuria are commonly found and there is an inability to concentrate the urine normally. There is usually a reduction in the power to excrete phenolsulfonphthalein and an increase in the blood nonprotein nitrogen, chlorides and uric acid levels. The history of long-standing kidney disease before the onset of skeletal symptoms is usually the most helpful diagnostic criterion. The association of kidney disease with bone demineralization does not necessarily mean secondary parathyroid hyperplasia because in parathyroid adenoma there may be eventual renal insufficiency due to nephrocalcinosis. Making the distinction between these two conditions may tax the talents of the most able diagnostician.

The stimulation of the parathyroid glands to excessive secretory activity is probably the result of a long continued low serum calcium content. The exact cause of the low calcium level is not known. It may be due to the incompetence of the renal tubules to synthesize ammonia with a resulting substitution of the serum base ions of which calcium is one of the most important. The serum calcium may be thus expended along with other ions such as sodium and potassium. In chronic nephritis the damaged glomerular filter results in retention of phosphates. It has been presumed by some that under normal conditions there is physiologic saturation of the serum with the calcium and phosphorus ions and that the addition of one above this saturation level necessitates a fall in the other. It has been shown by other workers that an increase in one of the components elevates the solubility product and causes a precipitation of calcium phosphate that is deposited in the tissues and in motile blood phagocytes. There being a superabundance of phosphorus ions, this level is not critically affected but the available calcium stores are thus depleted. The usual serum calcium level in renal osteodystrophy is normal or slightly depressed; the phosphorus may be normal but is often elevated. The changes in ion levels are almost never as dramatic as those in parathyroid adenoma and idiopathic spontaneous parathyroid hyperplasia. The most important distinguishing feature is the high calcium level in the primary parathyroid diseases and the low or normal level in renal disease. The serum phosphorus and alkaline phosphatase levels are usually high in the latter.

Metastatic calcification is not nearly as common in secondary parathyroid hyperplasia as it is in the primary parathyroid disturbances. But nephrocalcinosis may occur and even widespread calcific deposits possibly because of the increased solubility product related to excess phosphorus. When the kidney disease supervenes in parathyroid adenoma the serum calcium level may fall. Then the combination of kidney insufficiency, metastatic calcification, parathyroid hyperplasia and skeletal deossification makes it almost impossible to ascertain the correct nature of the disease unless there is a clear history of renal disease before the appearance of bone disease. It may be of significance, however, that the bone changes develop more slowly, are more chronic in nature and less severe in renal hyperparathyroidism with the exception of those cases that begin very early in life.

The bone changes in renal osteodystrophy depend upon the severity of the kidney disease, its duration and the stage of skeletal development at which it began. If the nephritis results in a profound uremia early, the patient succumbs before osseous changes occur. If the kidney insufficiency is moderate, beginning early but sparing the child for several years, the skeletal changes may become very severe by the time he reaches 7 to 10 years. In this type, dwarfism is usually the outstanding feature and the skeleton may show all the changes of advanced rickets, because there are insufficient calcium ions to produce enough calcium salts to mineralize the osteoid of growing bone. The more rapidly the skeleton grows, the greater is the mineral lack and the more severe the bone changes will be. In addition to the changes that are characteristic of rickets, one may find fractures with faulty healing such as those encountered in parathyroid adenoma. Late in the disease, subperiosteal cortical lysis, identical to that seen in parathyroid adenoma, is superimposed on the changes that characterize rickets.

If the disease is later in onset, dwarfism does not occur. Here the clinical findings are largely those of chronic renal disease and skeletal deformity such as that found in parathyroid adenoma. The normally formed skeleton becomes less rigid owing to demineralization and stress causes abnormal bending (Figs. 11–17 and 11–18).

Pathogenesis. The exact mechanisms
(*Text continued on page 359.*)

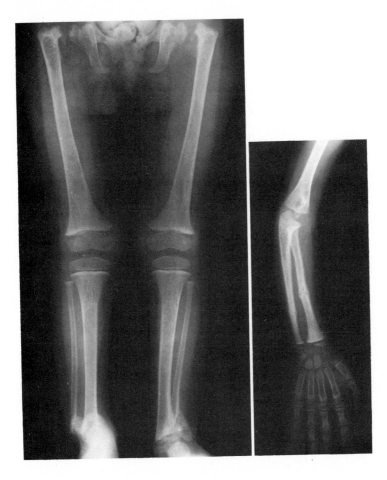

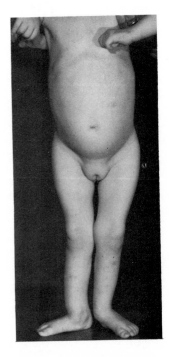

Figure 11-17 Hyperparathyroidism secondary to renal abnormality has resulted in skeletal demineralization and fractures of the proximal femurs and distal tibias and fibulas (left). Subperiosteal resorption of bone is evident in the phalanges (right). The lamina dura was absent. Gross rachitic changes are not present owing to failure of growth.

Figure 11-18 Renal osteodystrophy. The radiographs of this patient are illustrated in Figure 11-17. Note the prominence of the costal margin as well as the deformity of the ankles.

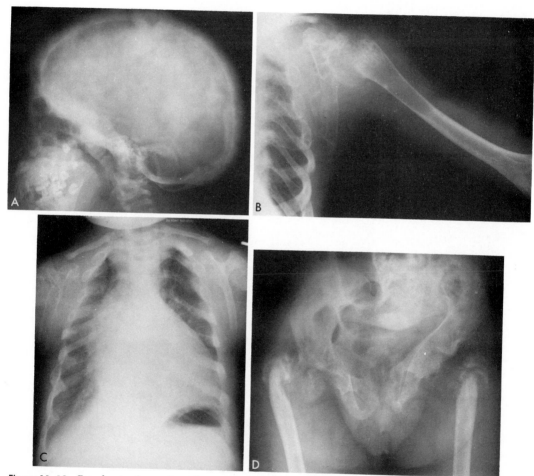

Figure 11–19   Renal osteodystrophy. The examination is of the same patient illustrated in Figures 11–17 and 11–18 at the age of 12 years (six years later). The deformities are severe with bone resorption of the proximal femurs and brown tumors expanding the scapulae, ribs, humerus and ilia. Granularity and thickening of the cranial bones and mandible are marked. The teeth are displaced.

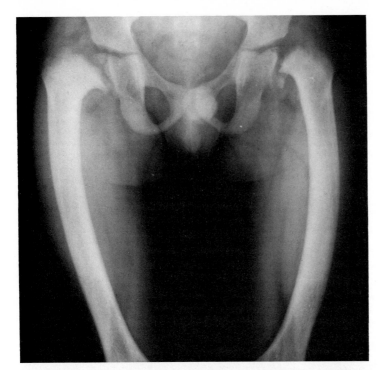

Figure 11-20 Renal osteodystrophy. There is bowing of the femurs in which there is a coarse, dense trabecular pattern. An acute slip of both the right and left femoral capital epiphysis has occurred; not an uncommon event in this condition.

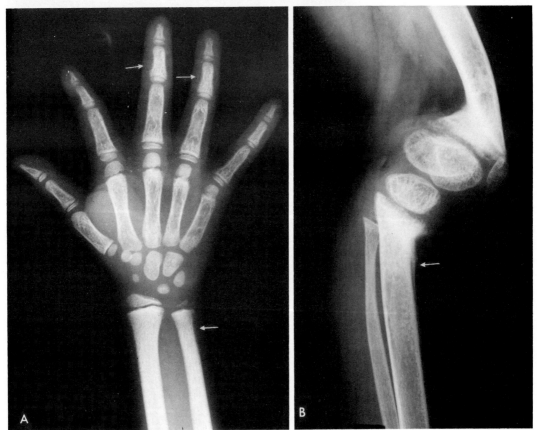

A   B

Figure 11-21 Renal osteodystrophy, female, 8 years of age. The trabecular pattern is coarse. Subperiosteal resorption is present in the phalanges (arrows) and along the medial aspect of the distal ulna (arrow, A). At the knee, there is marked bowing of the femur and of the tibia. Periosteal new bone (arrow) suggests that trauma played a role in the deformity. Rachitic changes are present (B).

of the processes that result in renal osteo-dystrophy have never been elucidated. It has been assumed that diminished glomerular filtration of phosphates causes the hyperphosphatemia. Concomitant tubule damage has been thought to produce a failure of base economy resulting in depletion of skeletal calcium and systemic acidosis.

Among other materials glucose, amino acids, organic acids and phosphates are reabsorbed from the glomerular filtrate by the cells lining the proximal convoluted tubules. It is in this portion of the tubule also that the hydrogen ion exchange mechanism takes place. This activity, an important device for controlling systemic pH, is concerned with the exchange of sodium ions of the filtrate sodium bicarbonate with hydrogen ions to form carbonic acid. The sodium is normally reabsorbed. As the carbonic acid descends the tubule it is dehydrated with diffusion of the carbon dioxide into the cells; thus both components of the sodium bicarbonate are conserved. Synthesis of ammonia and acidification of the urine take place in the distal tubule. When proximal tubule bicarbonate absorption is defective and an excessive amount in the distal tubules competes for hydrogen ions, there is a decrease in the urine ammonia and titratable acidity. Other available cations including calcium are utilized and the ultimate result is a lowering of the serum calcium level. Low serum calcium levels stimulate parathyroid activity, which mobilizes stored calcium from bones and further inhibits phosphate reabsorption by the tubule cells of the kidney. How much each facet of this complex mechanism contributes to the over-all disturbance is almost impossible to evaluate but it is obvious that when inadequate phosphorus or calcium or both are available for normal ossification, rickets or, later in life, osteomalacia must develop.

It is assumed by most that the drain on serum calcium has resulted in parathyroid stimulation. Because of recent changes in concepts of renal physiology, the assumed mechanisms of renal osteodystrophy may have to undergo revision. There is evidence that a factor, as yet unidentified, in chronic azotemia may interfere with osteoid mineralization. Yendt et al.[14] incubated rachitic rat cartilage in sera from 58 humans including normal subjects and those with various diseases in which there was alteration of serum calcium or phosphorus or both. They found that sera from non-azotemic subjects with a calcium-phosphorus ion product of 34 or greater almost always caused in vitro calcification, whereas that from azotemic patients, even though the ion product was higher, usually did not. Because magnesium is known to inhibit in vitro calcification they tested for this substance and found it increased more often in azotemic sera. Because it was not always elevated, however, they concluded that the magnesium ion was not the only, and probably not the important, factor.

Microscopy. Examination of the kidneys reveals maldeveloped or shrunken fibrotic organs. The appearance is usually that of the end stage of pyelonephritis often accompanied by a hydronephrosis. Microscopic sections show extensive disease in both the glomeruli and the tubules (Fig. 11–22). Often there are fine deposits of calcium salts in the supportive tissue of the tubules and even in the glomerular tufts.

When the parathyroid glands are dissected, all or the majority are usually found to be enlarged. Through the microscope the entire parenchyma is seen to be involved in a cellular hyperplasia. At times, this hyperplasia is entirely of chief cells, but usually some of the cells are somewhat enlarged and moderately clear (Fig. 11–23). Scattered single or aggregates of oxyphil and fat cells may be encountered. If the entire gland is composed of clear cells arranged along a fibrillar septum with a basal arrangement of the nuclei, the case is said to be one of idiopathic spontaneous hyperplasia and not of renal osteodystrophy. The difficulty for the pathologist comes in attempting to differentiate the glands of parathyroid adenoma and those of secondary hyperplasia on microscopy alone. In the majority of cases this cannot be done, because in both instances the components may be mixed and variable. If a rim of normal parathyroid tissue can be found this is a strong factor for parathyroid adenoma, because in secondary hyperplasia the entire organ is usually involved.

If sections are made through the epiphy-

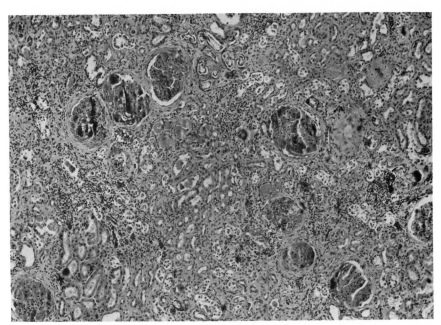

Figure 11–22   Kidney in secondary parathyroid hyperplasia (renal osteodystrophy). Both glomeruli and tubules show post-inflammatory scarring and calcium deposition. (× 25.)

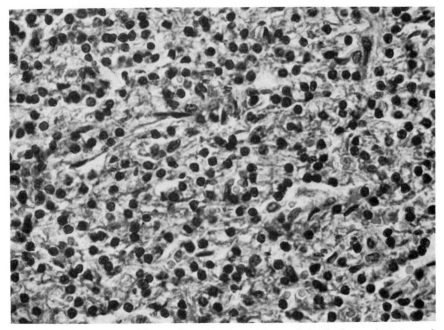

Figure 11–23   Secondary parathyroid hyperplasia (renal osteodystrophy). The hyperplasia is predominantly of the chief cell type. One can detect some tendency to clear cell transition. (× 455.)

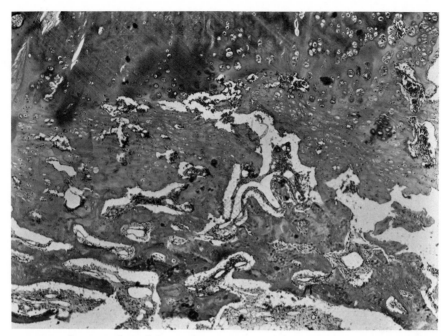

Figure 11–24 Secondary parathyroid hyperplasia (renal osteodystrophy). The epiphyseal line (above) shows a lack of scaffolding. The metaphysis contains large amounts of unmineralized osteoid. (× 25.)

seal plate and the metaphysis of a long bone in secondary parathyroid hyperplasia (renal osteodystrophy) the changes of vitamin D rickets may be found, because here too there is inadequate calcium to form sufficient calcium salts for mineralization (Fig. 11–24). The provisional line of calcification may be incomplete or irregular. Failure of chondroid bar mineralization may allow the mature cartilage cells to persist. They are pushed downward to form islands within the metaphysis. Because there is no disturbance in osteoid production, in growing bone this material is formed just as in true rickets though usually it is not as abundant. Because of the failure in provisional calcification and the persistence of chondrocytes a normal chrondroid lattice is not formed so that the osteoid is laid down in irregular masses or as seams along old bone spicules and abnormal cartilage islands. On comparing this section with one of true rickets a distinction cannot be made.

Sections through areas of intramembranous bone formation show less characteristic changes. Masses of fibrous hyperplasia replacing the disappearing cortex are the most obvious finding. Osteoclasts are abundant and there may be some narrow seams of new osteoid.

Prognosis. The prognosis in well developed renal osteodystrophy is eventually poor. The disturbances of bone growth and deossification can be arrested by raising the serum calcium level with high calcium and low phosphorus diet and by giving adequate vitamin D.[15] Special attention should be directed to the primary difficulty, the kidney disease. Renal insufficiency profound enough to cause bone disturbance will almost certainly result in fatal uremia but the patient may be carried along a number of years, sometimes well into adult life, until this ultimate event.

Renal Osteomalacia

Osteomalacia due to calcium loss— phosphorus retention glomerulonephritis, preferably known as renal osteomalacia— is actually a combination of calcium loss osteomalacia and secondary parathyroid hyperplasia. By definition, the disease can occur only after the epiphyseal ossification centers are closed so that bone growth is not affected.

The disease is considerably less common than renal osteodystrophy because the most common cause of the type of renal malfunction that results in disturbances of bone growth and maintenance is congenital malformation. In rare instances, however, a chronic glomerulonephritis may be severe enough to cause a long-standing low grade uremia yet spare the life of the patient for a number of years. With sufficient time the resulting calcium-phosphorus imbalance induces secondary parathyroid hyperplasia and the bone changes of excessive parathormone activity.

The symptoms are primarily those of chronic renal insufficiency on which are superimposed the bone symptoms of osteomalacia.

Microscopy. The microscopic features of hyperparathyroidism are bone destruction, fibrous replacement, hemorrhage and brown tumors. Those of osteomalacia are bone lysis and replacement with considerable amounts of osteoid, which remains unmineralized. There have been too few cases to date to allow a critical comparison of the material from cases of renal osteomalacia with that from true osteomalacia and osteitis fibrosa cystica. Until such comparisons have been made, it is impossible to say whether renal osteomalacia can be differentiated on the basis of bone tissue examination.

Hypophosphatemic–Vitamin D Refractory Rickets

In their monograph on the parathyroid glands and metabolic disease, Albright and Reifenstein mention and give a follow-up on their originally published case (1937) of rickets that was resistant to ordinary doses of vitamin D but that responded to massive therapy. Since that time, numerous reports have appeared describing cases of severe rickets that can be controlled only by giving enormous

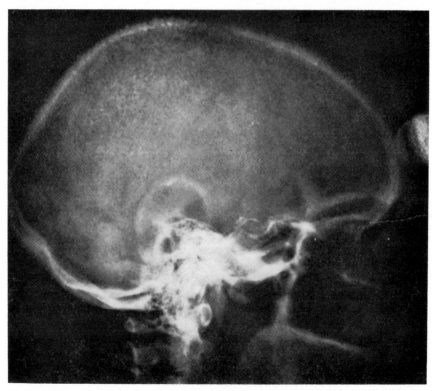

Figure 11–25 Renal osteomalacia. The granularity of the cranial bones is indistinguishable from the alterations of primary hyperparathyroidism.

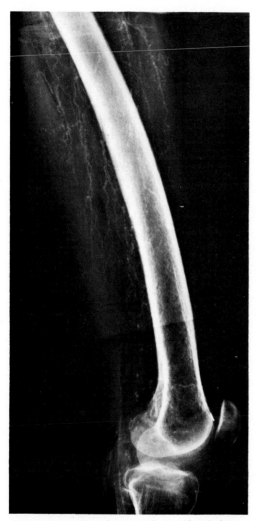

Figure 11–26 Renal osteomalacia. The skeleton is underminarilized. Extensive vascular calcification is present; it is more commonly associated with primary hyperparathyroidism.

amounts is the mediation of the absorption of calcium through the gut wall though it is now believed that one or more of the intermediate metabolic products of the original vitamin D_3 are the actual agent which is necessary for calcium ion transport. Massive doses over a long period result in a generalized deossification of the skeleton and it has been assumed that its action is directly upon the bone, very similar to that of the parathyroid hormone. For some time it has been suspected that massive amounts of vitamin D also have a controlling action upon the reabsorption of the phosphate ions by the renal tubules. This suspicion has been strengthened by several recent reports though definitive evidence is still wanting.

In 1933,[16] and again in 1956,[17] de Toni published papers describing cases of dwarfism in which there was renal dysfunction as a prominent clinical accompaniment. Since these papers there has developed a concept of a type of rickets that results from an inability of the proximal tubules of the kidney to reabsorb certain substances, particularly glucose, amino acids, phosphates and bicarbonates, from the glomerular filtrate. These cases were classified under the general heading of "de Toni-Debre-Fanconi syndrome" and in this country they were called the "Fanconi syndrome."

As newer and more accurate means of analysis were developed and as more cases were studied it became apparent that there are a variety of conditions in which the proximal tubules are either congenitally unable to reabsorb a number of substances or in which a number of toxic agents may induce this inability. When phosphorus, or less frequently calcium, is dissipated by this absorption deficit the skeleton develops the changes of rickets because of inadequate mineral salt for normal ossification. In the past these changes have been called "renal rickets," a term that caused confusion with the disease that we prefer to call "renal osteodystrophy." Most authorities in this field agree that the mechanisms of these various diseases have not been clearly defined as yet. Dent[18] did much of the early work that resulted in our present concepts of the conditions and more recently Fraser and

doses of vitamin D. Because the symptoms, signs and bone changes are the same as those of ordinary rickets, it was almost inevitable that this condition should receive the name of vitamin D refractory rickets. It was assumed that the tissue threshold for vitamin D effect was higher in these patients than in the normal and indeed, because the several facets of vitamin D metabolism have not yet been certainly delineated, this cannot be denied unequivocally though other mechanisms have been proposed that quite satisfactorily satisfy the known facts. There is ample evidence to show that the main activity of this vitamin in physiologic

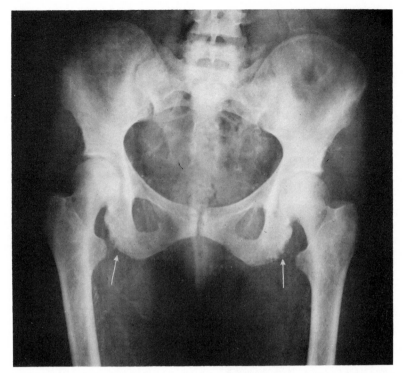

Figure 11–27 Renal osteomalacia. The bones are more lucent than is normal. Resorption is present along the ischia (arrows) and the sacroiliac joints. There are vascular calcifications.

Salter[15] and later Fraser[12] have attempted to classify these diseases. Their classification will be used in this discussion with the realization, expressed by these authors, that as more information is gathered it may be necessary to make revisions. However, some classification is necessary to guide our thinking through this jungle of morbid physiology. Easier paths can be established when we have mapped the general area.

In the following types of rickets it is currently believed that a defective reabsorption mechanism in the proximal convoluted tubule is a factor, in most instances etiologically related, in the development of the disease. Among other materials glucose, amino acids, organic acids and phosphates normally are reabsorbed from the glomerular filtrate by the cells lining the proximal convoluted tubules. When phosphate reabsorption failure occurs, often associated with failure of reabsorption of one or combinations of several other substances, rickets is the inevitable result. It is therefore a phosphorous deficiency type of rickets.

Hypophosphatemic–vitamin D refractory rickets consists of the following types:

Type I—vitamin D resistant rickets

Type II—with aminoaciduria

Type III—with aminoaciduria and acidosis

Type IV—cystine storage disease

Type V—with hyperglycinuria

Type VI—Lowe's disease (oculocerebrorenal syndrome)

The cause of the reabsorption defect appears to vary. In some instances it is apparently due to a congenital enzymatic deficiency. In others it may be due to a congenital malformation of this portion of the tubule. In still others it may be due to a number of toxic agents acting upon the tubule lining cells of this area. These include an agent (Bence Jones protein?) produced in plasma cell myeloma, as well as copper (Wilson's disease), lead, uranium, cadmium, lysol, maleate and cystine (cystinosis). The abnormal activity may be secondary to excess glycogen storage.

A number of structural changes in and about the proximal convoluted tubules have been reported. These include lining cell atrophy, hypertrophy, vacuolization and degeneration. Other investigators have reported peritubular, focal fibrosis, tubule dilatation with flattening of the lining cells, intracytoplasmic granular inclusions and lack of alkaline phosphatase. Clay et al.[19] microdissected the kidneys in two cases and found a peculiar bending of a narrowed tubule, "swan neck," connecting the convoluted portion to the glomerulus, a shortening of the convoluted portion and a thinning and atrophy of the distal tubule. Other investigators have failed to find these changes consistently and it appears probable that they are secondary to the functional alteration, that there are a number of causative structural changes that vary from case to case or that all the "findings" are simply normal variations. As a greater experience illuminates the subject the last begins to appear the most reasonable.

Vitamin D in massive doses improves kidney function in all but a few of these cases. The exact site of its action is not clearly defined. In Type I its major effect may be in increasing the absorption of calcium through a congenitally "resistant" gut wall. This idea was originally proposed by Albright and co-workers,[9] later largely abandoned by other writers and then suggested again by some recent work in which it has been shown that not vitamin D_3 but one of its metabolites formed in the kidney may be the agent which controls the calcium absorption. In the other types the site of action is either in the proximal tubules in which vitamin D quite possibly increases the absorption of phosphates or in the glomerulus where it decreases phosphate filtration. Evidence for the latter in a few cases is quite convincing but the most popular hypothesis is the enhancement of phosphate reabsorption by the tubule lining cells.

Pedersen and McCarrol[20] reported 25 cases of hypophosphatemic rickets and found involvement in 10 parents. They concluded that there is a strong hereditary and familial incidence. Because dwarfism is the outstanding feature of the disease and because these patients do not respond to average doses of vitamin D, it is possible, as these workers suggest, that numerous cases of hypophosphatemic rickets are masked at present as congenital chondrodystrophic dwarfism. These cases may be diagnosed, when suspected, by blood chemical analysis and therapeutic trial. Doses of as high as one million units of vitamin D daily have been used though considerably smaller doses are usually effective.

TYPE I – HYPOPHOSPHATEMIC–VITAMIN D REFRACTORY RICKETS (SIMPLE TYPE). This type is the most common of all the cases of rickets due to tubule insufficiency. It has a familial incidence and is a sex-linked dominant. It occurs in both males and females. Manifest dwarfing and bone distortion usually begin early, at about the commencement of weight bearing. The changes as they develop are those of advanced rickets of the ordinary type. All the clinical signs are associated with the deficient mineralization of the skeleton because there is no glomerular disease and therefore no uremia. There is hypophosphatemia and an elevated alkaline phosphatase. In some cases there is renal glycosuria. Serum calcium, blood urea and urinary amino acid excretion are normal. Because of the skeletal changes and the occasional renal glycosuria this type of rickets has been placed with the tubule reabsorption dysfunction diseases by most writers but the principal defect, excessive phosphate loss, conceivably might be due not to a reabsorption defect but to hyperparathyroid action. The latter could occur as the result of inadequate gut absorption due to the vitamin D refractory status. Unlike most of the other types of tubule reabsorption dysfunction rickets, the tubule disease does not extend to involve the glomeruli, uremia does not intervene and, therefore, life expectancy is not altered.

Treatment is usually carried out by gradually increasing doses of vitamin D to the maximal level without inducing signs of toxicity. The latter include lassitude, polydipsia, polyuria, irritability and weight loss. The serum calcium rises to 11.5 mg. per 100 ml. or higher. In this state the patient may enter hypercalcemic crisis or over a longer period develop nephrocalcinosis and kidney failure. Properly managed, these patients can live a normal, uncurtailed life, though a normal growth rate may never be achieved.

TYPE II—HYPOPHOSPHATEMIC–VITA-
MIN D REFRACTORY RICKETS WITH
AMINOACIDURIA. This type is much less
common than Type I. Though the onset is
earlier and the manifestations more severe,
the prognosis is probably better. This
type is differentiated from ordinary rickets
and Type I rickets by the presence of large
amounts of amino acids in the urine. Because there is no elevation of the serum
amino acids it is presumed that the urinary
acids are the result of an inability of the
renal tubules to reabsorb them. The disease appears in infancy and because this is
normally a rapid growth period the skeletal
alterations are dramatic. Disturbances in
amino acid excretion are frequently associated with juvenile cirrhosis of the liver
and it is probable that if these patients are
not diagnosed early and treated effectively
they may succumb of liver insufficiency.
Fraser and Salter[15] treated two patients
with large doses of vitamin D and obtained
rapid and complete healing of the epiphyseal lesions, normal serum calcium, phosphorus and phosphatase levels and disappearance of aminoaciduria. A third case
was diagnosed late (age eight) and developed cirrhosis and hepatoma.

TYPE III—HYPOPHOSPHATEMIC–VITA-
MIN D REFRACTORY RICKETS WITH
AMINOACIDURIA AND ACIDOSIS. This
type may appear at any time from infancy
to middle age. Its pathogenesis apparently
is very similar to that of Type II with the
addition of a dysfunction in the acid-base
regulatory mechanism. These cases must
be treated with large doses of vitamin D,
which reestablishes tubule phosphate reabsorption, but in addition basic cations
must be supplied in the form of alkalis to
spare the calcium and other fixed bases
and to restore a normal pH. These cases
have been too few for adequate evaluation and prognosis. Eventually, they may
be classified as a subtype of another
variety.

TYPE IV—CYSTINE STORAGE DISEASE
WITH RICKETS. It has been noted by
experimenters that tubule reabsorption
can be altered by abnormal quantities of
cystine passing through the kidney. It is
assumed by most, though not by all, that
the primary disease in this, Type IV rick-

ets, is a derangement in cystine metabolism with cystine damage to the proximal
convoluted tubules and consequent reabsorption dysfunction, which causes the
skeletal alteration of rickets. Worthin and
Good[21] have written an admirable account
of two cases of this condition. The disease
is familial and probably inherited by an
autosomal recessive mechanism. Crystals
of cystine can usually be found in the
corneas, the bone marrow and other
reticuloendothelial sites. Cystine may account for the doubly refractile intracytoplasmic substance that has been found in
the lining cells of the renal tubules.

The disease becomes manifest in childhood with severe rickets and dwarfing. As
in other types of tubule reabsorption dysfunction rickets there usually are hypophosphatemia and hyperphosphaturia,
aminoaciduria without hyperaminoaci-
demia, and glycosuria.[22] In addition, there
are hypokalemia and systemic acidosis.
Apparently cystine eventually is toxic to
the glomeruli as well as the tubules so that
chronic kidney insufficiency with uremia
is to be expected as an ultimate outcome.
Worthin and Good point out that variations
in reabsorption values are to be expected
because, with glomerulus damage, filtration rate may be reduced to a point at
which, because reabsorption rates are relative, they become normal. Treatment with
massive doses of vitamin D and potassium
citrate may improve the rickets but eventually these patients develop symptoms of
pan-nephritic disease and die in uremia.

TYPE V—HYPOPHOSPHATEMIC–VITA-
MIN D REFRACTORY RICKETS WITH HY-
PERGLYCINURIA. In 1956, Dent and
Harris[23] described four cases of osteomalacia that began in the second and third
decades of life in which muscle weakness
was an outstanding clinical feature. The
developing osteomalacia became very severe but eventually was controlled by
massive doses of vitamin D. The chemical
pattern of the serum and urine of these patients was similar to that in other cases of
tubule absorption dysfunction rickets except that the urine contained large quantities of glycine. The metabolism of other
amino acids appeared to be undisturbed.
Because of the late onset this disease has a

different clinical appearance and so may deserve a special heading in our classification.

TYPE VI—LOWE'S DISEASE (OCULO-CEREBRORENAL SYNDROME). Four cases of rickets with mental retardation and glaucoma were reported by Lowe et al.[24] in 1952. Tubule reabsorption dysfunction is an important part of the syndrome because there are hypophosphatemia, acidosis and aminoaciduria. Again the clinical picture is sufficiently different to warrant separate classification, at least until further cases are studied and an explanation found for this curious triad of symptoms.

Roentgenographic Manifestations. The radiographic manifestations of hypophosphatemic–vitamin D refractory rickets are those of rickets of any etiology because the underlying bony disturbance is that of inadequate mineralization of osteoid (p. 344). In this abnormality, however, the patient is apt to be older than the patient with vitamin D deprivation rickets and in most cases the osseous alterations at the end of the bone tend to be somewhat less severe. Because of the chronicity of the process, bowing and shortening of the long bones may be prominent features.

The long bones have a coarse trabecular pattern superimposed on moderate, but generalized, radiolucency. At the ends of the long bones the trabeculae assume a longitudinal direction. Bowing of the bones of the lower extremities laterally may be marked and associated with Looser zones. As a result of the bowing, the medial cortex is thickened because the line of stress is through it. The metaphyseal changes may not be florid but at the knee it is the medial aspect of the femoral and tibial metaphysis that is widest.

As in some adults with osteomalacia, the skeletal structures, especially the spine and pelvis, may show sclerosis as well as coarsening of the trabeculae.

If the disease is untreated, deformities of the spine, pelvis and ribs will be encountered in the older child and adult.

Microscopy. Sections through the metaphyseal areas of bones in hypophosphatemic–vitamin D refractory rickets are quite like those in vitamin D deficient rickets except that all the abnormal fea-

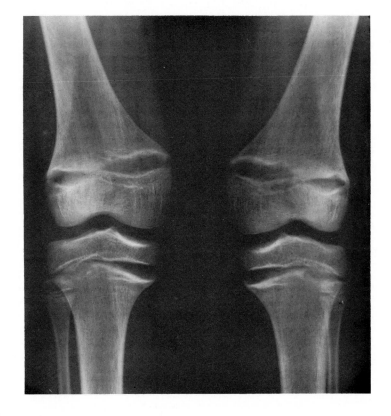

Figure 11–28 Vitamin D refractory rickets (hypophosphatemic). There is coarsening of the trabecular pattern in the metaphyses. The epiphyseal line is wide, particularly so medially. The femurs are bowed laterally.

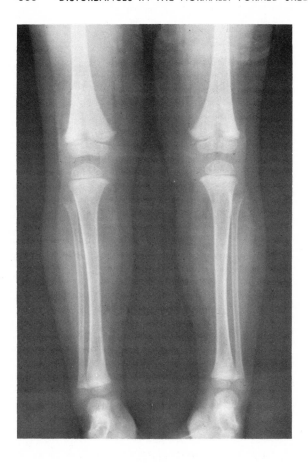

Figure 11–29 Hypophosphatasia. The radiograph of the knees of this male, 3 years of age, reveals indistinct zones of provisional calcification and triangular radiolucent defects in the metaphyses. These latter are frequently noted in this disease. (Courtesy of Dr. J. W. Hope, Children's Hospital of Philadelphia.)

tures are apt to be exaggerated. There is a failure of formation of the line of provisional calcification and a persistence of the unused mature cartilage cells. The latter form irregular masses deep in the metaphysis. Without chondroid mineralization there can be no normal lattice formation so that osteoid is laid down around anything in the metaphysis that will serve as a scaffolding. Irregular fields of unmineralized osteoid in patternless masses are the result. The lack of rigidity results in distortion of the epiphyseal line and the metaphyseal cortices. This is most notable in the areas of greatest stress, namely in the lower extremities.

Hypophosphatasia

This disease is presumed by some to be due to a lack of the enzyme alkaline phosphatase in the cells that normally contain

it and, as a result, a lowered phosphatase activity of the serum. Because it appears that alkaline phosphatase is necessary for normal mineralization of osteoid, the latter is formed but apparently cannot accept the mineral salts to form bone. The result is rickets in children and osteomalacia in the mature skeleton, the only type of these diseases presently known that is not caused by inadequate amounts of calcium or phosphorus in the fluid that perfuses newly formed osteoid. Rathbun recognized the disease as an entity in 1948. Fraser[26] reviewed the literature and reported three additional cases in 1957. Though the condition is still considered rare he was able to include 35 cases in his review.

Hypophosphatasia is an inborn error of metabolism with a genetic basis, probably inherited by an autosomal recessive gene. Evidences of the disease may be present at birth or even in utero or they may appear during childhood or in a few instances in adult life. The earlier the condition manifests itself the more severe its course is apt to be. If it develops in utero the patient probably will not survive 18 months, whereas in the older patient life expectancy may be normal. In the form appearing in young infants there are extensive skeletal lesions characterizing the changes of severe classic rickets. Because of the inability to mineralize osteoid, there is failure of bone development in the calvarium so that in the most severe cases the brain appears to be ensheathed in membrane (osteoid), with only small patches of ossification. Later there may be craniostenosis. This may be related to the lack of mineralization or, as Fraser suggests, due to inadequate or abnormal osteoid production. Mature chondroblasts and osteoblasts both lack alkaline phosphatase and because these cells are responsible for provisional calcification as well as osteoid production, this suggestion may be correct. Severe cases in the young group also manifest anorexia, vomiting, irritability and decline in growth rate. In most cases there has been premature loss of primary teeth. Death is apt to be due to suffocation because of a failure of ossification of the ribs.

A marked reduction in alkaline phosphatase levels in both serum and tissues is one of the cardinal features of hypophosphatasia. This occurs not only in sites of enchondral and intramembranous bone formation but in the viscera as well. The serum calcium levels are apt to be high but they fluctuate considerably. Serum phosphorus levels are normal. It has been shown experimentally that serum from typical cases of hypophosphatemia supports mineralization of rachitic rat cartilage in vitro and that cartilage from the epiphyseal area in cases of hypophosphatemia does not mineralize in serum of the normal human.

One of the interesting features of this disease is an excessive excretion of phosphorylethanolamine in the urine. The significance of this finding is difficult to interpret though it may mean that this substance is one of the normal substrates of alkaline phosphatase. It has been postulated that because it is hydrolyzed in vitro by alkaline phosphatase it may accumulate in excess in cases in which the

enzyme is deficient; however, when phosphorylethanolamine is injected into patients with hypophosphatemia it apparently is hydrolysed at a normal rate.

The histologic picture in hypophosphatasia is essentially that of very severe rickets. There is failure of mineralization at the line of provisional calcification and excessive cartilage proliferation in the metaphysis. The metaphysis is greatly widened by excessive production of osteoid, which remains largely unossified, and if there has been weight bearing there is the usual distortion of this area because of lack of rigidity.

Fraser has reported one case in which treatment with cortisone was highly successful. This therapy in other cases has not been beneficial.

Hyperphosphatasia

Caffey has described a small series of patients with hyperphosphatasia. These children characteristically display a large head with overhanging frontal bones, short neck and thorax, long arms and legs, lateral bowing of the femurs and anterior bowing of the tibias. They stand in partial flexion. The roentgenograms reveal thick cortices of long bones and a heavy skull suggesting Paget's disease (Fig. 11–30). The spine may show universal vertebra plana; the lamina dura may be lacking. A few biopsies have been reported to reveal the presence of primitive bone without haversian systems. Dr. Sue Mitsudo has been kind enough to show me sections prepared from autopsy material on a case of hyperphosphatasia, one of those, incidentally, of the series originally reported by Caffey. The microscopy in these sections was that of florid Paget's disease. The mosaic was as classic as any this author has ever seen. All patients with hyperphosphatasia have had high alkaline phosphatase levels in the serum comparable to those found in Paget's disease. Though many writers still deny a relationship between the two conditions there are many convincing features suggesting that hyperphosphatasia is indeed juvenile Paget's disease.

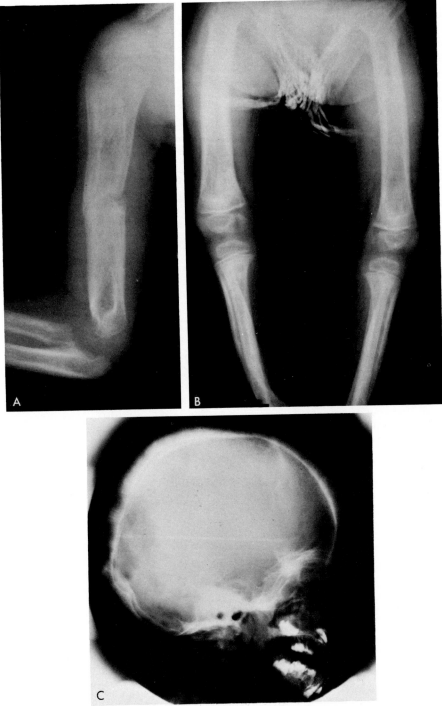

Figure 11–30 Hyperphosphatasia, female, 2 years of age. The long bones are increased in width (*B*); the cortex is dense in some areas (for example, the femurs) but striated in the humerus. The medullary canal is wide. There is a fracture of the humerus (*A*). The bones of the skull are thickened with irregular and poorly defined areas of sclerosis (*C*). (Courtesy of Dr. L. Verano, Hershey Medical Center, Hershey, Pa.)

DISEASES DUE TO AN INCREASED RATE OF BONE RESORPTION (OSTEOLYSIS)

We have very little definite knowledge concerning bone lysis. At present we know of only two mechanisms that cause bone resorption; one is by increasing the blood supply above the optimum and the second is through osteoclastic activity. A classic example of the former is the phantom clavicle or disappearing bone, which is caused by expanding or invading hemangioma. Infection causes bone lysis probably by an increased blood flow through granulation tissue. Pressure erosion and destruction by primary and secondary tumors is so poorly understood that there is little we can say about it. It has been noted that obese patients who are kept on a starvation diet develop a low grade acidosis and a negative calcium balance. It is assumed that calcium is withdrawn from the skeleton stores and that this withdrawal is not dictated by parathyroid control since this effect has been noted in hypoparathyroid patients. The easiest explanation for the negative calcium balance is the long continued lowering of the pH, a lowering which is so minimal that special laboratory methods are required to detect it. If chronic, low grade acidosis over a very long period does induce deossification, this mechanism might be used to explain certain instances of idiopathic osteoporosis.

Normal bone lysis, which is constant and continuous, is apparently accomplished by osteoclastic activity. The latter is controlled through the parathyroid glands. It has been suggested that the parathyroid route is the mechanism by which bone mass is reduced in hypervitaminosis D and Boeck's sarcoid.

Until relatively recently it was generally believed that senile osteoporosis was caused by a negative osteoid balance due to a decreased osteoid production rate that failed to keep pace with physiologic bone erosion, a wearing out of the skeleton with failure of osteoid replacement. But today we know that senile osteoporosis is a clinical symptom complex. Dietary deficiencies and inadequate stress quite certainly play a role by causing osteopenia (failure of osteoid production to meet the demands of physiologic erosion), but hormonal deficiency (estrogen or androgen) is probably even more important. The action of these hormones is usually said to be directly upon the osteoblasts. Recently it has been shown that the rate of osteolysis may be increased in certain cases of senile osteoporosis and even in pure postmenopausal (surgical castration) osteoporosis. This strongly suggests that estrogen and androgen act by antagonizing parathormone. Thus the reduction in bone mass in castrated young women could be purely osteolytic in nature.

Osteolysis by parathyroid activity is discussed in Chapter 12, Diseases Due to Endocrine Dysfunction. It may be due to parathyroid adenoma or to secondary parathyroid hyperplasia caused by a long continued low serum calcium value in cases of renal osteodystrophy. Primary parathyroid hyperplasia (clear cell hyperplasia) is still a dubious entity in the minds of the writers.

The role of thyrocalcitonin as yet has not been related to a disease entity. This hormone, elaborated by the acinar cells of the thyroid,[29] appears to inhibit release of mineral salts from bone. Apparently it also inhibits release of hydroxyproline and other organic matrix constituents. Its action may be mediated through the inhibition of the formation of osteoclasts from osteoblasts.

OSTEOPOROSIS

To this point in this chapter we have described types of reduction in skeletal mass due to osteopenia, osteomalacia and osteolysis. We have not discussed osteoporosis, a clinical symptom complex, the most important (from the standpoint of incidence) of the diseases characterized by skeletal mass reduction. It may be idiopathic but in most instances it is probably caused by a combination of the above mechanisms.

The most important type of reduction of bone mass from the standpoint of incidence is that seen in women, usually 60 years or older, a decade or more after the menopause; in men, perhaps a decade later. The usual complaint is back pain. The onset may be insidious or sudden following injury. The trauma may be disproportionately trivial in relation to the pain. The pain may be referred along the course of involved nerves, particularly down the posterior aspect of one or both legs. Eventually, the pain may spread to the pelvis, the thorax and the shoulders. If a vertebral body is weakened to the point of collapse there will be a kyphosis and loss of stature. This important disease of the skeleton, osteoporosis, is the most important factor in the incidence of hip fracture in the aged. Chemical analysis of the blood occasionally reveals a low alkaline phosphatase. Rarely there may be an excess of calcium in the urine. Estrogen levels are apt to be low.

This is the only type of reduction in bone mass that is properly called osteoporosis and the term osteoporosis properly refers to no other bone disease. The condition is a clinical syndrome rather than a pathologic entity. The pathogenesis is multiple and varied. Reduction in skeletal substance may be due to osteopenia (decreased rate of osteoid synthesis) because of dietary deficiency of proteins or vitamin C or absorption interference, or it may be the result of deficient stress stimulus. It may be caused by osteomalacia, a failure of proper mineralization of osteoid, or it may be caused by an abnormal rate of osteolysis due to parathormone stimulation of osteoclastic activity or possibly an insidious, long-standing, minimal lowering of blood serum pH. In reality most cases of true osteoporosis when carefully analyzed reveal evidence of osteopenia, osteolysis and sometimes osteomalacia.

Roentgenographic Manifestations. The roentgenographic manifestations of osteoporosis reflect the deficiency of organic matrix and parallel the gross pathologic findings. The cortices are thin and the trabeculae fine and sparse. The skeletal structures are therefore more radiolucent than normal. For the most part all of the skeletal structures are affected.

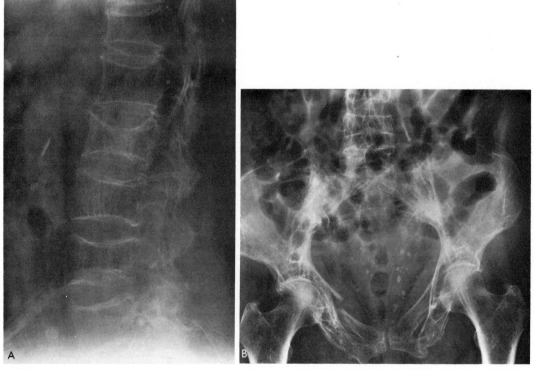

Figure 11–31 Osteoporosis. The bony structures are more radiolucent than normal. There are compression fractures of the lumbar vertebrae (A), and a fracture of the right pubic bone is evident in B. The cortices are thin and only the larger trabeculae are visible.

Fractures, particularly of the vertebrae and ribs, are not uncommon. The vertebral bodies may collapse anteriorly, producing loss of stature and a kyphotic deformity of the spine. Prominent vertical striae in the vertebral bodies may be an associated feature.

Morbid Anatomy. When the patient with advanced osteoporosis comes to autopsy the bone changes are quite obvious grossly. The ribs are as fragile and brittle as eggshell. They may be snapped with ease between the thumb and forefinger. When cylindrical bones are carefully examined it is noted that the silhouette is quite normal except where fracture and infractions have caused distortion. The compacta is greatly thinned, however, because of an enlargement of the medullary area. The thinning takes place from the inside so that the outer surface diameter remains constant. The vertebrae are most markedly involved and one or more may show wedge compression. If a vertebra is dissected and cut vertically in half, it is seen that the end plates are greatly thinned and cupped inward by the expanding intervertebral cartilaginous plates. The pelvic bones are next severely involved.

In cases in which the most important factor causing the osteoporosis is disuse (osteopenia), the skull bones are apt to be spared and the maximal thinning of long bones is found at the ends of the shaft.

When sectioned the bone tissue appears normal though there is too little of it. The haversian canals are widened and the compacta is thin (Fig. 11–32A). The trabeculae of the cancellous tissue are thin and often distorted by fracture. The ratio of bone mass to medullary soft tissue is greatly decreased so that the cancellous bone network under low magnification appears as a fine tracery in a matrix of fatty marrow (Fig. 11–32B). Osteoblasts are never numerous and are often entirely lacking.

The cause of the most common variety of osteoporosis, the postmenstrual or senile type, is often complex. The endocrine de-

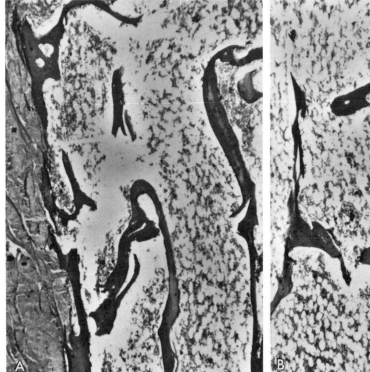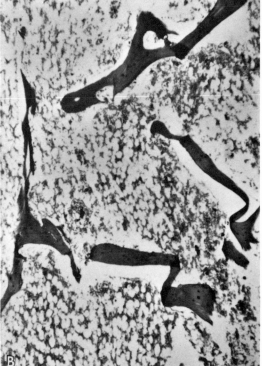

Figure 11–32   Osteoporosis. *A*, The cortex is markedly thinned and shows a fracture. *B*, The ratio of interspicular tissue to bone mass is greatly increased. The spicules are thin, delicate and easily fractured. There is no osteoblastic activity. (× 15.)

ficiency is the initiating and often the most important factor. These patients often look older than their age with atrophy of the skin and other features of senility. Frequently, a disuse atrophy complicates the picture. The muscles often show wasting. As these patients approach the sedentary age and as their bone pains appear they take to their rocking chairs and the normal stress stimulus for osteoblastic activity is decreased. Often they become fastidious concerning their diets. As their teeth become less efficient they take more to soft foods and avoid the tough proteins that are necessary for osteoid formation. As they lose interest in food the total caloric intake may be reduced to subadequate levels. Eventually, their diets may include too little calcium or phosphorus or both, and then a superimposed osteomalacia causes a melting away of the remaining skeleton to produce the most extreme weakening and bizarre distortion. The low serum calcium level probably causes increased secretion of parathormone, which increases the rate of osteolysis, again compromising any attempt to rebuild bone by increasing the rate of osteoid formation. Inefficient kidney function may cause an insidious acidosis so minimal as to be undetectable by ordinary laboratory methods. It is possible that this lowering of the pH may cause skeletal demineralization.

In cases in which the etiology of osteoporosis consists of several combined factors it is obvious that no one therapeutic agent will bring about a cure. These patients are usually treated with the deficient endocrine factor, given a high caloric, high protein diet, checked for adequate calcium intake and sufficient vitamin D to insure absorption and put on an exercise schedule. This regimen halts the progress of the disease and usually allays the symptoms but improvement in the roentgenograms is notably slow. It has been stated[29] that as much as half the bone mass of the skeleton may be dissipated in severe osteoporosis. This may amount to a mineral loss up to 3 pounds. Because only about 2 grams of calcium can be retained daily and that only with adequate newly formed organic matrix, to rebuild the skeleton would take two years or longer.

Posner, and later others, have shown that mineral is first deposited in osteoid in an amorphous form and the apatite crystal grows as the osteoid matures. The earlier phase is less stable. If fluoride is made available, it will replace a hydroxyl group of the amorphous form, stimulating the growth of the apatite crystal, thus converting an unstable form of osteoid to a stable form of bone. Hegsted[29] found that relatively high levels of fluoride in the water supply significantly reduce the incidence of osteoporosis. In many clinics throughout the country, osteoporotics are treated with 20 to 60 milligrams daily of sodium fluoride over an extended period up to 2 to 3 months. About 50 per cent of these patients attain symptomatic relief.

Osteoporosis after the age of 50 is a common condition. It should not surprise one that it is sometimes associated with certain catabolic or deossifying processes such as Paget's disease or parathyroid adenoma. When bone is rapidly broken down and there is no regenerative capacity because of the accompanying osteopenia, the clinical and roentgenographic pictures are greatly exaggerated. The serum alkaline phosphatase level, which is so characteristically elevated in these two diseases, may be normal because of the lack of osteoblastic activity making accurate diagnosis exceedingly difficult. When osteoporosis becomes combined with osteomalacia in its terminal stages it may be necessary to biopsy the bone to make a diagnosis. Though the clinical picture may be that of advanced osteomalacia, the lack of osteoblastic activity assures the pathologist that at least a part of the process is due to osteopenia.

Generalized plasma cell myeloma may give the same roentgenologic findings as senile osteoporosis. If the blood and urine chemistry is carefully considered, as it should be in every case of osteoporosis, a mistake in diagnosis will usually be avoided but in some cases a biopsy will be necessary.

References

SCURVY
1. Barlow, T.: Med. Chir. Trans., 66:159, 1883.
2. Hess, A. F.: J.A.M.A., 68:235, 1917.

3. Morris, G. E.: Am. Practit., 5:658, 1954.
4. Follis, R. H.: Bull. Johns Hopkins Hosp., 89:9, 1951.

RICKETS

5. Mellanby, E.: J. Physiol., 52:11, 1918.
6. Park, E. A.: Physiol. Rev., 3:106, 1923.

OSTEOMALACIA

7. McCrudden, F. M.: Arch. Intern. Med., 5:596, 1910.
8. Milkman, L. A.: Am. J. Roentgenol., 32:622, 1934.
9. Albright, F., Burnett, C. H., Parson, W., Reifenstein, E. C. and Roos, A.: Medicine, 25:399, 1946.
10. Engle, R. L. and Wallis, L. A.: Am. J. Med., 22:5, 1957.
11. Wallis, L. A. and Engle, R. L.: Am. J. Med., 22:13, 1957.

RENAL OSTEODYSTROPHY

12. Fraser, D.: J.A.M.A., 176:113, 1961.
13. Lucas, R. C.: Lancet, 1:993, 1883.
14. Yendt, E. R., Connor, T. B. and Howard, J. E.: Bull. Johns Hopkins Hosp., 96:1, 1955.
15. Fraser, D. and Salter, R. B.: Pediatr. Clin. North Am., 5:417, 1958.

HYPOPHOSPHATEMIC–VITAMIN D REFRACTORY RICKETS

16. de Toni, G.: Acta Pediatr., 16:479, 1933.
17. de Toni, G.: Ann. Pediatr., 187:42, 1956.
18. Dent, C. E.: Biochem. J., 41:240, 1947.
19. Clay, R. D., Darmady, E. M. and Hawkins, M.: J. Pathol. Bact., 65:551, 1953.

20. Pedersen, H. E. and McCarrol, H. R.: J. Bone Joint Surg., 33A:203, 1951.
21. Worthin, H. and Good, R.: Am. J. Dis. Child., 95:653, 1958.
22. Bickel, H., Smallwood, W. C., Smellie, J. M. and Hickmans, E. M.: Acta Pediatr., 42:27, 1952.
23. Dent, C. E. and Harris, H.: J. Bone Joint Surg., 38:204, 1956.
24. Lowe, C. U., Terry, M. and MacLachlan, E. A.: Am. J. Dis. Child., 83:164, 1952.
25. Reitz, R. E. and Weinstein, R. L.: N. Engl. J. Med., 289:941, 1973.

HYPOPHOSPHATASIA

26. Fraser, D.: Am. J. Med., 22:730, 1957.
27. Currarino, G., Neuhauser, E. B. D., Reyersbach, G. C. and Sobel, E. H.: Am. J. Roentgenol., 78:392, 1957.

HYPERPHOSPHATASIA

28. Progress in Pediatric Radiology. Vol. 4. Intrinsic Diseases of Bone. Kaufmann, H. S. (ed.), Basel, S. Karger, 1973.

OSTEOLYSIS

29. Hegsted, D.: Fed. Proc., 26:1747, 1967.

OSTEOPOROSIS

30. Deitrick, J. E., Whedon, G. D. and Shorr, E.: Am. J. Med., 4:3, 1948.
31. Stein, I., Stein, R. O. and Bellar, M. L.: Living Bone in Health and Disease. Philadelphia, J. B. Lippincott Co., 1955.

Chapter 12

DISTURBANCES DUE TO ENDOCRINE DYSFUNCTION

BONE CHANGES OF PITUITARY DYSFUNCTION

Giantism

The human growth hormone (HGH) or somatotropic hormone (STH) is a potent factor in the proliferation and perhaps maturation of the cartilage cells of the growth plate. It is generally believed by most writers, though largely on empirical evidence, that it plays a role in the development of all mesenchymal tissues including bone, periosteum, perichondrium and fibrous tissue. It is now regularly extracted from the eosinophilic cells of the anterior lobe of the pituitary gland. Its mechanisms are as yet not entirely understood, but experimentally and in humans it prolongs the growth period by providing a continuing crop of cartilage cells in the growth plate, thus keeping the ossification center open. Recent studies[1] have shown that HGH induces the formation of a secondary or intermediary growth promoting factor. This substance or probably class of substances has been given the generic name, somatomedin. Thus it seems likely that HGH functions and has its effects on cartilage via somatomedin. In certain instances of excessive growth during childhood and adolescence, tumor-like nodules of hyperplasia or a diffuse proliferation of the eosinophilic cells of the pituitary has been noted. This condition has been called pituitary giantism or gigantism.

As early as 1886, Marie called attention to abnormal stature in relation to the function of the pituitary gland but it was not until 1910 that Cushing hypothesized that it was the specific secretion of the eosinophilic cells that caused the remarkable overgrowth of the skeleton and soft tissues.

Giantism, which seems a better term than gigantism, is presumably caused by abnormally rapid growth during the normal growth period and often prolongation of the growth period. It is known that, in the experimental animal, HGH reestablishes active enchondral bone growth after the growth plate has ossified. Because the articular cartilage thus activated at the ends of long bones and at the boundaries of joints and synostoses now takes over the function of a growth plate, new bone growth may take place wherever articular cartilage is found. Though it has not been shown conclusively that HGH specifically delays systemic epiphyseal closure, it is known that gonadal hormones play a very important role in the establishment of the date of epiphyseal ossification, and that, in virilism due to excessive androgen stimulation, dwarfism may result from premature closure and cessation of linear growth. Because in some cases of giantism and often in acromegaly there appears to be inadequate gonadotropin secretion, it may be that the prolonged growth period in the former is at least partly due to delayed closure caused by hypogonadism.

Pituitary giantism is not a common condition. It has been defined as enchondral growth in excess of 6 feet 8 inches. This type of abnormal growth has resulted in statures that have exceeded 8 feet. It is relatively more common in males than females.

Because, by definition, giantism is excessive growth of bone, cartilage and fibrous tissue during the period of normal growth, often with some prolongation of this period, the active phase of giantism occurs during adolescence. The same process after the secondary epiphyseal centers have closed also results in excessive growth of bone, cartilage and fibrous tissue, but because the epiphyseal centers have been ossified, bone growth is different because it arises from the articular plate[2] rather than the enchondral plate and, therefore, the pattern of growth is quite distinctive. This condition is known as acromegaly.

Giantism presents a variety of patterns depending upon the stage of body development at which the condition begins. It should be kept in mind that the HGH stimulates growth mainly and perhaps only in mesenchymal derivatives. Thus, bone, cartilage and fibrous tissue are the principal tissues affected, but if the stimulus is applied early in their normal growth period the result is simply an exaggeration of the normal. Both length and mass of the skeleton are increased and concomitantly there is a proportionate growth in fibrous supportive tissue. The result is a huge but symmetric and well proportioned figure. There is some evidence to support the hypothesis that epidermal derivatives merely provide the necessary physiologic functions that support the mesenchyme. If this be true, it would explain the increased and balanced visceral size that accompanies mesenchymal growth. Because growth and maturation of the organic structure take place earlier in the brain than in other parts of the body, this organ is not involved in giantism or acromegaly.

In summary, if the effects of excessive HGH secretion begin before puberty, growth is balanced in all areas and the result is simply an exaggeration of the normal. But, periodically throughout adolescence, certain epiphyseal centers close and after closure enchondral bone formation in adolescent giantism is not normal in type. Consequently unbalanced growth takes place and the eventual product reflects the result of normal and abnormal bone growth. If the stimulus is applied after closure of all epiphyseal centers the picture, acromegaly, is quite different from giantism. If the stimulus continues throughout adolescence and into adult life the result is acromegaly superimposed on giantism.

The cause of abnormal skeletal growth in giantism is, as stated, an excessive production of HGH by the eosinophilic cells of the anterior lobe of the pituitary. Because HGH elaboration is stimulated by low serum sugar levels due to excess insulin, the two hormones are said to be antagonistic and HGH is diabetogenic. The cellular increase may be focal and well delineated (eosinophilic adenoma), diffuse (pituitary hyperplasia) or, as in a very few cases, giantism may be accompanied and presumably caused by an adenocarcinoma of the anterior pituitary lobe. In another few cases the pituitaries have been reported normal. There may be a functional increase without cellular hyperplasia.

The signs and symptoms of giantism fall into four groups: (1) those due to excessive HGH, (2) those due to stimulation by other hormones elaborated by the eosinophilic cells, (3) those due to the imbalance created by abnormal eosinophilic cell secretion and a deficiency of basophilic cell secretion because of basophilic cell destruction or atrophy by the eosinophilic cell hyperplasia, and (4) those due to the space-taking character of the lesion in the anterior pituitary lobe.

The excessive growth resulting from the elaboration of abnormal amounts of HGH involves all mesenchymal derivatives. The skeleton is large but so is the musculature. The viscera enlarge to accommodate the massive frame. This is especially true of the heart and kidneys. The latter show increased renal glomerular infiltration rate and proximal tubule activity.[3] Distorted growth takes place after the epiphyseal center closes so that in late adolescence the victim begins to take on the character of acromegaly superimposed on giantism. The increased height and weight sometimes lead to a thoracic kyphosis and to atrophic disturbances in the soft tissues of the feet.

Human growth hormone is the only known elaboration of the eosinophilic cells; however, a portion of its polypeptide chain acts as a lactogenic hormone. As previously stated, HGH is also diabetogenic.

The third group of symptoms is due to the suppression of function or the pressure atrophy of the basophilic cells. Because these cells are supposed to produce adrenal cortical stimulating hormone (ACTH) and other hormones, i.e., follicle-stimulating (FSH), luteinizing (LH) and luteotropic (LTH) hormones, one may find sterility in females and osteopenia in both males and females. The osteopenia, which is seen more often in acromegaly than in giantism, is presumably the result of a decrease in estrogens and androgens. In rare instances of excessive ACTH elaboration, cortical sugar active hormone may cause glyconeogenesis and rob the amino acid stores necessary for osteoid formation.

The fourth group of symptoms arises from the pressure effects of an enlarging, space-taking lesion within the cranial cavity. In most cases of giantism one finds a focal area of eosinophilic cell hyperplasia, termed eosinophilic adenoma. In some cases there may be several such adenomas or the hyperplasia may involve the entire anterior lobe. In a few cases no hyperplasia has been found. Whether minute nodules of eosinophilic cells were missed or whether there was a hyperactivity without increase in cell number is not known. In a very few cases an adenocarcinoma of the anterior lobe has been reported in giantism or acromegaly. The amount of increase in intracranial pressure depends, of course, upon the size of the lesion. Because adenomas are usually small and slowly growing, there may be no pressure symptoms or symptoms may not occur until many years after the somatic signs appear. Then erosion of the sella takes place. Headache is a frequent complaint. Extrasellar expansion of the lesion may result in pressure on the optic tract at the chiasm producing bilateral temporal hemianopsia.

Pituitary giantism must be differentiated from eunuchoid giantism. In cases of failure of proper descent and maturation of the testes or in males castrated before puberty, there is excessive growth of mesenchymal tissues. This phenomenon is comparable presumably to capon development in fowls. The body type is characteristic in eunuchoid giantism and growth never reaches the proportions of pituitary giantism. In the eunuchoid type the patient is always male, the lower half of the body exhibits greater growth than the upper half, there is failure of development of the external genitalia and the epiphyseal lines remain unossified for a prolonged period. This prolongation of the growth period due to deficient androgen elaboration is presumably responsible for the excessive size attained in areas that grow predominantly by enchondral ossification.

Morbid Anatomy. There has been a great paucity of material available for study in giantism. The patients rarely die before adult life when acromegaly supervenes and too little attention has been directed to the epiphyseal growth centers. Bone is increased in both length and thickness. Excessive chondroblastic growth maintains the epiphyses in proportion. Perichondrium and periosteum apparently share in the accelerated and prolonged growth activity. Most reports agree that the sites of enchondral ossification show no cytologic evidence of growth disturbance.

Prognosis. When giantism develops early in youth and persists throughout adolescence, the prognosis for normal life span is poor. The patients may die of their intracranial lesion or polyglandular dysfunction may lead to other conditions such as diabetes or hyperthyroidism. The patient usually develops sterility and often becomes impotent. Eventually a condition of hypopituitarism may intervene, presumably due to destruction or exhaustion of the hypophysis. There is weakness and loss of weight similar to that seen in Simmonds' disease. Most patients fail to reach middle age, and treatment—surgical eradication or irradiation of the adenoma and endocrine replacement therapy—may be beneficial but rarely curative.

Acromegaly

Acromegaly is the condition that results from excessive growth of mesenchymal tissues during adult life. It is caused by an abnormal secretion of HGH from the eosinophilic cells of the anterior pituitary. This increased secretion may be the product of an eosinophilic cell hyperplasia, one or more focal areas called adenomas or a diffuse multiplication throughout the lobe. In some instances it may be due to excessive secretion of a normal number of cells. A few cases have been reported accompanying adenocarcinoma of the anterior pituitary lobe.

Acromegaly may begin at any time during adult life or it may be superimposed on giantism that has developed during adolescence. The features that characterize acromegaly are the result of abnormal growth of cartilage, bone and fibrous tissues after the normal growth period has ended. Because the normal sites of enchondral bone growth, the epiphyseal lines, have been ossified, bone is formed from remaining cartilage deposits, the articular plates,[2] and from fibrous tissue, the periosteum. The first is enchondral in type and the second is intramembranous. Enchondral bone formation from the deep layers of the articular cartilage is slow and abnormal, leading to skeletal distortions that characterize the disease. Excessive intramembranous bone formation from the periosteum causes abnormal thickening of the cortices without proportionate longitudinal growth. At points at which the cartilage completely disappears in the course of closure of ossification centers no growth occurs, and, therefore, the over-all picture is one of disharmonious skeletal enlargement.

In areas in which considerable amounts of fibrous tissue are normally concentrated, growth at these points results in a curious type of enlargement. This accounts for the tufting of the fingers and toes, which resembles hypertrophic osteoarthropathy, and the bizarre thickening of the lips. There is a generalized thickening and sagging of the skin.

Where cartilage is not directly associated with bone, the chondroblastic hyperplasia increases the cartilage mass but does not go on to enchondral bone formation. This type of growth accounts for the enlargement of the nose.

Periosteal intramembranous bone growth not only causes generalized cortical thickening but it is accentuated at certain points. In the frontal area a supraciliary ridge is produced, and from the external occipital plate there grows a torus sometimes of considerable magnitude. The mandible is increased in length by enchondral growth from the cartilage remaining at the condyle, and its length is accentuated to grotesque proportions by the apposition of bone to the outer lamina of the anterior surface of the mandibular body. The huge jaw with dental malocclusion is one of the most characteristic features of the disease. The walls of the sinuses and mastoid become greatly thickened and the air spaces are enlarged. Despite this growth of bone in the cranial and facial areas there is no enlargement of the cranial cavity. This is probably because of the complete ossification of the centers of cranial growth before the onset of the disease.

Longitudinal growth of long bones is never proportional to the increase in thickness. Because reactivation of chondroblastic activity takes place at all sites of residual cartilage, the areas with the greatest number of articular cartilages exhibit the greatest increase in length. This is found in the disproportionate growth of the hands and feet where each of the digits has four units with seven articular cartilages.

The ribs are increased in diameter by periosteal apposition of bone and in length by enchondral bone formation at the costosternal junction. This increase in length anteriorly causes the characteristic chest deformity with an abnormal anteroposterior diameter.

The vertebrae enlarge by apposition of bone to the lateral and anterior surfaces of the body. This new bone is intramembranous in origin and forms a collar of cortical bone applied to the vertebra on three sides.

Thus the well advanced acromegalic acquires a typical facies and habitus. There is enlargement of the face due to the disproportionate growth of the masticatory skeleton. The mandible is widened and greatly lengthened. The lips are thick and prominent. The nose is large. There may be a prominent supraciliary ridge and an

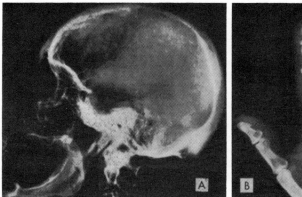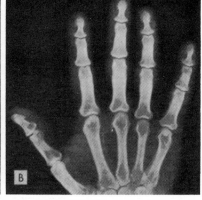

Figure 12–1 Acromegaly. The mandible is elongated, the frontal and maxillary sinuses prominent and the sella turcica enlarged and eroded (A). The phalanges are wide with thick cortices and enlargement of the tufts of the distal phalanges (B).

occipital torus. The skin is thick and coarse. The anteroposterior diameter of the chest is increased; there is often a thoracic kyphosis. The hands and feet are enlarged both in length and breadth with tufting of the distal ends of the digits.

Even more commonly than in giantism there is apt to be evidence of dysfunction in other endocrine glands, diabetes, exophthalmos and hyperthyroidism being most common. Males may exhibit testicular atrophy and loss of libido. Amenorrhea and sterility may develop in females.

As in giantism the prognosis is not very cheerful. The pituitary lesion may be removed surgically or an attempt may be made to reduce the eosinophilic cell secretion by irradiation. In either case the resulting endocrine disturbance is not easy to control.

Pituitary Dwarfism

Failure of the mesenchymal derivatives to attain a size within the limits of the normal variation results in dwarfism. The commonest variety of dwarfism is seen in achondroplasia, a congenital, hereditary condition of unknown mechanism. Failure of normal bone and cartilage growth in osteogenesis imperfecta and osteopetrosis may in the rare, severe cases result in statures of subnormal proportions. Inability to mineralize the organic matrix of bone because of insufficient calcium or phosphorus or both at the osteoid site may be encountered in advanced cases of renal osteodystrophy and hypophosphatemic–vitamin D refractory rickets. A deficiency in hormonal stimulation may result in slow or impaired growth and such cases are typified by cretinism and pituitary dwarfism.

The eosinophilic cells of the anterior lobe of the pituitary secrete the human growth hormone (HGH). When there is insufficient hormonal stimulus there is inadequate growth of fibrous tissue, cartilage and bone. Because it is obvious that the failure in hormonal stimulation must apply before growth has taken place, the active phase of pituitary dwarfism always occurs in childhood or early adolescence.

The deficiency in HGH may be due to a congenital lack of eosinophilic cells or to destruction. In instances in which the deficiency is congenital, most cases exhibit deficiencies of other pituitary hormones in a balanced ratio. The result is not only a failure of growth in stature but also a complete and synchronized lack of somatic development. The body may remain diminutive but well proportioned. There is a concomitant failure of maturation and sex development. This rare type has been called, appropriately, the Peter Pan type of dwarfism. These cases may be helped by therapy with human pituitary extracts. Extracts from animal pituitaries are not effective enough to warrant their use. The collection of cadaver pituitaries by the

American Pituitary Foundation has done much to alleviate deficiency states in this country.

Destruction of the normal eosinophilic cell complement is usually caused by tumors or tumor-like (lipid histiocytosis) processes. Here the destruction is usually selective and unbalanced and bizarre combinations of signs and symptoms including dwarfism emerge. These can be accurately diagnosed only by thorough and meticulous endocrine analysis. As such they are usually designated the problems of the endocrinologist rather than the orthopedist.

BONE CHANGES OF THYROID DYSFUNCTION

Hypothyroidism

A hormone elaborated by the thyroid gland plays an important role in the normal growth of the mesenchymal frame of the body. It may or may not be identical to the hormone that is concerned with iodine metabolism and the regulation of the metabolic processes within the cell. It is uncertain whether this hormone controls skeletal growth directly or whether its effect is achieved through its influence on the pituitary. It has been shown that when the thyroid is completely removed, the eosinophilic cells of the anterior pituitary lobe gradually become greatly reduced in number. It has been hypothesized, therefore, that the thyroid hormone stimulates the transformation of eosinophilic cells from the neutral chromophobe cell reserve. Because the eosinophilic cells produce the human growth hormone that regulates mesenchymal growth and maturation, this may be the mechanism by which the thyroid affects cartilage and bone formation. In support of this hypothesis is the report that HGH prevents dwarfism in athyroid patients but does not control myxedema and mental retardation. Still to be explained is the reported finding of increased intramembranous bone formation (judged by increased cortical thickness) in hypothyroid patients. Pituitary growth hormone is supposed to control both enchondral and intramembranous bone formation.

In order that skeletal growth may be retarded, the thyroid deficiency must be severe and occur early. Myxedema is the condition of hypothyroidism characterized by a curious increase in water-binding capacity of the ground substance of the fibrous collagen. The meaning of the term is enlarged to include the low basal metabolic rate and the mental lethargy that occur in this condition. In cases in which dwarfism and retardation of mental growth are a part of the picture, the disease is called cretinism. It is obvious that cretinism can occur only during the growth period, usually beginning in infancy or early childhood. Myxedema may occur in either childhood or adult life.

Cretinism or thyroid dwarfism is usually caused by a congenital lack of thyroid formation. It may be produced by complete or nearly complete removal of the thyroid gland in early childhood. The body appears immature for the chronologic age. Skeletal growth does not catch up with fetal cranial growth so that the head appears abnormally large and the extremities short. The disturbance in collagen function manifests itself early. There is apparently an increase in its water-binding capacity so that it swells and takes on a myxoid appearance. The excess water is not free as in ordinary edema so that it cannot be drained by incision or removed through the kidneys by reducing the sodium content. There appears to be a colloidal bond between the collagen protein and the fluid. Because the water cannot be displaced by pressure, pitting does not take place. This swelling of all collagenous structures accounts for many of the signs and symptoms of the condition.

The skin is dry and scaly. It and the subcutaneous tissue are much thicker than normal, giving the myxedematous appearance. The eyelids and tongue are greatly enlarged, causing disturbance in function. Mental growth is seriously retarded; at times the patient attains an intellect no greater than that of a 3 to 4 year old child. There may be failure of development of secondary sex characteristics with hypogonadism.

Skeletal growth is greatly inhibited. The fault appears to be in the conversion of cartilage to bone, i.e., in enchondral bone formation. Intramembranous bone formation progresses at a normal rate so that eventually the cylindrical bones become disproportionately wide for their subnormal length. The mechanism of inhibited enchondral bone growth may be through a failure of metaplasia of eosinophilic cells from chromophobe cells of the anterior lobe of the pituitary and thereby a subnormal elaboration of human growth hormone. The osseous nuclei within the cartilaginous epiphyses are late in appearing, so that in mapping the cretin skeleton it appears to be much younger than its chronologic age. Multiple centers may develop instead of a single osseous nucleus and later merge to form an irregular area of opacity. There is probably decreased chondroblastic replication in the enchondral plate because the mature cells at the foot of the epiphyseal columns are not actively dissipated, and if new, young cells were added at a normal rate in the depths of the plate the latter would soon become abnormally thick. This does not occur in cretinism.

Chondroblastic proliferation cannot be the sole disturbance, however, because there appears to be a slowing of mature chondrocyte utilization to produce the calcified cartilaginous lattice that is necessary for the initial deposition of osteoid. Indeed, a dome or end plate of osteoid that becomes normally mineralized to bone is laid over the cartilage surface, sealing it away from the metaphyseal tissues. Thus, it appears that there is no fault in collagen, chondroid or osteoid formation nor in mineralization of osteoid. Because chondroid is very similar to collagen in chemical constituency one is led to wonder if the same disturbance in water metabolism occurs here. And, if it does, if this affects the formation of the chondroid lattice for enchondral bone formation.

There is delay in eruption of the deciduous teeth and irregular and delayed shedding, which eventually leads to impaction of permanent dentition. The teeth, however, appear to be normally formed, suggesting that there is no disturbance in normal matrix formation or mineralization. Dental difficulties probably stem from the failure of normal growth of the jaw.

The cretin fails to grow in height. Because apparently fibrous and intramem-branous osseous growth is not disturbed, these persons appear heavier than normal. There is not only delay in appearance of the osseous epiphyseal centers but also delay of ossification of the enchondral plate. All enchondral bone growth is inhibited, resulting in dwarfism. The bones that enlarge predominantly by enchondral growth, particularly those of the extremities, are the ones most dramatically affected. The fontanelles, frontal sutures and synchondroses at the base of the skull remain unossified for prolonged periods. The vertebral discs appear to be thickened. This is probably relative because the bodies fail to achieve normal stature. The vertebrae also show abnormalities secondary to retarded maturation. The first lumbar vertebra is often hypoplastic and beaked anteriorly and a kyphosis is present in this area.

The serum cholesterol is usually elevated in cretinism and there is a hyperlipemia. As one would expect in decreased thyroid function, the protein-bound iodine is low. The diagnosis should not be difficult because other types of dwarfism—pituitary dwarfism and renal osteodystrophy—are not complicated by the changes of myxedema and other features of thyroid deficiency.

Roentgenographic Changes Associated with Hypothyroidism. The roentgenographic manifestations of hypothyroidism are related to the severity and duration of the condition and are present only in growing bones. The appearance of the centers of ossification is delayed (Fig. 12–2). When the centers do appear, they tend to be smaller than normal and are often irregular in outline and spotty in their ossification, particularly at the hips and shoulders (Fig. 12–3). The cortices may be thick at the expense of the medullary canal and irregularities of the epiphyseal line may mimic rickets. The tubular bones are shorter than normal. The retarded bone age may be ascertained by comparison of the radiographic appearance of the hands, wrists and knees with available standards.

The roentgen examination of the skull reveals the vault to be normal in size. The sutures are wide as a result of retarded ossification. Intersutural bones are com-

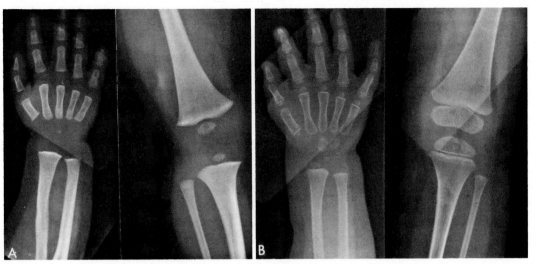

Figure 12-2   The hand, wrist and knee (*A*) of a female, age 2½ years, with hypothyroidism may be contrasted with those of a normal female (*B*) of the same age.

mon (Fig. 12–4). The sella turcica has been found to be larger in cretins than in the normal individual.[3] In later life there is poor differentiation of the diploic space and underdevelopment of the paranasal sinuses. The alterations in the lower dorsal and upper lumbar vertebrae characterized by kyphosis and antero-inferior beaking mimic those of Hurler's syndrome (Fig. 12–5).

Hyperthyroidism

Roentgen findings in hyperthyroidism are not commonly searched for. In children, chronic hyperthyroidism is associated with hyperplasia of the thymus,[4] accelerated osseous maturation and undermineralization of the skeleton.[5] In the adult the thymic alterations may be seen. Striations in the cortex, particularly of the

Figure 12-3 Hypothyroidism. The epiphyseal centers may be irregular in outline and show punctate areas of ossification.

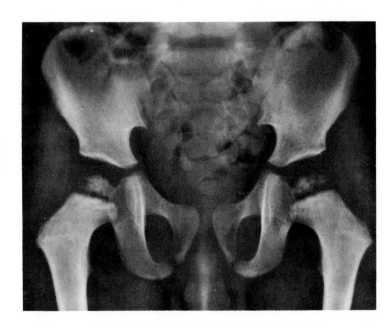

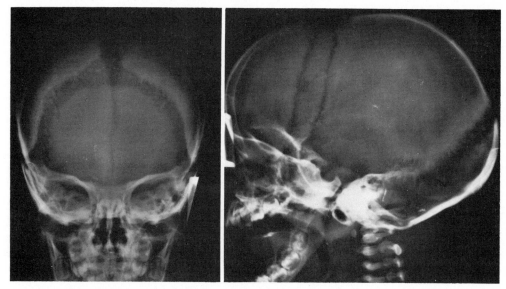

Figure 12–4   Hypothyroidism. The skull during early infancy is of normal size, but the sutures are wide and multiple intersutural bones are present.

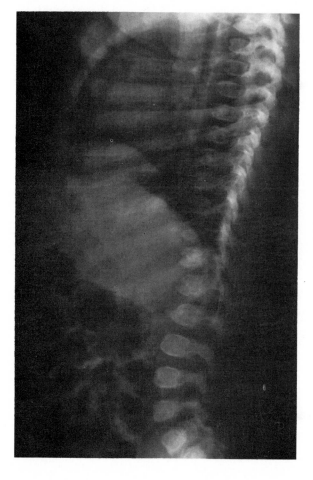

Figure 12–5 The lateral projection of the spine of a female, 9 months of age, with untreated hypothyroidism is illustrated. The bodies of the first and second lumbar vertebrae show antero-inferior beaking and a kyphosis is present in the same area.

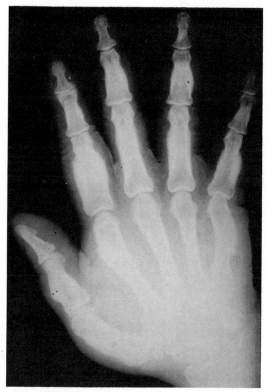

Figure 12–6   Thyroid acropachy. There is abundant new bone involving the phalanges and to a lesser extent the metacarpals. Soft tissue swelling is present.

metacarpals,[6] are often present and in a small percentage of patients a form of osteoarthropathy, thyroid acropathy, occurs (Fig. 12–6). This latter is characterized by soft tissue swelling and marked periosteal reaction, rough and irregular, of the long bones and phalanges.

BONE CHANGES OF PARATHYROID DYSFUNCTION

HYPERPARATHYROIDISM
   Parathyroid adenoma
   Parathyroid hyperplasia
      Secondary (renal osteodystrophy)
      Primary (idiopathic, spontaneous)

HYPOPARATHYROIDISM
   Secondary
   Idiopathic
      Spontaneous
      Pseudohypoparathyroidism

Hyperparathyroidism

PARATHYROID ADENOMA

Circumscribed hyperplasia of the secretory cells of one, rarely more than one, parathyroid gland is known as parathyroid adenoma. If these abnormal cells secrete an excessive amount of parathyroid hormone, and our knowledge is limited to those that do, this excess acts upon the skeleton and the kidneys to produce a condition called osteitis fibrosa cystica generalisata or von Recklinghausen's disease of bone. Because certain types of kidney disease may cause secondary parathyroid hyperplasia (renal osteodystrophy) and because the term osteitis fibrosa disseminata refers to a completely different condition (fibrous dysplasia), and osteitis fibrosa cystica localisata still another, and because von Recklinghausen's neurofibromatosis may affect bones but has no relation to von Recklinghausen's disease of bone, it seems best to sidestep this semantic nightmare and refer to the condition that is caused by adenomatous parathyroid hypersecretion as parathyroid adenoma. There is a distressing tendency to report cases of parathyroid adenoma under the title of "primary hyperparathyroidism," thus leaving the reader in a state of uncertainty whether the case is parathyroid adenoma or idiopathic primary hyperplasia.

Before discussing this disease, it would be well to review what is known and what is assumed concerning the parathyroid glands and their secretion.

These endocrine structures vary considerably in number, in size and in position. Any operative procedure calculated to accomplish their removal should take these variations into consideration. Usually the glands are four in number, the superior pair lying one behind the upper pole of each thyroid lobe, the inferior pair just below and behind the lower poles of the thyroid within the fibrous supportive tissue of the neck. One or more glands may be situated in the thyroid capsule, within the substance of the thyroid gland, at some distance from the thyroid or even in the mediastinum. These structures are usually moderately flattened anteroposteriorly, light tan in color, and have an average measurement of 5 by 3 by 3 mm. When sectioned and examined through the microscope they are found to consist of fields of polyhedral gland cells (chief cells) with very little tendency to acinus formation. Among them one often finds aggregates of larger cells, the cytoplasm of which stains poorly or not at all (clear cells). It is supposed by most that this variation in morphology is due to differences in secretory activity in the same cell type. At about puberty, large cells whose cytoplasm stains pink with eosin appear and increase in numbers with age (oxyphilic cells). These are about twice the size of chief cells. Some writers believe they represent chief cells in another phase of functional activity (Fig. 12–7); however, they do not appear until puberty and then they increase in numbers throughout the remainder of life. If they have a separate secretory function their product is still unknown. Electron microscopy studies[8] indicate that the chief cell, clear cell and oxyphilic cell are all the same cell type in various stages of activity. Mature fat cells begin to appear about the time of puberty

and increase in number until about the fifth decade. They are usually quite evenly dispersed throughout the section and eventually constitute about one half the bulk of the gland.[9]

A substance supposed to be the secretion of the chief and clear cells was extracted by Collip in 1925. It is known as parathormone. This hormone is assayed by its manufacturers for its direct effect upon bone (calcium activity) but not for its effect upon the kidney (phosphorus activity). Thus the Ellsworth-Howard test designed to measure the function of the parathyroid glands by the parathormone effect on the kidney must depend upon the uncertain quality of the prepared hormone that is used. A relationship between the physiology of the parathyroid glands and the skeleton was realized shortly after their discovery by Sandström in 1880, and Askanazy reported a parathyroid tumor and concomitant bone disease in 1904. Erdheim expressed the opinion in 1907 that the parathyroid enlargement represented a compensatory hyperplasia. MacCallum and Voegtlin[10] reported the relationship of parathyroid insufficiency and

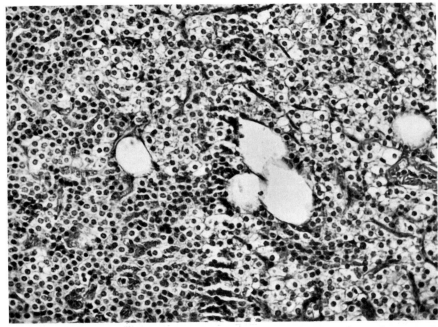

Figure 12–7 Normal parathyroid gland of a male in the third decade. Chief cells predominate. On the right there is some clear cell transition. Oxyphil cells are located in the left lower corner but are difficult to discern in a black and white photograph. (× 215.)

tetany in 1909. It was not until 1926, however, that proof of the relationship of excessive parathyroid activity and demineralizing disease of bone was reported by Mandl, who, believing with Erdheim that parathyroid hyperplasia was the result rather than the cause of osteitis fibrosa cystica, transplanted glands into such a patient. When the condition became worse he removed the transplanted glands, and dissecting the neck region found a parathyroid adenoma, which on removal caused reversal of the disease. Until 1891 the condition in the skeleton produced by parathyroid adenoma was widely confused with osteomalacia and certain other demineralizing diseases. In that year von Recklinghausen separated and described an entity that he called osteitis fibrosa cystica and that has since come to bear his name.

Today it is known that a focal hyperplasia of a parathyroid gland— adenoma— by secreting excessive amounts of parathormone will cause a demineralization of the skeleton, focal areas of bone destruction, brown tumors, a lowering of the serum phosphorus level, increase in serum calcium, which eventually produces metastatic and dystrophic soft tissue calcification, kidney stones and often nephrocalcinosis with insufficiency. The mechanism of the action of the hormone upon the bones is apparently through the osteoclasts, which increase in number and cause deossification.[11.] The hormone also antagonizes reabsorption of phosphates from the glomerular filtrate by the tubule lining cells, causing phosphaturia and hypophosphatemia.

The matter is exceedingly complex because both calcium and phosphorus are involved, because the controlling mechanism of parathyroid activity is not certainly known, because kidney dysfunction can be both the cause and the result of high serum mineral levels, and because the physiology of ossification is not completely understood.

The increase in the calcium level in parathyroid adenoma appears to be proportionate to the rate and severity of deossification. At a critical level, the serum calcium spills over the kidney threshold to cause hypercalciuria. The increase in urinary mineral content leads to the formation of kidney stones. If the stones obstruct the urinary passages, altered pressure plus infection may lead to overwhelming kidney damage and kidney insufficiency. The excess calcium in the serum is deposited first in collagenous tissues that have been damaged to become calcifiable—dystrophic calcification—and finally into normal tissues—metastatic calcification. Eventually it may produce nephrocalcinosis (Fig. 12–8) and this may lead to impaired kidney function. Impaired kidney function results in retention of phosphates and increased calcium loss. Now the low serum phosphorus level may rise to normal or higher and the high calcium level may fall. The resulting high ionization product may cause further metastatic soft tissue calcification.

The low serum phosphorus level is now generally believed to be the result of the action of parathormone upon the lining cells of the renal tubules. Here it apparently inhibits the reabsorption of phosphates from the glomerular filtrate, thus causing a phosphorus diuresis.

The tetany that has frequently been reported occurring immediately following the removal of a parathyroid adenoma is probably best explained on the basis of involutional atrophy of the uninvolved glands because of the reciprocal action of the high parathormone levels. This same type of atrophy has been described in other endocrine glands that are the seat of a functioning adenoma and in instances consequent to overenthusiastic endocrine therapy. Apparently the normal stimulus for secretion is inhibited by the excessive hormone and the unaffected glands undergo a disuse atrophy. After a period in which the low calcium levels must be controlled by therapy, the glands become reactivated and a normal balance is reestablished.

Parathyroid adenoma is approximately twice as common in women as in men. The incidence is highest in the middle years, but may occur in children and the aged. There is usually no gross evidence of the offending parathyroid mass. In all but two of the 19 cases reported by Castleman and Mallory,[12] the adenoma involved but one gland. In the other two, two glands revealed adenomatous proliferation.

It is now known that functioning para-

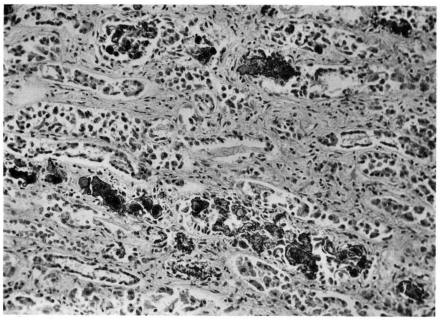

Figure 12–8 Nephrocalcinosis of parathyroid adenoma. The tubule lining cells and their supportive stroma are infiltrated with crystalline calcium salts. (× 125.)

thyroid adenoma manifests itself clinically in many ways and that the bone changes usually represent an advanced stage of the disease. Today most cases of parathyroid adenoma should be diagnosed before the onset of bone signs and symptoms. The symptoms may be divided into three groups: first, those caused by the effects of high serum calcium levels upon nerve cells and neuromuscular impulse conduction; second, those arising because of metastatic calcification of soft tissues; and, finally, those that occur as a result of bone destruction.

The disease usually begins insidiously with lethargy, somnolence, loss of muscle tone and weakness. Because the calcium ion acts as an "insulator" for nerve impulses, it may be assumed that motor impulses do not elicit a normal response. Visceral nonstriated muscles are affected as well as skeletal muscles and soon there are anorexia, abdominal distention and constipation, followed by nausea and often vomiting. In a few patients with prolonged elevated serum calcium levels, a deranged psyche may be noted. Symptoms referable to the urinary tract include polyuria,

nocturia, polydipsia, dehydration, nephrolithiasis and pyelonephritis.

Peptic ulcers have been reported in as high as 33 per cent in a series of male patients with hyperparathyroidism. Other writers[13] have found the incidence only slightly greater than in a normal population.

Symptoms of hyperparathyroidism with high serum calcium levels may supervene in chronic pancreatitis. Recently it has been shown that in alpha-cell hyperplasia with calcific pancreatitis there is a high serum glucagon level and that glucagon stimulates parathyroid activity.[14] The hypocalcemia frequently seen in acute necrotizing pancreatitis is thought to be due to saponification of fatty acids in necrotic areas.

As the skeleton is weakened by actual thinning, stress may cause bone pain. This is often misdiagnosed arthritis, though it is probably due to infractions. In perhaps a quarter of these patients, focal areas resembling bone tumors may develop (Fig. 12–9). These are usually seen at the ends of cylindrical bones. They represent the so-called "brown tumors" probably

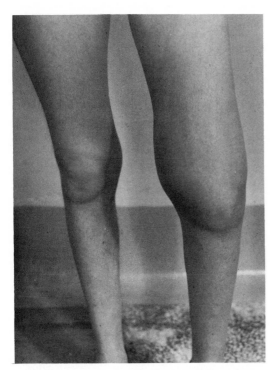

Figure 12-9 Parathyroid adenoma. A large brown tumor in the lower end of the femur. Other bones show similar masses.

caused by infractions in the thinned and weakened cortical bone, the tearing of vessel walls and the formation of intraosseous hematomas. We assume that the numerous giant cells (osteoclasts) can be attributed to the high parathormone levels. The teeth may become loosened owing to loss of the lamina dura. Eventually, fracture due to an insignificant trauma occurs and this focuses the attention of the physician on the disturbance in bone maintenance. Roentgenographic and chemical studies may then reveal the true nature of the disease.

Calcium salts may be deposited in many areas and types of tissues in the body, though metastatic calcification of soft tissues usually does not occur until late in the disease and after kidney damage has taken place. The most common related symptoms are those due to nephrolithiasis. Some authors have estimated that as many as 5 per cent of all kidney stones are due to parathyroid hyperactivity. It is true that all cases manifesting renal colic should be investigated for this possibility. Other signs of kidney involvement are polyuria and polydipsia. Eventually evidence of kidney insufficiency may appear. The levels of blood urea nitrogen, creatinine and chlorides rise and there is a decrease in carbon dioxide combining power. The patient develops a chronic uremia and a certain proportion succumb.

The clinical features of hyperparathyroidism in parathyroid adenoma may wax and wane. By some[15] this is thought to be caused by episodes of necrosis within the adenomatous nodules due to pressure upon vessels.

The diagnosis is usually made, or at least verified, by laboratory examination. The serum calcium should be above 12 mg. per 100 ml. and has been reported as high as 22. The phosphorus level is less constantly low, but averages 2.5 mg. per 100 ml. The serum protein should be estimated at the same time because in hypoproteinemia a high ionizable calcium level may be masked by the low protein-bound calcium content. Because in osteitis fibrosa cystica there is an attempt on the part of the osteoblasts to repair the destruction in the skeleton, the alkaline phosphatase levels are consistently elevated. During the active phase of bone demineralization abnormal amounts of calcium should be found in the urine. Hyperphosphaturia is almost constantly present until the kidneys are damaged.

A high serum calcium level makes it mandatory to rule out myeloma, metastatic carcinoma, sarcoidosis, vitamin D poisoning and the milk-alkali syndrome. It is of interest that in these cases adrenal steroids usually induce a prompt return of the elevated level to normal but do not affect the hypercalcemia of parathyroid adenoma.[15] Renal failure secondary to hyperparathyroidism is associated with acidosis, which is not present in other types of hypercalcemia.

Hypercalcemic crisis may occur at any time during the course of the disease. This condition apparently results from an excessively high level of serum calcium. In one of our cases it rose to 22. The patient is apt to succumb at levels of 18 or higher. The symptoms are nausea, vomiting, progressive drowsiness and coma.

Unless operative intervention with removal of the adenoma is accomplished directly, the patient is almost sure to die. Postmortem examination in one reported case has shown microscopic areas of focal necrosis in the heart, kidneys, duodenal mucosa and liver.[16]

It is generally agreed at present that the secretion of the parathyroid gland has two well defined and probably independent effects upon the body tissues. It acts locally upon bone to cause disintegration of the matrix, thus freeing the bone salts, and it acts upon the lining cells of the kidney tubules to inhibit reabsorption of phosphates from the glomerular filtrate. Many attempts have been made to clarify the mechanisms of the first activity. A paper by Ascenzi and Marinozzi[17] suggests the mechanism by which deossification occurs. Using a combination of modern modalities, microradiography, x-ray diffraction, polarizing microscopy and histochemical staining, they concluded that osteoclastic resorption is the only process responsible for the bone destruction of parathyroid adenoma. They believe that the osteoclast probably secretes some substance that dissolves the bone matrix. Moreover they believe that the osteoblast is somehow affected in this disease so that it is unable to form normal osteoid. The bone that is laid down as a reaction to the osteoclastic destruction reveals an organic matrix in which there is alteration of quality and pattern of collagen fibrils, defective lamellar structure and failure of haversian system formation. They believe the released bone mineral is deposited in tissues with a prominent mucopolysaccharide constituent and in tissues that have a tendency toward alkalinity—the kidneys, the lungs, the myocardium and the gastric mucosa.

Actually, parathyroid adenoma is an uncommon disease. It is important less from the standpoint of its incidence than from the fact that several demineralizing bone and kidney insufficiency conditions are commonly mistaken for it. One might hazard the guess that most tentative diagnoses of parathyroid adenoma are ultimately proved to be wrong. This only emphasizes the importance of understanding the condition thoroughly.

Roentgenographic Manifestations. The roentgenographic manifestations of hyperparathyroidism are characterized by deossification of the skeleton and localized areas of bone destruction, often expansile and the site of a pathologic fracture—brown tumors. Deossification may not be detected until later in the course of the disease but certain areas are apt to be abnormal when the skeleton in general appears to be normal. These are the lamina dura, the phalanges and the cranial bones. When mineral is removed from bone, finer trabeculae disappear and the larger ones diminish in size; the cortex thins and the skeleton becomes more lucent. In hyperparathyroidism the skeleton may become diffusely involved or the bones may show spotty, almost cyst-like areas of lucency.

Subperiosteal resorption of bone is an important radiographic manifestation of hyperparathyroidism. Lamina dura is the cortex about tooth sockets and normally is seen as a dense, opaque line surrounding the lucent socket. Disappearance of this cortex results from subperiosteal deossification and while it may be seen on routine radiography of the mandible, it is best appreciated by dental radiographic techniques. Irregular deossification of the mandible may also be evident.

The phalanges are characteristically the site of subperiosteal resorption as well. The radial aspect of the middle phalanges is apt to be involved first, but in time all will be affected. This alteration may be associated with endosteal resorption and cyst-like alterations. The tufts of the distal phalanges are often resorbed. Striations in the cortex of the metacarpals associated with subperiosteal resorption are probably best seen by the use of magnification techniques. The outer table or cortex of the cranial bones becomes indistinct and the diploë becomes coarse and granular with loss of trabecular detail. Other areas of bone resorption are the distal end of the clavicles and the concavities of long bones, i.e., the medial aspect of the proximal end of the tibia and of the humerus. The latter findings may be particularly evident in the child.

Localized destructive areas or brown tumors are most frequently encountered in tubular bones and are of the density of soft tissue of which they are composed. Their margins are indistinct and as they enlarge they become marginated by a thin shell of bone. Brown tumors vary in size but may be multiocular in appearance and at times extremely large suggesting overlay with aneurysmal bone cyst. Often they present as small radiolucent cyst-like areas (Fig. 12–12).

Other findings of significance are calcification of soft tissues, especially blood vessels and articular cartilage. Renal calculi may be present.

In growing bones, attempt at repair is evident at the metaphyses and results in large amounts of poorly ossified osteoid. Depending on the rate of growth of the patient, osteomalacic or rachitic alterations will be associated with the primary manifestation, bone resorption.

The radiographic manifestations of hyperparathyroidism as the skeleton is involved are the same in the primary and the secondary forms of the disease. Further illustrations will be found in Chapter 11.

Microscopy. The name osteitis fibrosa cystica was doubtless used for this disease because of the prominence of the proliferating fibroblastic tissue that characterizes the sections. This fibrous tissue replaces the bone that disappears under the influence of abnormal amounts of parathormone and fills in the intervals between the remaining bone spicules (Fig. 12–15). There is nothing unique about the appearance of this fibrous tissue but the cause for its growth is not understood. The weakening of the rigid bone structure leads to multiple infractions and these in turn cause hemorrhages. Wherever there is

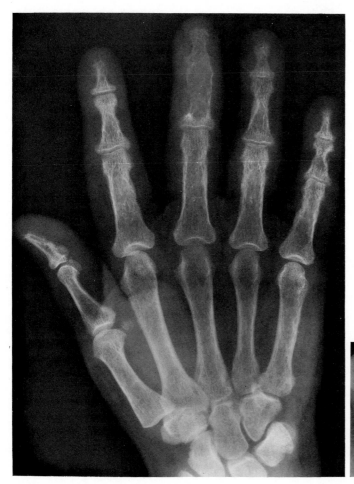

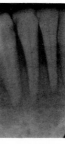
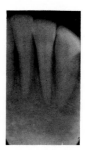

Figure 12–10 Hyperparathyroidism. Extensive subperiosteal resorption of bone is evident in the phalanges. There is resorption of the tufts of the distal phalanges and the diameter of the second, fourth and fifth middle phalanges is small. The cortices are thin and lacy in outline and a cystic lesion is present in the middle phalanx of the third digit. A dental radiograph shows the absence of lamina dura.

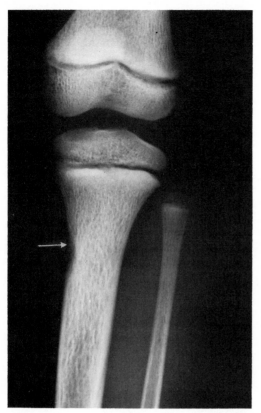

Figure 12–11   Hyperparathyroidism (renal osteo-dystrophy). Resorption of the medial aspect of the proximal tibia is evident (arrow).

tempt at repair, the deposition of new bone over old results in prominent cement lines. Because the pattern of destruction and replacement is not as confused as that in Paget's disease, the mosaic is rarely seen so prominently. Within the diaphysis new bone formation is never prominent[18] but in the metaphyses, particularly in growing bone, wide seams of recently formed osteoid are usually encountered (Fig. 12–16). Along the surfaces of these seams one often finds a row of active osteoblasts. This osteoblastic activity produces the increase in serum alkaline phosphatase. The presence of considerable amounts of osteoid may present a picture similar to that of rickets or osteomalacia. In sections of the metaphysis it may be impossible to distinguish these conditions, though in most cases osteoid production is not as florid or as irregular in parathyroid adenoma as it is in rickets and osteomalacia.

Dr. Max Westerman has made the diagnosis of parathyroid adenoma in several instances by finding even a very thin seam of new osteoid on the surface of a spicule removed by needle aspiration of marrow biopsy material.[19]

The sections through the brown tumor areas present a highly characteristic appearance. Here again, there is evidence of old hemorrhage with considerable amounts of hemosiderin. The matrix consists of a proliferation of fibroblasts. In it are thickly dispersed hundreds of giant cells (Fig. 12–17). The combination of giant cells and a fibrous matrix presents the problem of differentiation from giant cell tumor of bone. This is not always possible. Indeed, it is our opinion that a certain percentage of the lesions diagnosed "giant cell tumor" are, in fact, focal giant cell reactions of hyperparathyroidism. In brown tumor the giant cells are usually clearly separated from the stromal matrix by a space and the amount of hemorrhage also may be a helpful distinguishing feature.

The brown tumor is probably nothing more than an extravasation of blood into cancellous tissue, an intraosseous hematoma, caused by infraction in a weakened area due to osteoclastic deossification. Giant cells usually abound wherever

extravasation of blood into mesenchymal tissues fibrous proliferation is stimulated. There is ample evidence of old blood pigment in the lesions, and aggregates of giant cells, which accumulate especially about areas of hemorrhage, are one of the hallmarks of the disease. It is unknown whether this fibrous reaction is the direct response to hemorrhage or whether other factors as yet unknown play a role.

Outside the brown tumors, osteoclasts are always found in large numbers in the active phase of the disease. These are widely scattered throughout the skeletal tissues, even in areas that give no roentgenographic evidence of deossification. The presence of large numbers of osteoclasts in a section should always suggest the possibility of parathyroid adenoma or Paget's disease.

There is an actual decrease in bone mass, seen in both the spicules and the compacta. Because there is a constant at-

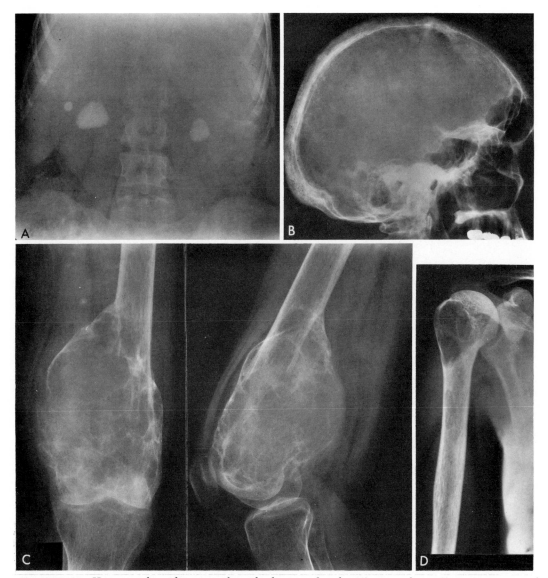

Figure 12–12 Hyperparathyroidism, parathyroid adenoma, female, 25 years of age. Large, opaque renal calculi are present (*A*). There is a diffuse granular pattern of the cranial bones and small, scattered cystlike areas of lucency (*B*). A brown tumor involves the distal femur; the shell of bone around it is quite thin; its upper margin is poorly demarcated (*C*). Several cystic areas are present in the proximal humerus; irregular endosteal thinning may be appreciated (*D*).

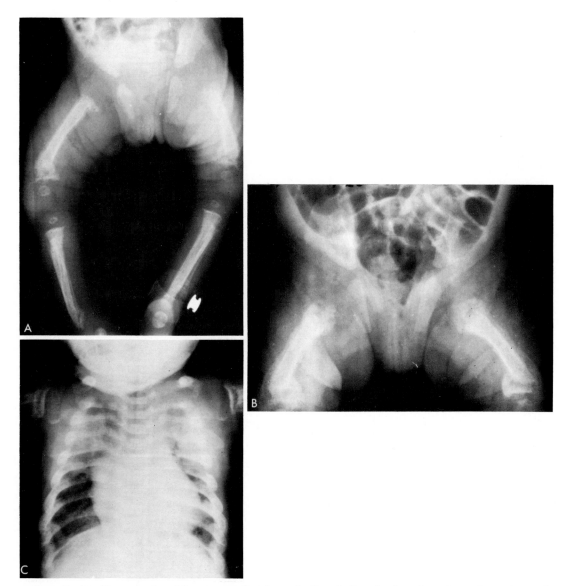

Figure 12–13   Hyperparathyroidism in an infant 1 month of age believed to have been born of a mother with hypoparathyroidism. The initial examination (*A*) revealed extensive bone resorption and metaphyseal deformity secondary to fractures. Healing (*B* and *C*) occurred as manifest by mineralization of the growing ends of the bones and by the appearance of periosteal new bone.

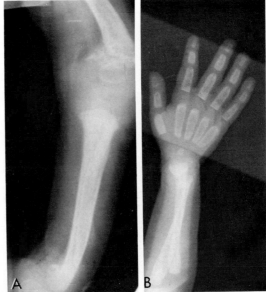

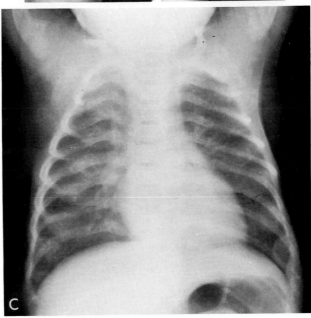

Figure 12–14 Hyperparathyroidism. This male, 8 months of age, has parathyroid adenoma. The bones are deossified; there is evidence too of bone resorption and rachitic changes. Deformities of the long bones are the result of fractures through the softened bone.

there is hemorrhage within bone; this feature is apparently greatly exaggerated under the influence of high parathormone levels. The remarkable expansion occurring in some brown tumors conceivably might be due to aneurysmal bone cysts because the latter, we believe, are frequently engrafted on bone hematomas.

The importance of differentiating a brown tumor from other giant cell lesions can hardly be overemphasized from the standpoint of the pathologist, because in the past, numerous patients have undergone surgical treatment for the former, a procedure that can hardly be construed as beneficial to the patient with parathyroid adenoma.

Microscopic diagnosis on parathyroid tissue alone also presents its problems. Usually the adenoma is composed largely of chief cells, but clear cell forms, transitional types and combinations of all of

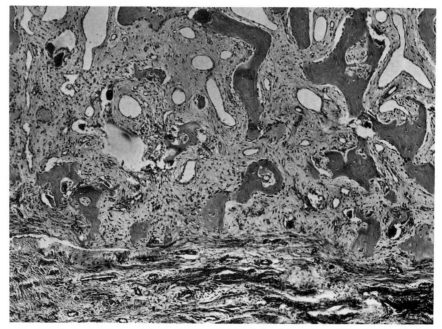

Figure 12-15   Parathyroid adenoma. Fibroblastic proliferation between the thinned bone spicules is usual. There is almost complete deossification of the cortex in this area. Note the numerous osteoclasts.

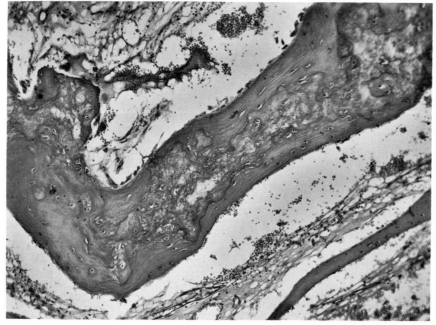

Figure 12-16   Parathyroid adenoma. The core of this spicule consists of the old, original bone. On both sides are wide seams of newly formed osteoid, which smooth out the irregularities of abnormal deossification. Along the upper seam is osteoblastic activity. ($\times$ 102.)

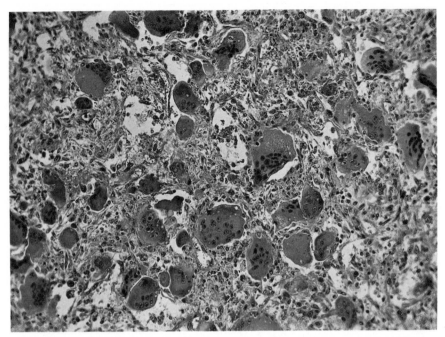

Figure 12–17   Parathyroid adenoma. Section of a brown tumor. Giant cells are prominent. They lie in a fibrous matrix that lacks the characteristics of neoplasia. (× 125.)

these are not unusual. At least one oxyphil adenoma has been reported that produced hyperparathyroidism.[20] Moreover, in adenoma, there is a tendency for the cells to form acini that often contain a colloid-like material, thus making difficult the distinction from thyroid tissue (Fig. 12–19). At times a margin of compressed but otherwise normal parathyroid tissue may be encountered at the periphery of a para-

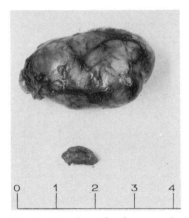

Figure 12–18   Parathyroid adenoma above compared with a normal parathyroid gland. The scale is in centimeters.

thyroid adenoma. This, when present, helps to distinguish the adenoma from secondary hyperplasia in which the entire gland is more likely to be involved. In secondary parathyroid hyperplasia, the cells are chief cells or mixed chief and clear cells. It is thus impossible on the basis of parathyroid sections alone to differentiate the two. In primary hyperplasia, if such occurs, the proliferation is of the clear cell type and, at this moment at least, this picture is considered by some to be pathognomonic of this condition.

Throughout this discussion the parathyroid lesion of osteitis fibrosa cystica has been referred to as "parathyroid adenoma." The subject should not be closed without mentioning that most oncologists no longer consider it a true neoplasm. It is a focal hyperplasia of functional cells that mature and secrete very much as normal cells. Their increase in number and their failure to respond to the stimulating and checking influences that govern normal cells result in excessive amounts of parathormone elaboration. The reason for this breaking away from normal control is not known because the para-

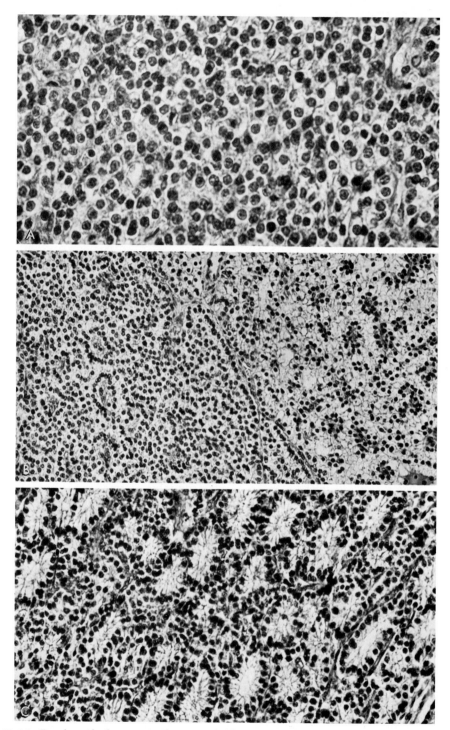

Figure 12–19   Parathyroid adenoma. *A*, The entire field is composed of chief cells. (× 350.) *B*, The left half of the illustration is composed of chief cells, the right half of clear cells. (× 170.) *C*, The adenoma cells may have an acinar arrangement. All three sections were taken from the same gland. (× 200.)

thyroids are apparently not affected by the secretions of other ductless glands. Such functioning "adenomas" also occur in the thyroid, adrenal cortex, pituitary and pancreas. In these, however, a complex hormone balance is involved, which may be responsible for their behavior.

The factors that govern the secretory activity of the normal parathyroid gland are not certainly known. Some are of the opinion that a high serum phosphorus level is the stimulating agent but most writers now concur with Albright that the initiating factor is a critical low serum calcium content. Most of the facts known about the clinical aberrations of this gland are consistent with this idea, though in those cases of hyperplasia that are known to be secondary (renal osteodystrophy) there is always an elevated serum phosphorus level. The secretory activity of most ductless glands is checked by a high level of their secretory product (feedback mechanism). For the present, at least, this may be assumed to be true of the parathyroid gland.

True tumors of the parathyroid have been reported but these are rather unusual, and because their cells are usually nonfunctional, these lesions do not pertain to this subject.

This subject has been presented primarily as a disturbance in parathyroid function rather than as an entity of skeletal disease. Because the manifestations in bone are only signs of this disturbance and frequently late ones, this approach appears to be a logical one. Furthermore, because the therapy is directed toward the gland rather than the bones, the parathyroid adenoma should be emphasized. Its surgical removal should completely cure the disease. The hypercalcemia may be helped by diluting the serum with saline and the rate of calcium absorption through the gut wall may be diminished by feeding sodium phytates.

IDIOPATHIC (PRIMARY) PARATHYROID HYPERPLASIA

In 1935, Castleman and Mallory[12] reported the results of their study of 25 parathyroid glands removed from patients with demineralizing skeletal disease. In 19 cases they were able to make the diagnosis of parathyroid adenoma, a single gland being involved in 17 and two glands in two cases. In another case, there was ample evidence that the hyperplasia in three of the four glands involved was secondary to longstanding kidney disease. In the remaining five cases the cellular morphology and pattern was strikingly similar, having an appearance that was quite different from the other 20 cases. All of these five patients had kidney stones. In none was there clinical evidence of preceding, chronic renal disease. In three of the cases all four glands were involved; in one, three of the four; and in the fifth the only two glands found were enlarged.

They have suggested that three classes of hyperparathyroidism may be recognized: parathyroid adenoma, secondary parathyroid hyperplasia due to renal disease and idiopathic parathyroid hyperplasia.

In the years since this report several cases of this third class have been reported, most of them presenting symptoms of nephrolithiasis but showing little evidence of the severe skeletal disturbance that characterizes parathyroid adenoma. The condition is now commonly called "primary hyperparathyroidism."

If the hyperplasia of these glands is truly "primary," of necessity it must be of neoplastic nature. This would suggest that the parathyroid glands are not autonomous in relation to other ductless glands but that normal secretion is part of endocrine balance, and that "primary" hyperplasia is the result of breaking away from the normal control just as the multiple nodules of the thyroid in nodular hyperplasia establish independent activity. Because the serum chemistry appears to be the same as that in parathyroid adenoma and because preceding renal disease has not been reported in these cases, there is much to be said for this hypothesis. It should also be noted that instances of idiopathic hyperplasia have been reported to have been accompanied by adenomas of the pancreas, pituitary and adrenal cortical hyperplasia.

On the other hand, the multicentric foci and the diffuse involvement of all or most of the parathyroid tissue have led some to insist that this is a secondary hyperplasia of unknown cause. To avoid a term that suggests the mechanism, it is probably best to refer to the condition as idiopathic parathyroid hyperplasia.

An insufficient number of these cases has been studied to give a clear picture of the clinical, roentgenologic and pathologic aspects. It is said that most cases are initially admitted to the urologic service because their most prominent symptoms are those of kidney stones. An analysis shows the serum phosphorus to be below 3 mg. per 100 ml. and the calcium level is above 12.5 mg. A skeletal x-ray survey may or may not reveal deossification though it may be assumed that the bone stores of calcium are being utilized in order to maintain the high serum level. To date, no means of separating this entity from parathyroid adenoma has been suggested other than microscopic examination of the parathyroid glands. These authors have been waiting for over 30 years for a bona fide case of "primary" parathyroid hyperplasia. None has appeared. Others of our acquaintance have had a similar experience. One must eventually begin to have serious doubts that such an entity exists.

Microscopy. According to the reports, sections of the parathyroids in the classic case reveal such a unique picture that even the novice should recognize the condition (Fig. 12–20). The entire architecture of the normal chief, clear, oxyphilic and fat cells is replaced by monotonous sheets of large cells with distinct limiting membranes and cytoplasm that is almost devoid of opacity. This appearance has led to the term clear cell or wasserhelle hyperplasia. The nuclei are comparable to those of normal chief cells but appear relatively small. The cells are grouped by thin, linear strands that traverse the section and the nuclei are placed in the portion of the cell in contiguity with its septum. We have seen at least two parathyroid glands in which the sections appeared quite typical but in which the clinical data were those of secondary hyperplasia. We have never encountered a case in which the microscopic appearance and the clinical features were typical of idiopathic, primary or clear cell hyperplasia. Apparently this experience has not been unique with us.[15]

In secondary hyperplasia the entire gland may be composed of chief cells but usually there is an intermixture of other

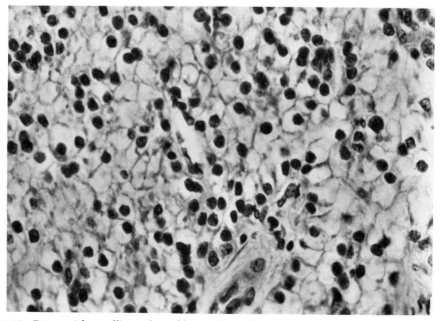

Figure 12–20 Primary (clear cell) parathyroid hyperplasia. The cells are large, the cytoplasm clear, the nuclei darkly staining and arranged along linear trabeculae. (× 412.)

normal elements and in some fields the appearance may be that of clear cell hyperplasia. Such is also the case in parathyroid adenoma and these two conditions cannot usually be differentiated on cytologic grounds alone. Unless the sections are composed entirely of clear cells, the diagnosis of idiopathic (primary) hyperplasia should not be made.

Several cases of idiopathic hyperplasia have been treated by removal of all or the major portion of the hyperplastic gland tissue. In those that have been reported, the serum calcium and phosphorus levels have reverted to normal within a few days. If the diagnosis of hyperparathyroidism is reasonably certain, if the serum phosphorus level is low and the calcium high and if primary chronic renal disease and fat absorption disturbance can be ruled out, surgical exploration of the neck should be undertaken. If an enlarged parathyroid is found, it should be removed and immediately sectioned by frozen technique. If it is composed of chief cells or a variety of transitional types the condition is probably one of parathyroid adenoma and nothing further need be done. If the sections reveal a clear cell hyperplasia the remaining glands must be dissected and removed. If the preponderance of the abnormal tissue is excised, the calcium and phosphorus levels should revert to normal and the disease should be arrested.

We have analyzed the few cases in our material that might be idiopathic hyperplasia. The data gathered are confusing. We have found glands with a mixed picture, chief cell hyperplasia in one gland and clear cell hyperplasia in another of the same patient, and instances of obvious clear cell hyperplasia associated with longstanding renal disease. To date we have not been impressed with the histologic criteria for idiopathic hyperplasia though perhaps our material is too scant for a final conclusion.

THYROCALCITONIN. In 1961 Copp et al.[21] reported the existence of a hormone that reduces serum calcium levels in dogs. They believed this hormone was the product of the parathyroid glands. In 1963 Hirsch et al.[22] reported a substance extracted from rat thyroid that had the same action and in 1964 Foster et al.[23] reported the same hormone from the goat thyroid but not from the parathyroid. The substance eventually was refined to a single chain polypeptide and was found to be synthesized in or stored by the thyroid acinar cells.[24] It was not found in the intra-acinar thyroglobulin. This substance is now known as thyrocalcitonin. The mechanism by which it reduces serum calcium is not completely understood as yet but it is at present believed that it slows the rate of mineral withdrawal from bone. It appears to have a reciprocal action with parathormone in regulating the serum calcium level.

A great deal of work is still needed to determine the actions and therapeutic value of this hormone. At this writing it is being used in the treatment of Paget's disease[25] and early reports are most cheerful.

Hypoparathyroidism

CHRONIC HYPOPARATHYROIDISM

The exact action, the sites and mechanisms of the secretory product or products of the parathyroid glands are not known. Whereas it has been assumed that a single hormone was elaborated, some evidence has been presented to indicate that there are more than one.[26, 27] Because the glands are composed of more than one morphologic type of cell, this seems a reasonable hypothesis. Most writers agree that the parathyroid hormone has at least two actions. It lowers the serum phosphorus level by inhibiting reabsorption of phosphates through the renal tubules, thus causing phosphorus excretion in the urine. It acts upon the organic matrix of bone, probably through osteoclasts, causing lysis of the matrix and freeing calcium salts, which are then washed into the blood. These two actions may be accomplished by the same hormone or they may be caused by two different hormones, and no one can be sure that the glands have only these two activities.

On the assumption that these two activities are valid, we might expect in hypoparathyroidism a failure of phosphorus excretion in the urine and an inability to move stored calcium from bone to replenish a falling serum level. The serum phosphorus level, therefore, should be high and the serum calcium low in cases in which the parathyroid glands secrete inadequate parathormone or have been removed. This is precisely what is found in cases in which the glands have been removed accidentally in thyroidectomy, called secondary hypoparathyroidism. It occurs also in cases in which no known damage to parathyroid function can be found and this is known as idiopathic hypoparathyroidism. In a few of these cases investigation has shown the apparent lack of the glands or their replacement by fat. This type has been called spontaneous hypoparathyroidism. In other cases, the glands are histologically normal or hyperplastic. This type is known as pseudohypoparathyroidism.

The commonest type of deficient parathyroid function is secondary hypoparathyroidism in which the glands have been removed at surgery. The second commonest type is spontaneous hypoparathyroidism of which about 60 cases have been reported.[28] The least common type in the literature, totaling less than 20 cases, is pseudohypoparathyroidism.[29]

Regardless of the type, the signs and symptoms of hypoparathyroidism are much the same. Since the report of MacCallum and Voegtlin[10] in 1909, it has been known that a deficiency in parathormone secretion results in tetany. The serum calcium level falls and the phosphorus content rises. The muscle spasms that occur, in the larynx (laryngospasm), the wrists and ankles (carpopedal spasm) and in severe cases of the entire skeletal musculature (convulsions), are widely accepted as being caused by a deficiency of calcium ions in the peripheral nerves, sympathetic ganglia, the myoneural end plates and perhaps the intracerebral pathways where nerve excitability is increased. In cases in which the patient gives a history of thyroidectomy with onset of tetany soon after, these symptoms are readily recognized and controlled with proper therapy. In cases in which no such history is ob-

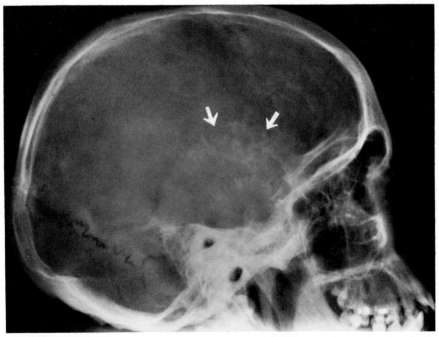

Figure 12–21 Hypoparathyroidism. Calcification of the basal ganglia is evident (arrows). The bones of the skull are normal in thickness.

tainable a diagnosis of epilepsy may be made, and because in longstanding, chronic idiopathic hypoparathyroidism there may be dwarfism, skeletal changes and metastatic calcification of the cerebral basal ganglia, the cases may be confused with orthopedic diseases.

The first case of idiopathic spontaneous hypoparathyroidism was reported by Albright and Ellsworth in 1929. Since that time a considerable number of adequately studied cases have accumulated. The diagnosis is made in patients who have muscle cramps, spasms or convulsions. The serum calcium level is low and the phosphorus high. The alkaline phosphatase level may be elevated. Many patients suffer from opacities of the lenses. The Chvostek and Trousseau tests are positive, the latter being the manifestation of ischemia in the presence of hypocalcemia. There are often multiple defects in the ectodermal structures including scant scalp and body hair, dryness and coarseness of the skin, flecking and cracking of the nails, and poor development and early loss of the teeth. Symmetrical areas of calcification occur in the cerebral basal ganglia and in a few cases symptoms of parkinsonism have developed. In several cases, mental deterioration has occurred along with headache and papilledema. These signs have led to the misdiagnosis of an expanding intracranial lesion. They are thought to be due to an accompanying cerebral edema. Candidal infection of the skin, nails and mucous membranes has been reported in a number of cases.

An increase in the density and width of the cortices of the long cylindrical bones and, less frequently, the calvarium has occurred in some patients. This is not a constant finding and, indeed, some patients have shown generalized osteopenia and in others the skeletal roentgenographic survey is normal. The Ellsworth-Howard test depends upon an increase in urine phosphates following the injection of parathormone. It has been shown that, performed as originally outlined, this test may be misleading particularly if parathormone has been used therapeutically. However, if the previously mentioned signs and symptoms are present and if renal disease and a fat absorption defect can be ruled out, a positive Ellsworth-Howard test indicates the patient has chronic idiopathic hypoparathyroidism; i.e., there is too little parathyroid tissue to supply adequate amounts of hormone, or the tissue may be normal in amount but incapable of secreting adequate hormone. Most cases respond fairly well to sustained therapy with dihydrotachysterol and vitamin D, showing a gradual rise in serum calcium and fall in phosphorus levels.

PSEUDOHYPOPARATHYROIDISM

In 1942 Albright, Burnett, Smith and Parson[30] reported three cases of idiopathic hypoparathyroidism that did not respond to parathormone injection and considered them cases of pseudohypoparathyroidism. They believed that in these cases the parathyroid glands were normal but that the target organs were nonresponsive. They believed that these cases were examples of what they called the "Seabright bantam" syndrome. The Seabright bantam cock bears the plumage of the hen because, it was thought, the target organ, in this case the feather follicles, were unresponsive to gonad secretion. It has since been shown that upon castration this particular animal does become responsive to male hormone stimulation; therefore, the term "Seabright bantam syndrome" has become meaningless. However, numerous cases of hypoparathyroidism that are refractive to parathormone stimulation have been reported. In addition, the patients are apt to be dwarfed, with heavy stature, round face, a curious deformity of the hands and calcified or ossified nodules in the soft tissues about the joints. The deformity of the hands, and less often the feet, is due to a failure of normal growth and an early closure of the epiphyseal growth centers of the first, fourth and fifth metacarpals and metatarsals. Thus, the index and third fingers are apt to be much longer than the others (Fig. 12–22).

MacGregor and Whitehead point out that dwarfism and the moon face are unsafe criteria, but that if there is hypoparathyroidism in the absence of fat absorp-

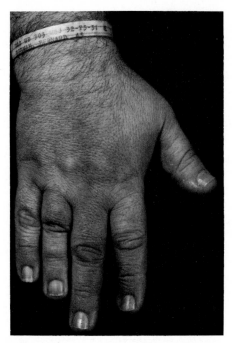

Figure 12-22 Pseudohypoparathyroidism. The first, fourth and fifth metacarpals are shorter than normal.

ism is now believed to be a clinical entity in which the glands are normal or moderately hyperplastic in appearance. The symptoms are those of chronic hypocalcemia with localized muscle contractions, laryngospasm or carpopedal cramps, or generalized convulsions. The patient is apt to be of short stature with a moon face, stubby, misshapen hands due to one or more short metacarpals (Figs. 12–23 and 12–24) and with a convergent strabismus. He may have cataracts and faulty dentition. There may be mental retardation and calcification of basal ganglia. There are often areas of subcutaneous calcification in the extremities (Fig. 12–24). Candidiasis has not been reported. Serum calcium levels are low; phosphorus levels are high. Parathormone does not cause the renal tubules to excrete more phosphorus in the urine but the blood chemistry reverts to normal and symptoms are relieved by therapy with dihydrotachysterol and vitamin D.

tion defect or renal disease and if the patient fails to achieve a normal serum calcium level within one week of treatment with at least 200 U.S.P. units daily of parathormone, the case is one of bona fide pseudohypoparathyroidism.

In summary, pseudohypoparathyroid-

Pseudo-Pseudohypoparathyroidism

As cases of pseudohypoparathyroidism were collected, it was noted that some patients with the same clinical manifestations as the group consistently had normal serum calcium and phosphorus levels. It was inevitable that these

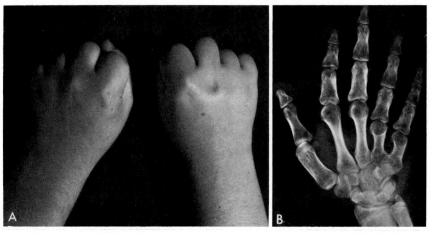

Figure 12-23 Pseudohypoparathyroidism. A concavity in place of a convexity is evident at the knuckles when the patient clenches the hands (A). This is a reflection of short metacarpals, particularly the first, fourth and fifth (B).

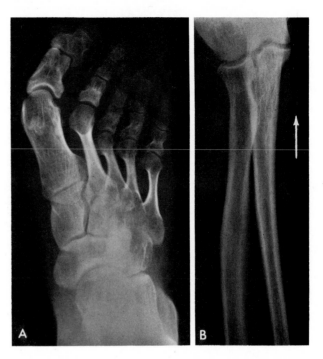

Figure 12–24 Pseudohypoparathyroidism. *A,* There is hallux valgus deformity and shortening of the metacarpals, except the first. *B,* Subcutaneous calcification is evident adjacent to the ulna (arrow).

cases should be called pseudo-pseudohypoparathyroidism. At first it was thought that this condition was a distinct entity but as more cases were collected it became evident that the two conditions were the same basic disturbance of varying degrees of intensity. When siblings of patients with pseudohypoparathyroidism are examined, some are found to have pseudo-pseudohypoparathyroidism. Some of these, when followed over a long period, were observed to develop into cases of true pseudohypoparathyroidism. The hypocalcemia apparently is most apt to develop during the period of most rapid skeletal growth.

Evidence is now accumulating suggesting that the disease is a Mendelian dominant rather than a recessive as formerly believed. Because it is about twice as common in females and there are no reported cases of male to male transmission, this evidence is against an autosomal dominant, suggesting transmission is probably sex linked.

Kolb and Steinbach[31] have reported two cases of what they have called pseudohypo-hyperparathyroidism. These cases had clinical manifestations of hypoparathyroidism with roentgenographic evidence of parathyroid adenomatous effect upon the skeleton, subperiosteal resorption, mottling of the calvarium and absence of the lamina dura. They explained this paradoxical situation by suggesting that the low serum calcium level of pseudohypoparathyroidism (in which the glands are supposedly normal) stimulated the parathyroids to hypersecretion, that the kidney tubules remained resistant to high parathormone levels (Seabright bantam syndrome) but osteoclastic stimulation did occur. They failed to explain the mechanism for the continued low serum calcium.

References

BONE CHANGES OF PITUITARY DYSFUNCTION

1. Van Wyk, J. J., Underwood, L. E., Lister, R. C. and Marshall, R. N.: Am. J. Dis. Child., *126*: 705, 1973.
2. Weinmann, J. P. and Sicher, H.: Bone and Bones. Ed. 2. St. Louis, C. V. Mosby Co., 1955.
3. Gershberg, H., Heinemann, H. and Stumpf, H.: J. Clin. Endocrinol., *17*:377, 1957.

BONE CHANGES OF THYROID DYSFUNCTION

4. Franken, E. A., Jr.: Radiology, *91*:20, 1968.
5. Bonakdarpour, A., Kirkpatrick, J. A., Renzi, A. and Kendall, N.: Radiology, *102*:149, 1972.

6. Meema, H. E. and Shatz, D. L.: Radiology, 97:9, 1970.
7. Silverman, F.: Am. J. Roentgenol., 78:451, 1957.

BONE CHANGES OF PARATHYROID DYSFUNCTION

8. Engfeldt, B., Hellstrom, J., Ivemark, B., and Rhodin, J.: Nord. Med., 61:558, 1959.
9. Roth, S.: Arch. Pathol., 72:495, 1962.
10. MacCallum, W. and Voegtlin, C.: J. Exper. Med. 11:118, 1909.
11. Chang, H.: Anat. Rec., 106:266, 1950.
12. Castleman, B. and Mallory, T.: Am. J. Pathol., 11:1, 1935.
13. Ostrow, J., Blanshard, G. and Gray, S.: Am. J. Med., 29:769, 1960.
14. Paloyan, E., Lawrence, A., Straus, F., Paloyan, D., Harper, P. and Cummings, D.: J.A.M.A., 200:97, 1967.
15. Howard, J.: Trans. Stud. Coll. Physicians Phila., 30:53, 1962.
16. Thomas, W., Wiswell, J., Conner, T. and Howard, J.: Am. J. Med., 24:229, 1958.
17. Ascenzi, A. and Marinozzi, V.: Arch. Pathol., 72:297, 1961.
18. Jaffe, H.: Arch. Pathol., 16:63, 1933.
19. Westerman, M.: Personal communication.
20. Selzman, H. and Fechner, R.: J.A.M.A., 199:359, 1967.
21. Copp, D., Davidson, A. and Cheney, B.: Proc. Can. Fed. Biol. Soc., 4:17, 1961.
22. Hirsch, P., Gauthier, G. and Munson, P.: Endocrinology, 73:244, 1963.
23. Foster, G., Baghdiantz, A., Kumar, M., Slack, E., Soliman, H. and MacIntyre, I.: Nature, 202:1303, 1964.
24. Hargis, G. and Arnaud, C.: Science, 152:73, 1966.
25. Haddad, J., Berge, S. and Avioli, L.: N. Engl. J. Med., 283:549, 1970.
26. L'Heureux, M., Tepperman, H. and Wilhelmi, A.: J. Biol. Chem., 168:167, 1947.
27. Stewart, G. and Bowen, H.: Endocrinology, 51:80, 1952.
28. Robinson, P. K., Carmichael, E. A. and Cumings, J. N.: Q. J. Med., 23:383, 1954.
29. MacGregor, M. E. and Whitehead, T. P.: Arch. Dis. Child., 29:398, 1954.
30. Albright, F., Burnett, C. H., Smith, P. H. and Parson, W.: Endocrinology, 30:922, 1942.
31. Kolb, F. and Steinbach, H.: First International Congress on Endocrinology, Copenhagen, 1960, p. 475.
32. Haymovitz, A.: Pediatrics, 45:133, 1970.

Chapter 13

MISCELLANEOUS DISEASES OF THE SKELETON

PAGET'S DISEASE

Paget's disease, named osteitis deformans by Sir James Paget[1] in 1877, is a disease of bones in which repeated episodes of osteolysis closely followed by excessive attempts at repair result in a weakened, deformed skeleton of increased bone mass. In its advanced and symptomatic stage it is rarely seen before the age of 40 though at least one case has been reported as early as 18 years. We have seen one case strongly suspected of being Paget's disease in a woman aged 28 and a case of advanced monostotic Paget's disease in a man of 29. The disease that is sometimes called juvenile Paget's disease, hyperostosis corticalis generalisata or Van Buchem's[2] disease may or may not be a pathologic entity. Descriptions of the few cases reported may include hyperphosphatasemia (which may be juvenile Paget's disease), Caffey's infantile cortical hyperostosis or that group which we have classified as diaphyseal sclerosis (Camurati, Engelmann, Ribbing).

Because the roentgenogram is reasonably characteristic in the majority of cases, considerable numbers of asymptomatic, monostotic or solitary focus Paget's disease may be discovered on skeletal studies carried out for other reasons. Many of these lesions never manifest themselves symptomatically; others progress into clinically obvious Paget's disease. In its florid state most of the bones of the skeleton may be involved, with crippling or complete invalidism of the patient. Numerous and severe complications, most often involving the cardiovascular system, may lead to a fatal termination.

Paget's disease is usually slowly progressive over a period of months and years. It starts as a small focus and gradually spreads to involve large areas of both cylindrical and flat bones. At first there is a demineralizing process, which causes skeletal radiolucency and a coarsening of the trabeculations. But as it progresses, areas of density appear, which may eventually overshadow in opacity the surrounding normal bone. Even though the bone mass ultimately may be increased, the repair is not normal in lamellar stress lines, so that pathologic fracture is a common occurrence. These fractures often heal poorly with excessive, poorly distributed callus. In long bones the ends are usually involved first but the process may spread to involve the entire bone.

Several reports have emphasized the greatest incidence in the bones subjected to the greatest stress. Thus in Schmorl's reported studies[3] on autopsied cases, the sacrum was the most common site of the disease and the related structures, upper femur, lower spine and pelvic bones, were almost as often affected. The skull, too, is frequently involved for a reason that is harder to explain. The over-all incidence of the disease probably approaches 3 per cent, but if all instances of radiologically presumed cases were included the figure would be somewhat higher.

In cases in which the focus is solitary and in only one bone, the condition may remain silent indefinitely. As the lesion progresses it may cause pain and a sensation of stiffness. Eventually this may be severe enough to bring the patient to his physician or, if the bone is sufficiently weakened, minor trauma may cause fracture. If a skeletal survey is done at this time other smaller and probably younger lesions are often found.

In cases in which large areas of numerous bones are affected the deformity and symptoms are quite characteristic. There is a slowly progressive deossification, which appears to begin along the inner cortical surfaces. As it continues, the substance of the bone disappears. It becomes weakened and distorted under pressure. Collapse of the anterior portions of the vertebral bodies causes a typical kyphosis of the thoracic spine, which thrusts the head forward and downward. The femurs bend outward to produce bowing and this deformity is accentuated by an outward and forward bowing of the tibias. These various curvatures cause shortening of the stature. Softening of the femoral necks results in coxa vara. The bones of the feet are usually spared but in cases in which they are involved there is collapse of the arches and plantar elongation. The feet appear to enlarge, requiring bigger shoes.

Flat bones are involved as often as cylindrical bones. Softening of the sacrum and the iliac bones, together with the coxa vara, causes a waddling gait. The ribs and sternum also may be involved in severe cases. There is a lateral flattening of the thorax with increase in the anteroposterior diameter. This deformity with the kyphosis interferes with the lifting of the ribs in normal respiration. This feature may play at least a part in the respiratory difficulty that these patients experience. Poor ventilation may add to the increased work load of the heart. The forward curvature of the spine causes the belly to protrude.

The weakening of the normal bone structure is doubtless due in large measure to the progressive deossification process. But, some time in the course of the disease, probably when the deossification is fairly well advanced, an attempt at repair sets in. There are no data available that prove unquestionably that the bone destructive process is transitory and cyclic with interspersed periods of repair. One gets the impression on examination of the bones in advanced Paget's disease with a hand lens that irregular areas are destroyed throughout the entire thickness of the cortex, and that around the fragments that remain a poorly constructed and disoriented substitute is laid down. The resulting cortex is thicker than the original but it is coarser, less dense and obviously not as strong, because fractures continue to occur during this stage.

Sometime during this period the cambium of the periosteum begins to form coarse primitive bone, which is arranged in spicules more or less vertical to the outer cortical surface. When long bones bend from weakening, infractions occur along the convex surface and the periosteum lays down new bone on the opposite side to strengthen the member. The periosteal osteogenesis, whether it occurs in cylindrical or flat bones, is additive in effect, causing widening of the bone as a whole without decreasing the medullary volume. If the medullary area is decreased, and it sometimes is (Fig. 13–1), the narrowing is due to the replacement of the original cortex with one that is thicker and more porous than normal. Thus, the cranial capacity and the marrow space are rarely greatly intruded upon by the increasing bone mass, though the latter may be invaded by fibrous proliferation at the expense of hematopoietic tissue.

A concept of the Paget's process may be gained by examining the sawed edges of the calvarium by means of a hand lens. In the normal bones of the calvarium one sees an inner and outer table of dense cortical bone, which together approximately equal in thickness the middle layer of more porous bone. The calvarium in Paget's disease shows an outer layer of cortical bone that is more porous and often thicker than the combined three layers of the normal (Fig. 13–2). The dural surface is quite smooth and normal in appearance.

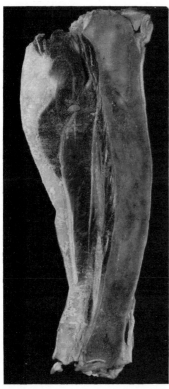

Figure 13-1   Paget's disease. Sagittal section of the tibia reveals anterior bowing and replacement of the cancellous tissue with compact bone.

What was previously the outer table is extremely rough and irregular. Applied to this "surface" is a much thicker layer of very porous bone, which apparently has been laid down by the periosteum. It is so coarse that it has much the appearance of pumice. The outer surface is irregularly scarred and pitted. Occasionally, a thin layer of more dense bone may be found immediately beneath the periosteum.

Attempting to reconstruct the process that results in the final appearance, there is first destruction of the normal cortex in widely disseminated but finely patchy areas, then there is replacement about the irregular fragments that remain by osteoblastic proliferation within the remaining cortex, and sometime during the process an addition of a very poor and primitive type of bone on the outer surface by periosteal activity.

Anemia has been reported in Paget's disease and it may be severe. However, it is certainly not common, and if one examines the normal hematopoietic areas one wonders why a greater incidence is not found, because there is usually a considerable amount of fibrosis in these regions. The reason may lie in the fact that

Figure 13-2   Paget's disease. *A*, A Paget's calvarium on the right, and on the left a normal specimen. The cranial cavities are about equal in volume but the bone thickness is enormously increased in the Paget's skull. *B*, Higher magnification of a Paget's calvarium. Note that the inner table is fairly normal. Apposed to this is a thick layer of coarse bone. The outer surface is rough and pitted.

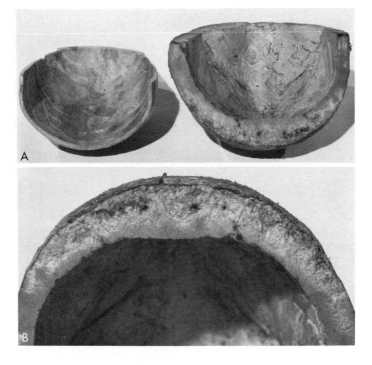

during the decades in which Paget's disease is found, only a relatively small proportion of the medullary area is utilized for hematopoiesis. The remainder is filled with fat. But this fat may shift back to hematopoietic tissue if the demand arises, so that the compensatory reserve is usually adequate to make up for the fibrosis.

In areas in which periosteal bone formation impinges upon the foramina of emerging cranial and spinal nerves, pressure may interfere with nerve function. Impaired vision and deafness have been ascribed to this cause. The squeezing of other cranial and spinal nerves may result in both motor and sensory disturbances.

The weight of the brain and the enlarged skull may cause the softened bones at the base to flatten. The plane of the foramen magnum becomes inclined dorsally and the odontoid process is thrust up into the posterior fossa. Thus, the brain stem must bend over the odontoid and ventral margin of the foramen magnum,[4] the olivary processes sink into the cervical canal and there is tension on nerve roots.

The mechanism of the pigmented corneal degeneration and the choroidal atrophy and pigmentation that has been reported in Paget's disease is not clear unless they are etiologically associated with pressure atrophy of the optic nerves. Because a large number of patients with Paget's disease eventually develop hypertension, this may be responsible in part.

A few cases of mental deterioration have been reported with the far advanced disease. Because Paget's and arteriosclerotic cerebral disease occur in the same age group, the association may be coincidental though there are a few reports of alteration in the capacity of the brain box.

Cardiovascular disease is listed as the most common cause of death in advanced, generalized Paget's disease. There are several factors, each of which probably plays a role. The cervico-thoracic kyphosis and the impaired motion of the ribs result in a limited ventilatory capacity. This in turn may increase cardiac output and cause right-sided hypertrophy and eventual right heart failure.[5] The incidence of hypertension, arteriosclerosis and

valvular disease is reported to be higher in generalized Paget's disease than in the average population of comparable age. These complications may be related to the observation that the cardiac output in Paget's disease is considerably elevated.[6] It has been known from almost the first observations of the disease that the affected part is warmer than the normal. Surgeons have noted that during the active stage the tissues bleed abnormally, and microscopists have frequently mentioned the unusual vascularity of the fibrous proliferation that forms a matrix for the abnormal bone. It has been supposed either that there are multiple small arteriovenous aneurysms or that the large vascular sinuses in some way create their effect. If such is the fact, the increased cardiac output might be so explained, and it is conceivable that the arteriosclerosis, the valvular and coronary calcification and eventually even the hypertension might be related, but the actual mechanisms of these complications are still unexplained.

One would expect the serum calcium level to be elevated in generalized Paget's disease in the destructive phase. Yet this is not usually true, and perhaps any elevation that occurs may be the result of disuse atrophy in patients who are incapacitated by the disease. A hypothetical explanation for the lack of high serum calcium levels may be offered. In the natural course of the disease new osteoid is laid down and mineralized in the wake of the destructive process. This new bone may utilize most of the mineral that is liberated except in cases in which a lack of the stress stimulus causes slowing down or failure of osteoblastic activity. Excessive quantities of alkaline phosphatase are found in the serum. In active, severe, generalized Paget's disease the levels may be very high. When one sees the flamboyant display of osteoblastic activity that is occasionally encountered in Paget's disease one is not surprised. The serum phosphorus level remains normal.

The pathogenesis of Paget's disease is an enigma. Though there is abnormal vascularization of bone tissue and increased cardiac output it is impossible to interpret the structural alterations in the bone lesions with these functional changes. Horses fed a bran diet develop "big head" disease, which may be analogous to Paget's disease of the skull in man. Bran contains a high phosphorus component. It has been noted that in geographic areas in which dietary phosphorus is low, there is a decreased incidence of Paget's disease. Patients given aluminum to remove the phosphorus from their diets are often relieved of the pain of Paget's disease and the same has been reported by giving parathormone, which causes phosphorus diuresis. No one seems to understand the mechanism by which aspirin relieves this disease.[7]

Recently suggested modes of treatment (see therapy and prognosis) may lead to a better understanding of the pathogenesis of this important and interesting disease. Calcitonin (inhibition of mobilization of bone calcium), mithramycin (reduction of osteoclasts probably due to RNA inhibition), and diphosphonate compounds (slowing of bone resorption by stabilization of hydroxyapatite crystals) all have been reported to have caused improvement in Paget's disease.

Roentgenographic Manifestations. The roentgenographic manifestations of Paget's disease reflect osteolysis and excessive repair, alone or in combination. Thus areas of radiolucency and opacity result. The trabecular pattern is prominent and coarse. The smaller trabeculae are not evident, but the larger ones in the line of weight bearing increase in size. Particularly do the bones of the pelvis show this alteration in trabecular pattern. The long bones may be thick and opaque but pseudofractures and bowing belie the apparent strength of the bones.

The destructive or osteolytic phase is often most characteristic on radiographs of the skull. The radiolucent defect slowly enlarges and is in sharp contrast with the normal surrounding bone. The cortex, particularly the external cortex, becomes indistinct and hazy in outline. The term osteoporosis circumscripta has been applied to this demineralization. As the disease progresses, areas of opacity appear within the radiolucent region and then excessive new bone becomes evident with thickening of the cranial bones. The radiograph shows coarsely granular cranial bones reflecting areas of osteolysis and excessive new bone formation. Involvement of the mandible and maxilla is most marked in relation to the tooth sockets. There is lysis, which results in absence of lamina dura. Later malocclusion results from overgrowth of bone. As involvement of the base of the skull progresses, basilar invagination occurs.

The involved tubular bones increase in size. Most of the new bone is produced by the periosteum so that the cortex is thickened externally with no encroachment on the medullary canal. At times, however, the canal may be narrowed by the excessive repair. Lytic areas are seen in the long bones as well as in the skull, and such an area often terminates in a point or V. Osteolysis and new bone formation are seen in combination resulting in radiolucency and opacity of a most bizarre nature. Immobilization of affected bones appears to accentuate the osteolytic phase. In response to weight bearing, bowing of the femurs (laterally) and tibias (anteriorly) occurs. Fractures may occur in relation to the abnormal curvature, particularly avulsion fractures at the site of attachment of muscles. Acetabular protrusion may accompany the pelvic alterations.

Coarse trabeculations in affected vertebral bodies are common. These tend to be horizontal and accentuate the margins of the body. Compression fractures are not uncommon and result in narrowing of the vertebral body anteriorly. Almost homogeneous opacity of a vertebral body may be evident without fracture or coarse trabeculae (Fig. 13-7).

Microscopy. The mosaic pattern described by Schmorl remains the hallmark of the full-blown, mature Paget's picture. When an osteone is formed, that is, a haversian canal with its complement of ensheathing lamellae, the external surface of the outermost layer acquires a peculiar staining quality. It takes the hematoxylin stain more avidly than do related tissue areas so that when the osteone is cut in cross section it is seen to be delineated by a heavy blue line called the cement line. Thus the province of one osteone can be distinguished from that of its neighbor.

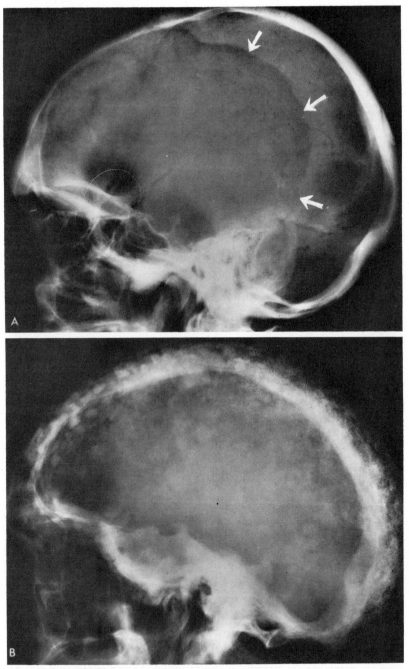

Figure 13–3 Paget's disease. *A*, Osteoporosis circumscripta is apparent in the frontoparietal region. The margin of this area of radiolucency is well defined posteriorly (arrows) by normal bone. Areas of thickening of the cranial bones are associated with irregular destruction in *B*. The inner aspect of these bones is well defined. Deformity at the base of the skull, basilar invagination, is the result of softening of the bone in this region.

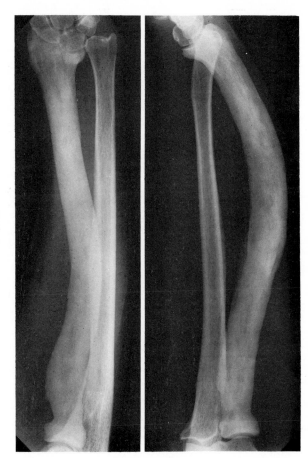

Figure 13-4 Paget's disease. Deformity of the entire radius is apparent. The bone is thickened and opaque, the medullary canal obliterated, and there is bowing.

In Paget's disease portions of osteones are irregularly gnawed away. To this rough and erratic surface new osteoid is applied by the repairing osteoblasts. But the new bone is never annealed to the old as are the lamellae of an osteone and consequently, when cross sectioned, a crazy quilt pattern of areas of all sizes and shapes is outlined by the cement lines that are formed (Fig. 13-8). This does indeed look like a mosaic done by an artist who had forgotten his objective. These irregular areas have been called breccie.

In cases in which these irregular breccie dominate the microscopic section there can be little doubt of the diagnosis. However, Paget's disease does not show the mosaic pattern in all phases and any condition in which there is irregular bone destruction and immediate osteoid apposition may mimic this picture to some degree. Then the histologic diagnosis becomes more difficult. A mosaic pattern simulating that of Paget's disease is most apt to be encountered in parathyroid adenoma, hyperphosphatasia and chronic osteomyelitis.

The new osteoid is laid down by osteoblastic activity and it is not unusual to see the entire length of an irregular fragment of bone solidly surfaced by these cells. In other areas a fibroblastic proliferation dominates the picture, and in the midst of such a field one may find a coarse-fibered osteoid and obvious fibro-osseous metaplasia. In the phase of deossification large numbers of osteoclasts are often encountered (Fig. 13-9). Sometimes one finds them nestled against a spicule, the opposite surface of which is being built up by osteoblasts. Large numbers of osteoclasts in a section of adult bone should always make the microscopist think of

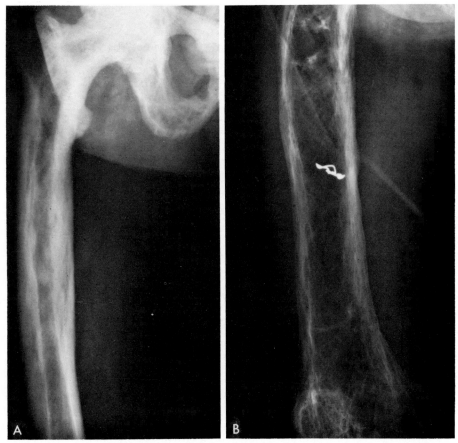

Figure 13-5 Paget's disease of the femur. In both *A* and *B*, the bone is increased in diameter. In *A*, excessive repair is evident; in *B*, there is extensive osteolysis.

Paget's disease and parathyroid adenoma. Eventually, both osteoblasts and osteoclasts disappear leaving a spongework of massive spicules demonstrating the mosaic pattern. The fibrous matrix eventually may be converted to fat.

The feltwork of fibrous tissue that forms the background for the irregular bone spicules may show numerous, large, thin-walled vascular sinuses along with evidence of blood extravasation and an incidental sprinkling of exudative inflammatory cells. If numerous arteriovenous sinuses exist, however, ordinary technique does not show them. Moreover, it is difficult to account for the changes visualized by microscopy on the basis of an increased blood supply. Bone appears to demineralize when exposed to abnormal quantities of arterial blood, but the bizarre changes

seen in Paget's disease do not then materialize. It is probably best to admit that the cause and mechanism of Paget's disease are still unknown. If increased vascularity plays a role, we must await a more convincing demonstration of this phenomenon.

Prognosis and Therapy. It is exceedingly difficult to predict the behavior of Paget's disease. As mentioned earlier in this chapter, it is almost certain that some monostotic lesions remain asymptomatic throughout life. Others progress and a small percentage become generalized, cardiovascular and respiratory complications develop and the patient almost certainly dies in a state of heart failure, but the course of the disease may run for many years.

One of the most interesting complications of the condition is the superimposition of malignant mesenchymal tumor, usually in an area previously affected by Paget's disease. The sarcoma may be osteosarcoma or fibrosarcoma, and in our material a chondrosarcoma developed (Fig. 13–10). Though these cancers run approximately the same course that they do in younger patients, they are much more apt to occur in the bones of the pelvis and other flat bone sites that would be unusual in the younger age group.

There has been considerable controversy concerning the incidence of this tragic complication. Jaffe[8] states that the figure may be set at about 4 per cent of all symptomatic Paget's disease. In our material a very high percentage of osteosarcomas and fibrosarcomas in patients over 45 has occurred in the pelvic and other flat bones, and a considerable number of these have shown microscopic or radiographic evidence (Fig. 13–11 A), or both, of concomitant areas of Paget's disease. Some authors have made the statement that approximately one third of the osseous and fibrous cancers of the older age group are superimposed on Paget's disease. When multiple samples were taken from various levels an incidence of

(*Text continued on page 419.*)

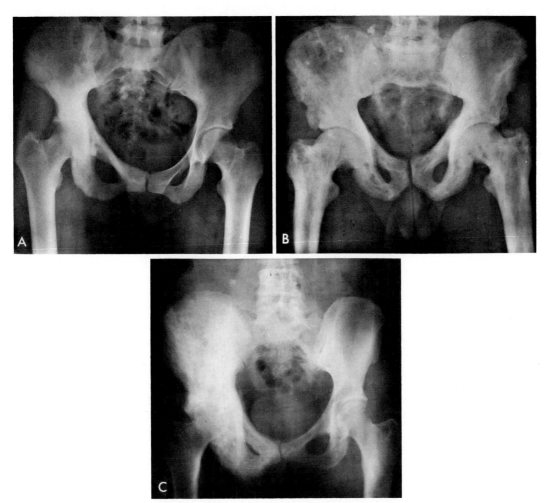

Figure 13–6 Paget's disease. The lesions involving the bones of the pelvis in the region of the right acetabulum are almost uniformly opaque. A. In B, the involvement of the pelvis is diffuse and the lesions are both osteolytic and sclerotic. C, There is marked thickening of the right side of the pelvis with extensive periosteal new bone involving the ischium and to a lesser extent the pelvic bone. The hip joint is narrow.

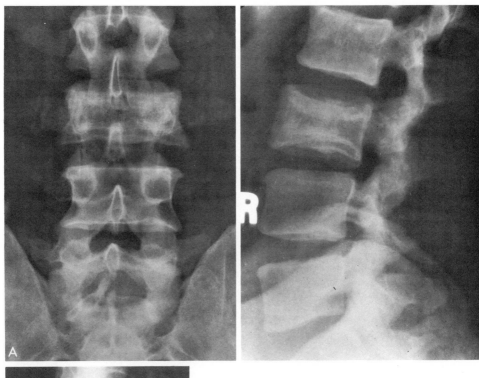

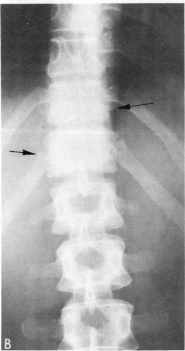

Figure 13–7   Paget's disease. *A*, The third lumbar vertebra is compressed. Horizontal opaque lines parallel the superior and inferior surfaces of the body. *B*, The body of T_{11} and T_{12} is dense and homogeneous in a male 52 years of age.

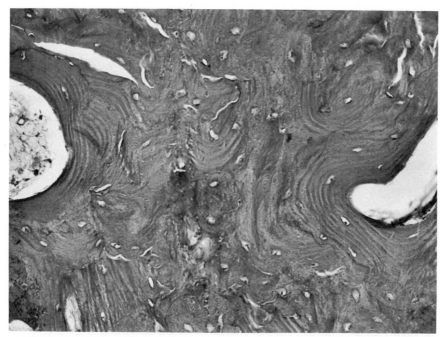

Figure 13–8   Paget's disease. Irregular osteones are fitted together without respect to the haversian pattern. This produces the mosaic appearance. (× 170.)

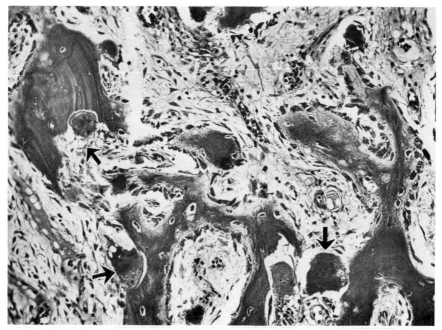

Figure 13–9   Paget's disease. There is brisk osteoblastic activity in a fibrous matrix. Abnormal numbers of osteoclasts (arrows) are usual (× 150.)

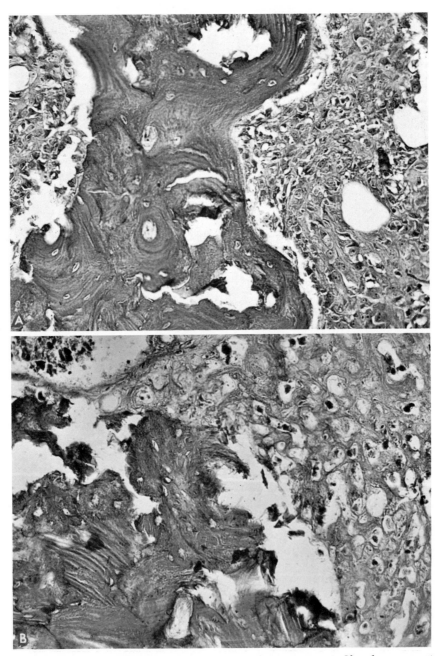

Figure 13-10 Paget's disease with secondary sarcoma. *A*, Osteosarcoma. *B*, Chondrosarcoma. (× 186.)

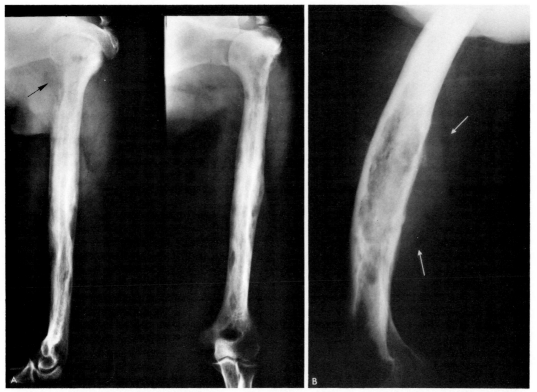

Figure 13–11   Osteosarcoma superimposed on Paget's disease. While the tumor in the humerus involves much of the diaphysis as manifest by localized areas of destruction, the cortex at the proximal end is interrupted where the sarcoma has broken through (A). In the femur of another patient (B), there is a large lytic area of destruction on the mid-diaphysis with interrupted periosteal new bone and a soft tissue mass posteriorly (arrows).

associated Paget's disease, either generalized or monostotic, of nearly 60 per cent of all primary bone sarcoma (except those arising from marrow cells) in patients over 40 years of age was found in our material.

Until quite recently the treatment of Paget's disease was purely symptomatic and supportive. With the discovery of calcitonin and the availability of the porcine type, it was inevitable that this hormone, which apparently controls the release of mineral from the bone stores, be tried. There are now several reports which record its effect. Haddad et al.[9] reported the treatment of three cases with a decrease in cardiac output in one, decrease in serum alkaline phosphatase levels in all three and decreased hydroxyprolinuria in two. The evidence of decreased bone turnover persisted for four to five weeks after withdrawal. Some authors have noted a fall in serum calcium

and consequent stimulation of parathyroids with resultant hyperparathyroidism. After several months there was cessation of improvement or even regression with increased amounts of immunoreactive parathormone as well as antibodies to calcitonin. Ryan et al.[10] treated 55 patients with Paget's disease with mithramycin, an RNA inhibiting factor extracted from *Streptomyces plicatus*. They found it highly effective in controlling symptoms and reducing the rate of bone turnover. Biopsy suggested that its action was accomplished through reduction in the number of osteoclasts. Diphosphonate compounds, which stabilize bone by binding the hydroxyapatite crystals, have also been used with good results. Limitation of dietary phosphates has been tried with encouraging evidence of improvement in symptoms and reduction in bone turnover rate.

HYPEROSTOSIS CORTICALIS

In 1955 Van Buchem and Hadders described what they believed to be a new pathologic entity and called it "hyperostosis corticalis generalisata." In 1962 Van Buchem and his colleagues reported[2] seven cases. The condition is now generally referred to as "Van Buchem's disease." They describe a skeleton in which there is cortical thickening of the ribs and clavicles. The diaphyseal cortices are wide and there is a dramatic sclerosis of the skull and lower jaw with pressure effect on emerging nerves leading to facial paralysis, deafness and blindness. The serum calcium and phosphorus levels are normal but there is a high serum alkaline phosphatase. Clinical aspects are somewhat different from those of hyperphosphatasia, Caffey's infantile cortical hyperostosis and that group of lesions (Camurati, Engelmann, Ribbing) which we choose to call diaphyseal sclerosis. In exactly which category Van Buchem's disease belongs is still a question in the minds of most but it appears to these authors to be a subgroup of one or more of the above conditions rather than a clinical-pathologic entity. Its high serum alkaline phosphatase level suggests a relation to hyperphosphatasia and thus there may be some rationale for considering it to be juvenile Paget's disease.

EPIPHYSIOLYSIS

Epiphysiolysis, slipped epiphysis, epiphysiolisthesis or epiphyseal coxa vara is a condition in which there is a separation of the epiphysis from the metaphyseal diaphysis along the lattice line. This separation may or may not progress to a displacement of the epiphysis in relation to the diaphysis in a manner that suggests a sideways slipping. Though several epiphyses have been reported to demonstrate this curious behavior, the condition is relatively so much more frequent in the superior femoral epiphysis that in cases in which the site is not specifically designated one assumes the lesion to be in this region. In areas other than the capital femoral epiphysis the so-called "slipped epiphysis" is probably always due to acute trauma.

Epiphysiolysis was described nearly a century ago but the pathology of the early cases was unknown and the condition was confused with a number of other diseases of the hip of a variety of etiologies. Monk's report, in 1886, was probably the first nontraumatic case the identity of which is unmistakable. Sprengel correctly demonstrated the pathology in 1898, and in the same year Poland reported a thorough search of the literature. The best modern reviews of the subject are those of Key[11] and the later report of Howorth.[12]

Epiphysiolysis is not a rare condition. The busy orthopedist is apt to encounter two or three cases each year. The lesion is more common in males, the proportion varying in different series from four to one to a "slight preponderance." When it occurs in females the onset is usually one or two years earlier than in males. The disease begins and runs its active course during adolescence, between the ages of 10 and 18. This age incidence is so common that the process is sometimes called epiphyseal coxa vara of adolescence. Slipped epiphysis probably never begins after the closure of the superior femoral epiphysis.

The preponderance of these adolescent patients in whom no frank and significant history of trauma can be obtained is heavier than average; indeed, some are frank cases of Fröhlich's adiposogenital dystrophy. The association is so common that should one encounter persistent hip pain of recent onset and inability to properly abduct and externally rotate the thigh in a child after puberty who is fat and manifests an underdevelopment of the genitals, the diagnosis of epiphysiolysis must be assumed until disproved.

The disease runs its active and healing course in one to three years. It is bilateral in about 15 per cent of the cases. It begins with a widening of the epiphyseal line of the capital femoral epiphysis. It is apparent that the epiphysis is now loose upon the proximal end of the neck. If there be no unusual strain or trauma it may remain here, held in place apparently by the ensheathing periosteum and perichondrium. Eventually, the epiphysis begins to shift downward and backward, usually with some rotation. The periosteal-perichondrial covering is first stretched and twisted and then torn. As the head slides downward and backward the postero-inferior margin of the end of the neck penetrates into the substance of the epiphysis and the anterosuperior margin is bared. This change in relationship of the femur with the pelvis causes some outward rotation of the thigh, a slight degree of flexion and a small amount of shortening.

The onset of the disease is usually accompanied by pain, which may be minimal or quite severe. There is usually a limp that at first is due to the pain, but after the disappearance of the pain that usually persists for several months, the disability remains, presumably owing to alteration in the mechanics of the joint. When examined, the leg is found to be externally rotated, slightly adducted and a little shortened. The trochanter is slightly elevated and prominent. There may be a minimal atrophy of the thigh. There is frequently a permanent flexion of 15 degrees or more and flexion limitation to

about 80 or 90 degrees. Abduction and internal rotation are also limited.

Without intervention the epiphysis remains in its abnormal position and eventually becomes fixed there by fibrous tissue and callus formation. This permanent fixation is accomplished in two or three years. The process has usually become static by the time of normal epiphyseal closure. The limp and disability may in a few cases completely disappear, may persist unchanged or become progressively worse as atrophy of the acetabulum and neck and new bone formation take place in response to changed trajectory lines. Later, an osteoarthritis is apt to set in because of the altered weight-bearing surfaces.

Roentgenographic Manifestations. The roentgenographic manifestations of slipped femoral capital epiphysis depend on the degree of displacement of the femoral head. If the examination is made early in the course of the process only widening of the epiphyseal line is apparent. Minimal displacement of the epiphysis may not be appreciated in the anteroposterior projection because the

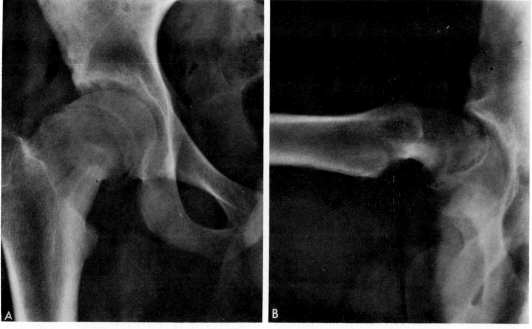

Figure 13–12 Epiphysiolysis. The deformity of the femoral neck and the femoral capital epiphysis is evident on both the anteroposterior (A) and lateral (B) projections. The widened epiphyseal line is best seen on the lateral projection. New bone is most evident at the postero-inferior aspect of the femoral neck adjacent to the epiphyseal line.

displacement is downward and posterior, but it is apparent on the lateral projection. When the displacement is more severe, the abnormality is appreciated on both projections.

Because the process is a slowly progressive one, adaptive changes take place in the neck of the femur. New bone is formed at the postero-inferior aspect of the neck and bone is resorbed at the exposed anterosuperior margin. Anterior bowing of the neck is common, as a result of which the neck appears short and broad on films exposed in the anteroposterior projection. The femoral head maintains its relation with the acetabulum; it is the femoral neck that is actually displaced. Changes in the joint in untreated patients are manifest early by narrowing of the joint space, presumably secondary to necrosis of cartilage.

Traumatic slipped femoral capital epiphysis is, of course, a rapidly occurring event and may be differentiated from the spontaneously occurring lesion by virtue of displacement of the epiphysis and the absence of new bone formation and adaptive changes in the neck of the femur. Slipped femoral capital epiphysis is common in children with renal osteodystrophy (see Fig. 11–17).

Pathologic Morphology. The gross appearance of slipped epiphysis depends, of course, upon the degree of displacement of the femoral head. Cases may now be diagnosed in the pre-slipped stage so that there is little alteration of the gross anatomy when the surgeon approaches the region. Or the epiphysis may slide downward and backward until a considerable portion of its subchondral surface becomes applied to the postero-inferior surface of the neck. In the nontraumatic cases the progression is usually slow and there is considerable reparative tissue proliferation by the time the lesion is fully developed. The denuded portion of the end of the femoral neck becomes covered

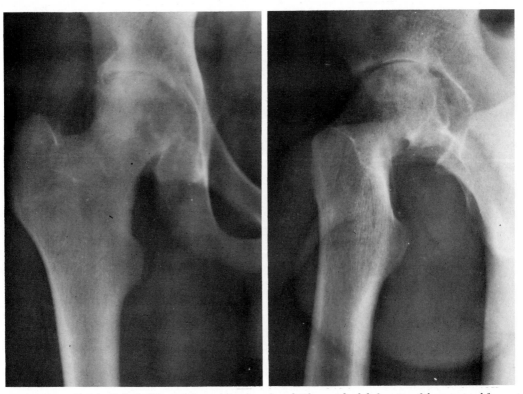

Figure 13–13 Epiphysiolysis. The epiphyseal line has closed. The residual deformity of the proximal femur is apparent as is the marked narrowing of the joint space. This was an untreated case and the abnormality of the joint reflects mechanical factors secondary to the deformity of the femur.

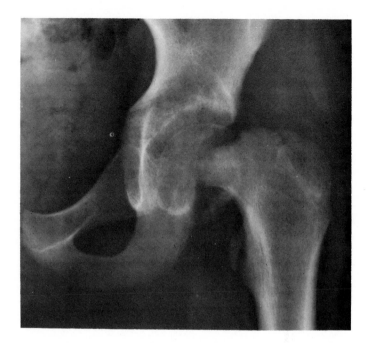

Figure 13-14 Traumatic epiphysiolysis. Note the lack of new bone formation adjacent to the epiphyseal line. There is no deformity of the femoral neck.

with a thick layer of densely collagenized fibrous tissue. In the interstices between the convex outer surface of the cortex of the neck and the subchondral surface of the epiphysis there is a proliferation of fibrous scar tissue and callus with irregular masses of cartilage and later bone. When the epiphysis at last comes to rest, the stress lines of cortical and cancellous bone are altered to the local topography by absorption and re-formation of bone lamellae. Corresponding changes take place within the acetabular cup to accommodate the new position of the articular surface.

The microscopy of slipped epiphysis in sections taken at various periods of the process fails to give a clue to the etiology of the disease. Nothing is found on microscopic examination that cannot be accounted for on the basis of traumatic loosening and eventual displacement of the epiphysis. The early changes all take place along the line of separation. The cartilage cells of and on both sides of the line of provisional calcification become deranged and distorted by pressure. The degenerative changes in this region are probably secondary to the disturbance in the normal vasculature. The osseous nucleus of the epiphysis remains intact

until impingement by the neck or altered stress lines cause changes. The granulation that first appears, then the fibrosis and callus formation and eventually the active osteogenesis are all normal responses to bone injury. If there is interruption of the epiphyseal arteries in consequence of the epiphyseal migration, an epiphyseal ischemic necrosis may result with eventual collapse of the osseous nucleus and flattening of the articular cartilage.

Pathogenesis. The mechanisms of epiphysiolysis are now quite clear thanks to periodic roentgenograms taken during the course of the process and a correlation with the gross and microscopic pathology. The cause of the disease is still unknown. In the earliest accounts it was thought to be a type of tuberculosis and later of rickets. Today, we can be definite in stating that neither infection nor a bone salt deficiency is associated with the typical case of epiphysiolysis. Other causes that have been proposed and warmly supported, at least for a time, are arthritis, osteomalacia, chondrodystrophy and nutritional disturbances. In our present state of knowledge there is nothing to support any of these contentions. It is well known that acute trauma may dislodge the epiphysis from the femoral head but most cases fail to give a history of a single episode of frank trauma commensurate with the lesion, and besides a single episode of trauma does not account for such other features as the age incidence in adolescence, a tendency for bilateral involvement, the male preponderance and the characteristic obese body type. Yet the closest scrutiny of the lesion both grossly and microscopically fails to reveal evidence for a cause other than trauma. Curiously, there is a definitely increased incidence of epiphysiolysis in renal osteodystrophy.[13]

All or most of the features that characterize slipped epiphysis are satisfied in the hypothesis that excessive stress in a conditioned structure may produce the lesion. The excessive stress may be accredited to the abnormal weight found in a large number of subjects. The conditioning may be the result of the normal changes that take place at the site about the time of puberty. If one sections any actively growing long bone longitudinally one finds the weakest point in the cortex immediately beneath the line of provisional calcification. At this level only the cancellous bone is well formed; the cortex is paper thin because there has not been sufficient time for the deposition of intramembranous bone by the periosteum. The periosteum and perichondrium probably play an important role in holding the epiphysis fast to the shaft. The junction of the head and neck of the femur is one of the several points of great stress in the skeleton. The last hurdle in the chronic trauma or stress hypothesis is the consistent occurrence of slipped epiphysis during adolescence.

One might ask why slipped epiphysis does not occur with equal frequency during the first decade. Key contends that, until osseous union of the epiphysis with the shaft, the surrounding periosteum is much thicker and more dense than it is after epiphyseal closure, and that in the years immediately preceding closure it atrophies to assume the postclosure thickness. If this be true, excessive stress due to overweight or unusual activity or frank trauma at a stress point (the femoral epiphyseal line), at a time when the normal cortical thickness has not been attained and the supportive periosteum is weakened, might result in a lesion or lesions with all the clinical and pathologic features of the disease, epiphysiolysis. Such, at present, appears to be the most logical explanation.

Lathyrism

For a number of years it has been known that experimental animals (growing rats) fed a meal made of sweet peas (*Lathyrus odoratus*) develop, among other lesions, a characteristic defect in their epiphyses that resembles epiphysiolysis (slipped epiphysis) in the human. A considerable amount of experimental work has shown that a substance in pea meal, beta-aminoproprionitrile, interferes with osteoid production by altering the constituents of the mucopolysaccharide ground substance.[14] More recently Andren and Borgstrom have noted a correlation between the incidence of epiphysiolysis in Swedish children and the season during which cows are allowed to graze. The hypothesis has been made that cows may ingest lathyrogenic substances, which are transmitted to patients in milk. Lathyrogenic substances may interfere with osteoid formation in the active metaphysis, weakening this area to allow twisting and slipping of the epiphysis in rapidly growing patients in whom the area is exposed to strain; for example, in Fröhlich's syndrome or obesity. We examined sections of the metaphyses of rats fed aminoproprionitrile. There is indeed a deficient osteoid production. The relationship to human epiphysiolysis is, of course, conjectural.

ANEURYSMAL BONE CYST

Aneurysmal bone cyst is a curious, solitary lesion of bone which has been so named because typically it causes a bulging of the overlying cortex, bearing some resemblance to the saccular protrusion of the aortic wall in true aneurysm. The name has caused a good deal of confusion because the lesion is vascular and therefore has been interpreted as an aneurysm of a bone vessel, which it may be, but which implication is not intended by the descriptive name applied.

Ewing, in his first edition (1919) of *Neoplastic Diseases*, alludes to two lesions in bone that are probably aneurysmal bone cysts, but he classifies them as hemangiomas of bone. In his third edition (1928) he uses the term "malignant bone aneurysm" as a synonym of telangiectatic osteosarcoma and also describes an aneurysmal variant of giant cell tumor that almost certainly is an aneurysmal bone cyst or an aneurysmal bone cyst superimposed on a giant cell tumor. Until quite recently a number of papers have appeared giving recognizable descriptions of this lesion, but they were always interpreted as vascular variants of other conditions. In 1942, Jaffe and Lichtenstein in their paper on solitary cyst of bone[15] devoted considerable space to the description of two of their cases, each manifesting a large cyst of bone filled with a spongy mass of blood channels. They coined the term "aneurysmal cyst." Eight years later, both had collected sufficient cases to recognize the lesion as an entity and to present their material in separate papers.[16, 17] More recently Dahlin et al.[18] have published a series of 26 cases, which were seen at the Mayo Clinic in the period from 1905 to 1952. Most of these cases were misdiagnosed both radiologically and by tissue examination because the features of the lesion had not yet been described. It is obvious that the incidence of this condition is still unknown, but it is probable that it is considerably more common than we have suspected, even in the recent past.

Aneurysmal bone cyst has been found in patients of almost every age over 3 and under 50, but about three quarters of them occur in the second decade and most of the rest in the third. Though there has been a female predominance in some series, as more adequate figures are collected it appears that there is no sex predilection. Many of the earlier cases involved the bodies, neural arches and spines of the vertebrae and for a time it appeared that these were the sites most frequently affected, but now it is known that aneurysmal bone cyst probably involves any bone of the skeleton and that vertebral lesions probably constitute less than 10 per cent of the cases.

Aneurysmal bone cyst usually causes pain. It may be of several weeks' or several months' duration. In cases in which a vertebra is affected, severe muscle spasm may be responsible for most of the symptoms or, if there is compression of the cord or nerve roots, the pain may be referred. Though the lesion rarely invades the joint structures, it may occur in the end of a long bone near a joint and thus cause joint pain and disability. Usually before diagnosis is made there is swelling of the area. This has been variously interpreted but the enlargement is actually due to "expansion" of the cortex that overlies the medullary soft tissue mass. The "swelling" is usually accompanied by tenderness. If intervention is delayed, aneurysmal bone cyst may grow to huge proportions. Because it causes lysis of the bone in which it resides and erosion of contiguous bone structures, destruction severe enough to necessitate amputation may eventuate. In the late cases, this disproportionate anatomic distortion makes the diagnosis of malignant bone tumor plausible. In almost every reported series at least one case has been so diagnosed and amputation has been performed as a last resort. For this reason alone it is mandatory that all orthopedists, radiologists and pathologists learn the diagnostic features of this innocuous lesion.

Aneurysmal bone cyst usually begins in cancellous or medullary structures. Occasionally it may arise between the periosteum and cortex, often following trauma. It is assumed that this is the conversion of a subperiosteal hematoma into an aneurysmal bone cyst. It may arise at any point in the shaft but it most often affects the ends of the diaphysis, often very close to the epiphyseal line in cases in which it involves cylindrical bones. Whether it begins centrally in the medullary tissues and expands further in one direction than another or whether it always begins beneath the compacta is impossible to say, because it cannot be identified on the roentgenograms until the cortex is involved. It apparently has a remarkable lytic propensity because the overlying compacta melts away before it as it expands. The contiguous periosteum is pushed outward and reacts by laying down a thin shell of bone, which must be continuously replaced as its inner layers are eroded away (Fig. 13–15). Thus, a bulky structure soon protrudes beyond the uninvolved cortical surface, pushing soft tissues before it and eroding other bones on contact. This appearance and behavior has given rise to the name aneurysmal bone cyst. In cases in which large cylindrical and flat bones are affected the lesion has a saccular, eccentric structure. In shorter or more slender bones the entire circumference is involved and the lesion has a fusiform shape.

Aneurysmal bone cyst is a disturbance of the vasculature of marrow tissue. As such it never begins in the cartilaginous epiphysis. After the epiphysis is ossified it may be involved in the process but it is unusual for the lesion to transgress the articular plate and invade the joint cavity. The lesion may grow to a huge size (Fig. 13–16). Aneurysmal bone cysts more than 20 cm. in diameter have been described.

Regardless of the size of the cyst the periosteum manages to maintain a covering shell of bone but eventually this thin shell fractures and the bloody contents of the lesion extravasate into the soft tissues. Now the lesion becomes much more difficult to recognize because it is essentially a

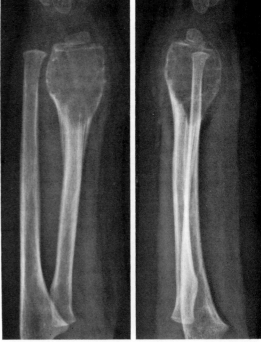

Figure 13–15 Aneurysmal bone cyst. The distal end of the radius has been expanded by the lesion, which is covered by a thin shell of bone. Multiple layers of periosteal new bone are evident proximal to the lesion.

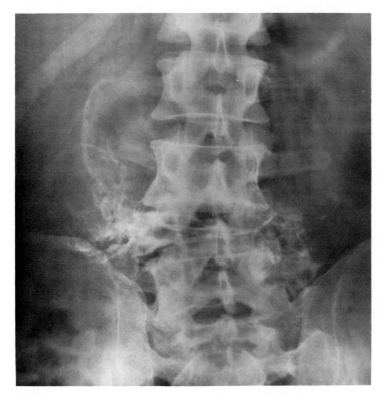

Figure 13–16 A huge aneurysmal bone cyst arising from a vertebra. The body has been destroyed and the cortex has been expanded to produce a sac-like structure, which protrudes into the abdominal cavity. A mistaken diagnosis of inoperable malignant tumor was made and the patient was watched until the cyst ruptured and the patient bled to death.

massive hematoma accompanied by the usual reaction of muscle, fat and fibrous tissue to the presence of free blood. The advent of rupture may result in an alarming increase in the rate of growth, inspiring the clinical diagnosis of malignant neoplasm. Excessive lysis may weaken the bone to the point of fracture, and erosion of neighboring bones may give the appearance of invasion. Thus, the radiologist is apt to fall into the same trap as the clinician. If the pathologist fails to recognize the lesion for what it is or if the surgeon fails to obtain diagnosable tissue, the condition is almost certain to be misdiagnosed and an amputation may be performed. If a high index of suspicion were maintained and all irregular features of the clinical, radiologic and pathologic aspects carefully considered, this tragedy would occur less often.

Roentgenographic Manifestations. Radiographically an aneurysmal bone cyst presents as a radiolucent area with the density of soft tissue within which are multiple fine, often incomplete septa. It is an expanding lesion with sharply demarcated scalloped borders. The lesion erodes bone and after cortical destruction has occurred it is covered by a shell of periosteal new bone. At times, rupture and disruption of this thin shell of bone may occur with only fragments of the shell being visible.

The typical aneurysmal bone cyst begins in cancellous tissue. It may be centrally or eccentrically located in either the mid-diaphysis or near the end of the shaft of a long bone. The lesion has been described as parosteal in location[19] with the bulk of the tumor in the soft tissues and only slight underlying cortical erosion. When a vertebra is involved, it is usually the neural arch that is the site of the lesion; there may be extension into the spinal canal (Fig. 3–19).

Correlation of the radiographic examination with the microscopic examination is most important. Inadequate biopsy of a

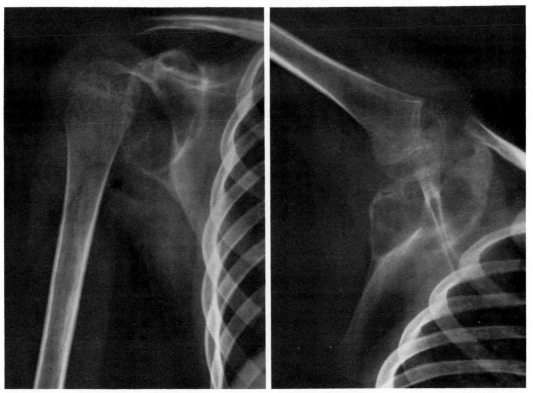

Figure 13–17   Aneurysmal bone cyst. This lesion has involved the scapula (glenoid) of a 7 year old white boy. The glenoid is enlarged by the expanding radiolucent lesion. Note the incomplete septa within it, and its scalloped borders. Periosteal new bone defines its extent.

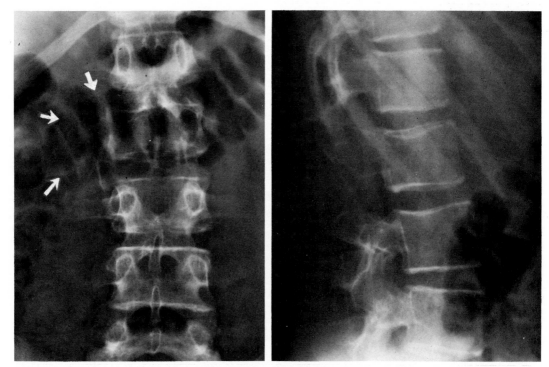

Figure 13–18   Aneurysmal bone cyst. The right lateral and posterior portions of the second lumbar vertebra are involved. There is partial collapse of the lateral portion of the body, the pedicles and lamina are destroyed and the lesion extends well beyond the confines of the vertebra. It is covered by a thin shell of bone (arrows).

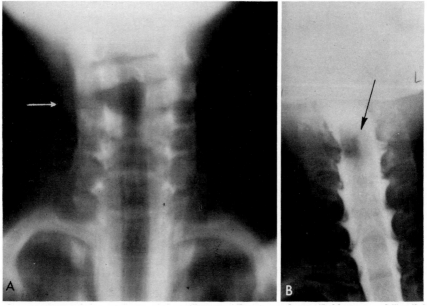

Figure 13–19   A large aneurysmal bone cyst has destroyed the right lateral portion of the fourth cervical vertebra (arrow) with loss of stature (A). There is an intraspinal component visible on the myelogram (arrow, B).

lesion that is clearly malignant by radiographic criteria may reveal only "aneurysmal bone cyst" and not the underlying abnormality. (See page 432.)

Morbid Anatomy. Aneurysmal bone cyst is an aggregate of thick-walled channels carrying streams of blood. Judging from the color of the lesion the blood is probably venous rather than arterial. One important feature to be kept in mind is that the blood is not a stagnant pool but unclotted and in motion, so that there must be a constant supply at one end and a continuous drainage at the other. A second feature is that the channels that contain this stream of blood are not true vessel walls because they contain no elastic or muscle lamina and in most areas are not even lined with endothelium.

The name aneurysmal bone cyst is misleading in more ways than one because the lesion is not a true cyst. It only appears to be a cyst on the roentgenogram. Actually, it is a spongelike structure. An excessive blood supply to the area probably accounts for the remarkable deossification of normal bone, which characterizes the process.

When the surgeon removes a portion of the covering bony shell he usually finds what appears to be a well of blood that bleeds freely and steadily. There is no pulsation. When probed, however, what appears to be a pool is found to be partitioned by tissue walls. Hemorrhage may be exceedingly difficult to control because tangible structures concealed in blood are elusive, retreating into a formless mass as they are approached. The blood spaces are frequently larger in the central portion of the lesion. Sometimes there is considerably more solid matter separating the blood sinuses and then the structure resembles a sponge soaked in blood. When the tissue has been removed and drained, it is found to constitute only a fraction of the mass that filled the exposed cavity. The walls may continue to bleed steadily. At times the fibrous walled channels may constitute an inconspicuous component of the lesion. They may be replaced by large masses of collagenous tissue, the channels appearing as irregular clefts in dense fibrous scar tissue (Fig. 13–20A). This may represent the late stage of an aneurysmal bone cyst in which there has been considerable blood extravasation and resultant reactive fibrosis. The vascular elements may be so diminished that bleeding at surgery is not a feature. This should be remembered by the surgeon who has read elsewhere that unless his operative site bleeds profusely the lesion is not an aneurysmal bone cyst.

Within the bone the lesion is moderately well circumscribed. If rupture into soft tissue has taken place, the reaction to extravasated blood conceals the margins of the process and makes the selection of representative tissue for biopsy exceedingly difficult. In the area of bone destruction about the periphery of the sinus mass and sometimes within it there are apt to be solid areas of soft tissue. The surgeon is tempted to select these for biopsy. These areas are usually the product of reaction of the injured bone and fibrous tissue rather than the culprit that is causing the injury. Thus, the issue may be confused by the pathologist who must read what he sees rather than what is left behind.

Through the microscope, the aneurysmal bone cyst may appear to be a mass of communicating spaces containing fluid blood surrounded and supported by fibrous walls of varying thickness (Fig. 13–20 B). There is no organized elastic lamina and if muscle fibers are present they are lost in the collagen of the fibrous tissue, which is the main constituent of the walls. Often, slender, smooth spicules of bone are found in the partitions, apparently the product of fibro-osseous metaplasia (Fig. 13–21). Hemosiderin granules are frequently prominent. Giant cell reaction occurs wherever there has been spillage of blood and large masses of giant cells usually constitute the most outstanding feature of the lesion. In areas, whole fields have a fibrous matrix and sufficient giant cells to suggest the diagnosis of giant cell tumor or brown tumor of parathyroid adenoma. These fields are usually the solid areas about the periphery of the sinus mass. This appearance accounts for the all too frequent diagnosis of eccentric or subperiosteal giant cell tumor. In an attempt to repair bone defects and infractions there may be a brisk proliferation of new bone and cartilage. The appearance of active osteoblasts or chondroblasts may mislead

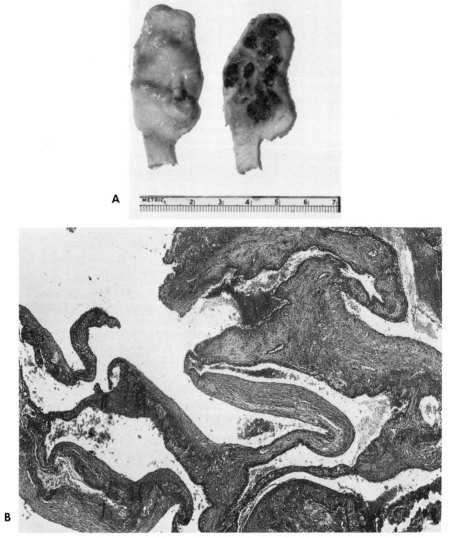

Figure 13–20   *A*, Aneurysmal bone cyst, proximal phalanx of thumb. Left, outer expanded cortical surface; right, cut surface showing large irregular vascular channels in collagenized matrix. *B*, Section through the spongy portion of an aneurysmal bone cyst. Since the blood has drained away, the sinuses have collapsed but their fibrous walls are apparent. (× 30.)

the pathologist into the diagnosis of osteo-sarcoma or chondrosarcoma. If the lesion is described by the radiologist as a cyst, and if this is not corrected by the surgeon who fails to obtain sinus material for microscopic study, the pathologist has but one choice of diagnosis, solitary cyst, because the tissue lining a solitary cyst and that surrounding an aneurysmal bone cyst are often identical.

There are few clues to the cause and mechanism of aneurysmal bone cyst. It is

not a neoplasm because it does not have the microscopic constituents of a true tumor. It has been suggested that an altera-tion in circulatory dynamics has produced a mass of varicosed venous channels. Against this is the lack of venous wall structure and the bone-lysing propensities of the lesion, the latter suggesting that the excess of blood is active rather than pas-sive. Hypothetically, an arteriovenous communication through a plexus of fibrous channels would supply most or all of the criteria found in aneurysmal bone cyst. Congenital arteriovenous fistulas are found in various tissues of the body including bone. They usually result from a failure of complete differentiation of arteries and veins. True congenital aneurysms may form because of a failure of development of the arterial muscle coat. Arteriovenous fistulas are usually associated with varicosities of the associated veins.

Against this hypothesis as the cause of aneurysmal bone cyst is the frequent occurrence of pulsation in congenital fistula (not reported in aneurysmal bone cyst); birthmarks of the skin are frequently associated and though there are no reports of gasometric analysis of the blood in aneurysmal bone cyst, it appears to be no more highly oxygenated than ordinary venous blood. Also the tubular structures said to be the pathognomonic feature of aneurysmal bone cyst are found in lesions that clinically and radiologically are quite obviously not aneurysmal bone cysts.

The most constant microscopic feature of the lesion is the presence of large fields of giant cells in a collagen-producing matrix in which one usually finds consider-

able quantities of hemosiderin pigment. Though this type of reaction occurs in other bone lesions, i.e., solitary cyst and non-ossifying fibroma, it probably is most characteristic of an old intraosseous hematoma. One might rationalize the pathogenesis of aneurysmal bone cyst as a hematoma that has eventually established one or more arteriovenous fistulas. In instances in which fistula formation does not occur and instead the hematoma becomes encapsulated and undergoes liquefaction resolution, the lesion becomes a solitary cyst. If it completely collagenizes it then becomes a non-ossifying fibroma. At a certain transitional stage in the formation of the last, giant cells, so often found in the presence of extravasated blood in cancellous tissue, might dominate the section accounting for their presence in all three entities.

In reality there is too little factual evidence to make the previous statements anything more than an attractive hypothesis to account for the pathogenesis of three very common skeletal lesions. We have encountered numerous lesions in bone, however, in which a history of trauma was undeniable and in which sections of the

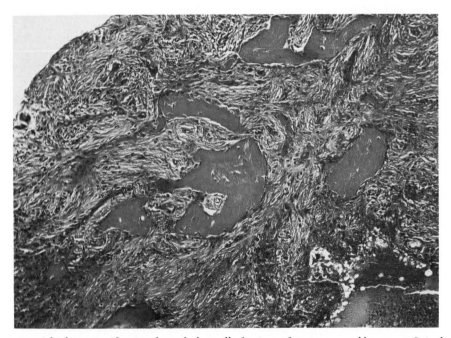

Figure 13–21   A higher magnification through the wall of a sinus of an aneurysmal bone cyst. Spicules of bone are often seen.

biopsies disclosed only masses of giant cells. The pseudotumor of hemophilia may have all the radiographic features of a typical aneurysmal bone cyst. Biopsy material on these lesions has been inadequate, understandably, for conclusive opinion on the nature of the tissue involved. It is our belief that in certain, probably rare, instances trauma may cause a hematoma that is converted to a mass of collagenizing tissue thickly infiltrated with giant cells. This does not mean that all giant cell lesions are the result of traumatic (or nontraumatic) hemorrhage nor that the occurrence of trauma in the history must be considered a significant etiologic factor.

Lindbom et al.[20] have reported a highly vascular appearance in the arterial phase of angiograms with patchy opacification in the venous stage. They state that angiograms of giant cell tumor (osteoclastoma) are less patchy and more opaque though the difference is probably not sufficient to make a distinction on the basis of angiograms alone.

An analysis of 95 cases of aneurysmal bone cyst seen at the Mayo Clinic[21] resulted in a conclusion that none showed any acceptable evidence of a precursor lesion. This is in sharp variance with the findings of ourselves and others. Biesecker et al.[22] in a later report analyzed 66 cases and concluded that 32 per cent had an accompanying benign lesion of bone, among the most frequent of which were nonosteogenic fibroma, chondroblastoma, giant cell tumor and osteoblastoma. Our own material constitutes nearly 100 cases. Scrutiny of the clinical, radiologic and microscopic features of these suggests an association of either a benign or a malignant lesion in almost 50 per cent. Of these, osteoclastoma occurs most commonly, though osteosarcoma is not rare. Recurrence of solitary cyst after curettage on careful reexamination will, in perhaps all cases, be found to be aneurysmal bone cyst.

Pathogenesis. It must be admitted that the pathogenesis of aneurysmal bone cyst is still unknown but during the past 30 years much circumstantial evidence has been collected to suggest that it is an aggregate of arteriovenous communications which arise consequent to developmental fault or hemorrhage from hemangiomas, spontaneous, idiopathic hemorrhages in cancellous bone or secondary to bone injury. The injury rarely may be trauma; more often it is a primary bone lesion benign and innocuous in itself or neoplastic and malignant. Arteriography supports this explanation as do the few available manometric readings.[22] The concurrence of a multiple variety of primary lesions at the site can be interpreted only as a causative factor in the pathogenesis of aneurysmal bone cyst. The exact mechanism of the reaction to the primary injury which results in multiple arteriovenous fistulas cannot as yet be described, nor the reason why the incidence of this occurrence in cancellous bone tissue is greater than in extraosseous soft tissues. However, such seems to be the case; the explanation will doubtless appear when sufficient cases have been studied with the proper objectives in mind.

In summary, aneurysmal bone cyst is a noncystic lesion of bone, which has been produced by the flow of blood through a spongelike network of fibrous walled channels. These channels may represent a tangle of congenital arteriovenous fistulas or they may evolve from the organization of a hematoma within cancellous bone tissue. The hematoma may have arisen as the result of leakage from a congenital hemangioma, from trauma or from any other disease or lesion of bone that may injure its vasculature. These include bone tumors (aneurysmal bone cyst is frequently superimposed on osteosarcoma) and hamartomas. A high proportion of solitary cysts appears to be transformed into aneurysmal bone cysts by fracture or surgery apparently secondary to hematoma formation. We believe that many osteoclastomas are complicated by aneurysmal bone cyst in their late phase. One frequently encounters an osteoclastoma that in repeated radiographs appears to progress slowly, and then suddenly to explode into a wildly destructive lesion. Samples of the tumor may disclose accompanying aneurysmal bone cyst. The giant cell reaction of the latter intermingled with the giant cells of osteoclastoma make the histologic picture exceedingly difficult to interpret. If the giant cells of osteoclastoma are derived from vessel endothelial lining cells as we believe they may be, the association of these two lesions is not surprising.

Prognosis. The destruction of bone in aneurysmal bone cyst appears to be the consequence of an excessive supply of blood to a localized area. Anything that reduces that supply to the normal level should arrest the progress of the disease. This has been found to be true. The lesion may be treated surgically and occasionally by irradiation.[23, 24] The former has usually been used because by the time the diagnosis is made the protruding mass is best handled by excision. It has been shown that even a partial curettement with no attempt to remove all of the vascular tissue has resulted in a cure. There has been recurrence in a number of our cases suggesting that a hematoma remained after curettage. The pathologist should always keep in mind that the aneurysmal bone cyst is often superimposed upon another lesion that may have an even more serious implication. Recurrence has been reported in as high as 21 per cent of cases.[21] This incidence is much greater than in our own material and in other reported series.

SOLITARY CYST OF BONE

Solitary cyst (solitary unicameral cyst) is an entity, distinct from other cystic and fibrous lesions of bone, occurring for the most part at the ends of the large cylindrical bones of the extremities in the growing skeleton.

The term "bone cyst" has been used loosely in the past and still is used, regrettably, in designating a wide variety of bone lesions whose roentgenograms reveal sharply delineated, smooth-walled areas of radiolucency. A cyst is a collection of gas or fluid enclosed in a capsule. Because the radiograph cannot distinguish between fluid and soft tissue, numerous proliferative lesions that contain no opaque bone salts are casually categorized as "bone cysts." This leads to unnecessary confusion and misunderstanding between the roentgenologist and the pathologist. The clinician is sometimes at a loss to know what either is talking about.

Cystic lesions characteristically occur in few other bone diseases—parathyroid adenoma (osteitis fibrosa cystica) and less often fibrous dysplasia—but the "cysts" are merely areas of degeneration in proliferative processes and though they contain fluid they should be designated as areas of liquefaction necrosis rather than cysts. The lesion which we have chosen to call "posthematoma cyst" is a true cyst (see later description) probably arising in a walled, liquefied hematoma as does that curious entity called "subchondral cyst" or "ganglion cyst" of bone. The latter closely resembles solitary cyst[27] except that it occurs in an older age group, usually in the vicinity of the ankle, is juxta-articular and contains a thick mucinous substance. Its pathogenesis is unknown, though some feel that it is related to the subchondral cysts of degenerative joint disease. The solitary cyst is the only other true cyst of bone.

Solitary cysts have been described in the skeleton since the days of Virchow but it was not until the early part of the present century[25] that it was realized that they are an entity apart from osteitis fibrosa cystica and, later, fibrous dysplasia. The more recent account of Jaffe and Lichtenstein[26] adequately summarizes the modern concept of the condition.

Solitary cyst is a disease of the growing skeleton. In the Jaffe-Lichtenstein series of 19 cases, 15 patients were between 3 and 14 years of age. One was 42. In our own material there are 89 patients. All but 10 range between 3 and 19 years of age. In almost all series there has been a male preponderance. Of our cases, only 25 of the 89 are females.

It has been said that solitary cyst occurs only in cylindrical bone and there can be no argument that the large bones of the extremities are the ones most consistently involved. Among our cases four diagnoses of bone cyst were made on lesions in the os calcis (Fig. 13–22), one in the tarsal navicular, two in the clavicle, one in a rib, one in the mandible and one in the ramus of the pubic bone. Admittedly, neither the microscopy nor the roentgenograms of solitary cyst are absolutely specific but in cases in which these features are combined with the gross appearance of a fluid-containing bone cyst lined with a thin layer of soft tissue, almost no other diagnosis may be con-

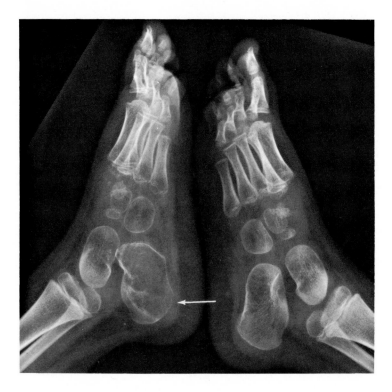

Figure 13-22 Solitary cyst. The right os calcis has been expanded by a lesion that proved at biopsy to be a solitary cyst. A fracture involves the inferior aspect of the bone (arrow).

sidered if posthematoma cyst and ganglion cyst can be ruled out. One of the os calcis lesions occurred in a medical student who has been followed for 12 years after conservative therapy. It seems highly improbable that the diagnosis is in error.

It is noteworthy that the majority of the cysts occurring elsewhere than the ends of the shafts of large cylindrical bones were in patients older than 18 years. This suggests to us that these cysts may have a different pathogenesis from the usual typical solitary or unicameral bone cysts. We encountered a series of these in the ribs in young adults, many of whom gave a significant history of trauma, and concluded that solitary cysts may be produced in adult bone as a result of the lysis of a hematoma of cancellous tissue. On several instances cysts occurred in adult epiphyses, a site at which ordinary solitary cysts never arise. We suggest that if these atypical cysts contain a thin, watery, amber fluid they may be classified as posthematoma cysts (see p. 324), whereas, if they are filled with a clear, glairy, mucinous material they be called subchondral or ganglion cysts (see following).

Lesions in the proximal humerus, the ends of the femur and the proximal tibia account for approximately nine tenths of the cases of typical solitary cysts. The incidence is probably in the order named, with the proximal humerus being the commonest site.

Because solitary bone cyst develops very slowly, it rarely, if ever, of itself causes pain. Pain ensues when the overlying cortex is thinned to the point of pathologic fracture. Consequently, though pain is the usual presenting symptom, a roentgenogram most often reveals a fracture through the wall of an already well established bone cyst. If no fracture lines are apparent it is probable that one or more undemonstrable infractions have involved the periosteal sensory structure.

Because these lesions are symptomless until fracture there has been little opportunity of studying them in the early phase of their development. Occasionally a bone cyst is discovered in radiographic surveys done for another reason. The lesion probably always begins in the spongy bone of the metaphysis, either in contiguity with or near the epiphyseal line. It expands slowly, widening until it occupies the entire diameter of the medullary region and extending through the shaft toward the mid-diaphysis. As it enlarges it first abuts against the surrounding compacta and then slowly erodes it from the inside. As the cortex thins, some appositional bone is laid down on the exterior surface by the periosteum so that the cortex becomes expanded, but apparently the stimulus for periosteal bone formation is so gentle that external new bone formation does not keep pace with inner erosion and the expanding wall becomes thinner and thinner until fracture occurs.

Though most lesions are confined to the metaphyseal region and contiguous portion of the shaft, a few very large cysts (Fig. 13–23) may expand to involve more than half the entire diaphysis. This probably accounts for those rare cysts that are found occupying the mid-third of the shaft; i.e., they probably started in the metaphysis and extended to involve that half of the bone, then crossed the midpoint to involve the mid-diaphyseal portion of the remaining half. Because the cysts heal from the metaphyseal pole, the unhealed residuum would eventually come to lie within the middle third of the diaphysis. If this is in fact what happens, this would contradict the most widely accepted theory of pathogenesis, i.e., that of osteogenic defect in the epiphyseal line. However, large "cysts" of the middle third of the shaft, particularly if they are expanding and in the second decade, are more apt to be aneurysmal bone cysts.

In its typical form the cyst occurs in the end of a large cylindrical bone in the extremity of a patient between the ages of 3 and 17. It may have caused some expansion of the overlying cortex and this "eggshell" covering often has the slate or bluish discoloration of the blue-domed cysts of the breast. There is almost always a zone of normal bone interposed between the cyst and the epiphyseal line.

Because the cyst begins in the metaphysis, possibly immediately contiguous to the epiphyseal line, the zone of normal tissue represents the amount of longitudinal bone growth since the establishment of the lesion. As the bone continues to grow, an illusion of drifting of the cyst toward the mid-diaphysis is created. Attempts have been made to judge the age of the lesion by its distance from the epiphyseal line. It has been stated that cysts that appear very near the line are still actively growing and that therapy at this time is more apt to result in a recurrence than if it is in the "latent phase" more deeply situated in the shaft.[28] It is difficult to evaluate this hypothesis but the evidence is probably insufficient to warrant postponement of therapy and risk of further fracture and deformity. A few very large cysts have been observed to impair normal bone growth.

When a window is cut in the cyst wall, it is found to contain fluid though it need not be filled. Sometimes incision through the thin, expanded cortex results in a fountain of fluid that may actually spout a centimeter or more because of the intracystic pressure. Usually the fluid is amber though

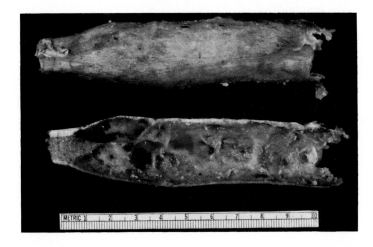

Figure 13–23 Solitary cyst. The outer cortical surface is shown above. Note expansion of cortex. A sagittal section is shown below. The fluid contained enough protein to coagulate in the fixative.

it may be almost clear or have the appearance of pure blood, and occasionally it may be clotted. The cyst is lined with a thin layer, often not more than a millimeter in thickness, of red, brown or less often pale membrane. The cyst is unilocular and the wall is usually quite smooth, though it may be traversed by narrow ridges of bone. The lining may be curetted away leaving a more or less complete wall of bone.

Roentgenographic   Manifestations. The roentgenographic manifestation of a solitary cyst of bone is a radiolucent defect usually involving the spongiosa near the end of a long bone. The defect is round or oval and is of the density of soft tissue because it has a wall of soft tissue and contains fluid. The distance between the cyst

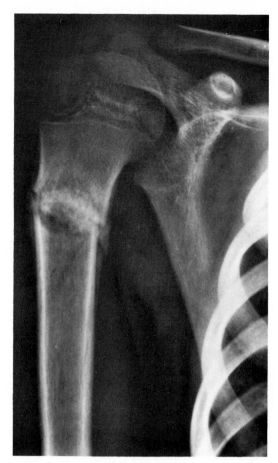

Figure 13-25   Healing fracture of the humerus that has occurred through a solitary cyst.

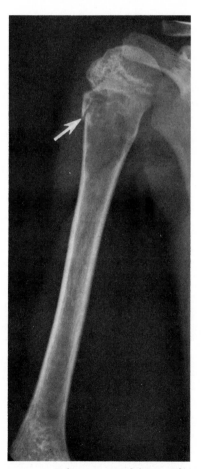

Figure 13-24   Solitary cyst of bone. The ovoid radiolucent defect is evident in the proximal humeral diaphysis. Bone separates its superior aspect from the metaphysis. No septa are evident within the lesion. There is a fracture (arrow) through the thinned cortex.

and the metaphysis varies, probably depending upon the duration of the process. Although expansion of the shaft may occur, the defect is usually no wider than the adjacent metaphysis and uncommonly expands the bone in a localized area. The size of the cyst varies considerably, but the limits of the cyst are usually well defined.

Periosteal new bone is not a feature of this lesion even though the cortex may become quite thin because the migration and erosion of the cyst are so slow. There is little bone reaction about the cyst. Its outline is evident by virtue of contrast between bone and the fluid and soft tissue of the cyst.

Fracture through the cyst is common. In this instance, the integrity of the cortex over the lesion is lost and deformity may be present. Periosteal new bone is seen as the fracture heals (Fig. 13–25). Irregular sclerosis follows surgical treatment in which bone has been placed within the cyst (Fig. 13–26).

Microscopy. The microscopic sections only corroborate the clinical and roentgenologic diagnosis. There are no pathognomonic features about the tissue that is curetted from the bony walls. It usually consists of a more or less definite membrane of moderately young fibrocytes of a rather loose texture intermixed with masses of more deeply staining fibrin (Fig. 13–27A). The amount of collagen varies considerably. At times it is quite densely collagenized or it may consist almost wholly of quite young granula-

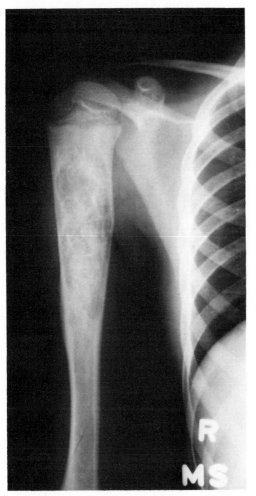

Figure 13–26 Postoperative appearance of a large solitary cyst. Thick trabeculae and irregular fragments of bone (graft) are visible so that the area of the cyst is irregularly dense.

tion. Considerable amounts of granular, yellow-brown pigment are usually in evidence within macrophages and scattered through the intercellular areas. Most of this pigment is hemosiderin and takes the Prussian blue reaction. Its erythrocytic origin is often obvious because of the aggregates of red cells in various stages of degeneration. Pools of recently extravasated blood are sometimes seen. Xanthoid cells whose cytoplasm is swollen and pale with quantities of lipid may occur singly or in small groups. In some areas this material may collect in the intercellular spaces to form masses of fusiform, sharp-pointed crystals. These dissolve in the processing fluid to leave characteristic clefts usually surrounded by collagen.

Giant cells occur in varying numbers, their cytoplasm sometimes containing lipid, pigment or cell debris (Fig. 13–27B). They may be clustered about an area of hemorrhage or diffusely scattered throughout the granulation matrix. The presence of these cells surrounded by young fibrocytes has led to the contention that this lesion is a variant of the giant cell tumor of bone. If the material is scant, as it often is, and predominantly composed of this type of tissue, it may be exceedingly difficult to differentiate the cyst wall from the solid masses of giant cell reaction that occur in the metaphyseal region in response to bone injury and hemorrhage, a lesion that is often mistakenly called benign giant cell tumor. The gross description usually makes the diagnosis obvious because of the lesion's cystic nature. It should be remembered that a giant cell reaction is to be expected whenever there is extravasation of blood in the end of a long bone but, with the exception of the posthematoma cyst, these lesions are not cystic. Bone tissue is usually lacking in the sections but there may be a few irregular fragments of the compacta, which have been dislodged by the curet or even some spicules of immature bone from a fracture site or from the subperiosteal region. Osteogenesis is usually not prominent enough to suggest the possibility of osteosarcoma. The diagnoses of non-osteogenic fibroma, subperiosteal cortical defect and, in some instances, aneurysmal bone cyst cannot be eliminated on the appearance of the sections alone.

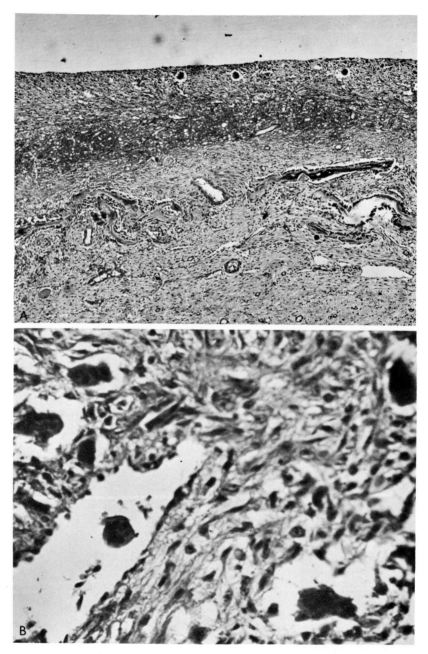

Figure 13–27   *A*, Low magnification (× 40) through the wall of a solitary cyst. There is a fibrous wall containing a few spicules of new bone in its deeper portion. In the superficial layer (above) there is a layer of blood, perhaps the residuum of the original hematoma, and a covering of fibrin. *B*, Higher magnification (× 396) showing a fibroblastic reaction with several giant cells.

Pathogenesis. The pathogenesis of solitary cyst of bone has been the subject of concern of a number of writers. When at last solitary cyst was separated from osteitis fibrosa cystica (parathyroid adenoma) it was reclassified as a variant of giant cell tumor. When rescued from this group it became tempting to speculate on the cause and mechanism of its development. Mikulicz suggested that because the lesion occurred in growing bone it was probably the result of mechanical trauma to an area of bone growth in the epiphyseal line, creating a defect at the point at which enchondral bone formation failed to occur and resulting in a hiatus, which presented as a cyst. Jaffe and Lichtenstein supported this theory and there is much in favor of it, particularly the age group affected. The evidence that appears to contradict this idea is found in cysts that cross the mid-diaphyseal point. If the cyst is a defect resulting from failure of bone formation in an area of one epiphyseal line, the defect could involve only the portion of the diaphysis normally formed by that epiphyseal structure. Admittedly, the two epiphyses of a cylindrical bone are not necessarily responsible for an equal amount of the intervening shaft, but in unusual cases in which the cyst has involved two thirds or more of the diaphysis it is probable that the lesion could not be caused by a defect at one end.

Pommer suggested that the solitary cyst is the result of a hemorrhage into the growing metaphysis. In organization a fibrous wall forms about the extravasated blood, which clots and then undergoes liquefaction. The surrounding fibrous capsule acts as a semipermeable membrane and if the osmotic pressure of the intracystic content is higher than that of the surrounding tissue, water is drawn into the cyst. As the pressure within the wall increases the cyst expands, causing pressure erosion on the surrounding cancellous tissue and then cortex. Eventually, the extra- and intracystic densities are equalized and the process stabilizes and is now said to be in its latent stage.

This above theory is attractive for the following reasons. Such expanding cysts are fairly common following subdural hemorrhage. Sections of the bone cyst wall are compatible with the appearance of the capsule about old hemorrhage; there are fibrosis, cholesterol, giant cells, pigment and degenerating red cells. The contained fluid is characteristic of liquefied hematoma. There is sometimes increased pressure within the cyst wall. Sometimes the cyst content is frankly bloody. The age incidence and prevalent sites are harder to explain. In the growing bone the metaphysis is more vascular and probably less sturdy than after the epiphysis is ossified. It is probably worthy of mention that these areas in the lower extremities may be traumatized by traction when infants are lifted by the feet in changing diapers and in the upper extremities when they are held by the arms in learning to walk.

Against the theory is the apparent fact that patients with hemophilia, in which one expects a high incidence of intramedullary hemorrhage, do not show a high incidence of solitary bone cysts, although we have encountered two such instances and wonder if more complete study would reveal more. Also, though the hemorrhages that occur in parathyroid adenoma may produce areas of cystic degeneration, the brown tumors of this disturbance are quite different from solitary bone cyst. It is quite possible, of course, that the age at onset and the level of parathyroid hormone may account for these differences.

The occasional cyst that occurs in the adult is difficult to explain. Some of them probably represent the residuum of a lesion that developed during childhood or adolescence. The reasons for their quiescence for several to many years probably vary with each specific case and usually remain unknown. Others are more likely old posthematoma cysts and a few may be subchondral or ganglion cysts.

Prognosis. If the cyst lining is adequately curetted, the lesion almost always heals with replacement by new bone. Recurrence is seen in a small percentage for reasons that are often not apparent. We have encountered 13 cases of what we were reasonably sure were solitary cysts that after fracture or surgical intervention became aneurysmal bone cysts. It is impossible, of course, to be sure that these were not aneurysmal bone cysts from the outset but we prefer to believe that the latter developed as the result of hemorrhage into the original lesion, which in organizing developed arteriovenous fistulas and consequent aneurysmal bone cyst. In those cases of solitary cyst that are curetted and that recur as aneurysmal bone cysts (this is not an unusual event), we suggest that incarcerated blood consequent to oozing after closure may organize and form the arteriovenous fistulas that constitute aneurysmal bone cyst. It is said that cysts that undergo pathologic fracture may heal spontaneously. Some of them doubtless do but a favorable result should not be expected in the majority. Very large cysts may cause distortion of bone and inhibit bone growth. Bone cysts do not predispose to neoplasm. Radiotherapy has no proven value in this condition and should not be used.

SUBCHONDRAL CYST

In 1956 Hicks described three cases of bone cyst in adults. They were all located within the fused epiphysis beneath the articular plate. They were lined by what appeared to be modified synovia and contained a mucinous material. He suggested that they were synovial in origin. Several other such cysts have been reported. Because of the nature of the contents they have been called ganglion cysts[27] implying a relation to the soft tissue cysts of that name. More recently Nigrisoli and Beltrami[29] have written a review of the 32 cases reported in the world literature. These cysts occur at any age after the fusion of the epiphysis with the diaphysis. The ankle region—the distal end of the tibia, the two malleoli and the astragalus—is the most common site. These cysts are located in the subchondral area, suggesting the name given by these authors. They are lined by a membrane which may or may not resemble synovia and they contain a mucinous material which is quite different from the content of solitary cyst or posthematoma cyst. In two of the four cases which they reported they found communicating sinuses to the nearby joint space. These communications have been found by others.[30] A likely explanation is that a break, traumatic or otherwise, occurs in the overlying articular plate. The hydraulic pumping action of weight bearing probably forces synovial fluid through the break and into the subchondral cancellous bone tissue. The joint synovium attempts to heal this breach and itself is herniated into the bone cavity eventually lining the space. It secretes the mucinous content which characterizes the lesion.

Thus "subchondral cyst" appears to be a more accurate and appropriate name than "ganglion cyst." Though these cysts may be identical with those seen in degenerating joint disease (but not with those occurring in rheumatoid arthritis) the adjacent joint is otherwise normal.

There are but five true cysts of bone. The best known is the solitary cyst which occurs in the epiphyses of growing children. Another, rather rare, is probably related etiologically to the solitary cyst but occurs at any bone site and at any age. We have chosen to call this posthematoma cyst. The third variety, also rare, occurs in the fused epiphysis probably as a herniation of the joint cavity. The remaining two are related to the common types of arthritis, degenerative joint disease and rheumatoid arthritis. They will be described under their proper headings.

INFANTILE CORTICAL HYPEROSTOSIS (CAFFEY)

The cause of this curious disease is still equivocal. It is often placed among the inflammatory diseases of bone because it has all the clinical attributes of such, though careful search on numerous occasions for an etiologic agent has been fruitless and the disease does not respond to the usually effective anti-infection type of therapy.

Cortical hyperostosis is a disease of infants, usually making its appearance before the sixth month of life, but cases have been reported as late as a year and a half. However, cases occurring after the sixth month are so unusual that one should question the diagnosis. It runs an irregular course, often with remissions, and usually subsides within one year. Radiographic alterations almost always disappear within three years.

Caffey and Silverman described a small series of cases[32] in 1945, and provided a name for the condition. Since then it com-

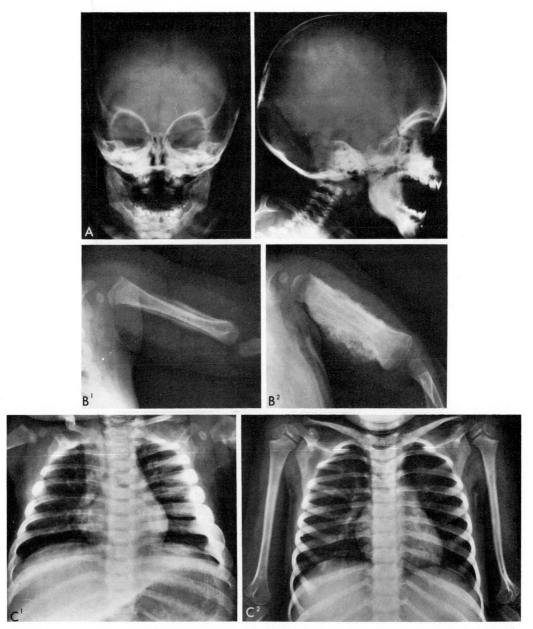

Figure 13–28 Infantile cortical hyperostosis. *A*, Abundant new bone is evident about the entire mandible. There is also prominence of the soft tissues (13 weeks of age). *B¹*, The humerus (11 weeks of age) shows new bone about the diaphysis. This progressed over the following two weeks (*B²*). *C¹*, The left ribs (3 through 8) are involved. *C²*, A radiograph exposed at the age of 3 years reveals no residual enlargement of the humerus or of the ribs.

monly has been referred to as "Caffey's disease." More than 100 cases were reported in the following decade; therefore, it is apparent that the condition is not rare.

The onset is usually suggestive of a systemic infection. There are fever, leukocytosis and an increase in the erythrocyte sedimentation rate. The child is irritable and obviously unwell. In a matter of days or weeks soft tissue swellings are noted over flat bones, particularly the mandible and clavicle, and the shafts of long bones. These masses are often firm, even brawny and obviously tender. They are not red or hot. Bone changes may be present at this time or they may be lacking but appear when the apparent acute phase of the disease is subsiding. When the swellings have disappeared the child may seem to have recovered but the same process may then recur at another site. Lesions have been described in every bone of the skeleton except the vertebrae. They are apparently rare in the small bones of the hands and feet. The serum alkaline phosphatase level is said to be elevated in most instances.

It was once thought that the mandible was always involved but it is now known that though usual it is sometimes lacking. Residual alterations in bone which remain throughout life have not been adequately emphasized.[33] Persistent facial asymmetry, synostoses between ribs, radius and ulna and tibia and fibula have been reported.

Roentgenographic Manifestations. Infantile cortical hyperostosis is manifest radiographically by marked proliferation of bone by the periosteum. The metaphyses and epiphyses of the tubular bones are spared. The periosteally produced bone surrounds the shaft and, as the process progresses, this new bone is produced in larger amounts so that its external surface may be quite coarse and irregular in outline. Early in the course of the process the underlying cortex is usually visible but later it blends with the surrounding newly formed bone. At this time, swelling of the surrounding soft tissues may be evident. The diameter of the involved bones may become quite large. When healing commences, the new bone becomes lamellated and over a period of months the bone resumes a normal contour.

In longstanding cases after remissions and exacerbations, the involved bones may show a large medullary canal and thin cortices as healing progresses. In time, however, the bone usually returns to a normal contour and the cortex becomes normally thick. Bridging between the radius and ulna, tibia and fibula and occasionally between ribs may occur when involvement is severe.

Pathology. Because infantile cortical hyperostosis is a self-limiting disease and because the diagnosis is usually made on the clinical findings and the roentgenograms, there is inadequate material for conclusive descriptions of the organic changes. There is always subperiosteal bone formation. Fine spicules of new bone

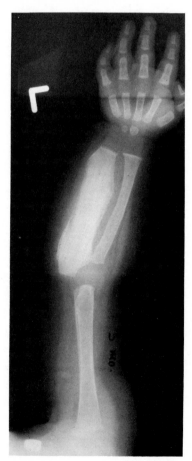

Figure 13–29 Infantile cortical hyperostosis. At 5 months of age, the diaphysis of the radius is involved in its entire length. The new bone is homogeneous in nature and smooth in outline in this instance. The metaphyses are spared.

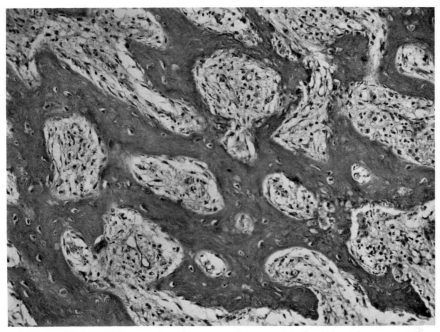

Figure 13-30   Infantile cortical hyperostosis. A section of tissue taken from the subperiosteal area of the midshaft region. This bone has been laid down by the cambium and apposed to the normal cortical surface. Between the bone spicules is a fibroblastic reaction. Note the lymphocytes scattered throughout the latter. (× 124.)

are laid down by the cambium on the outer cortical surfaces. In our limited material the arrangement is orderly, the axes of the spicules at right angles to the axis of the bone (Fig. 13–30). Several microscopists have failed to find the expected inflammatory reaction in these tissues. In at least one of our cases there were very definite aggregates of lymphocytes, which gave the impression of a low-grade chronic productive periostitis. The roentgenograms in this case were classic and the clinical course was in every way compatible with the diagnosis of cortical hyperostosis. At least one report describes degeneration and fibrosis of the overlying muscle tissue.

Several recent reports have suggested the possibility of a hereditary factor in the pathogenesis of infantile cortical hyperostosis. One of these reports 11 cases in two generations of one family.[34]

The clinical aspects of this curious disease at its outset are those of infection. Though bacterial and viral cultures have been consistently negative, it is conceivable that the lesions have not been cultured early enough. Certain it is that the earlier a lesion is biopsied the more dramatic are the inflammatory features. Hypersensitivity has been suggested as the mechanism of the recorded alterations. Though this possibility cannot be denied, the usual course of the disease with complete healing and no recurrence in later life contradicts this explanation. Though the disease may be familial there are no other hereditary features and this characteristic of the process may support the hypothesis of infection rather than genetic alteration.

The greatest difficulty in this disease is the exclusion of other entities, such as hypervitaminosis A, syphilitic periostitis, trauma and scurvy. Careful analysis of the roentgenograms and of the history is usually adequate for differentiation. The rare entities, progressive diaphyseal sclerosis (Englemann, Ribbing) may be more difficult to exclude. Indeed, there is in our files a case that was debated for months by numerous orthopedists, roentgenologists and pathologists without sufficient agreement to include it under either category.

HYPERVITAMINOSIS D

Hypervitaminosis D is a clinical entity caused by an excessive intake of vitamin D, usually D_2, resulting in a high serum calcium level and eventual deossification of the skeleton. The latter occurs usually without symptoms, but the prolonged high serum calcium level produces (1) symptoms referable to its effect on peripheral nerves, muscles, both skeletal and visceral, and probably the brain, and (2) metastatic calcification of numerous tissues, particularly the kidneys.

The term "hypervitaminosis D" is probably inexact because almost all cases reported have been due to an excess intake of vitamin D_2, though vitamin D_3 has caused the condition in infants.[35]

The disease is rarely encountered now because of the general awareness that vitamin D is a toxic agent in massive doses and because more effective therapy has been found for the conditions in which it was used. Two or three decades ago, vitamin D in daily doses of 50,000 I.U. and more was commonly used in the treatment of rheumatoid arthritis, tuberculosis, Boeck's sarcoid and certain allergic conditions. With the discovery that irradiation and electrical activation of such substances as ergosterol produced therapeutic agents of great potency, it became possible to prescribe massive doses of vitamin D at relatively small expense and inconvenience to the patient.

The variations in dosage and in the time required to produce the disease are considerable, ranging from 50,000 to one million I.U. daily and from a few days to six years.[36] Because in very few of the reports is the specific type of the offending preparation noted, it is impossible to be sure whether these variations are due to the chemical constituents of the agent or the resistance of the patient. There is some evidence to show that if a high calcium diet accompanies the excessive vitamin D dosage, the disease is brought on more rapidly. It might be presumed that if the diet contains large amounts of a chelating agent such as the phytates found in the roughage cereals, the opposite might be true.

A knowledge of this disease helps to understand the mechanisms of the action of vitamin D. The enhancement of the absorption of calcium through the gut wall is universally accepted. The action of vitamin D upon the renal tubules is still debated. The evidence garnered from study of cases of vitamin D toxicity suggests that this agent, in large doses at least, increases reabsorption of phosphates from the glomerular filtrate.

The possibility that vitamin D has a parathormone-like action directly upon the bone, causing deossification, has long been suspected. Massive doses of vitamin D in the human cause a sustained, high serum calcium level even with a low calcium intake. This seems to verify the preceding suspicion, particularly since the source of the calcium is apparently the skeleton, which synchronously undergoes demineralization.

Recently acquired data[37] are enlarging our concepts of action of vitamin D. This vitamin may be hydroxylated by the liver to form a hormone, 25-hydroxycholecalciferol (25 HCC), which acts directly upon bone to release mineral salts. It in turn may be further hydrolysed by the kidney to produce a second hormone, 1,25-dihydroxycholecalciferol, which is probably necessary for calcium ion transport across the gut wall. Its mechanism for the promotion of kidney phosphate conservation, if such it has, is still unknown.

The symptoms of an abnormally high serum calcium content are much the same as those in hyperparathyroidism and the latter condition is the most difficult to differentiate. The sense of profound fatigue and weakness is often the first to manifest itself and probably reflects the action of calcium ions upon the peripheral nerves and myoneural junctions. The diarrhea, abdominal pain, anorexia, nausea, vomiting and eventual weight loss are doubtless due to comparable effects on the smooth muscle of the gastrointestinal tract. Paresthesias are sometimes encountered. The mental depression, psychoses, headache and vertigo may be the direct effects of the excessive calcium in the fluid that perfuses the nerve cells of the central nervous system, or they may be caused by the cerebral edema that has been reported in hypercalcemia. The altered electrocardiogram, with a shortened QT interval, also may be a neuromuscular phenomenon.

Metastatic deposits of calcium salts

within collagen are particularly common in hypervitaminosis D. This incidence is presumably the consequence of the combined high levels of both calcium and phosphorus. It is found in hyperparathyroidism also but less constantly, perhaps because here there is a parathormone action upon the renal tubules, which causes a phosphorus diuresis, thus maintaining a normal or low serum phosphorus content. In vitamin D poisoning, calcium deposits have been reported in almost every conceivable area including the corneas, meninges, skin, capsules of joints and bursas, tendon sheaths, blood vessels, gastric mucosa, heart, lungs, thyroid, pancreas and kidneys.[38] Deposits in the skin may give rise to pruritus, in the cornea to a "band keratitis."

Nephrocalcinosis is the most important sequel of the disease because it may lead to permanent kidney damage, uremia and eventual death. The evidences of kidney insufficiency are found in rising nonprotein nitrogen and albumin levels, casts and red cells in the urine. The specific gravity remains low. Polydypsia and polyuria have been severe enough to arouse the suspicion of diabetes insipidus. Eventually, there is a normocytic, normochromic anemia.

The calcific deposits in the periarticular tissues are considered characteristic though they have been reported in the various types of hyperparathyroidism. The joint capsules, tendon sheaths and bursas are particularly prone to calcification. Because most cases of vitamin D toxicity have occurred in treatment of rheumatoid arthritis, the question is pertinent whether the regional selectivity involving the joints may be due to the changes in the collagen incident to the disease being treated. These masses of calcium may be very large, measuring up to 10 cm. in diameter. When opened, they are found to contain a pale grumous material like that found in gout, or they may be cystic and contain a fluid that closely resembles milk. The calcium salt deposits have been of particular interest to the roentgenologist.

The skeletal demineralization that occurs is generalized, resembling that of osteopenia. In early or mild cases this change may not appear. In some instances focal areas of bone destruction have oc-

curred, but it is likely that this finding was the result of the disease that was being treated and not of the action of vitamin D. The occurrence of deossification strongly suggests a direct action of vitamin D upon the bone, because the parathyroid glands are not involved and the high serum calcium level forestalls any need for withdrawal of the calcium stores.

Chemical evaluation of the serum is most helpful in hypervitaminosis D. The calcium content should be above 12 mg. per 100 ml. and has been reported as high as 16. The phosphorus is often normal but is more apt to be slightly elevated. The serum alkaline phosphatase is usually high normal or slightly raised, depending upon the stage of activity and degree of severity of the disease. The phosphorus level may be particularly helpful because usually the most difficult differential problem is hyperparathyroidism, which should produce a low normal or subnormal level.

Other differential possibilities are nephritis, diffuse bone tumor (myeloma) or neoplastic bone metastasis, myelogenous leukemia, osteoporosis and less commonly certain cases of osteopetrosis. All of these except nephritis should have accompanying signs and symptoms that are foreign to vitamin D toxicity. An accurate history with specific questioning concerning the taking of vitamin D is, of course, of the greatest help. It is not enough to know that the patient is not taking vitamin D at the moment. Cases have been reported in which termination of therapy had occurred as long as two months before the patient presented himself for diagnosis.

Roentgenographic Manifestations. The radiographic manifestations of hypervitaminosis D in the adult are those of demineralization of skeletal structures, focal or diffuse, and soft tissue calcification. Because the demineralization produces the picture of osteopenia and because osteopenia of disuse may result from the disease for which vitamin D was administered, this manifestation may be difficult to appreciate except in cases which are focal. The soft tissue calcification may present as periarticular, irregular masses of opaque material. Joint capsules or vessels may be visible by virtue of calcification. Renal calcification is often evident.

In contrast, the radiographic manifesta-

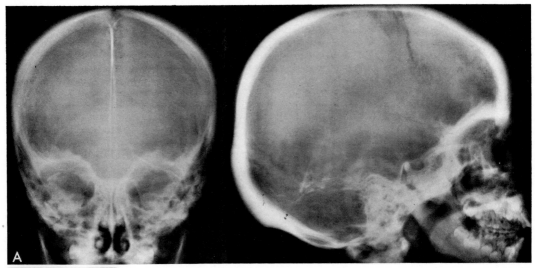

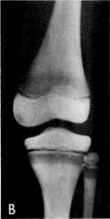

Figure 13–31 Hypervitaminosis D. The cranial bones are thick and opaque; there is extensive calcification of the falx and the tentorium (*A*). Radiolucent zones are present across the metaphyses of the bones of the knee (*B*); these are symmetric.

tions of excessive vitamin D intake during childhood consist of an increase in the opacity of skeletal structures except for symmetrical areas of radiolucency adjacent to the zone of provisional calcification. The epiphyseal centers may be ringed by a dense opaque band and the bones of the skull may be more opaque than the normal. Calcification of soft tissues, such as the kidneys, falx cerebri and tentorium, may be seen. In cases in which renal damage occurs, renal osteodystrophy may complicate the total picture.

Microscopy. Nothing is known of the microscopic appearance of the bone in hypervitaminosis D. The so-called "calcium cysts" have been removed surgically and examined. The masses of calcium salts apparently cause tissue necrosis. The area may break down and liquefy, producing a milklike fluid, or it may remain as an inspissated, chalky mass that is positive with the calcium stain. There is a stimulation of a fibrous reaction around the calcium deposits to form a heavy, collagenous capsule. There is usually a giant cell foreign body reaction in this capsule and in contiguous tissues.

Prognosis. The condition is treated by withdrawing vitamin D and placing the patient on a low calcium, high fluid diet. There is a gradual but progressive dissolution of the calcified areas, though if they are massive they may not completely disappear. Cases of well defined kidney insufficiency have been reported to recover normal function over a period of months on this regimen.

IDIOPATHIC HYPERCALCEMIA

Reports of a condition, called in Great Britain "idiopathic hypercalcemia," began to appear in 1951. In the mild form the patients were all less than 11 months of age. There was sudden onset of anorexia, vomiting, polydipsia, hypotonia, pruritus, constipation and dehydration. The level of serum calcium was 12 mg. or above, often in the range of 15 or 16, and the level of serum phosphorus was normal or slightly elevated. Some cases progressed to manifest hematuria, casts and azotemia. It was soon realized that this was the acute form of cases with the following symptomatology: falling hair, fissuring of the lips, unremitting pruritus, thick sagging lips, arrested cerebral development, depressed nasal bridge and a curious facies that was called the "elfin face." These children had constantly elevated serum calcium levels and roentgenograms revealed an increased density of their skeletons, particularly the bones of the face. Mental deterioration progressed to idiocy and the patients developed chronic uremia due to nephrocalcinosis.

The histories of a few of these patients showed that they had ingested large amounts of vitamin D. It was assumed that these were cases of vitamin D poisoning and that those who gave no history of excessive intake were hyper-responsive to the drug in normal doses. This hypothesis may account for a few of the cases but a more plausible explanation comes from a more critical analysis of the total diets of these children.[39] Today, vitamin D is added to many products, especially canned milk and flour. These additions have in the past been less carefully controlled in Great Britain than in the United States. The incidence of idiopathic hypercalcemia has been considerably greater in England than in this country. Recently, the British have limited the use of vitamin D in foodstuffs and the incidence of the disease has fallen dramatically. Formerly it was thought that 25,000 units per day was necessary to induce symptoms of toxicity, but today it is known that vitamin D poisoning may be induced by much smaller amounts, probably in the range of 4000 to 5000 units. These amounts may be attained by children, who drink more milk than adults.

Roentgenographic Manifestations. The radiographic manifestations of idiopathic hypercalcemia parallel those of hypervitaminosis D and consist of opacity of the skeletal structures and soft tissue calcification. The cranial bones, particularly those at the base of the skull and those of the orbits, are opaque and thick. In our experience, thickening of the bones of the orbits reduced the size of the optic foramina to cause optic atrophy in one pa-

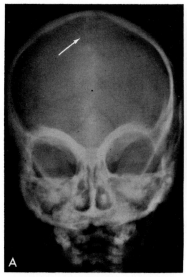
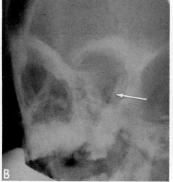
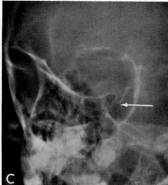

Figure 13-32 Idiopathic hypercalcemia. The bones of the skull, particularly those of the orbits and at the base, are thick and opaque (A). Calcification of the falx (arrow) is evident. Optic atrophy was present and the small, deformed optic foramen (arrow, B) may be compared with one of normal size (arrow, C).

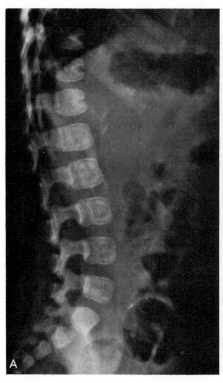
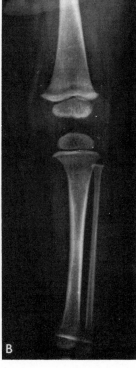

Figure 13–33 Idiopathic hypercalcemia. Opaque lines within the vertebral bodies parallel the cortex (*A*). The zones of provisional calcification are thick and opaque and are paralleled by bands of radiolucency and opacity. There is failure of modeling of the long bones (*B*).

tient (Fig. 13–32). In the long bones there is failure of normal modeling so that the metaphyses are wide. The zone of provisional calcification is thick and dense, and alternating bands of radiolucency and opacity are apparent across the metaphysis. Similar bands are found in the vertebral bodies and epiphyseal centers. Most of the opacity of the long bones is secondary to thickening of trabeculae, not of the cortex; at times this may not be a prominent feature, depending on the degree of hypotonia and hence disuse osteopenia that results.

Calcification may be demonstrated in the kidneys, meninges, brain and blood vessels.

The osseous changes may not be apparent during the first months of life, but appear over a period of time. As the disease progresses there may be early closure of the cranial sutures, particularly the sagittal suture.

Therapy. Treatment is based on withdrawing vitamin D therapy and all foodstuffs containing vitamin D and lowering the calcium content of the diet. Even thus

treated it may take several weeks for the serum calcium level to fall, and to avoid nephrocalcinosis cortisone may be used to bring the level to normal more quickly.

HYPERVITAMINOSIS A

Hypervitaminosis A, almost always caused by taking excessive amounts of certain proprietary agents, is manifested by changes in the skin and mucous membranes, the skeleton and the central nervous system. Acute and chronic forms have been reported in both children and adults. Because the bone changes are similar to those of infantile cortical hyperostosis (Caffey included two cases of hypervitaminosis A in his early series of cortical hyperostosis), a discussion of the subject is germane to the consideration of orthopedic pathology.

We are indebted to the studies of Wolbach[42] for our knowledge of the action and mechanisms of vitamin A in the growth of bone in the experimental animal. He showed that this substance is necessary for the normal replication, growth and maturation of the epiphyseal chondroblasts and, therefore, plays an important role in enchondral bone growth. He believed that vitamin A is also a factor in the modeling of bone, stimulating osteoclastic activity in areas in which changes in conformation of bone mass are taking place. We know that certain amounts of this vitamin are necessary for normal epithelium and for optimal growth,[43] and to prevent night blindness. Apparently there are no toxic effects as long as ingestion is limited to the carotinoids. It is unknown whether a deficiency affects the growth of bone. It is apparent, however, that an excess of vitamin A causes an abnormal subperiosteal bone proliferation, one of the principal findings in chronic vitamin A toxicity. Abnormalities of the growth plate and shortening of long bones have been reported following prolonged ingestion of massive doses of this vitamin.[43a]

Arctic explorers have known for nearly a century that the liver of the polar bear contains a toxic substance which, when eaten, induces an acute episode of headache, nausea, vomiting, dizziness and drowsiness. In 1943, it was shown that the substance in the liver responsible for these symptoms is vitamin A, concentrated to the extent of 18,000 U. per gram.[44] In 1944, Josephs[45] reported a case of hypervitaminosis A in a child. Following this, numerous cases in children have been reported, including a series of five by Caffey[46] and an extraordinary case in an adult reported in 1954.[47]

Chronic hypervitaminosis A has been reported most commonly in children between the ages of 1 and 3 years, a period in which they are dosed with vitamins and in which less attention is paid to the exact measurement. It has not been reported in infants under 1 year, probably because the infant does not absorb the oily medium as efficiently and because some time must elapse to establish high storage levels and to develop the symptoms. Acute hypervitaminosis A may occur at any age from the ingestion of a million or more units. Frontal headaches, bulging fontanelles in infants and drowsiness indicate the sudden increase in intracranial pressure. Desquamation may begin within 36 hours and becomes severe. There are no changes in the bones.

Chronic hypervitaminosis A begins with anorexia, weight loss and finally causes nausea and vomiting. There are numerous signs and symptoms referable to the nervous system, most of which can be accounted for on the basis of an elevated intracranial pressure due to an increase in the amount of cerebrospinal fluid. It is not known whether this increase is due to an excessive formation or a decreased absorption. Headache appears early and is severe. Irritability, dizziness, fatigue and insomnia have been reported. Signs referable to the eyes are exophthalmos, strabismus, nystagmus and papilledema.

The skin becomes dry and there is a furfuraceous desquamation. Eventually the palms may become thickened, cracked and scaly. Pruritus may be a troublesome feature. The mucous membranes are dry and fissures appear in the lips. The hair becomes dry and coarse and there is epilation of both scalp and body areas, including the eyebrows and the lanugo.

Bone pain is a constant finding in chronic hypervitaminosis A. This has been severe enough to cause complete invalidism. Firm tumefactions may be noted over the midshaft regions of the long bones and ribs. Almost any bone may be affected though there are no reports of involvement of the mandible. Roentgenograms reveal a subperiosteal proliferation of bone, which is thickest in the center of the diaphysis and fades off toward the epiphysis, giving the shaft a fusiform shape. The metatarsals and the ulna are the bones most commonly reported affected.

The serum calcium and phosphorus levels are normal. The serum alkaline phosphatase level may be moderately elevated. The serum vitamin A and carotene levels must be high to confirm the diagnosis.

Because of the roentgenograms these cases are frequently misdiagnosed as cortical hyperostosis. Caffey[46] notes the following distinguishing features. In cortical hyperostosis the onset is within the first six months of life, there is accompanying fever, the radiographic outline of the lesion is more irregular, lesions of the jaw are usual and in the metatarsals rare;

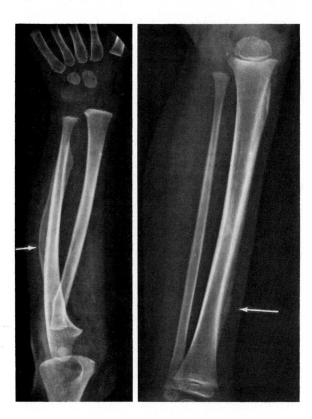

Figure 13–34 Hypervitaminosis A. Areas of wavy cortical thickening involve the ulna and the tibia (arrows).

there are no accompanying signs of skin and central nervous system involvement. When the intake of vitamin A is such that longitudinal growth is affected, the most involved area is the bones at the knee. Here, cupping of the metaphysis with narrowing of the growth plate occurs. This latter may mimic the long-term effect of infection or trauma in the same area.[47a]

The most helpful finding is, of course, a history of excessive vitamin A ingestion. It is usually taken in the form of one of the proprietary agents such as oleum percomorphum. Because the concentrations are high, large doses may be taken in a relatively small amount of medium. These accidents usually occur because the patient or his parents have not been instructed that overdosage with vitamin A can result in a state of toxicity.

Microscopy. Very little is known of the tissue changes that are produced by hypervitaminosis A. Biopsies of the skin and bone were made in the adult case reported by Gerber, Raab and Sobel.[47] The skin showed hyperkeratosis and parakeratosis.

There was appositional new bone formation by the periosteum.

Prognosis. The treatment for hypervitaminosis A is withdrawal of the causative agent. When this is done, the bone pain is relieved within a week and the patient becomes asymptomatic in about a month. The roentgenographic changes fade more slowly but in children the skeleton resumes a normal appearance within a year.

URTICARIA PIGMENTOSA

In 1952, Sagher, Cohen and Schorr[48] reported the association of urticaria pigmentosa and areas of osteosclerosis of a variety of bones. Jensen and Lasser[49] have more recently reported the seventh instance of such association and today most radiology clinics recognize and look for bone involvement in adult cases of this disease.[50]

Urticaria pigmentosa is a systemic disease characterized by macular or nodular areas of pigmentation in the skin, enlarged liver, spleen and lymph nodes, and pancytopenia of the peripheral blood. Diffuse (macular) or focal (nodular) masses of mast cells are found in the skin. Stroking these areas with a blunt instrument initiates the appearance of urticaria, presumably due to the release of histamine from the mast cells. The pigmented areas are produced by an increase in the melanin in the basal epidermal layer over the lesions.

Diffuse or focal areas of radiopacity occur in both flat and long bones. This has been described as a ground glass appearance and as an increased trabecular prominence. Cortical thickening and stippling have also been described. The mechanism of the osteosclerosis is unknown.

Radiographically, the lesions of urticaria pigmentosa in bone may be of two types, destructive or productive. The radiolucent lesions of bone destruction represent areas in which the accumulations of mast cells have resulted in disappearance of trabeculae. These lesions may be circumscribed or diffuse. When the lesion is diffuse, the trabecular pattern of the spongiosa appears coarse. The nature of the formation of new bone is not understood, but new bone production is manifest by thickening of trabeculae, thickening of the cortex or localized areas of sclerosis within the spongiosa.

In a review by Poppel et al.[51] the bulk of the osseous abnormalities was found in the long bones in children and in the skull, ribs, spine and pelvis in adults. This distribution parallels the position of the active marrow and reticuloendothelial system in the two age groups.

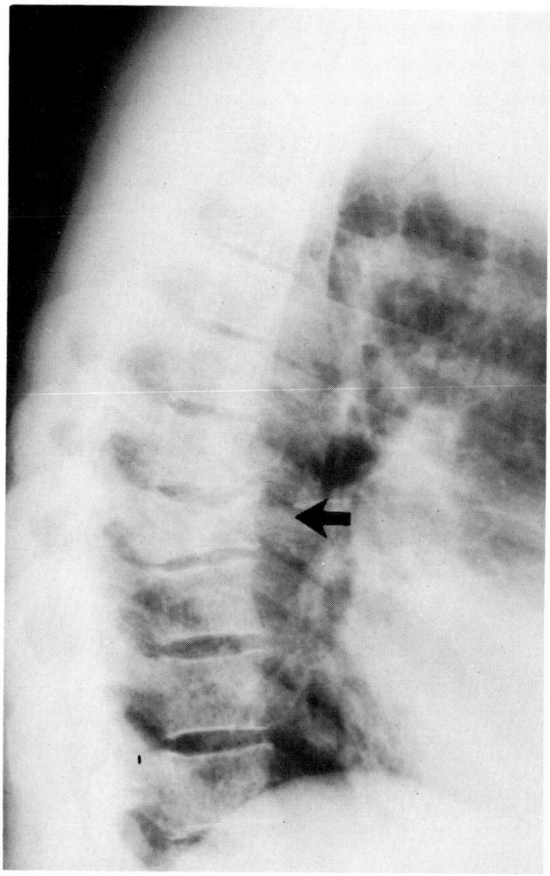

Figure 13–35   Mast cell disease. The lower dorsal vertebrae are osteopenic with tiny sclerotic areas (trabeculae?). There is loss of stature of one vertebral body (arrow).

CHROMOSOMAL ABNORMALITIES

The normal human cell contains 22 pairs of somatic chromosomes and two sex chromsomes, a total number of 46. The sex chromosomes are identified as XX, female, and XY, male. In order to identify the chromosomal pattern or the karyotype, it is necessary to prepare a culture of cells, to stop mitosis when the cells are in metaphase, to separate the chromosomes, to photograph the preparation (Fig. 13–36), and finally to pair and arrange the chromosomes into their respective groups. The grouping is according to the length of the chromosome and the position of the centromere. The usual grouping is as follows: Group A (1 to 3), Group B (4 to 5), Group C (6 to 12), Group D (13 to 15), Group E (16 to 18), Group F (19 to 20) and Group G (21 to 22) and the sex chromosomes XX or XY (Figs. 13–37 and 13–38).

Only gross chromosomal abnormalities are noted by examination of the karyotype. One looks for abnormalities in number or structure of chromosomes. In the autosomal trisomy syndromes that have been recognized, there is an extra chromosome related to either the 13 to 15, 16 to 18, or 21 to 22 groups. In these instances the total number of chromosomes is 47.[52, 53] In syndromes related to abnormalities of the sex chromosomes, one finds a normal

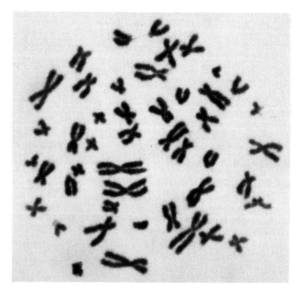

Figure 13–36   Preparation of chromosomes before grouping and arrangement of karyotype.

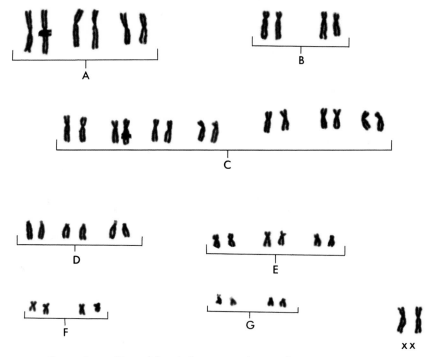

Figure 13–37   Normal female karyotype; the sex chromosomes are XX.

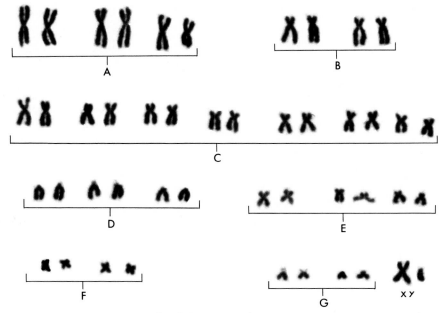

Figure 13–38   Normal male karyotype; the sex chromosomes are XY.

number of autosomal chromosomes but an absent X or extra X or Y chromosome.[54]

TURNER'S SYNDROME

A syndrome in females characterized by sexual infantilism, short stature, webbed neck and cubitus valgus was described by Turner in 1938. It has been determined in recent years that most patients lack sex chromatin material in their nuclei (Barr body). The karyotype of such a patient reveals a total number of 45 chromosomes of which there are 44 autosomes and only one sex chromosome.

There is gonadal aplasia, the "ovary" being only a primitive streak in the broad ligament. In addition to the clinical findings, there is primary amenorrhea and in some patients, hypertension and coarctation of the aorta.

Radiographically, the principal features are found in the hands and wrists, knees and spine (Fig. 13–39). The fourth metacarpal is apt to be short so that a line tangent to the ends of the fifth and fourth metacarpals impinges upon the distal end of the third metacarpal (metacarpal sign). The carpal angle is more acute than in the normal individual. At the knee, there is enlargement of the medial femoral condyle with flattening of the opposing tibial plateau. The medial aspect of the proximal epiphysis and metaphysis of the tibia is deformed. There may be a second center of ossification adjacent to the flattened medial aspect of the metaphysis so that with growth, the epiphysis appears to overhang the medial aspect of the metaphysis. This latter configuration bears some resemblance to the deformity associated with Blount's disease. In the spine, scoliosis may be present. There is often hypoplasia of the posterior arch of C_1.[54]

KLINEFELTER'S SYNDROME

This syndrome is characterized by primary hypogonadism and an abnormal complement of sex chromosomes, XXY. The physiognomy is male. In addition, the testes are small, gynecomastia is evident in adolescence, eunuchoidism may be present and most patients are sterile. By puberty, the level of urinary gonadotropins is elevated.

Skeletal abnormalities are inconstant; a

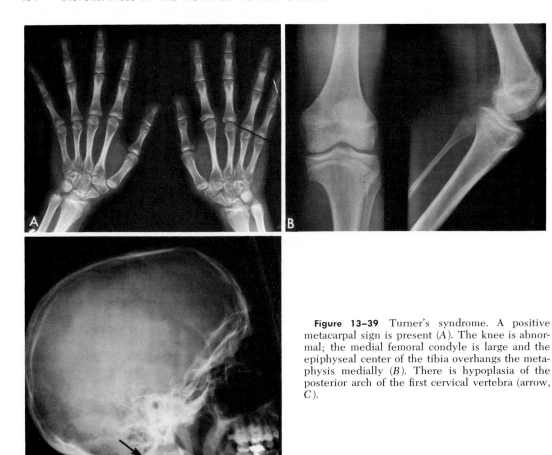

Figure 13-39 Turner's syndrome. A positive metacarpal sign is present (*A*). The knee is abnormal; the medial femoral condyle is large and the epiphyseal center of the tibia overhangs the metaphysis medially (*B*). There is hypoplasia of the posterior arch of the first cervical vertebra (arrow, *C*).

short fourth metacarpal has been noted in some patients. However, there are patients with this syndrome in whom there are even additional X chromosomes, e.g., XXXXY. In these individuals, skeletal abnormalities are apt to be present and include scoliosis, radioulnar synostosis and short upper extremities.[55]

AUTOSOMAL TRISOMY SYNDROMES

Mongolism or Down's syndrome — trisomy 21 — is the most commonly encountered of the trisomy syndromes. There is an extra G chromosome. A variety of skeletal abnormalities have been described, the most consistent being the configuration of the pelvis during the first year of life as described by Caffey and Ross.[56] The iliac bones flare laterally and the osseous roof of the acetabulum is flatter than normal (Fig. 13-40). These abnormalities can be quantitated by determination of the acetabular and iliac angles as well as the iliac index. The iliac index is the sum of the two iliac angles and the two acetabular angles divided by 2. In general one finds these angles to measure less than normal but to have a range that overlaps the normal. For example, the acetabular angle varies from 7 to 25 degrees with an average of 16 degrees as compared to the normal range of 12 to 37 degrees with an average of 28 degrees.

Near the end of the first year of life, the ischia become noticeably elongate. At about the same time, one begins to note valgus deformity of the proximal femurs.

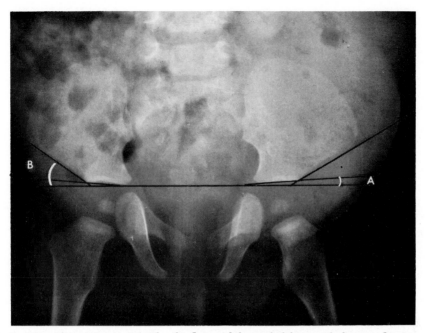

Figure 13–40   Mongolism (trisomy 21). The ilia flare and the roof of the acetabulum are flat. Lines are drawn to demonstrate the acetabular (A) and the iliac (B) angles. The ischia are slender and elongate.

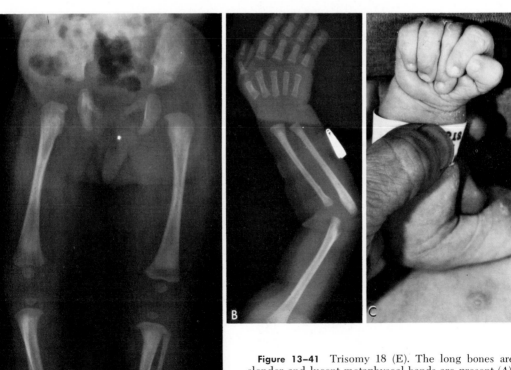

Figure 13–41   Trisomy 18 (E). The long bones are slender and lucent metaphyseal bands are present (A). There is ulnar deviation of the fingers (B). The second finger overlaps the third (C), a characteristic clinical finding.

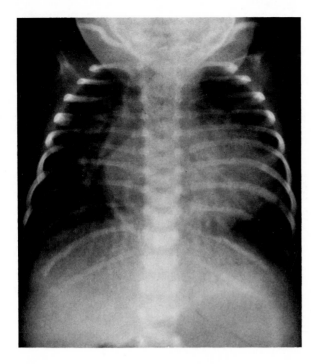

Figure 13–42   Trisomy 18 (D). The heart is enlarged; there is evidence of a shunt to the lungs. The ribs are slender; there are 11 pairs of ribs.

Hypoplasia of the middle phalanx of the fifth finger is not uncommon. The lumbar vertebral bodies tend to be square rather than rectangular in shape as seen in the lateral roentgenogram of the area. Two centers of ossification in the manubrium are more common in this group of patients than in the normal population. There may be 11 pairs of ribs. Congenital heart disease is common, particularly defects of the interventricular and interatrial septa. In the skull the base is short, there is delayed development of the paranasal sinuses and the nasal bone is small.

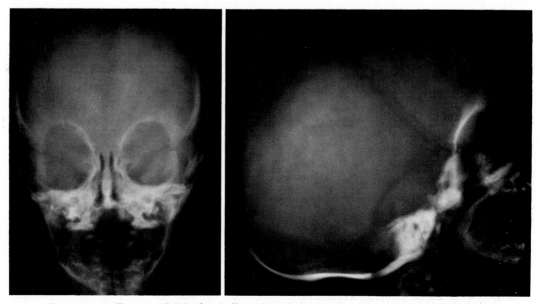

Figure 13–43   Trisomy 18 (E). The skull is relatively long and narrow; the mandible is small.

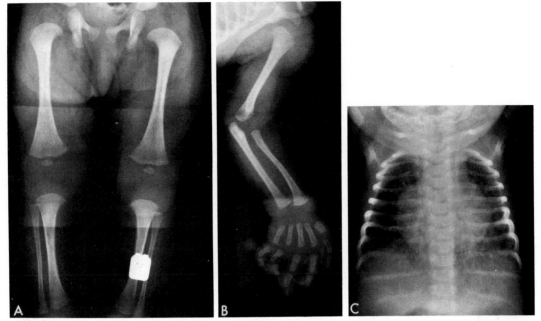

Figure 13–44   Trisomy 13–15 (D). The long bones are relatively normal (A). Polydactyly is present as well as flexion deformities of the fingers (B). There are 11 pairs of ribs. The heart is enlarged and there is a shunt to the lungs (C).

The trisomy 18 syndrome is characterized by an extra E chromosome, the total number of chromosomes being 47. These patients usually die in infancy. No radiographic findings are diagnostic of this syndrome; however there are features that are commonly encountered. Clinically there is a curious flexion deformity of the fingers in which there is overlapping of the second digit on the third and ulnar deviation of the fingers (Fig. 13–41). Rocker bottom feet are common. The long bones may be slender and often show metaphyseal alterations associated with stress. The ilia appear narrow in the anteroposterior projection; the acetabula are normal. The ribs are slender and the sternum is often hypoplastic. Congenital heart disease is frequent. The skull tends to be long and narrow and the mandible hypoplastic.

The trisomy 13–15 syndrome is characterized by an extra D chromosome. As in the other trisomies, the total number of chromosomes is 47. There are fewer osseous abnormalities in this group of patients as compared to the others. Polydactyly and flexion contractures of the hands are common (Fig. 13–44). The long bones tend to

be normal; 11 pairs of ribs are commonly encountered. The pelvis may have a mongoloid configuration. There is apt to be congenital heart disease, particularly intracardiac shunts and patent ductus arteriosus. Clinically, ocular defects such as coloboma, cataracts and microphthalmia are very frequent and should alert one to the presence of this trisomy.

References

PAGET'S DISEASE

1. Paget, J.: Trans. Roy. Med. Chir. Soc. London, 60:37, 1877.
2. Van Buchem, F., Hadders, H., Hansen, J. and Woldring, M.: Am. J. Med., 23:387, 1962.
3. Schmorl, G.: Virchows Arch. path. Anat., 283:694, 1932.
4. Wycis, H. T.: J. Neurosurg., 1:299, 1944.
5. Sornberger, C. F. and Smedal, M. I.: Circulation, 6:711, 1952.
6. Edholm, O. G., Howard, S. and MacMichael, J.: Clin. Sc., 5:249, 1945.
7. Henneman, P.: Trans. Stud. Coll. Physicians Phila., 31:10, 1945.
8. Jaffe, H. L.: Arch. Pathol., 15:83, 1933.
9. Haddad, J., Berge, S. and Avioli, L.: N. Engl. J. Med., 283:549, 1970.
10. Ryan, W. and Schwartz, T.: Ann. Intern. Med., 74:824, 1971.

EPIPHYSIOLYSIS

11. Key, J. A.: J. Bone Joint Surg., 8:53, 1926.
12. Howorth, M. B.: J. Bone Joint Surg., 31A:734, 1949.
13. Shea, D. and Mankin, H.: J. Bone Joint Surg., 48A:349, 1966.
14. Bean, W. B. and Ponseti, I. V.: Circulation, 12: 185, 1955.

ANEURYSMAL BONE CYST

15. Jaffe, H. L. and Lichtenstein, L.: Arch. Surg., 44:1021, 1942.
16. Lichtenstein, L.: Cancer, 3:279, 1950.
17. Jaffe, H.: Bull. Hosp. Joint Dis., 11:3, 1950.
18. Dahlin, D. C., Besse, B. E., Pugh, D. G. and Ghormley, R. K.: Radiology, 64:56, 1955.
19. Sherman, R. S. and Soong, K. Y.: Radiology, 68:54, 1957.
20. Lindbom, A., Soderberg, G., Spjut, H. and Sunnquist, O.: Acta Radiol., 55:12, 1961.
21. Tillman, B., Dahlin, D., Lipscomb, P. and Stewart, J.: Mayo Clin. Proc., 43:478, 1968.
22. Biesecker, J., Marcove, R., Huvos, A. and Miké, V.: Cancer, 26:615, 1970.
23. Dabska, M. and Buraczewski, J.: Cancer, 23:371, 1969.
24. Nobler, M., Higinbotham, N. and Phillips, R.: Radiology, 90:1185, 1968.

SOLITARY CYST OF BONE

25. Bloodgood, J. C.: Ann. Surg., 52:145, 1910.
26. Jaffe, H. and Lichtenstein, L.: Arch. Surg., 44: 1004, 1942.
27. Sim, F. and Dahlin, D.: Mayo Clin. Proc., 46:484, 1971.
28. Baker, D.: Clin. Orthop., 71:140, 1970.

SUBCHONDRAL CYSTS

29. Nigrisoli, P. and Beltrami, P.: Lo Scalpello, 1:65, 1972.
30. Crane, A. and Scarano, J.: J. Bone Joint Surg., 49A:355, 1967.
31. Hicks, J.: Aust. N.Z. J. Surg., 26:138, 1956.

INFANTILE CORTICAL HYPEROSTOSIS

32. Caffey, J. and Silverman, W.: Am. J. Roentgenol., 54:1, 1945.
33. Staheli, L., Church, C. and Ward, B.: J.A.M.A., 203:96, 1968.

34. Tampus, J., Van Buskirk, F., Peterson, O. and Soule, A.: J.A.M.A., 175:491, 1961.

HYPERVITAMINOSIS D

35. Christensen, W. R., Liebman, C. and Sosman, M. C.: Am. J. Roentgenol., 65:27, 1951.
36. Chaplin, H., Clark, L. D. and Ropes, M. W.: Am. J. Med. Sci., 221:369, 1951.
37. DeLuca, H.: Trans. Stud. Coll. Physicians Phila., 39:1, 1971.
38. Adams, F. D.: N. Engl. J. Med., 244:590, 1951.

IDIOPATHIC HYPERCALCEMIA

39. Fraser, D.: J.A.M.A., 176:281, 1961.
40. Shiers, J. A., Neuhauser, E. B. D. and Bowman, J. R.: Am. J. Roentgenol., 78:19, 1957.
41. Singleton, E.: Radiology, 68:721, 1957.

HYPERVITAMINOSIS A

42. Wolbach, S. B.: J. Bone Joint Surg., 29:171, 1947.
43. Yaffe, S. and Filar, L.: Pediatrics, 48:655, 1971.
43a. Peace, C. N.: J.A.M.A., 182:980, 1962.
44. Rodahl, K. and Moore, T.: Biochem. J., 37:166, 1943.
45. Josephs, H. W.: Am. J. Dis. Child., 67:33, 1944.
46. Caffey, J.: Am. J. Roentgenol., 65:12, 1951.
47. Gerber, A., Raab, A. P. and Sobel, A. E.: Am. J. Med., 16:729, 1954.
47a. Caffey, J.: Am. J. Roentgenol., 108:451, 1970.

URTICARIA PIGMENTOSA

48. Sagher, F., Cohen, C. and Schorr, S.: J. Invest. Dermatol., 18:425, 1952.
49. Jensen, W. and Lasser, E.: Radiology, 71:826, 1958.
50. Klaus, S. and Winkelmann, R.: Mayo Clin. Proc., 40:923, 1965.
51. Poppel, M. H., Gruber, W. F., Silber, R., Holder, A. K. and Christman, R. D.: Am. J. Roentgenol., 82:239, 1959.

CHROMOSOMAL ABNORMALITIES

52. Singleton, E. B., Rosenberg, H. S. and Yang, S. J.: Radiol. Clin. North Am., 2:297, 1964.
53. Warkany, J., Passarge, E. and Smith, L. B.: Am. J. Dis. Child., 112:592, 1966.
54. Keats, T. E. and Burns, T. W.: Radiol. Clin. North Am., 2:297, 1964.
55. Nelson, W. E.: Textbook of Pediatrics. Ed. 9. Philadelphia, W. B. Saunders Co., 1969.
56. Caffey, J. and Ross, S.: Pediatrics, 17:642, 1956.

TUMORS AND TUMOR-LIKE PROCESSES

Chapter 14

GENERAL CONSIDERATION
OF TUMORS

The most important section in orthopedic pathology is that dealing with tumors. The incidence of primary bone tumors does not compare with that of the carcinomas of the breast, cervix, lung and stomach, yet, excluding the leukemias and lymphomas, the primary bone tumors constitute the most important single group in patients under the age of 20 years.

Also, a thorough knowledge of the primary bone tumors is absolutely essential because the differential diagnosis arises in practically all lesions that cause focal bone destruction. Because the malignant bone tumors must be treated radically, often necessitating amputation, it is paramount that the diagnosis be made early and correctly in order that the patient may have the maximal chance for survival in the case of tumor and in order that a needless sacrifice of a part be avoided in non-neoplastic lesions.

The number of entities usually classified under the heading of bone tumors is uncommonly large. The most valuable asset in consistent diagnostic accuracy is a thorough knowledge of the possibilities. Thus, every clinician, radiologist and pathologist must be familiar with this rather formidable array of lesions and their features that apply particularly to the specialty. The following discussion is a general survey of the entire field including a classification. Following this survey each of the cytogenic groups will be considered in greater detail.

The term "primary bone tumor" cannot be satisfactorily defined at present because as yet we cannot define either a tumor or the various so-called types, benign and malignant. At best we can only say that a primary bone tumor is one that arises in one of the various tissues that compose the skeleton. But the definition is not strictly accurate because we include the myelomas as bone tumors and do not include the leukemias, which may form tumor masses within the marrow tissue. The definition of tumor is even less informative. In the name of accuracy the word "neoplasm" has been suggested to separate the true tumors from inflammatory and traumatic masses. The substitution does not materially ease the dilemma because no one has been able to define neoplasm satisfactorily.

To shorten a discourse in semantics one may say there are three types of new growth. We may have an excessive reparative proliferation of cells that ultimately mature, as exemplified by the keloid. This group of lesions we may designate as A—the reactive processes. Or we may have a "spontaneous" proliferation of cells in which maturation is incomplete at the time of observation. Such is the nature of the lesions that we call fibroma, the desmoids and fibromatoses. These appear to have the capacity to invade their surrounding tissues, but this appearance is probably deceiving. It is less invasive than an involvement of the collagenous supportive tissues that are indigenous to the affected tissues. In cases in which this process involves cartilage we call the lesion enchondroma. In cases in which it involves enchondral bone formation the product is known as osteochondroma. This entire group we designate as B—the hamartomas. Finally, there is the nonmaturing hyperplasia of cells that not only invade but also have the ability to set up independent growth, metastases. The inability of a group of cells to achieve maturity probably implies progression. A progressive hyperplasia is one that proceeds, though not necessarily at a constant rate, until intervention by some agent whether it be surgery, irradiation, chemotherapy or, in rare instances, alteration of the blood supply. This last group obviously falls in the category C—neoplasia.

The progressive, invading, metastasizing hyperplasia is obviously a true tumor, or neoplasm. How far one may extend this category to the non-invading or even nonprogressive groups depends upon the inclination of the writer. We choose to include in the category of neoplasm only lesions that are at least progressive, believing that our knowledge of the etiology of malignant tumors implies that the hereditary pattern of a cancer cell has been changed unalterably, causing it to reproduce before it reaches maturity, thus setting up an endless chain of reproduction —progressiveness. Those spontaneous growths that produce an excessive number of cells beyond the normal, which cells reach maturity and cease to reproduce except for the normal replacement caused by necrobiosis, are called hamartomas. Hamartomas exceed the normal limits of growth but eventually cease growing because their cells mature. A true tumor has the potential of infinite growth as long as its host can supply it nourishment. In short, it is progressive.

The criteria for judging a group of cells maglignant are still more nebulous. All microscopists agree that increased nuclear-cytoplasmic ratio, irregularity of nuclear border, excess chromatin particularly if it is found in rough aggregates, the prominence of the nucleolus and an increase in mitotic figures are features that accompany malignant behavior. Yet every experienced microscopist has found some or all of these features in normal, young, rapidly growing cells whose growth has been altered by inflammation, environment or change in blood supply. This constitutes the greatest hazard for the orthopedic pathologist who at times must judge a lesion on the basis of the microscopic sections alone, because injury and repair in skeletal tissues may mimic every feature of malignant tumor.

The line that separates malignant from benign tumors, if it exists, is especially vague. The microscopy of a tumor is immensely helpful in this respect but it must be admitted that all the morphologic features of malignancy may be found in tumors that do not metastasize and in a few that are non-invasive. There is a modern school that is of the opinion that all true tumors are malignant, though demonstrating variable degrees of malignancy, and that there is no such thing as a benign tumor. The latter they would classify as hamartomas, choristomas or simply hyperplasias of known or unknown etiology such as the viral papillomas. There is much to be said for this contention but our knowledge is as yet too incomplete to make more than presumptive statements in this field.

In the search for the cause of cancer we have learned much concerning its physiology. A basic understanding of these mechanisms is fundamental to a working concept of bone tumors. A digression into the theories of the cause of general cancer may be warranted at this point.

Though there is still disagreement on the subject, most oncologists believe that the characteristics of cancer are transmitted from one cell to its offspring through the genetic equipment in the nucleus. It is probable that the heredity pattern is dictated by the arrangement of the molecular constituents of the genes and the spatial relationship of their molecules. It has been shown that deoxyribonucleic acid is the principal fabric of the gene. Its constituents, the most important of which are adenine, thymine, guanine and cytosine, are probably arranged in a double helix allowing a variability in pairing patterns. These patterns apparently establish the template for the copying process, which dictates the genetic equipment of the new cell.

The deoxyribonucleic acid of the nucleus is synthesized through ribonucleic acid in the cytoplasm. Here, enzymatic activity manufactures the nuclear requirements and passes them on to the nucleus in preparation for cell division. It is probable that the genetic equipment of a nucleus, once mature, is stable and constant until it is being prepared for division. Thus the offspring of a normal cell must be normal cells but as the genes are constructed in the latter, abnormal enzymatic activity in the cytoplasm may result in abnormal molecular patterns in the gene. This cell is still a normal cell for practical purposes as long as it does not divide but, in dividing, its offspring are different cells and one of the probably many different types that may result is a cell that undergoes replication before it matures, a cancer cell.

It is apparent then that cancer can arise from any cell or group of cells whose genetic equipment bears a certain type of abnormal structure. The cancer stigma may lie latent until the cell divides, either in the course of normal tissue replacement or secondary to an outside influence. The abnormal gene may have come from the parent, primary hereditary factor, or it may have been constructed by abnormal enzymatic activity of the cell that it replaced, somatic factor. The activity of the enzymes may be influenced by viruses, which are themselves very similar to enzymes, by metals that may inhibit enzymes, by any substance that competes for enzymatic activity or by cancerogenic agents. A number of chemical substances including radioactive calcium and beryllium have been used to produce osteosarcomas in the ex-

perimental animal. A knowledge of these mechanisms is helpful in building a classification of bone tumors.

It was stated earlier in this chapter that the greatest help in making a diagnosis is a knowledge of the possibilities. The very essence of such knowledge is a classification, one that is simple enough to remember yet complete enough to embrace all possible entities. The only perfect classification is the one constructed by its author, but certainly some are more useful than others even though fathered by strangers.

Until approximately 20 years ago all malignant bone tumors arising from the fibroblastic stem cell, i.e., those of the osteogenic, chondrogenic and collagenic series, were usually classified as osteosarcomas. This has made it most difficult to use the older literature because in many instances the reader cannot be sure which entity is being discussed. In 1939, Ewing constructed a classification for the Bone Sarcoma Registry but, though it was an improvement on the older system, it was soon realized by nearly all who tried to use it that it was hopelessly inadequate. Several better classifications have been prepared by individual writers. The one offered here is a modification of these and, though seemingly complex is, we believe, the easiest to use and retain. Actually two classifications are given here (pp. 464 and 468). Because several of the entities included in the standard classifications are reactive lesions or hamartomas, they are so entered in the second classification.

Bone tumors are best divided into four

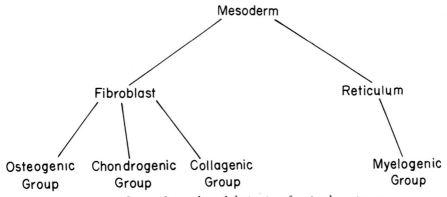

Figure 14–1   Schema of mesodermal derivatives forming bone tumors.

groups, each group arising from one of the four stem cell types that are derived from the mesoderm. Figure 14–1 is a schema indicating these lines of derivation. The primitive fibroblastic cells (see Chapter 1) come from the mesenchyme, which also gives rise to fat and muscle. The fibroblasts are so named because they are the progenitors of three types of cells each of which is related to a specific type of intercellular substance, the osteoblasts to osteoid, the chondroblasts to chondroid and the collagenoblasts (fibrous connective tissue cells) to collagen. All of these intercellular substances, though exhibiting markedly different physical properties, are chemically very similar. Each consists of a feltwork of collagen fibers in a mucopolysaccharide ground substance. Each tumor group is made up of a number of entities each of which is characterized by the type of ground substance of the group. The members of the fourth group, the myelogenic tumors, probably come from the various derivatives of the marrow reticulum.

CLASSIFICATION OF PRIMARY BONE TUMORS

A. Osteogenic series
   1. Osteoid osteoma
   2. Benign osteoblastoma
   3. Osteoma
   4. Osteochondroma
   5. Osteosarcoma
   6. Parosteal sarcoma
B. Chondrogenic series
   1. Enchondroma
   2. Benign chondroblastoma
   3. Chondromyxoid fibroma
   4. Chondrosarcoma
C. Collagenic series
   1. Non-osteogenic fibroma
   2. Subperiosteal cortical defect
   3. Angioma
   4. Aneurysmal bone cyst
   5. Fibrosarcoma
   6. Angiosarcoma
D. Myelogenic series
   1. Plasma cell myeloma
   2. Ewing's tumor

3. Reticulum cell sarcoma
4. Lymphoma of bone
5. Hodgkin's disease

THE OSTEOGENIC SERIES

Six lesions are usually classified in this series. All but the last two, osteosarcoma and parosteal sarcoma, always produce an intercellular substance that, though it may be abnormal, is recognizable as osteoid. Osteosarcoma usually produces at least some osteoid but it is our contention that it need not, thereby allowing the inclusion in this class of a group of tumors whose cells have the appearance of osteoblasts and whose behavior is like that of osteosarcomas. To place these tumors among the fibrosarcomas because they produce no osteoid is to resort to a completely morphologic classification without consideration of the effect the tumor has upon the patient. Fibrosarcomas are slowly growing tumors, invasive and frequently recurrent, but they metastasize late and the metastases, like the primary neoplasm, grow slowly. Osteosarcoma grows rapidly and in most instances has sown seeds of metastasis before diagnosis is made. Metastatic deposits grow rapidly and therefore the fatal outcome is earlier and the mortality rate higher than that of fibrosarcoma. The behavioral rather than the morphologic characteristics should dictate the classification of these tumors, accounting for inclusion of the rapidly growing, non-osteoid–producing tumors in the osteogenic series.

The parosteal sarcoma occurs much less commonly than the osteosarcoma. It appears to arise from cells within or near the periosteum. These cells apparently have the capacity to form collagen, osteoid or cartilage and in most instances produce all three in the same lesion. When such is the case they might be called mesenchymomas of bone, following the precedent set by Stout for the name he applies to tumors in soft tissues that are made up of a variety of mesenchymal derivatives. But to do so would introduce a new name into the already crowded terminology of the field and the importance of this tumor probably does not warrant it. Admittedly, the lesion might be placed in the collagenic or chondrogenic series with as much logic as it is placed in the osteogenic group. Because it is frequently mistaken for an osteosarcoma, perhaps its contiguity in classification with that tumor may serve to emphasize their differences. A limited experience with 34 cases of parosteal sarcoma has convinced us that this tumor is the malignant analogue of the osteochondroma. It is doubtful that it always originates as the benign lesion but some parosteal sarcomas are almost certainly malignant transitions of their benign counterpart.

The osteoblastomas are conceived by Lichtenstein,[1] who provided their name, as a nebulous group, embracing all the "benign" bone-forming lesions whose characteristics do not conform to those of other bone-forming lesions. Dahlin emphasized the similarity of this lesion to osteoid osteoma and named it giant osteoid osteoma. Others noted its resemblance to the ossifying fibroma of the jaw. It is not a common lesion but we now have made the diagnosis of benign osteoblastoma 10 times in lesions involving the vertebral axis. Many of these occur following trauma and appear to be a reaction to a hematoma peculiar to these tissues. We have also encountered eight similar lesions elsewhere in cylindrical as well as flat bones. We have concluded that this lesion is a reaction to bone injury of one type or another. Its microscopic as well as its clinical and radiologic features in some cases appear to merge imperceptibly with those of osteoid osteoma. Whatever it may be, it is not a true neoplasm but, like osteoid osteoma, a peculiar reaction to bone injury of unknown type.

The osteoma is a hamartomatous production of bone by periosteum. The bone is always formed by intramembranous ossification and represents a simple exaggeration of a normal, physiologic process. The formation of this lesion is quite different from the progressive, invasive proliferation of cells that characterizes true tumor; therefore this lesion cannot logically be accepted in a tumor classification.

Like the osteoma, the osteochondroma is a hamartomatous overgrowth. But in this instance the excess bone is formed by enchondral ossification. The body pedicle is laid down in much the same manner as the primary cortex of a normal cylindrical bone in the metaphyseal region, the cartilaginous cap serving as the enchondral plate. Most osteochondromas mature and cease growing at the time the nearest ossification center closes. Their growth is orderly and limited and so they must be considered hamartomas rather than tumors. A small percentage serve as the sites of true neoplastic growth arising in one or another of their cellular components. These tumors are not a part of the original process and represent a neoplastic accident superimposed on an aberrant growth process. The commonest of these, in our opinion, is parosteal sarcoma. The fact that the incidence of tumor development is higher in osteochondroma than in normal bone can be explained by comparing this incidence with that of tumor formation in other ectopic tissues.

The nature of the osteoid osteoma has been much debated. To some it appears to be an inflammatory reaction caused by an unknown etiologic agent. Others have described it as a disturbance in bone caused by an alteration in blood supply. Whatever its exact nature it does not have the qualifications of a tumor. Its productive pattern is regular and its growth period is limited. Because we cannot yet define the morbid physiology that results in this lesion it is best to include it among the reactions to bone injury. It probably should be classified as a variant of osteoblastoma or vice versa.

Thus, in the standard classification of tumors of bone that form osteoid we have two hamartomas (osteoma and osteochondroma), two idiopathic bone reactions (osteoid osteoma and benign osteoblastoma) and two true bone tumors (osteosarcoma and parosteal sarcoma).

THE CHONDROGENIC SERIES

The only entity in the standard classification of the cartilage-forming tumors that is unequivocally a true neoplasm is the chondrosarcoma. There is much evidence to suggest that the benign cartilage-forming lesions that are called chondromas are in reality a mixed group, some being cartilage-forming hamartomas like the enchondroma, and the others, chondrosarcomas that lack the cellular characteristics of malignancy. The clinician has learned to distrust the microscopist's diagnosis of benign chondroma because so many of these tumors have eventually shown the aggressive behavior of malignancy. It is easy to explain this behavior by assuming that the malignant tumor represents a superimposed change on the benign one. If the pathologist admits that not all malignant tumors have the cytologic characteristics of malignancy, some malignant tumors may be posing as hamartomas. A more careful analysis of the clinical features of these lesions, the age incidence and the skeletal region involved may help us to clarify this matter.

The enchondroma is a true hamartoma, i.e., an excessive proliferation of cells, which eventually reach maturity and cease to reproduce. The enchondroma obeys the laws of body growth and usually becomes static at about the time the bone involved reaches its maximal size. It remains static for the duration of life unless some stimulus for neoplastic growth changes its character. Only then can it be included in a classification of true tumors.

The benign chondroblastoma and the chondromyxoid fibroma are lesions about which more knowledge is needed before they are designated a permanent place in the classification of bone tumors. Some of these lesions have given us the impression that they too are hamartomatous cell proliferations, but in each group a few have shown the aggressive characteristics of true tumor. For that reason they are being placed here in the category of cartilaginous neoplasms. Certain similarities (both clinical and microscopic) suggest that they may be closely related or perhaps even the same entity conditioned by the area in which the lesion arises. The chondroblastoma always arises in the epiphysis or in relation to it, whereas the chondromyxoid fibroma arises in the metaphysis or shaft. The term fibroma for the latter tumor is probably inappropriate because the cartilage that it produces is one of its most distinctive features. A better name for it would be fibromyxoid chondroma, but this

may be treading too heavily the halls of academic propriety.

In the standard classification of cartilage-producing tumors there are five entries; one of these is unquestionably a tumor (chondrosarcoma), one (chondroma) we believe is a mixture of hamartomas and low grade chondrosarcomas, two are probably tumors (chondroblastoma and chondromyxoid fibroma) and one (enchondroma), a hamartoma. In the classification offered here we choose to delete the term chondroma because our practical experience of the past several years has led us to doubt its existence. We believe that, omitting the chondroblastoma and the chondromyxoid fibroma, a cartilage-forming lesion of bone is either an enchondroma or a chondrosarcoma. We expect to be criticized for this seemingly radical stand but when we critically review our own material collected over the past 30 years we find that many of the lesions that we called chondrosarcomas now can be diagnosed enchondromas. Two lesions diagnosed chondrosarcoma on the basis of the sections alone have eventually proved to be fracture with callus and proliferation of cartilage in a Charcot joint. Review of the sections still calls forth the diagnosis of chondrosarcoma by most pathologists who see them.

Other lesions diagnosed chondroma, after years of almost imperceptibly slow growth, have taken on the clinical attributes of chondrosarcoma. One of these now displays a progressive growth with invasion of the soft tissues far beyond its bony origin, meanwhile maintaining a microscopic appearance as innocent as that of the ordinary enchondroma.

Unless the microscopic features of a cartilaginous lesion are either obviously and unequivocally malignant or nonmalignant we prefer to weigh the radiologic, clinical and gross features more heavily than the microscopy, a position that pathologists are not apt to regard with much enthusiasm.

THE COLLAGENIC SERIES

This group includes six entries, two of which are probably reactive lesions in bone, one of which is a hamartoma (the hemangioma); one, the aneurysmal bone cyst, is a lesion of uncertain pathogenesis and the remaining two are true neoplasms.

The non-osteogenic fibroma is no longer considered a neoplasm by most clinicians and roentgenologists. By some it is considered a type of ischemic necrosis. Whatever it is, it is quite certainly not a true tumor and until its exact nature is known should be classified as a type of bone tissue reaction. The subperiosteal cortical defect is probably the same lesion as non-osteogenic fibroma except that it occurs along the outer surface of the cortex rather than the inner.

The ossifying fibroma, sometimes included in this classification, is the term used for a group that has been a scrap basket for a variety of lesions. If there be such an entity as the benign bone-forming lesion called benign osteoblastoma, it has been included until recently under this head. The bone-producing fibrous lesions of the jaw are reparative reaction to injury in most instances.

The angioma and the aneurysmal bone cyst are placed in the collagenic series because they originate from the fibroblastic cell that may produce connective tissue of blood vessels depending upon its environment and stimulus. The angioma of bone, like the angioma of soft tissues, is a hamartomatous multiplication of vessel units. Angiomas are often multiple throughout a variety of tissues including bone, are often congenital and obey the laws of growth of the part that they affect. Angiosarcoma rarely develops from a preceding hemangioma.

The aneurysmal bone cyst is an entity produced by an unproven mechanism. The osteolysis and reparative shell of newly formed bone may be caused by an excessive supply of blood to the area. The extra blood may be the result of alterations of pressure gradients or of congenital or acquired arteriovenous fistulas. Whatever the mechanism the process is not a tumor and is rarely classified as such. It is placed in the following classification among the hamartomas because it consists of an abnormal mass of vascular channels. It could probably be placed just as accurately among the reactions to bone injury.

In the past the giant cell tumor usually has been classified in the collagenic series. The term "giant cell tumor of bone" has been used over the past half century to designate a number of quite distinct pathologic lesions. In 1940, we undertook an analysis of all the cases so diagnosed in our files. By critically examining the roentgenograms and clinical records of these patients as well as the microscopic sections, and considering the follow-up histories, we concluded that only half the diagnoses were correct. In their paper published in 1940, Jaffe, Lichtenstein and Portis[2] reported essentially the same experience in analyzing their cases.

Since 1942, six entirely new bone lesional entities have been defined. These include benign chondroblastoma, non-osteogenic fibroma, aneurysmal bone cyst, chondromyxoid fibroma, endosteal villonodular synovitis and benign osteoblastoma. In addition, another lesion, solitary cyst, has been definitively described and named. It is not unusual to find giant cells in a fibroblastic matrix in all seven lesions. In addition, other conditions may display a prominent giant cell reaction. These are hematoma of bone, fibrosarcoma and osteosarcoma.

It is widely accepted that the tissues that constitute the skeleton commonly react to bone injury of a variety of types by an extravagant proliferation of giant cells in a fibroblastic matrix. Lacking a better diagnosis we believe that pathologists have frequently used the term giant cell tumor to designate these lesions. It seems safe to assume that of the recently defined lesions previously mentioned, those with prominent giant cell reactions were called giant cell tumors prior to their definition.

It seems to us that the benign giant cell tumor, grade I, of Jaffe, Lichtenstein and Portis is no more than a variety of innocuous giant cell reactions to bone injury. The grade II giant cell tumor may include the most active and florid examples of the previously mentioned lesions and perhaps some true giant cell tumors. The difficulty in evaluating this lesion and the dangers inherent in prognosing its behavior are well known to any pathologist who has made the attempt. And, finally, the grade III (frankly malignant) giant cell tumors may be the rapidly progressing giant cell (non-osteoid–forming) osteosarcomas. It is certainly best to allow the physician who must deal with the matter to come to his own conclusions. Though it is not always possible to find another diagnosis in cases that seem to have the microscopic criteria for giant cell tumor, if these cases are set aside while all aspects of the lesion are studied and the course of the disease observed, in most, if not all cases, the correct diagnosis eventually emerges. Some of these most certainly will prove to be bona fide giant cell tumors or, as we prefer to call them, osteoclastomas.

THE MYELOGENIC SERIES

The five entities of this group are all malignant tumors. The exact cell of origin is known in none of them though various cytogenic theories have been offered. From rather sketchy data it appears to us that the Ewing's tumor may arise from the most primitive cell of the osteoblastic series, probably a derivative of the endothelial lining cells of capillary blood vessels. The reticulum cell sarcoma probably arises from an attenuated derivative of these cells in an older age group. The exact cytogenesis of the plasma cell myeloma is unknown. Some have suggested that it may come from a forerunner of the erythrocyte. It seems more probable, considering the alteration in serum protein elaboration, that the tumor cell is indeed a plasma cell. It is probable that all five types are derived eventually from the marrow reticulum as is the lesion of Hodgkin's disease.

REVISED CLASSIFICATION OF BONE TUMORS AND TUMOR-LIKE LESIONS

I. Reactive Bone Lesions
   A. Osteogenic
      1. Osteoid osteoma
      2. Osteoblastoma
   B. Collagenic
      1. Non-osteogenic fibroma
      2. Subperiosteal cortical defect
II. Hamartomas Affecting Bone
   A. Osteogenic
      1. Osteoma
      2. Osteochondroma
   B. Chondrogenic
      1. Enchondroma
   C. Collagenic
      1. Angioma
      2. Aneurysmal bone cyst
III. True Tumors of Bone
   A. Osteogenic
      1. Osteosarcoma
      2. Parosteal sarcoma
   B. Chondrogenic
      1. Chondroblastoma
      2. Chondromyxoid fibroma
      3. Chondrosarcoma
   C. Collagenic
      1. Fibrosarcoma
      2. Angiosarcoma
   D. Myelogenic
      1. Plasma cell myeloma
      2. Ewing's tumor
      3. Reticulum cell sarcoma
      4. Hodgkin's disease
   E. Osteoclastoma

If one insists that a true tumor must, by definition, be progressive, i.e., that the replication of its cells is due to a fundamental alteration in its genetic character, only the entities entered in category III can be accepted as actual neoplasms. Thus the standard classification of bone tumors becomes immensely simplified. By excluding the hamartomas, the reparative reactions to bone injury and other idiopathic lesions of unknown mechanism, the number of primary bone tumors becomes relatively few and easy to remember. Such simplification, we believe, provides a clearer concept of the subject and a more, workable classification for diagnoses.

A more interesting concept of bone tumors has been proposed by Johnson.[3] It is based on the premise that the morphology and behavior of this group of neoplasms are dictated not only by the cell of origin but by the area within the bone affected, the region of the skeleton and the age of the host at the time of growth. It concedes that the primary bone tumors arise from a variety of cells, the osteoblasts, chondroblasts, collagenoblasts (fibroblasts), marrow cells and osteoclasts (a transitional stage of osteoblasts), but suggests that all these cells have a common denominator, the stem cell from which they arose, the mesenchymal cell. These cells may be divided broadly into three groups. Those that normally produce an extracellular substance that is composed predominantly of a "collagenic" material include the reticulum cell, collagenoblast (fibroblast) and osteoblast. Those that normally produce a predominantly glycoprotein substance, the marrow cells (apparently excluding the reticulum cell), make up the second group, and finally cells that are predominantly osteolytic in function, the osteoclasts, are placed in a third group. The metabolism of the tumors that arise from these cells, i.e., the chemical constituents of their cellular products, is determined by the cell of origin, but because the cells are all related by a common ancestor, the functions, perverted by neoplastic alteration, may become mixed with wide overlapping.

Because morphology is closely related to metabolic activity the appearance of any one tumor may show variations that characterize other types. This kinship is enhanced by the normal predominant activity of the area involved; matrix synthesis dominates the subepiphyseal metaphysis, and osteoclasis preparatory to bone reconstruction occurs towards the shaft. As a tumor enlarges and spreads from one area to another, its morphology is correspondingly changed. Tumor incidence and rate of growth are influenced by what Johnson calls the metabolic gradient within the bone and the position of the bone in the skeleton. Metabolic activity is lowest in the epiphysis, next in the mid-diaphysis and becomes greater as the subepiphyseal metaphysis is approached. Moreover, this activity is greater in a cylindrical bone at the end of maximal growth—lower end of the femur, upper end of the tibia, upper end of the humerus and lower end of the radius. Also, the activity rate declines in direct proportion to the distance from the vertebral axis. The metabolic activity is also influenced by the age, being high in the last "reconstruction spurt" of adolescence and decreasing thereafter.

Johnson's concept is boldly comprehensive and refreshingly new. Whatever may be said about it, his approach disregards a burdensome mass of preconceived ideas and starts afresh with behavior rather than morphology as the correlating feature. Such a concept will be hard for morphologists to accept or even to contemplate but this does not necessarily make it erroneous. In our material, the frequency and the age and site incidence are compatible with Johnson's thesis. Also the association of growth rate and the relation of nonneoplastic lesions and superimposed tumors are consistent. The hypothesis fails when one attempts to find the variety of forms within a single neoplastic lesion. A rare tumor from a very early stem cell may diverge into numerous morphologic types but this is the exception, and most evidence of diversity within a single lesion can usually be accounted for on the basis of reparative response of injured tissue. The chondroblast in certain instances may resemble a plasmacyte to some extent, but similarity in appearance does not justify the conclusion that there is similarity in metabolic activity. Moreover, though the interrelationship of tumors deserves more emphasis than it has had in the past, "over-lumping" may blur the sharp focus of identity, which is so important for diagnostic acuity. The behavior of bone tumors varies according to type. In most instances this behavior, if the tumor is correctly diagnosed, is predictable. To deemphasize this predictability would be unwise. However, whatever its merit, everyone interested in bone tumors should read Dr. Johnson's paper carefully.

TUMORS METASTATIC TO BONE

The great preponderance of the metastatic tumors in bone are of epithelial origin. A few sarcomas manifest this behavior. Ewing's tumor metastasizes to one or more bones in less than half the cases. There is a type of osteosarcoma that characteristically involves several bones. It is unknown whether it is multicentric in origin or whether it metastasizes to other bones from a primary site. It is rare; there are but six cases in our material. It is usually encountered in children. It is usually of the sclerosing variety. Bone involvement may be found in less than one quarter of the cases of leukemia, malignant lymphoma and Hodgkin's disease.

Practically any tumor, with the exception of the primary tumors of the central nervous system, may occasionally metastasize to bone, but this phenomenon is unusual in some instances, as in squamous cell carcinoma of the skin, and highly characteristic in others, as in cancers of the breast and prostate. From a half to two thirds of the latter two carcinomas, some time in their course, metastasize to bone. Other cancers that frequently develop secondary deposits in bone are those of the thyroid, kidney and lung. Bone metastasis is also very common in neuroblastoma.

Emboli of viable tumor cells are carried by both the blood vascular and lymphatic systems. Because the latter method is exceedingly common in breast and prostate cancers the pattern in these lesions is often highly suggestive. The thoracic vertebrae, the ribs, sternum and clavicles are most commonly involved in breast cancer, whereas the lumbar and sacral vertebrae and the pelvic bones are the ones usually affected in carcinoma of the prostate. In cases in which transport is by the systemic arterial circulation the metastases may occur anywhere in any bone, but in most cases the flat bones are more often involved than cylindrical bones and metastases in bones distal to the elbows and knees are somewhat unusual.

The principal symptoms and signs of metastatic bone tumor are pain and pathologic fracture. The pain may be insidious at the onset with periods of remission but eventually it usually becomes extreme. The layman's concept of cancer as a disease of agonizing pain is largely derived from the cases with multiple bone metastases. Most metastatic carcinoma causes bone lysis so that it is not surprising that pathologic fracture is common. The fracture may be the first evidence of neoplastic involvement, either metastatic or primary. This is especially true of carcinoma of the prostate. Fracture may stimulate the remaining normal skeletal tissues to produce callus and eventually achieve healing even in the presence of the tumor that caused the fracture. Secondary deposits of breast cancer may lie quiescent within the bone for years. It is not highly unusual to find bone metastases suddenly manifesting themselves 20 symptomless years after a radical mastectomy for breast cancer.

Some metastatic tumors produce characteristic changes in the serum chemistry. The most important of these is the elevation in acid phosphatase that occurs in bone metastasis of prostate cancer. Acid phosphatase is produced by the cancer cells but for some as yet unsatisfactorily explained reason the serum levels are not appreciable until metastasis has occurred, or at least until the cancer has invaded the prostate capsule. It would seem logical that the amount of acid phosphatase in the blood is directly proportional to the number of cancer cells that produce it. A cancer confined to the prostate gland apparently is not large enough to cause a significant elevation in total serum acid phosphatase. However, with L-tartrate inhibition of nonprostatic acid phosphatase, the increase in prostate acid phosphatase may be appreciated. Invasion of the capsule probably means that the tumor has actually spread elsewhere, and though the early bone deposits cannot be demonstrated the cells are sufficient in number to produce a measurable increase in the total enzyme.

Any cancer that destroys a considerable amount of bone may initiate sufficient osteoblastic reparative activity to produce a rise in the serum alkaline phosphatase. This is particularly true of prostatic cancer, which is often of the osteoblastic or sclerosing type. Excessive amounts of mineralizing osteoid are characteristically produced in response to the presence of carcinoma of the prostate and less often in other cancer types, especially those from the breast. The serum alkaline phosphatase level may sometimes be used as a guide in treating these metastases. Because alkaline phosphatase is excreted by the liver, abnormal serum levels may mean liver disease rather than osteoblastic activity. Considerable difficulty is encountered in this respect in cases in which the liver is the site of metastatic growth as it so frequently is in adenocarcinomas.

Blood calcium levels may be altered in extensive skeletal metastases. This may be due to actual bone destruction and the freeing of bone salts into the blood and it may be enhanced by disuse atrophy secondary to pain. High serum calcium levels may lead to metastatic calcification of soft tissues. Nephrocalcinosis is especially prone to occur in these situations. The excess calcium may spill into the urine and urine calcium levels may be indicative of the progress of the disease. In osteoblastic metastases sufficient calcium may be taken up by the excess osteoid to keep the serum level normal or even lower than normal. In rare instances dangerously low calcium levels may be induced by this mechanism. Excessive osteoid production is usually induced by the tumor but irradiation and hormone therapy may also stimulate new bone formation.

The Radiology of Tumors Metastatic to Bone

The radiographic manifestation of tumor metastatic to bone is related to destruction of bone. Sometimes, as with metastatic carcinoma of the prostate, the destruction is obscured by the osteoblastic response provoked by the tumor. In contrast, carcinoma of the breast usually causes frank destructive, radiolucent defects but may at times cause an associated osteoblastic response with resultant areas of opacification. Metastatic neuroblastoma results in small destructive foci, usually in the long bones, which grow rapidly and which may be associated with periosteal new bone overlying the involved cortex. In any event, radiographic appearance of the osseous lesions of metastatic malignancy does not permit positive differentiation of metastatic neoplasms from primary neoplasms of bone, nor is it specific for any given primary site of origin of the metastatic disease. The location of a metastatic focus may suggest the site of the primary tumor; e.g., peripheral metastases are not uncommon from the lung, kidney or esophagus. A fracture through a bone weakened by metastases may be the first manifestation of metastases or, at times, of the primary neoplasm.

The surrounding trabeculae are destroyed by the emboli of neoplastic tissue

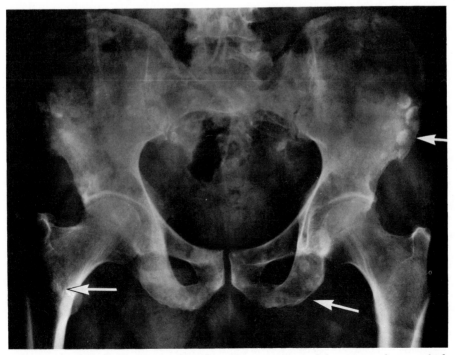

Figure 14–2 Metastatic tumor in bone. Metastases from carcinoma of the prostate have evoked an osteoblastic reaction in bone. Multiple rounded opacities are evident (arrows) as well as thickening and diffuse opacity of the right ischium.

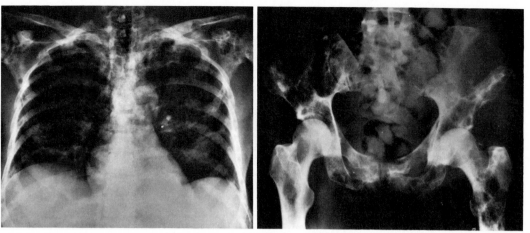

Figure 14–3 Metastatic tumor in bone. There are diffuse areas of radiolucency secondary to carcinoma of the breast. The lesions vary in size but tend to be round or ovoid with no surrounding bone reaction.

that grow in the marrow. Metastatic neoplasms that are confined to the marrow are thus associated with round or ovoid areas of radiolucency without associated reactive bone. In metastatic carcinoma of the prostate, the osteoblastic response results

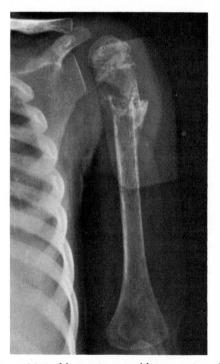

Figure 14–4 Metastatic neuroblastoma. A pathologic fracture has occurred through the proximal end of the humerus. Multiple small areas of destruction are evident in the cortex and medullary cavity. There is involvement of the pleura by metastatic tumor.

in round or ovoid areas of opacification that are homogeneous but fuzzy in outline. In the pubic bones, the slowly growing metastases of carcinoma of the prostate may result in actual widening of the bone as the periosteum is stimulated to lay down new bone. This appearance may be confused with that of Paget's disease.

Bones may be eroded and invaded by direct extension of carcinoma involving the adjacent tissues. The cortex is then irregularly destroyed from without, with little or no periosteal reaction. Before there is involvement of the cortex, considerable destruction of trabeculae may be present and not visible by standard roentgen techniques (Fig. 14–8). Bone scans may be most helpful in the determination of metastases (Fig. 14–9). When extensive invasion has occurred, the appearance may be identical to that of a growth originating in the medullary cavity and extending outward through the cortex.

Pathology of Bone Metastases

Tumor emboli may be deposited anywhere within bone but the hematopoietic marrow appears to be most fertile for survival and growth. In the cancellous tissue the metastatic tumor must reach sufficient size to destroy considerable spicular or cortical bone before it can be appreciated. Thus, we must presume that most meta-

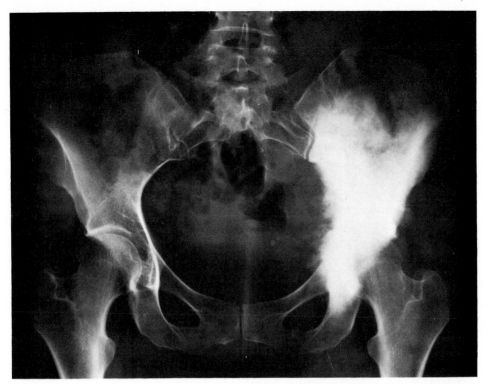

Figure 14–5 Metastatic carcinoma of the left ilium has evoked an osteoblastic reaction.

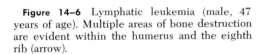Figure 14–6 Lymphatic leukemia (male, 47 years of age). Multiple areas of bone destruction are evident within the humerus and the eighth rib (arrow).

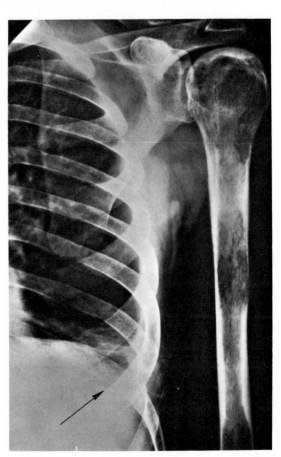

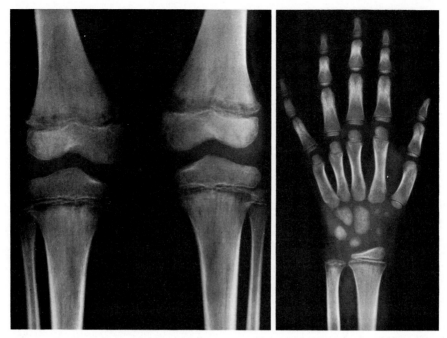

Figure 14–7 Lymphatic leukemia (male, 7 years of age). Radiolucent bands are evident in the metaphysis adjacent to the zone of provisional calcification. These areas reflect destruction by aggregates of leukemic cells as well as interruption of normal growth of bone in the area.

static deposits in bone are present for some time before they are apprehended. Most metastases are focal, destroying bone by pressure and by interfering with its blood supply. At times viable tumor cells may be seeded diffusely throughout an entire bone or the major portion of the skeleton. The general deossification that occurs then may be hard to distinguish from osteoporosis or diffuse myelomatosis.

Diagnosis of metastatic tumor should always be made by microscopic section even though there is a history of primary cancer and the roentgenograms are typical. Many instances of expected metastases have been found to be innocuous, coincidental lesions, thus altering the prognosis and allowing a more intelligent attack on the primary neoplasm. Biopsy by open surgical approach may seem unjustified in the face of the clinical evidence for metastasis. Here the needle aspiration method is invaluable. One of a variety of needles with a cutting edge may be used and numerous samples removed by multiple punctures if necessary. If the procedure is properly done and the material correctly handled, the efficiency of the method is high and may sometimes yield results after an open biopsy has failed. The slides are relatively easy to interpret even though minute quantities of tissue are withdrawn. Most osseous metastases are carcinomas made up of cells that are entirely foreign to the normal tissue area. Even a few of these cells can give the microscopist assurance of the presence of metastatic tumor.

The reason for osteosclerosis in several types of metastatic carcinoma is not known. Osteoid may be laid down in a highly irregular pattern producing osteones of great variation in size and shape. Consequently the microscopist must rule out osteoblastic metastatic carcinoma when he encounters the mosaic pattern that is regarded to be so characteristic of Paget's disease. Perhaps the tumor growth within the non-expansile cortex may gradually diminish the blood flow, thus provoking a slowly mounting ischemia. This mechanism may account for the excessive osteoid formation. Why metastatic prostatic carcinoma is more apt to produce this phenomenon more often than any other type of cancer is unknown.

Because adenocarcinoma is the com-

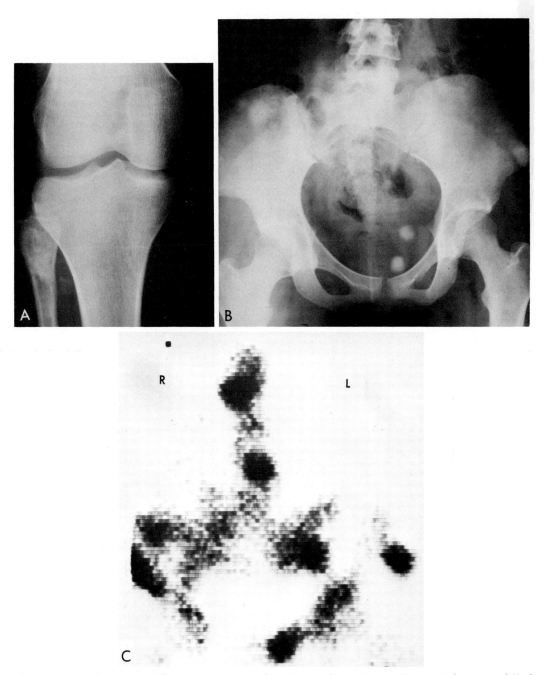

Figure 14–8 Osteosarcoma. The primary tumor in this patient, who is 16 years of age, is in the proximal fibula (*A*). The bone scan reveals the metastatic lesions apparent on the radiograph of the pelvis as well as two foci in the spine (*B* and *C*).

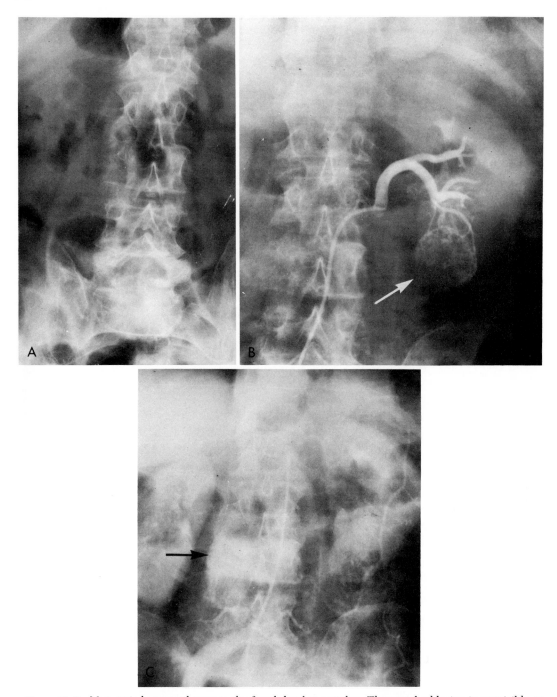

Figure 14–9 Metastatic hypernephroma to the fourth lumbar vertebra. The vertebral lesion is not visible on the plain radiograph *(A)*. The angiogram delineated the primary tumor *(B)* and by chance the metastatic focus in the spine *(C)*.

monest tumor type metastasizing to bone and because the primary lesion may arise in any epithelial or glandular tissue in the body, it is quite often impossible for the pathologist to name the site of origin from examination of material removed from bone. One exception is the tubule lining cell carcinoma primary in the kidney. The metastatic deposits usually faithfully reproduce the original and because of the distinctive cellular morphology and pattern, can be readily identified. Carcinomas from the prostate frequently present cells that show none of the nuclear characteristics of malignant tumor. Carcinomas from the intestinal tract usually show some evi-

dence of mucin production within the cells. The metastatic neuroblastoma may be impossible to distinguish from the Ewing's tumor on microscopic sections alone. Metastatic tumor from the thyroid may be identified if its cells are sufficiently differentiated to take up radioactive iodine.

References

1. Lichtenstein, L.: Cancer, 9:1044, 1956.
2. Jaffe, H., Lichtenstein, L., and Portis, R.: Arch Pathol., 30:993, 1940.
3. Johnson, L. C.: Bull. N.Y. Acad. Med., 29:164, 1953.

Chapter 15

TUMOR-LIKE PROCESSES

REACTIVE
    Osteogenic
        Osteoid Osteoma
        Osteoblastoma
    Collagenic
        Non-osteogenic Fibroma
        Subperiosteal Cortical Defect

HAMARTOMAS
    Osteogenic
        Osteoma
        Osteochondroma
    Chondrogenic
        Enchondroma
    Collagenic
        Angioma
        Aneurysmal Bone Cyst

REACTIVE LESIONS IN BONE

The microscopist should constantly remember that the mesenchymal tissues that constitute the skeleton have the capacity to react in only a limited variety of ways to a much greater variety of noxious agents that produce bone injury. By bone reaction to injury we mean specifically the attempt by bone-forming cells to repair the damage incurred by trauma, hemorrhage, ischemia, infection, chemical agents, allergy or neoplasm. The injuring agents vary greatly in their mode of action but the bone response may reveal little or no specificity to the agent that prompts it. This is the reason for the difficulty frequently encountered by the microscopist in attempting to diagnose bone disease on the basis of the sections alone. But if he realizes that the reaction at the periphery of a rapidly destructive neoplasm can have all the features of a chronic infectious process, he is more cautious about assigning a diagnosis until the clinical and radiologic features have been weighed. Or if he realizes that

the cells producing reparative collagen, crude chondroid or osteoid can in some instances reveal all the nuclear features of malignant neoplasm he may save himself the embarrassing mistake of overdiagnosing an innocuous lesion, and may better understand why the authors insist on a tumor classification that clearly separates the reactive processes from the neoplasms. Or if the microscopist learns that one of the commonest reactions of bone tissues, especially that of or about the metaphyseal area, is a proliferation of spindled cells producing variable amounts of collagen in which are embedded multinucleated giant cells, he will appreciate the fact that the diagnosis of giant cell tumor is often only an easy "out" for a more occult disease.

Without any proof whatsoever we believe it entirely possible that an injury to bone that is associated with extravasation of blood may be responsible for a number of reactive lesions frequently classified as tumors, depending upon how the tissues respond to the hematoma. If encountered at the time when (early) and the place in which (the metaphysis) there is a florid giant cell reaction, the lesion may be diagnosed giant cell tumor. If a capsule is formed about the hematoma, as is the case in the subdural hematoma, and the central portion undergoes liquefaction, it may represent a solitary cyst. If collagen-producing fibroblasts penetrate the hematoma converting it to a mass of scar tissue, as may occur in soft tissues, it would be a non-osteogenic fibroma. If this collagenoblastic tissue matured to the point of osteoid production it could form an osteoblastoma. And finally, if the injury resulted in the formation of a post-traumatic arteriovenous fistula, perhaps an aneurysmal bone cyst would be formed.

We are certainly not contending that intraosseous hemorrhage is the cause of all these various bone lesions. We are merely suggesting the possibility in order to emphasize the importance of recognizing bone reactive processes and separating them from neoplasms.

OSTEOID OSTEOMA

The osteoid osteoma is a small (usually not greater than 2 cm. in diameter), circumscribed lesion occurring within bone or very much less frequently between periosteum and cortex. It is characterized clinically by pain out of proportion to its size, radiologically by a translucent sphere surrounded by an exaggerated zone of sclerosis and pathologically by a nidus of osteoid surrounded by a network of fine, new-bone trabeculae in a vascular fibrous matrix.

Henry Jaffe recognized the lesion as a distinct entity, suggested the name "osteoid osteoma" and gave a thorough and lucid description of five cases in 1935.[1] Several more recent papers have cited instances of earlier descriptions, but, with the exception of Bergstrand's cases reported in 1930, they were thought to belong to other bone disease categories. Bergstrand considered the lesion non-inflammatory and non-neoplastic and by exclusion arrived at the conclusion that they were congenital rests. Five years later Jaffe defined the lesion as a benign neoplasm and his beautiful descriptions and illustrations established the criteria for its diagnosis. More recently several workers have expressed dissent from the theory of neoplastic genesis but there can be no doubt that osteoid osteoma is a clinical, radiologic and pathologic entity.

Osteoid osteoma is a rather common bone lesion. More than 300 cases have been reported and most active orthopedic clinics can cull 15 or more cases from their files. It has been reported in almost every bone of the skeleton though about half the lesions are found in the bones of the lower extremity and most of these in the femur. In at least one series[2] the vertebrae were involved in 25 per cent of the cases. Unlike most bone lesions, osteoid osteoma may occur anywhere in the bone rather than just in the metaphysis. The diaphysis is usually involved but at least one case has been reported in the epiphysis. It may be surrounded by cancellous bone, it may lie against the inner cortical surface, it may be located entirely within the compacta or, as in a few cases,[3] it may be found on the outer cortical surface directly beneath the periosteum. We have seen 15 cases of the last.

The most important clinical characteristic of osteoid osteoma is pain. The patient first becomes aware of a minor, nagging discomfort and frequently attributes it to muscle stiffness, joint disease (if the lesion is at the end of a cylindrical bone), or previous trauma (about 25 per cent). At first the discomfort is usually intermittent but in time it becomes more persistent and sharply defined. After weeks or sometimes months the pain often becomes intense and point tenderness develops. As in many other bone lesions the pain is usually worse at night. Many patients volunteer the information that aspirin is effective in relieving the symptoms. Usually the pain is at the site of the lesion but if the osteoid osteoma is in the upper end of the femur, particularly the neck, it may be referred into the leg and pose as a herniated intervertebral disc.

Diagnosis is rarely made before several months of symptoms have elapsed, and because diagnosis depends upon roentgenographic evidence, this suggests that symptoms antedate demonstrable morphologic change. It has been estimated that pain usually antedates radiographic alteration by six months to one year. Pain in a few instances has become severe enough to cause threats of suicide and it has been known to persist for as long as six years. Often there is disability and disuse atrophy of muscle. Eventually, a swelling or mass due to bone thickening may become obvious but the lesion does not achieve the redness and heat of an infectious inflammation.

Osteoid osteoma is somewhat more than twice as common in males. The age group of predilection is 10 to 26. In a series of 30 cases reported by Jaffe and Lichtenstein,[4] all but 5 were in this age group, and in a series of 33 cases studied by us 17 cases were within this group. But in the same series there is a case at 4 years and one at 54 years, so that neither youth nor age precludes the diagnosis though they may make it unlikely.

Roentgenographic Manifestations. Because the osteoid osteoma is relatively constant in its pathologic features, one can expect the radiographic manifestations to be relatively uniform. The nidus of osteoid tissue in a vascular fibrous matrix produces a radiolucent zone that contrasts sharply with the surrounding sclerotic, opaque bone; if the osteoid tissue calcifies, an opacity may be visualized within the radiolucent nidus. The sclerotic bone about the lesion is lamellated and in cases in which the lesion involves the cortex, multiple layers of new bone may be apparent. More frequently, however, the lamellations are not apparent and the dense sclerotic bone casts a homogeneous shadow, which may be responsible for eccentric thickening of the shaft. The nidus may not be seen unless multiple projections or planigraphy of the involved area are made. Angiography may demonstrate abnormal vascularity within the lesion. If the lesion arises in spongy bone, peripheral sclerosis tends to be less marked than when compact bone is involved. In either instance the diameter of the bone in the area involved may be greater than normal.

In cases in which the lesion is located superficially just beneath the periosteum and particularly in the neck of the femur, only slivers of periosteal new bone may be evident (Figs. 15–5 and 15–6). A subperiosteal osteoid osteoma located near a joint may be associated with regional deossification of bone as well as effusion into the joint.

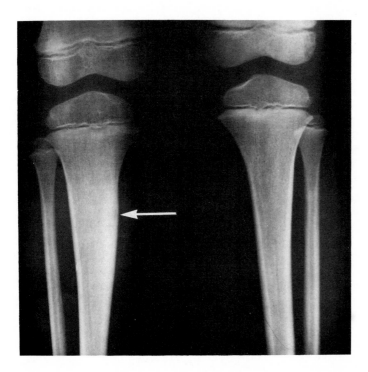

Figure 15–1 Osteoid osteoma. There is marked thickening of the cortex on the medial aspect of the right tibia. A central radiolucent nidus (arrow) is evident.

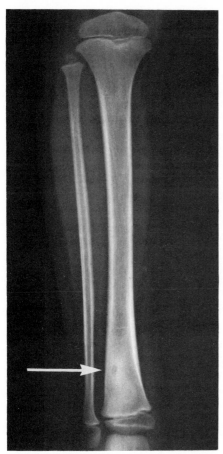

Figure 15–2 Osteoid osteoma. The lesion involves medullary bone; sclerosis is not marked, but a nidus (arrow) is evident and the diameter of the tibia is greater than is normal in this region.

Morbid Anatomy. The osteoid osteoma is a sharply circumscribed, spheroid or ovoid lesion that usually does not reach a diameter greater than 2 cm. (Fig. 15–7). The term "giant osteoid osteoma" has been used to designate an osteoid-forming lesion that is often larger than the classic 2 cm. osteoid osteoma.[5] The microscopy may be remarkably similar even to the inclusion of a "nidus" of calcified osteoid. The lesion usually is not as well organized, however, as the typical osteoid osteoma and the clinical aspects in some reported cases have not been typical of that lesion. Lichtenstein[6] insists that Dahlin's giant osteoid osteoma is an entirely separate entity from true osteoid osteoma and that it belongs in the category of "benign osteoblastoma." In cases in which it occurs within bone it has certain morphologic features that make one hesitant to classify it with osteoid osteoma but in cases in which it is subperiosteal it is identical. The current trend is to consider the osteoblastoma an unusually large and atypical osteoid osteoma.

Many osteoid osteomas have been removed en bloc and studied both grossly and microscopically in their entirety. The principal mass consists of an aggregate of deep red, brown, purple or gray tissue with a decidedly gritty consistency, encased in a wall of massive spicules or nearly solid bone. The surrounding area of sclerosis may be many times that of the lesion proper, particularly if it lies within or contiguous to the compacta. If isolated in cancellous bone the lesion is usually surrounded by an aura of sclerosis but overlying cortical thickening is less impressive. When the lesion is curetted the wall of the remaining cavity is fairly smooth.

If full sections are made through the mid-center a highly characteristic microscopic morphology is apparent. The central area is made up of one or more nidi of irregular masses of osteoid (Fig. 15–8). It may or may not be calcified. The osteoid dominates the field but in the interstices between its ramifications there is a moderately loose, rather vascular matrix of elongated and spindled cells, which appear to be fibroblasts undergoing transition into the more cuboidal cells that form a layer of osteoblasts over the solid osteoid nucleus (Fig. 15–9). As one progresses toward the periphery the crude osteoid merges into a network of very fine spicules of more mature bone. Osteoblastic activity is often quite apparent about these structures. These miniature spicules are arranged radially around their respective nidi. At the extreme edge they appear to press against but usually do not merge with the massive spicules of lamellated bone that run in the opposite direction to surround the lesion (Fig. 15–10).

In the peripheral zone, measuring approximately one third of the radius, one may find fairly normal appearing osteoclasts and the spicules are even more delicate than those toward the center. There is little or no evidence of fat and no hema-

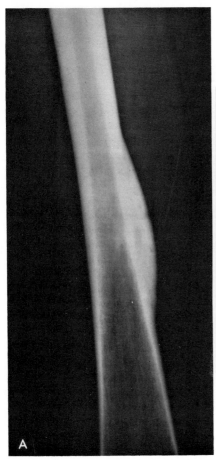

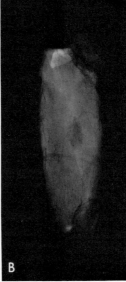

Figure 15-3 Osteoid osteoma. The surgical specimen (B) may be compared with the preoperative radiograph (A). Sclerosis is marked.

topoietic marrow. The density of the matrix tissue varies but it is never highly collagenized. There may be a few scattered lymphocytes, suggesting a mild inflammatory reaction, but never enough exudate to imply infection. Cartilage appears to play no role in the genesis of this lesion. Here and there one may find granules of hemosiderin but there is not enough to suggest hemorrhage as a factor. The pat-

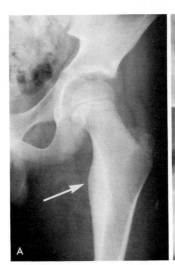

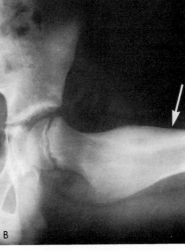

Figure 15-4 There is a large osteoid osteoma involving the anteromedial aspect of the femur (arrows, A and B). The head and neck are undermineralized and the capsule of the joint bulges because of fluid in the joint.

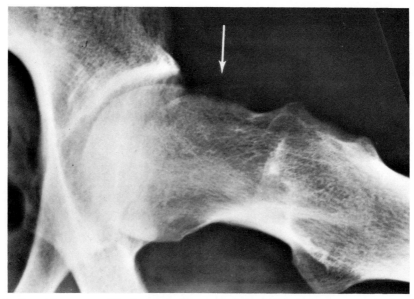

Figure 15–5   Osteoid osteoma. The lesion in the neck of the femur (arrow) is superficial and marked by slivers and spicules of new bone.

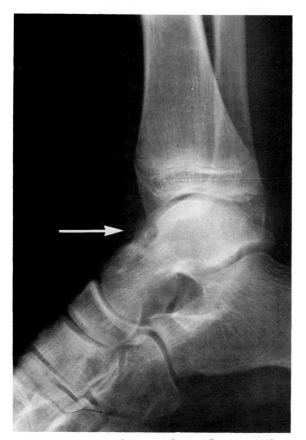

tern is rigidly dictated and, except for the apparent confusion in areas in which the alignment around one nidus intrudes upon that of another, in cases in which multiple nidi are present, the microscopy is marvelously consistent. When the lesion is removed intact and so sectioned the diagnosis is clearly apparent to anyone but the uninitiated. More often, however, the pathologist must depend upon sections

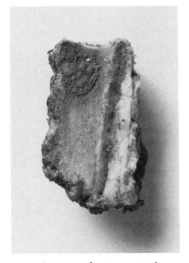

Figure 15–6   Subperiosteal osteoid osteoma. Close scrutiny of the neck of the talus reveals perilesional sclerosis and a calcified nidus (arrow). Demonstration of these lesions may demand the most exacting radiologic technique.

Figure 15–7   An osteoid osteoma in the upper end of the fibula. The lesion is round, about 1 cm. in diameter, sharply demarcated and gray-brown in color. Its sharp, regular delineation is almost pathognomonic.

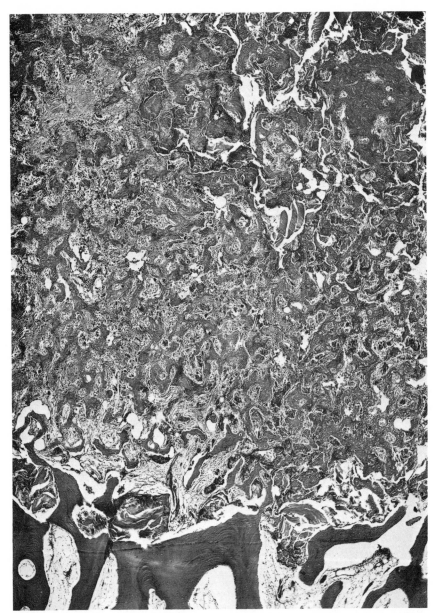

Figure 15–8 A quarter segment of a section through the center of an osteoid osteoma. The central nidus of mineralized osteoid is in the upper right corner, the peripheral zone of sclerotic cancellous bone is at the bottom. An orderly arrangement of microspicules forms a wide zone around the nidus. (× 20.)

made of curetted fragments of the lesion mixed with pieces of the surrounding bone and even marrow tissue. Under these unfortunate circumstances, unless the diagnosis has been strongly suggested by the clinician and roentgenologist, the nature of the lesion as demonstrated in the sections can only be surmised because a firm diagnosis depends so strongly on pattern.

The subperiosteal osteoid osteoma is an interesting lesion that occurs either within the cortical compacta or between this layer and its periosteum. It develops the same microscopic features as the deeper lying variety. There are one or more nidi of osteoid from which radiate an organized system of microspicules. (Fig. 15–11). The periosteum is usually elevated over the

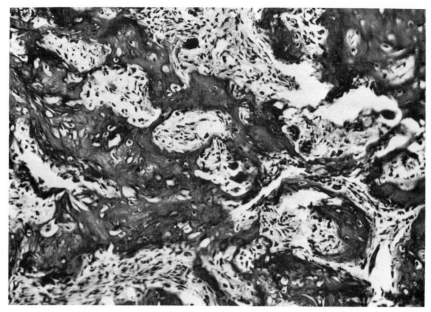

Figure 15–9 A higher magnification of the central osteoid nidus seen in Figure 15–8. (× 130.)

protruding mass. At times a thin shell of appositional bone is laid down to surround the lesion. Curiously, we have not seen the remarkable subperiosteal sclerosis that characterizes the deeper lesions. These superficial osteoid osteomas give rise to the same symptoms as the orthodox variety and they respond to the same treatment.

The lesions are almost certainly identical with the periosteal osteoblastoma. Indeed it has been suggested that when the lesion occurs in or within the cortex it is an osteoid osteoma; when it is extracortical it is an osteoblastoma. This may be true in many cases but we regard the osteoid osteoma, whether within cancellous tissue,

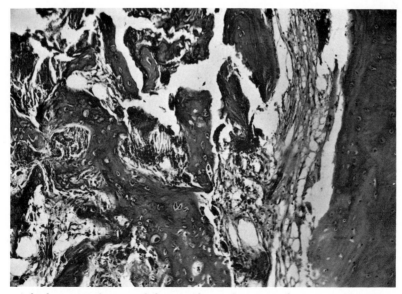

Figure 15–10 A higher magnification of the periphery of an osteoid osteoma. The surrounding zone of sclerotic cortex is seen on the right. The microspicules approach the encasing shell but in most places are separated from it by a zone of granulation. (× 115.)

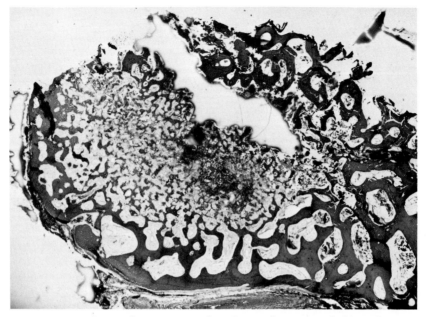

Figure 15–11 Subperiosteal osteoid osteoma. A nidus of osteoid is surrounded by radiating microspicules, which in turn are surrounded by a layer of sclerotic bone. The periosteum is seen along the bottom of the figure. (× 25.)

the cortex or the periosteum, as a reaction to some specific though idiopathic noxious agent. There are other general reactions to bone injury in the same locations that are not osteoid osteomas. These also have been classed as osteoblastomas.

Of the 15 cases of periosteal osteoid osteoma in our collection all but two arose from the cortical surfaces of the small bones of the hands or feet, four of them from the neck of the talus (see Fig. 15–6). Two arose from the neck of the femur at a point at which the capsule rather than the periosteum ensheaths the cortex. We have been informed that the capsules of the joints of the wrists and ankles serve the same function at certain areas. It is also noteworthy that vertebral osteoblastomas which are probably identical to subperiosteal osteoid osteomas, are usually located where the dura of the spinal cord serves as a bone covering.

Pathogenesis. The pathogenesis of osteoid osteoma is unknown. Before the definitive paper by Jaffe in 1935, it was categorized as traumatic, as infectious, as ischemic and as a congenital rest. Jaffe marshaled the facts against these theories

and concluded that the lesion was none of these and, therefore, it must be neoplastic. Whether one accepts this hypothesis depends upon one's concept of true neoplastic growth. Most oncologists today believe that a cell becomes neoplastic only after its nuclear hereditary mechanism becomes unalterably changed so that ultimate maturation can no longer occur. Thus, the cells must divide and their daughters divide until some mechanical or metabolic influence causes their death. Therefore, a true neoplasm cannot, by definition, reach a static growth plateau and all lesions that do are not true neoplasms.

If one accepts this definition, osteoid osteoma is not a neoplasm. There is serious question in our mind whether the classic osteoid osteoma grows at all. It is a most difficult point on which to gather dependable data but it appears that after a diagnosis is made radiologically, the lesion proper does not enlarge. On the contrary, it sometimes appears to diminish in size. This suggests that it appears, full blown, like an infarct or a fracture and then, though reaction about it may develop and seemingly enlarge the area, the lesion does not increase in volume or mass. There is no evidence at present to suggest that osteoid osteoma is the result of either fracture or infarction but failure of growth is strong evidence against a neoplastic genesis.

Another bit of evidence supports this thesis. Several writers have followed an increasing number of cases that have undergone spontaneous healing. The first of these[7] reported two cases that regressed to a healed state in seven years and others[8] described a similar behavior. Admittedly, more data are needed because an ultimate diagnosis can be made only on section, and section eradicates the lesion. But the remarkably consistent clinical and radiologic features coupled with a familiar behavior pattern are rather convincing.

Finally, there is one more characteristic about osteoid osteoma that makes its classification as a neoplasm unacceptable by the present authors. The microscopy of the lesion describes a set and predictable pattern that is decidedly unlike that of the random growth of a tumor. This pattern suggests that something happens to a circumscribed area of bone. In an attempt at repair a mass of osteoid, microspicules and granulation are substituted for the affected normal tissue. The central area appears younger and more active, suggesting that the lesion heals centripetally. If this is the case it would explain why the primary lesion does not grow in size. The cause of the surrounding zone of sclerosis is equally debatable. Perhaps, as Golding suggests, it may be due to pressure causing a relative ischemia, this in turn causing a laying down and mineralization of an abnormal amount of organic matrix.

On the basis of appearance and behavior the osteoid osteoma could be caused by virus infection. A few attempts have been made to isolate a virus without success. A much more thorough approach should be made before the idea is abandoned.

Prognosis. Osteoid osteoma may be a self-limiting disease. There is some evidence, previously quoted, that such is the case. But spontaneous healing is a long-protracted and painful process and no surgeon would knowingly impose this type of management upon his patient. The almost instantaneous relief of pain following excision of the lesion is ample testimony of the virtue of early surgery.

Osteoid osteomas have been known to recur and it is said that this may be expected if the nidus is not removed. If the surgeon wishes to comfort himself with the assurance that the lesion has been removed in toto, he may take radiographs of the removed block and find on the film the nicely delineated nidus. When the primary focus is removed, the patient may expect complete and absolute recovery.

OSTEOBLASTOMA

Until Lichtenstein's paper[6] was published in 1956, this lesion was variously known as ossifying fibroma, osteogenic fibroma, osteoid fibroma, fibrous osteoma and giant osteoid osteoma.[9] Even today many observers believe that no such specific entity as osteoblastoma exists and others believe that it is a particularly florid type of osteoid osteoma. At least one of the reasons for this state of confusion is that a variety of bone lesions, neoplastic, reactive, vascular and metabolic, are characterized by microscopic similarities. Though the clinical and radiologic features of these conditions may differ widely, the poor pathologist, who rarely has the opportunity of examining all aspects of the case, has had a tendency to lump together a variety of entities because of similarities in microscopy. As a result it is almost completely futile to obtain a lucid concept of the lesion that we describe here by analysis of the literature.

It is probable that many of these lesions have been in the past and perhaps still are being diagnosed osteoid osteomas. The age and bone site incidence of the two lesions are the same, and though the clinical aspects may be somewhat different and the radiologic features most certainly are, there is sufficient similarity between the two lesions to make differentiation difficult in most and impossible in some cases. We have been able to collect 34 cases that conform to the classic description of osteoblastoma. These exclude our 15 cases of periosteal osteoid osteomas. They include 17 cases involving the neural arches of the vertebral column which are so uniform in symptomatology, radiology and pathology that one is tempted to consider them a specific clinicopathologic entity. Of the remaining 17 cases, 6 involve the small bones of the hands or feet and 11 the large cylindrical bones. All of these show the same microscopy, a reparative bone reaction with prominent osteoid production and little or no chondroid.

The term ossifying fibroma continues to confuse some observers. This name is usually applied to a fibrous lesion within the maxilla or mandible. It may manifest osteoid production or the fibrous matrix may disclose numerous small, irregular deposits of calcium salts within a collagenous matrix. In our experience most of these occur in males in or about the third decade of life. There is often a history of an extracted tooth. It is our opinion that these lesions present a different microscopic anatomy from that of benign osteoblastoma and many, perhaps most, are poorly defined cementomas. Many lesions of the jaw so diagnosed are doubtless cases of monostotic fibrous dysplasia.[10] Others are probably instances of post-extraction reparative

granuloma. Though we have seen one case of benign osteoblastoma of the skull and know no reason why it should not occur in the jaws, we know of no such lesion as yet reported.

The benign osteoblastoma is usually defined as a benign neoplasm. There may be bone destruction suggestive of neoplastic progression. Also, the sections may reveal a very active and irregular osteogenesis by osteoblasts whose appearance suggests the possibility of sarcoma. But the thoughtful microscopist with a considerable experience in bone pathology will realize that the osteoblastic activity that characterizes this lesion is strikingly similar to that seen in bone repair. The presence of giant cells enhances this similarity. Moreover, though a history of trauma can be obtained in a large percentage of all bone lesions, in our experience the relationship appears more consistent and pertinent in benign osteoblastoma. And, finally, benign osteoblastoma is probably a self-healing lesion though its duration is long, like that of osteoid osteoma, and after its symptoms arise it is apt to be painful. It is our opinion that benign osteoblastoma is not a true

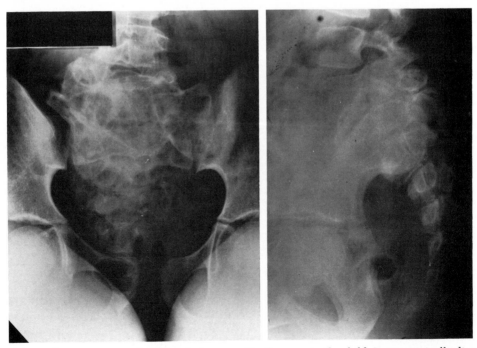

Figure 15–12 Roentgenogram of a lesion that occurred in the sacrum of a child. It was originally diagnosed osteosarcoma. Treated conservatively it healed and the patient is well after 13 years. Sections of the lesion (Fig. 15–16) analyzed with our present knowledge show it to be a benign osteoblastoma.

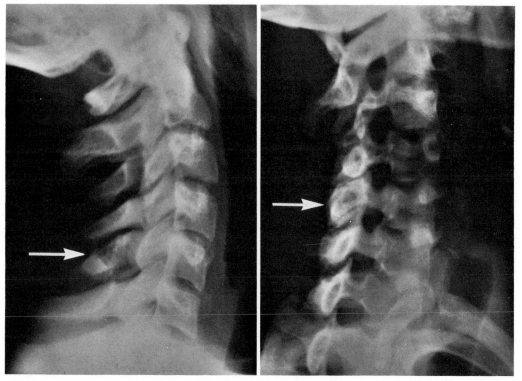

Figure 15–13   Benign osteoblastoma. The spinous process and neural arch on the right of the fifth cervical vertebra are involved (arrows). There is an area of destruction and slight expansion but minimal sclerosis.

neoplasm and, until we known more of its pathogenesis, it should be classified with the bone reactive processes.

Benign osteoblastoma is apparently an uncommon lesion. Only a few series have been published and these are small. We have collected 34 cases. The lesion occurs most frequently between the ages of 10 and 25. In our material the youngest patient was 6 and the oldest 38. The most common site of involvement is the neural arches of the vertebral column. Thus, 17 of our 34 cases arose in the vertebral axis, eight of them in males, and nine of them between the ages of 8 and 28.

The lesion causes pain. In our material the degree and type of pain revealed no differentiating features from that of osteoid osteoma. In one of our cases, relief with aspirin was striking. Tenderness is not mentioned prominently in the histories. In vertebral lesions the osteoblastoma frequently penetrates the cortex and causes pressure upon a spinal nerve or the cord itself. Benign osteoblastoma must always enter into the differential diagnosis of a young patient with radiating pain, backache, paresthesias or paraplegia.

Roentgenographic Manifestations. The radiographic appearance of the benign osteoblastoma is that of an expanding radiolucent lesion in which varying amounts of opacity are evident. A surrounding rim of sclerosis may be present. The radiolucency reflects the intercellular material and the opacity, the degree of mineralization of the osteoid that is present.

If the expanded cortex is perforated a soft tissue mass may be apparent in relation to the osseous abnormality. In this situation the radiographic aspects may mimic those of an osteosarcoma.

In cases in which osteoblastoma involves the neural arches, particularly in the cervical spine, it may present the appearance of aneurysmal bone cyst precisely. The distinction can be made only by biopsy.

Pathology.   The benign osteoblastoma

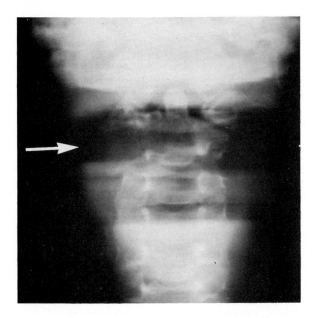

Figure 15–14 Benign osteoblastoma. Planigraphy of the cervical spine demonstrates the large lucent defect in the lateral mass of C_2 (arrow).

is usually not much larger than osteoid osteoma but in some instances it has been reported more than 10 cm. in diameter. It is a destructive lesion or it replaces an area of bone that has been destroyed, and though there may be some sclerosis of surrounding bone it does not provoke the degree of sclerosis that characterizes osteoid osteoma. Also, unlike osteoid osteoma it has a tendency to penetrate bone and may produce a small, soft tissue, tumor mass.

The microscopic appearance of benign osteoblastoma is similar enough to that of osteoid osteoma in most cases to make differentiation a problem. The principal feature of osteoblastoma is the remarkable number of osteoblasts. These are usually lined up along a surface of an osteoid or bone spicule, sometimes more than one cell in depth (Fig. 15–15). Sometimes they are found in solid aggregates with no osteoid in the field. These may represent tangential sections of a cluster of osteoblasts on a bone surface that lay beyond the section.

The intercellular material varies greatly in amount and in degree of maturation. There is great variation between cases and between different sections of the same case. This heterogeneity is to be expected because osteoblastoma is probably only the reparative reaction of bone tissue to a great variety of injuring agents. Sometimes this material is composed of the youngest and crudest osteoid with no evidence of mineral deposition. In others, fairly adult bone with lamellation and even haversian system formation is noted. There may be a rather delicate network of well formed spicules or heavy masses and irregular sheets of osteoid or bone with almost no interspicular matrix. This variation in microscopic character makes the lesion difficult to recognize. An occasional osteoblastoma reveals almost no mineral in its osteoid (Fig. 15–15 *B*). More often the spicules are at least partly ossified. Giant cells are a frequent component (Fig. 15–15 *C*). They may be sparsely scattered or occasionally thickly aggregated. These have been interpreted as osteoclasts by some writers and some of them unquestionably are. Elsewhere they have all the morphologic features of the multinucleated giant cells one finds so commonly in reactive processes. Old hemorrhage is apparent in many areas, usually represented by foci of hemosiderin pigment. Collections of giant cells are usually more prominent in the vicinity of extravascular blood or its derivatives.

The microscopist may find it difficult to differentiate benign osteoblastoma from osteoid osteoma and osteosarcoma. Osteoblastoma is apt to contain more bone,

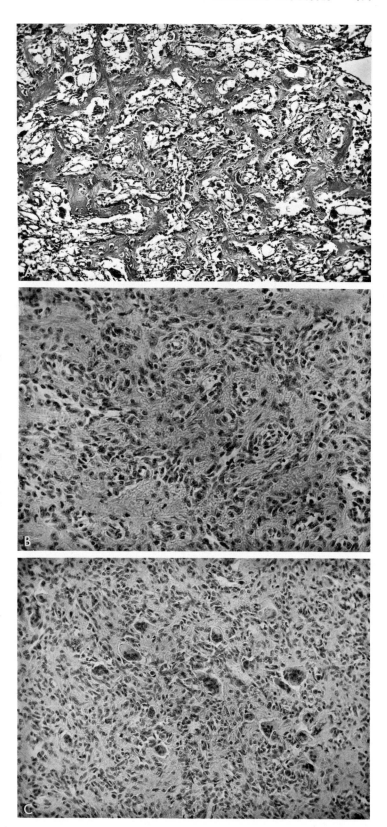

Figure 15–15 Benign osteoblastoma. *A,* Great numbers of osteoblasts are the most characteristic feature of the sections. Here they are producing coarse spicules of fiberbone. (× 175.) *B,* In some lesions, sheets and irregular masses of osteoid are formed. This may or may not be mineralized. (× 300.) *C,* Giant cells are often found in some areas of osteoblastoma. When bone is present they may have the appearance of osteoclasts. (× 275.)

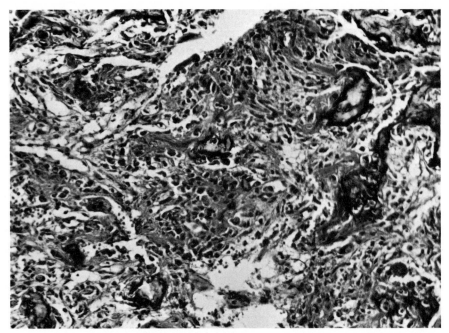

Figure 15–16 Benign osteoblastoma. This is a section of the lesion shown in Figure 15–12. Many benign osteoblastomas were called osteosarcoma, thus invalidating the survival statistics of that tumor in some series. (× 200.)

the osteoblastic activity should be more apparent and the radiating pattern of spicules less obvious than in osteoid osteoma. The cells of osteosarcoma should be more pleomorphic and mitotic figures more common (Fig. 15–16). Osteoid is rarely as well developed in the malignant tumor.

In summary we believe the osteoblastoma is a mishmash collection of reparative bone reactions. A goodly number, though probably not all, are large and atypical osteoid osteomas. Those that involve the neural arches appear to arise from vascular injuries within the dural sheath of bone. If the name "osteoblastoma" is to be retained it probably should be confined to this group. The rest of the lesions squeezed into this category are probably nothing more than a florid reparative reaction to an undemonstrated cause of bone injury. It matters little what we call them; however, this particular name, osteoblastoma, implies that they are neoplasms and so mislead the naive to treat them as such. One instance of osteoblastoma occurring in the spine of an adolescent was treated with cancericidal doses of x-ray, a therapy which can hardly be ex-

pected to cure the lesion or be beneficial to the future health of the patient.

Prognosis. Like the chondromyxoid fibroma, the benign osteoblastoma has not been recognized long enough and in sufficient numbers for one to be quite sure of its ultimate behavior. Today it is usually treated conservatively with curettage, sometimes followed by moderate amounts of irradiation. There appears to be no justification for the latter. To date there is no suggestion that the lesion is apt to recur and no evidence of progression in the manner of neoplasm.

NON-OSTEOGENIC FIBROMA

The non-osteogenic fibroma is a focal area of deossification replaced by collagenous fibrous tissue. It is difficult to estimate its incidence because more than half of the known cases have been symptomless and discovered only on skeletal surveys done for other reasons. It, with subperiosteal cortical defect, constitutes the most common type of delineated translucency found in the skeleton. The name "non-osteogenic fibroma" was applied by Jaffe and Lichtenstein in 1942[11] in their paper in which they established the identity of this lesion. They believed it was a neoplasm and classified it with the fibromas of bone. Because it is self-healing, often multiple and occasionally bilaterally symmetrical and usually asymptomatic, it is difficult for us to accept it as a true tumor and, therefore, it is considered more fully in another section. (See p. 308.) A brief summary is included here only because it is still classified in some texts as a tumor.

So-called "non-osteogenic fibroma" occurs most commonly in the age group 10 to 15 years, though characteristic lesions are not uncommonly found in younger children and less often in young adults. It occurs with greatest frequency in the large bones of the lower extremity, the femur being most often affected. Other parts of the skeleton may be involved, however, and it has been seen, though rarely, in flat bones.

It makes its appearance in the meta-physis a few centimeters from the epiphyseal line. It usually begins at the inner surface of the metaphyseal compacta and causes lysis of the contiguous cortical and cancellous tissues. It expands slowly over a period of months to reach a diameter of 3, 5 or even more centimeters. Because its growth is slow, the normal tissue along its advancing frontier manifests a reaction sclerosis, which sharply delineates it on the radiograph from the adjacent cancellous bone (Fig. 15–17). It erodes the overlying cortex from within and the periosteum responds by laying down a lamina of bone on the outer cortical surface, thus producing the picture of eccentric expansion. In slender bones it may occupy the entire diameter and cause a fusiform enlargement.

Because the process is so insidious there is no pain unless the cortex becomes so thinned that infractions occur or minor trauma results in a pathologic fracture. Practically all the symptomatic lesions are diagnosed on this basis.

Morbid Anatomy. When the surgeon removes the thin shell that often covers the non-osteogenic fibroma, he finds a mass of yellow, gray or brown soft tissue without spicules of bone. This tissue has a rather tough, stringy character.

When sectioned, it is found to consist of fields of spindled cells resembling moderately immature fibroblasts. There is a tendency for them to weave irregularly in a broad pattern, often producing whorls of poorly palisaded forms (Fig. 15–18 A). Intermixed, one can usually find, either singly or in aggregates, large macrophages whose cytoplasm contains lipid granules and vacuoles. This lipid apparently lends the yellow color to the lesion as it is seen grossly. Hemosiderin granules are usually quite prominent and if they are present the lesion may be brown. The fourth feature of note is the appearance of giant cells (Fig. 15–18 B). Intercellular collagen is usually present but rarely dominates the picture. If osteoid is found in the sections the lesion cannot be designated "non-osteogenic fibroma." However, some lesions which clinically and radiologically appear to be non-osteogenic fibromas will reveal small or even considerable amounts of osteoid in the sections. It is not at all improb-

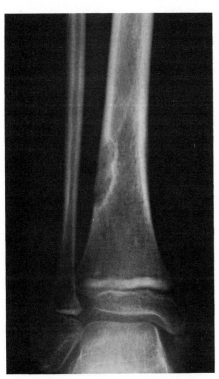

Figure 15–17 Non-osteogenic fibroma. Lesion in the distal tibia of a child. The eccentric position and the scalloped border of sclerotic bone are classic.

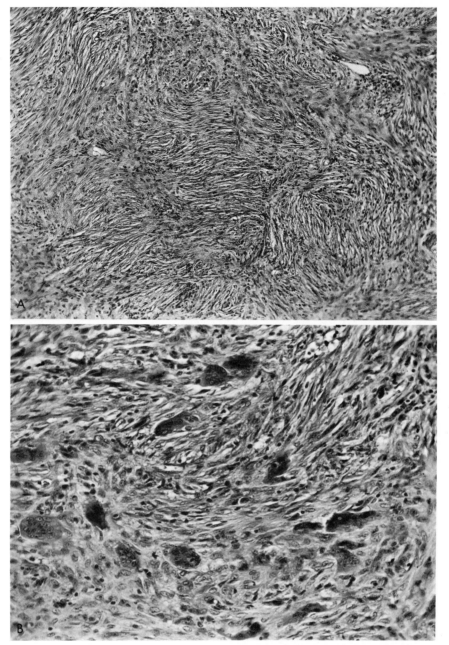

Figure 15-18   Non-osteogenic fibroma. *A*, Whorls of poorly palisaded cells are characteristic. (× 100.) *B*, Giant cells are often found scattered throughout the sections. (× 200.)

able, however, that non-osteogenic fibroma is a reparative lesion that cannot form bone, whereas osteoblastoma is the same type of lesion that can.

The microscopy is not pathognomonic because many types of reaction to bone injury produce an identical picture. The pathologist should have the advantage of viewing the roentgenograms or knowing the clinical diagnosis before he commits his diagnosis of non-osteogenic fibroma. If the lesion is young and the fibroblastic reaction florid, one may be misled into a diagnosis of fibrosarcoma, but the xanthoid reaction, the pigment, the collagen and the giant cells usually save the pathologist from this pitfall. The differential diagnosis of solitary cyst, giant cell tumor, fibrous dysplasia, histiocytosis, chronic osteomyelitis and bone infarct is dealt with in another section. (See p. 313.)

SUBPERIOSTEAL CORTICAL DEFECT

The lesion that we choose to call "subperiosteal cortical defect" appears to be an erosion of the outer cortical surface of the ends of long, cylindrical bones in children and adolescents. It is seen with such frequency in roentgenographic surveys of otherwise normal skeletons that one suspects it is a variation in normal bone growth. The importance of correctly recognizing the lesion stems from the danger of mistaking it for a process with a more serious prognosis and consequently overtreating a quite innocuous alteration. Should it be diagnosed as sarcoma, and at least one such lesion has been so diag-

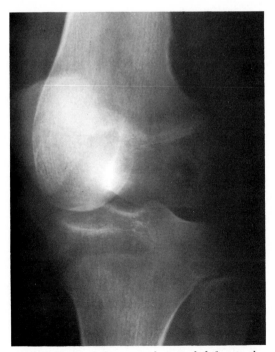

Figure 15–19 Subperiosteal cortical defect in the distal end of the femur. The lesion erodes the cortex from without and its advancing edge is delineated by an arc of sclerosed bone.

nosed, the mistake may lead to the tragedy of a needlessly amputated extremity.

Subperiosteal cortical defect is not a tumor. It is considered in this section only because it is most important that it be differentiated from a tumor. A more complete discussion may be found in another section. (See p. 314.)

The condition affects males about twice as often as females. It occurs most commonly in the first six years of life and less frequently up to the age of 15. To date, it has been reported only in cylindrical bones, usually in the lower extremity. The most common sites of involvement are the posterior and medial surfaces of the distal end of the femur. The next most common sites are the posterior and anterior surfaces of the proximal end of the tibia.

The lesion probably always starts at or near the epiphyseal line. As the involved bone grows, the affected area appears to pull away from the epiphysis and to drift into the metaphysis. There may be more than one area in a single bone but more commonly a second lesion is found on the opposite side involving an analogous situation.

On roentgenograms the affected area appears as a dishlike erosion beneath the periosteum (Fig. 15–19). The deep and advancing edge of the lesion may reveal a limiting zone of sclerosis and the overlying periosteum may produce a thin layer of bone, which roofs the cortical defect.

Morphology. When the periosteum is reflected or the eggshell-like roof is removed, a disc of yellow, gray or reddish brown tissue is found filling a concave defect in the compacta. This tissue is apt to be tough and fibrous. When sectioned it is found to consist of a fibrous stroma often with a suggestion of trabeculation. Scattered through this matrix one can usually find xanthoid cells, giant cells and hemosiderin pigment. In the limited material at hand (these lesions are infrequently biopsied) we have found small masses of osteoid and primitive cartilage. It is difficult to ascertain whether these components are the products of the lesion itself or the result of periosteal reaction.

The microscopy appears to be, within the limits of variation, that of non-osteogenic fibroma. This leads to the interesting speculation that together they constitute a single lesion type, one occurring within the metaphysis and the other outside. The radiology of the two lesions supports this thesis, because unless the roentgenograms are taken at various projections by rotating the part, it may be impossible to differentiate them.

The etiology and pathogenesis of subperiosteal cortical defect are unknown. It may be an ischemic lysis of bone, which is then replaced by the cheaper fibrous stroma, or it may be a reaction in the periosteal cambium, which brings an abnormal supply of blood to the part and thereby deossifies the area. One can make a very reasonable case by supposing that the lesion represents the repair of a subperiosteal hematoma. It is probable that the lesion from the outside may perforate the cortex and enter the cancellous metaphysis and that the non-osteogenic fibroma may progress in the reverse manner, making it impossible to state where such lesions started.

Prognosis. Subperiosteal cortical defect is a self-limiting condition. A number of cases have been followed throughout the course of the process and have eventually healed in two to five years.[12] At least one lesion is reported to have been excised and later recurred deeper in the metaphysis at the site at which it would have been had it been allowed to remain. Because the lesion is almost always symptomless its only importance is in recognizing it for what it is, rather than as a condition that would necessitate therapy.

HAMARTOMAS

The hamartoma differs from the bone reactive process. The latter is an attempt at repair in an area that has suffered injury. The former is a spontaneous disturbance in growth in which the cells of a circumscribed area outstrip those of the tissue surrounding it. Excessive proliferation interferes with pattern because of lack of room, and this in turn interferes with function. The cells mature just as normal cells do but they continue to exist as a useless cell mass, their presence in excess sometimes interfering with normal cell function. The cells of the hamartoma differ from those of the neoplasm because the cells of the latter do not mature and continue to proliferate; i.e., they are progressive. The question that logically follows is whether there is such a thing as benign neoplasm. Many of us believe that this question cannot yet be answered with assurance. If there are benign neoplasms, they must certainly be rare in a classification that recognizes the hamartoma in a separate class.

OSTEOMA

The osteoma is usually classified as a bone-forming tumor. Actually, it is no more than a localized exaggeration of intramembranous bone formation. It is a mass of bone tissue that is laid down on the surface of its host bone, matures and becomes static and can be considered an idiopathic hyperplasia or osteogenic hamartoma. Because it is strictly intramembranous in origin it is never complicated by the formation of cartilage and is found only in areas in which bone is normally produced directly by periosteum. Thus we may expect to find osteomas involving bones that are formed predominantly by intramembranous ossification, and such is the case. Most osteomas are found on the inner or outer surfaces of the head bones, though occasionally they arise from the bones of the extracranial skeleton.

The term osteoma has been applied to any excrescence or protuberance of fibrous or cartilaginous tissue that becomes ossified and predominantly bony. Such usage should be discouraged. Osteophytes are formed by the calcification and later ossification of tendinous tissue at the site of its insertion. This process is known as dystrophic calcification and is caused by a chemical or physical change in collagen that increases its affinity for calcium salts. Pointed "stalagmites" or ridges are thus formed, but the mechanism of formation is

quite different from that of osteoma or osteochondroma. Proliferating, reactive fibroblasts may acquire the ability to form
bone but here again these are not osteomas
but osteoid osteomas or benign osteoblastomas.

True osteomas usually occur on the
inner or outer tables of the bones of the
calvarium or bones of the face or mandible.
In certain conditions such as hyperostosis
frontalis interna and senile hyperostosis
they may be multiple. More often they occur singly and in cases in which they arise
on the outer surface of the skull they may
constitute a torus.

Osteomas are usually symptomless unless they protrude into a paranasal sinus or
its drainage channel (Fig. 15–20), or are located on the hard palate where the lesion
may interfere with a dental prosthesis, on
the internal surface of the mandible where
it may handicap the movement of the
tongue, or in the orbit.

Osteomas are formed by the apposition
of osseous tissue upon the surface of the
host bone. As the compacta is thickened
there may be resolution of the normal cortex with the formation of massive spicules
of lamellated bone, which forms the cancellous tissue of the protruding mass (Fig.
15–21). The ratio of bone mass to interspi-

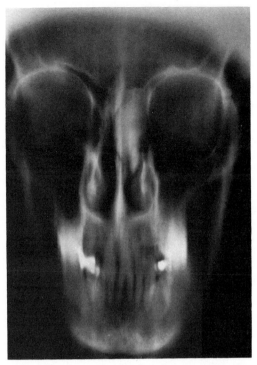

Figure 15–20   A planigraphic demonstration of an
osteoma in the outlet duct of the frontal sinus.

cular space is greatly increased over normal. Hematopoietic marrow may form in
the spaces or the latter may fill with fibrous tissue. The outer surface may be

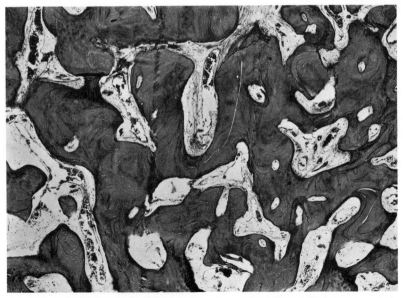

Figure 15–21   A section from the center of an osteoma. It consists of cancellous tissue composed of massive
spicules. This is covered with normal appearing compacta. (× 20.)

bosselated. It is always covered by a layer of periosteum.

Osteomas may form at any age but they are usually discovered some time during adult life. Once formed they remain without evidence of activity. They have never been known to exhibit truly neoplastic growth. They should be removed only if they intrude upon and disturb the function of nearby normal parts.

OSTEOCHONDROMA

The solitary osteochondroma is identical in every respect to the lesion that in multiple form constitutes osteochondromatosis (hereditary multiple exostoses). For a more general discussion see page 121. The abnormality is essentially a perversion in growth direction. It always arises at or near an epiphyseal line and protrudes at a right angle to the long axis of the host bone. Osteochondromas are always formed by enchondral growth, and because the bone substance produced is normal in every respect it may be considered not a tumor but rather an enchondral hamartomatous hyperplasia.

The cartilaginous portion of the osteochondroma acts as the growth plate for this abnormal growth. It persists only as long as there is growth activity and then becomes dissipated by the utilization of its chondrocytes to form a thin layer of hyaline cartilage over the top. The mature portion of the lesion consists of bone and therefore it should not be called a chondroma, or in its truest sense even an osteochondroma. A better name would be enchondral osteoma to associate it with the intramembranous osteoma, which is its counterpart.

The osteochondroma may be a solitary manifestation of osteochondromatosis (hereditary multiple exostoses) or more likely, because there appear to be no hereditary features involved, it may be an accidental occurrence of the same forces that are inherited in the general disease.

It may occur on any bone that is predominantly formed by enchondral ossification. A bit of the periphery of the growth plate of a normal bone apparently becomes separated from the main epiphyseal mass and retains its growth potential. It forms an epiphysis of the parasite lesion and is similar in all respects to the normal epiphysis except that it has no osseous nucleus. An irregular epiphyseal line is established and bone is laid down over a chondroid lattice. The cartilaginous cap is pushed outward over a cylinder of normal cortical bone that surrounds a "metaphysis" of cancellous tissue coextensive with that in the normal metaphysis. Interspicular hematopoietic marrow is formed with the same regulation as normal marrow. The same laws of growth that govern the normal skeleton also apply in the osteochondroma. Hamartomatous ossification slows and stops at the same time as normal ossification at the nearest epiphyseal line. At this point most of the lesions remain static. If they impinge on tendon movement, bursae form over them. A bursitis may develop or they may press upon vessels or nerves and thus give cause for removal.

Because of a failure of modeling of the host bone the metaphysis may remain wider than normal, giving a characteristic roentgenographic picture. If viewed perpendicularly a circle of translucency representing the defect in the cortex at the base of the lesion may appear on the film surrounded by a ring of opacity caused by the pedicle. Unless taken at another projection this may lead to confusion in diagnosis. For a more complete description of the radiographic findings, see page 124.

Morbid Anatomy. The osteochondroma is a cylindrical bony projection from the outer cortical surface of a normal bone. Its metaphysis is continuous with the cancellous tissue of the host. It is usually fin-shaped, flattened from side to side and leans toward the diaphysis and away from its epiphyseal center of origin. During its growth period its cartilaginous cap often extends down over the epiphyseal margin of the pedicle, a finding to be taken into consideration if surgical removal is contemplated because a certain percentage recur, perhaps because the germinal cartilage has not been completely removed.

When sections are made one finds the structure to consist of normal cortical and cancellous bone covered with a growth plate and a simulated epiphyseal line. One can judge whether the lesion is progressing or quiescent by the degree of activity in this area.

Prognosis. The fate of osteochondroma depends in part upon the site. A small lesion involving the large long bones may remain static and symptomless throughout a lifetime. Conversely, we have seen one arising from the acetabular articular plate that caused severe crippling. Rose and Fekete[13] reported one arising from the odontoid process that caused sudden death.

The osteochondroma should cease growing at the time of maturation of the nearest epiphyseal center. The great preponderance then remains inactive throughout adult life. Occasionally reactivation occurs and the reason is usually not apparent. There may be a history of trauma with fracture of the pedicle (Fig. 15–22). In cases in which renewed growth occurs the lesion must be considered a sarcoma until proven otherwise. It should be remembered that the cartilage and bone of osteochondroma are ectopic and like misplaced tissue anywhere in the body—em-

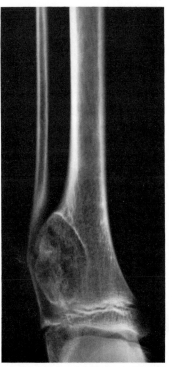

Figure 15–23 Osteochondroma. The lesion in this instance is sessile, but has widened the tibia and has resulted in adaptive changes in the fibula.

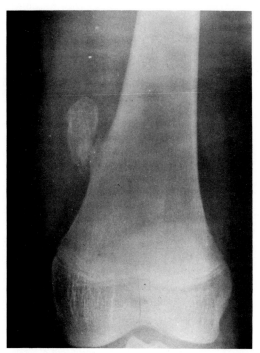

Figure 15–22 Osteochondroma. There is fracture of the pedicle due to trauma. Injury of this nature may reactivate the lesion and lead to transition to malignant neoplasm.

bryonal rests, undescended testis—are prone to take on a neoplastic character. It is assumed that a foreign environmental influence is responsible for this new growth potential. Because the three types of fibrous tissue are involved, the tumor may be a chondrosarcoma, osteosarcoma or fibrosarcoma. Or it may be made up of all three fibroblastic derivatives and as such produce a parosteal sarcoma. Indeed, it is our opinion that parosteal sarcoma is the malignant analogue of osteochondroma.

ENCHONDROMA

The solitary enchondroma is a circumscribed mass of cartilage cells occurring in the metaphysis of cylindrical bones. Both radiologically and cytologically the lesion is the same as that of enchondromatosis. (See p. 116.) Solitary enchondroma is rarely seen in children and in our own material of 79 patients there were only 14 under the age of 20 years, with an average

age incidence of 35. Of 23 patients with enchondromatosis, there was but one over the age of 26 with an average age of 14. These data suggest that the solitary enchondroma is not a congenital lesion. Because it is morphologically and behaviorally identical to the lesion of enchondromatosis, one must assume that it is an accident of bone development, which in enchondromatosis occurs in a congenital pattern, probably beginning in utero.

Solitary enchondroma begins in childhood or adolescence. A group of cartilage cells from the epiphysis apparently is not utilized in the process of chondroid lattice formation and is bypassed by the advancing epiphyseal line until it becomes isolated in the metaphysis. One might hypothesize that these are epiphyseal cells that fail to mature and, lacking the glycogen and enzymatic complements that are necessary for utilization in the line of provisional calcification, are ignored by the normal process of enchondral ossification and end up, viable and proliferating, in the metaphysis. They multiply slowly and it takes a long time for them to produce a mass sufficient to displace enough metaphysis to be identifiable on the roentgenogram. Eventually, they may occupy enough space to erode the cortex from within and to cause the overlying periosteum to compensate with an apposition of bone on the outer surface, giving the appearance of expansion. Occasionally they penetrate the cortex and then grow out into the soft tissue. When they do, the ectopic cartilage cells acquire the ability to form an epiphyseal line and stimulate osteoblastic activity. The process is thus converted into an osteochondroma.

The great preponderance of solitary enchondromas are found in the short, cylindrical bones of the hands and feet. Here they may cause lysis and replacement of the entire medullary tissue of the host bone. Less often they occur in the large, long bones of the extremities, the humerus and femur being most commonly involved. Solitary enchondromas may occur in the flat bones such as the ribs and ilium, but they are rare and any abnormal aggregate of cartilage cells within a flat bone should be regarded as a true neoplasm until disproved by adequate biopsy. Enchon-

dromas almost always begin near a cartilaginous epiphysis but we have encountered one within an unossified epiphysis. A cartilage mass in the mid-diaphysis should always arouse the suspicion of the diagnostician. It may be a benign neoplasm or a chondrosarcoma but it is almost certainly not an enchondroma and cannot be expected to behave like one.

Morphology. The solitary enchondroma is a spheroid mass of cartilage that replaces cancellous tissue and may erode the cortex. Because it grows so slowly it almost never produces symptoms until the overlying compacta becomes so thin that infractions or pathologic fracture occurs. Grossly it appears as a pale, bluish, glistening, resilient substance often with a lobulated or scalloped periphery. It never invades bone but pushes it aside or by pressure causes its lysis. Almost always one can find areas of sticky, semi-liquid or gelatinous material within its substance and sometimes the major portion of the lesion may have this consistency. This suggests that the normal cartilage cell function of chondroid production is deranged and the so-called "myxomatous material" is the best that it can produce.

Through the microscope one finds fields of chondroid in which are caught the chondroblasts. Their nuclei are small, uniform, darkly staining and young in appearance. Some fields may consist almost entirely of cells, other fields may be entirely chondroid and always the arrangement of the cells is much less regular than that of normal cartilage. Mitotic figures are usually lacking and if nucleoli are found they are small.

Prognosis. To foretell the behavior of an enchondroma from its microscopy alone is difficult or impossible, the reason being that the appearance of the cartilage cell, at least by present-day staining methods, gives us only an imperfect idea of what the cell is doing. In final analysis, the behavior of a tumor is far more important in its classification than its morphology, the latter being only a means, and often a poor one, of prognosing the former. The chondrosarcoma is, obviously, a true tumor; the enchondroma is a hamartoma. That we as yet have no means of absolutely differentiating the two lesions does not dispute this fact. It is possible that a chondrosarcoma begins in the metaphysis as often as elsewhere in bone, and when it does it is diagnosed as an enchondroma and its behavior denigrates the reputation of the latter. On the other hand, perhaps the enchondroma alone begins in the metaphysis and, being ectopic to the area, has a penchant for changing into a true neoplasm. Of the 79 enchondromas in our material, 10 had apparently undergone change to chondrosarcoma, an incidence of just under 13 per cent.

To our knowledge there is no means by which the clinician, the radiologist or the pathologist may be absolutely sure whether he is dealing with a neoplasm or a hamartoma, though there are certain features that are helpful. If the lesion is in a small bone of the hands or feet, it is almost surely an enchondroma. If it is in the metaphysis of a large, cylindrical bone, in the middle third of any bone or in a flat bone, it is more apt to be a chondrosarcoma. If the microscopist can demonstrate invasion, or evidence of rapid growth (numerous mitoses) or cellular pleomorphism, a diagnosis of neoplasm is warranted. In most instances the problem remains a problem until subsequent behavior of the lesion defines its character. Consequently it is justifiable to treat a problematic case more radically than one would recommend for a known enchondroma.

ANGIOMA OF BONE

The capillaries and the small afferent and efferent channels in relation to them are made up of a variety of cell constituents. Lining the vessel is a single layer of endothelial cells supported by a thin layer of fibrocytes. Spiraling about the latter are the hemangiopericytes of Zimmermann, curious cells, which like muscle have the capacity of contracting. These three cell types apparently have a common stem cell genesis, mesenchymal fibrous tissue. In newly formed granulation one can see evidence of transition of fibroblasts into endothelial cells and the reverse, and it is assumed that the hemangiopericytes have a like origin. The morphology and activity of the three types of cells appear to depend upon environment and functional demand. It should not surprise us, therefore, that developmental and neoplastic alterations in the components of vessels produce a variety of lesions. These lesions fall into two large classes, the neoplasms and the hamartomas. Because both arise from fibrous tissue they are placed in the collagenic group for the sake of convenience.

The appearance of the vasculature neoplasms depends upon the type of cell that is predominantly involved. If the proliferation is largely endothelial, these lesions are best called hemangioendotheliomas (Stout), if the fibrous element predominates they may be called hemangiosarcomas (Kaposi) and if the hemangiopericyte is principally concerned they are best called hemangiopericytomas (Stout).

The developmental lesions of vessels are less simply classified. Usually all structural elements are represented so that recognizable vascular channels form the unit of the lesion. If the channels are large and thin-walled they are called cavernous hemangiomas, if small and thick-walled, capillary hemangiomas. If the channels become obliterated by fibrous tissue they are called sclerosing hemangiomas. In the skin they may be called vascular nevi or birthmarks. All of these are simple overgrowths of tissues native to the part and as such are true hamartomas. The lesions enlarge at the rate of growth of the surrounding tissue and cease to grow at maturity. Because they are not progressive they should not be considered neoplasms.

A cumbersome nomenclature of eponyms has grown up to designate various complexes of vascular lesions of developmental nature. Various combinations of skin, visceral and brain involvement have been designated as Sturge-Weber disease, Rendu-Osler-Weber disease and von Hippel-Lindau disease. A combination of multiple hemangiomas and enchondromatosis is sometimes called Maffucci's syndrome.

Vascular hamartomas called angiomas have been found in practically every tissue of the body. They are often multiple. In the cavernous type the arteriovenous communications (referred to in some areas, particularly the lungs, as arteriovenous

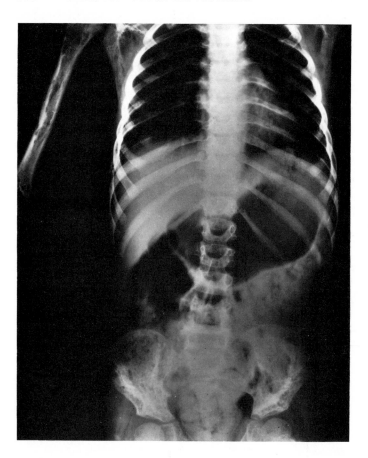

Figure 15–24 Hemangioma of bone. Extensive skeletal involvement is evident. The bones are less opaque than normal with many areas of circumscribed radiolucency. Both compact and spongy bone are involved.

fistulas) may be sufficient to cause hypertrophic osteoarthropathy, cyanosis and polycythemia. One of the hazards of these lesions if they involve an internal surface is hemorrhage.

Angiomas occur in muscle and bone. No one knows the incidence of the latter because apparently the majority are symptomless and can be found only on sectioning the bone. Others produce areas of bone lysis large enough to be seen on radiographs that have been taken for other reasons. Still others produce bone destruction and give rise to symptoms. These last are quite unusual.

The mechanism by which bone angioma produces lysis is unknown but one can presume that because there may be arteriovenous communications, an excess of arterial blood flows through the part. This alteration in other lesions produces a leaching of the bone involved and the same mechanism may apply in angioma.

Symptomatic angiomas may occur in any bone but they are rare in bones other than the vertebrae and skull. They are usually found in children and adolescents. Massive involvement of a vertebral body (Fig. 15–27) may eventuate in collapse with pressure upon the cord or the nerve roots. The pattern of bone destruction and reaction is often sufficiently characteristic to allow a diagnosis from the roentgenogram. An unusual lesion most apt to affect a bone of the calvarium is an infiltrating hemangioma, which causes a mushroom-like growth of bone from the outer cortical surface. This gives a dramatic sunburst effect on the roentgenogram.

There is a condition that has been called massive osteolysis, Gorham's disease,[14] acro-osteolysis, disappearing bones, acute absorption of bone or phantom clavicle (Fig. 15–28) in which, usually following trauma in adolescents and young adults, there is a progressive resorption of one or more bones in a skeletal area. The clavicle is most often involved but the scapula, jaw, pelvis, femur and bones of the hands and feet have been reported.[15] All or a major

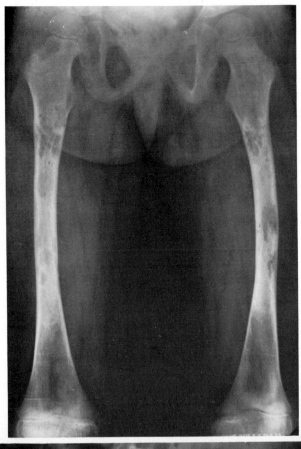

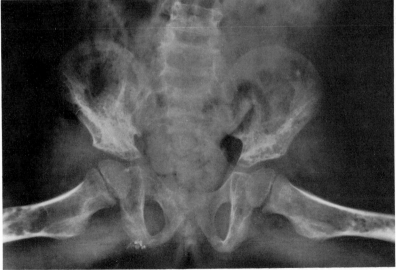

Figure 15–25   Hemangioma of bone. Same patient as in Figure 15–24 to illustrate better the individual lesions and the general abnormality of architecture and density.

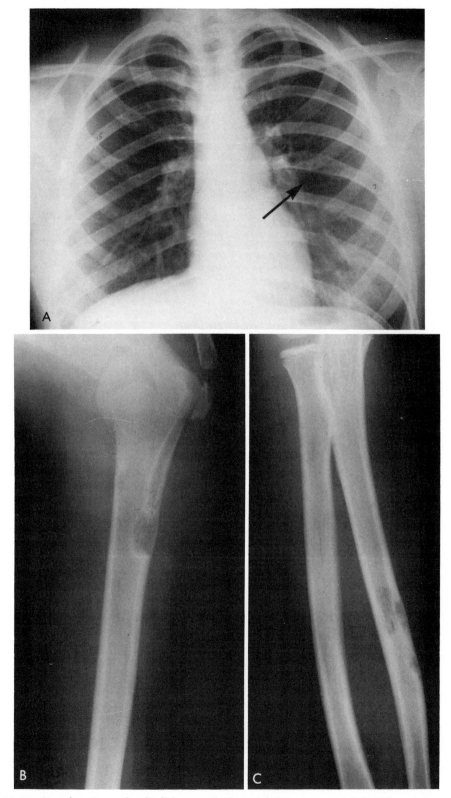

Figure 15–26   Lymphangioma of multiple bones. The lucent defects are associated with serpiginous sclerotic trabeculae and often a sclerotic border. The cortex may be involved (*B* and *C*) and the bone may be expanded (*A*).

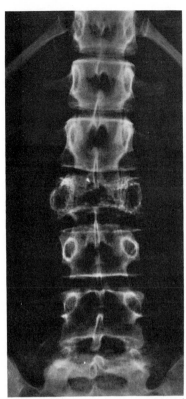

Figure 15-27 Hemangioma of vertebra. The third lumbar vertebra is more radiolucent than is normal with coarse striations (vertical). There is loss in stature of the body.

portion of an entire bone may gradually disappear from the roentgenograms over a period of months and years.[16] Only a few cases have been adequately studied but in some of these[17] the bone has been found to be involved in what is called angiomatosis, i.e., a permeation by an excessive number of small, thin-walled capillary type of blood or lymphatic vessels. Because these lesions do not progress to neoplastic growth it is assumed that they are a type of hamartomatous angioma. The bone or several related bones may be converted to a residual fibrous band showing no evidence of the former normal structure.

Morbid Anatomy. The highly vascular nature of the angioma of bone and its capacity for hemorrhage on incision may give the surgeon considerable difficulty. There are reports of patients who exsanguinated on the operating table.

The diagnosis on the sectioned tissue is usually simple. Most of these lesions are cavernous hamartomas consisting of large, irregular spaces filled with red blood cells and surrounded by thin walls lined with endothelium (Fig. 15-29). There are a number of situations in which the microscopy may be imitated by telangiectasis or varicosities of otherwise normal vessels.

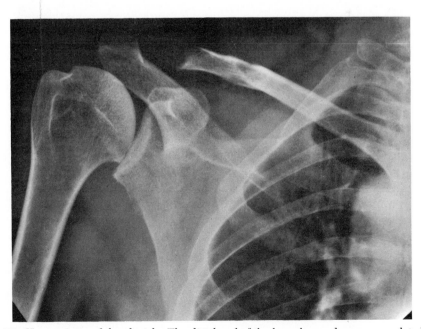

Figure 15-28 Hemangioma of the clavicle. The distal end of the bone has undergone complete lysis by the vascular hamartoma.

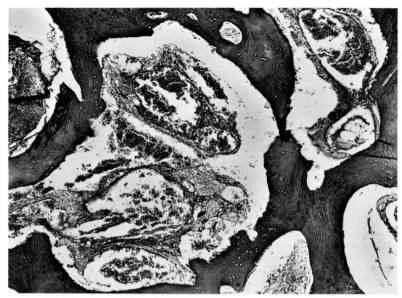

Figure 15–29 Section through a hemangioma of bone. Between the spicules of bone there are numerous large, thin-walled, vascular sinuses filled with blood. (× 27.)

Inflammatory granulation or highly vascular tumor may occasionally mimic angioma. If the lesion is not quite apparent the cautious pathologist should use restraint in making the diagnosis.

Prognosis. The angiomas may be vulnerable to irradiation therapy. If thrombosis can be produced, sclerosis may be initiated. The angiomas of bone are more difficult to reach than those of soft tissue

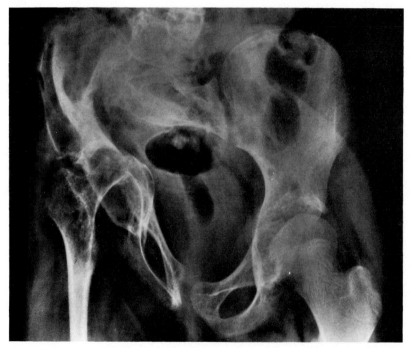

Figure 15–30 Angiomatosis involving the right pelvis and upper end of the femur. There is a congenital, hamartomatous proliferation of vessels, which inhibited normal growth. The left pelvis and femur have grown normally.

and the therapist must weigh the possibility of damage to the growth plates in growing bone.

True vasculature tumors of bone are exceedingly rare though hemangiosarcomas do occur. These usually run a rapid malignant course with fatal termination due to widespread metastasis.

Angiomas are often congenital and not infrequently multiple.[18] If several bones are involved the condition is known as angiomatosis of bone (Figs. 15–24, 15–25, 15–30). The lesions may be monomelic, unilateral or widely scattered and general. Any portion of the bone may be involved. Most patients with angiomatosis of bone reveal angiohamartomas in the soft tissues, especially the skin. Angiomas of the viscera, the eye, the mucous membranes of the pharynx and the coverings of the brain are apt to rupture and bleed. Other than large lesions of the vertebrae, most bone angiomas remain symptomless.

ANEURYSMAL BONE CYST

The aneurysmal bone cyst is a shell-like protrusion from the cortical surface of a bone, surrounding a mass of convoluted vascular channels bearing a blood flow in communication with the normal circulation. Because it causes bone destruction and a tumor-like mass it is frequently classified as a neoplasm. Neither its behavior nor its microscopy is that of neoplastic growth but it is a tumor-like mass; therefore, it deserves mention in this chapter. Some aneurysmal bone cysts probably arise in congenital arteriovenous fistulas and so can be considered hamartomatous growths. Others probably arise in organizing hematomas making them reactive processes. They are discussed more fully in Chapter 13 with the miscellaneous diseases of the skeleton.

Aneurysmal bone cyst, as an entity, has been reported only since 1950, though several accounts of the lesion may be found in the earlier literature under the title of aneurysmal cyst, bone hemangioma, aneurysmal giant cell tumor and telangiectatic osteogenic sarcoma. It differs from ordinary angioma of bone in that the sinuses are not true vascular walls

and the angioma does not produce the saccular outpouching of cortical bone.

Aneurysmal bone cyst has been reported over a wide age range from childhood to old age, but it occurs prevalently in the second and third decades. Both flat and cylindrical bones may be involved with perhaps one quarter of the cases occurring in the vertebrae, often involving the laminae or the pedicles.

The process almost always starts within cancellous or medullary tissue and erodes the cortex from within. The lesion has the peculiar and remarkable propensity of stimulating the periosteum to deposit bone over the affected area. Continuous erosion from within and apposition on the outside cause an expanding lesion whose silhouette is like that of a saccular aneurysm of the aorta—hence the name. Eventually stress or trauma is likely to cause fracture of the protective shell of bone and blood may be extravasated into the surrounding soft tissues. A hematoma with consequent organization, fibrosis, calcification and ossification may mask the primary lesion and produce a picture very similar to that in secondary myositis ossificans. Diagnosis of aneurysmal bone cyst before cortical outpouching takes place or after fracture and hemorrhage have occurred may be difficult or impossible. Misdiagnosis has all too frequently in the past resulted in overtreatment.

The only consistent symptom of aneurysmal bone cyst is pain, probably due to lifting of the periosteum, pressure upon contiguous normal structures or fracture. A firm mass may be palpated if the involved bone is superficial. Roentgenograms are frequently diagnostic though massive bone destruction and secondary hemorrhage may mask the saccular profile.

The morbid physiology of aneurysmal bone cyst is unknown. Because the structure is an alteration in vascular anatomy and because it is known that an excessive blood flow to a given region of bone causes lysis, one is tempted to use this mechanism as an explanation. The lesion has been so incompletely studied from the anatomic standpoint that confirming data are lacking. Perfusion x-ray studies would be most helpful but as yet an insufficient number have been reported to warrant firm conclusions.[19] It is unknown whether the lesion represents a congenital arteriovenous fistula, an organized hematoma with arteriovenous communications, an alteration in pressure dynamics, or perhaps all of these.

Gross and Microscopic Appearance. When the covering shell of bone is incised, a profusely and steadily bleeding mass of soft tissue is encountered. Much of the lesion consists of blood lakes traversed by a meshwork of fibrous walls in which are embedded larger, irregular fields of solid tissue. Sections of the latter show them to be basically fibrous, usually with large numbers of giant cells, xanthoid cells and degenerating blood pigment. This is the same microscopy that one finds wherever there has been extravasation of blood within bone. Frequently one encounters channels whose walls are composed of fibrous septa. It is impossible to say whether the lining cells are endothelial or merely swollen components of connective tissue.

Wherever a fluid-filled space is created within solid tissue one can find the surrounding fibrous tissue adapting itself, with the production of a lining of cells indistinguishable from those of normal vascular channels. In the walls one may find the same giant and xanthoid cells and hemosiderin granules that characterize the larger masses of solid tissue. In addition, there are often spicules of osteoid, which may be partially mineralized (Fig. 15–31). One must assume that the fibrous tissue is stimulated to produce bone in an environment that is supercharged with calcium salts being freed from the surrounding bone that is being destroyed. The channels are large and tortuous and the walls are often much thicker than those of normal vessels. The microscopist should always search diligently through numerous sections for the channels, but finding them does not guarantee the diagnosis of aneurysmal bone cyst. We have found channels that we believe identical in lesions that certainly were not aneurysmal bone cyst. Because they appear in less than half the cases in our material, failure to find them means little. The most consistent microscopic finding is a dramatic display of multinucleated giant cells (Fig. 15–32). The source of these cells is unknown but we assume them to be of histiocytic origin, perhaps in response to hemorrhage. If small bits of the solid tissue are obtained the appearance may be that of "giant cell tumor" or brown tumor of parathyroid adenoma.

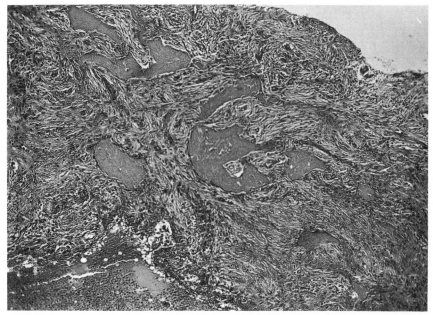

Figure 15–31 Aneurysmal bone cyst. Wall of a channel containing spicules of bone. Luminal surface is seen in upper right corner. (× 150.)

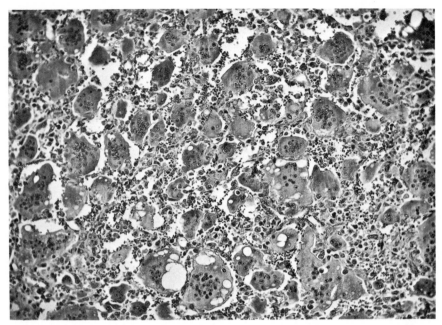

Figure 15–32 Aneurysmal bone cyst. Large masses of multinucleated giant cells constitute the most common finding. Usually these are most thickly dispersed about areas of hemorrhage.

Prognosis. The lytic activity of the lesion is apparently controlled if flow of blood through the sinusoids is prevented. This may be done by thrombosing and sclerosing the channels with irradiation (not usually practical) or mechanically interrupting the flow by curettage. Either method appears to be effective without completely destroying the lesion.

References

OSTEOID OSTEOMA

1. Jaffe, H. L.: Arch. Surg., *31*:709, 1935.
2. Sherman, M. S.: J. Bone Joint Surg., *29*:918, 1947.
3. Johnson, G. F.: Am. J. Roentgenol., *74*:65, 1955.
4. Jaffe, H. L., and Lichtenstein, L.: J. Bone Joint Surg., *22*:645, 1940.
5. Dahlin, D. C. and Johnson, E. W.: J. Bone Joint Surg., *36A*:559, 1954.
6. Lichtenstein, L.: Cancer, *9*:1044, 1956.
7. Moberg, E.: J. Bone Joint Surg., *33A*:166, 1951.
8. Golding, J. S. R.: J. Bone Joint Surg., *36B*:218, 1954.

OSTEOBLASTOMA

9. Dahlin, D. C. and Johnson, E. W.: J. Bone Joint Surg., *36A*:559, 1954.
10. Schlumberger, H.: Mil. Surgeon, *99*:504, 1946.

NON-OSTEOGENIC FIBROMA

11. Jaffe, H. L. and Lichtenstein, L.: Am. J. Path., *18*:205, 1942.

SUBPERIOSTEAL CORTICAL DEFECT

12. Sontag, L. W. and Pyle, S. I.: Am. J. Roentgenol., *46*:185, 1941.

OSTEOCHONDROMA

13. Rose, E. and Fekete, A.: Am. J. Clin. Pathol., *42*:606, 1964.

ANGIOMA OF BONE

14. Gorham, L. and Stout, A.: J. Bone Joint Surg., *37A*:985, 1955.
15. Torg, J. and Steel, H.: J. Bone Joint Surg., *51A*:1649, 1969.
16. Cheney, W.: Am. J. Roentgenol., *94*:595, 1965.
17. Gorham, L. W., Wright, A. W., Schultz, H. H. and Maxon, F. C.: Am. J. Med., *17*:674, 1954.
18. Halliday, D., Dahlin, D., Pugh, D. and Young, H.: Radiology, *82*:637, 1964.

ANEURYSMAL BONE CYST

19. Lindbom, A., Soderberg, G., Spjut, H. and Sunnquist, O.: Acta Radiol., *55*:12, 1961.

Chapter 16

OSTEOGENIC TUMORS

Bone is a complex of organic matrix, osteoid, in which are deposited crystals of mineral salts. The osteoid is elaborated in the presence of cells that we call osteoblasts. The exact mechanism of elaboration is unknown but the metabolic activity of these cells is somehow involved. We have no way of identifying osteoblasts until they become associated with osteoid but we assume they are derived from the more primitive type of cells that we call fibroblasts or in the metaphyseal area of growing bone, from vessel endothelial lining cells. Fibroblasts also provide collagenoblasts and chondroblasts and these three types of cells seem to have the ability to change from one type to another. In normal bone production the progression appears to be from collagenoblast to chondroblast to osteoblast. Osteoid production for the purposes of growth and maintenance apparently cannot occur without a nidus of cartilage or bone to support the osteoblast. Thus enchondral ossification is accomplished by means of a preformed cartilage lattice and intramembranous bone is laid directly on pre-existing cortical bone. Under abnormal conditions a peculiar type of osteoid may be produced by a process that has been called fibro-osseous metaplasia. This is the production of an osteoid-like substance by cells that retain the appearance of collagenoblasts.

All this becomes pertinent when we try to analyze what is happening in the growth of primary bone tumors. If the cell type has reached a stage of maturity that allows it to produce collagen alone, the tumor is a fibrosarcoma. Because it is the most mature of the three cell types this cell produces a tumor that grows slowly and is late to metastasize. Less mature cells produce collagen and chondroid. These tumors we know as chondroblastomas, chondromyxoid fibromas or chondrosarcomas. Finally, if the cells are so immature that they are capable of producing crude collagen, chondroid and osteoid or if a still younger form produces none of these, the tumor is an osteosarcoma, the most malignant variety of the three.

If the osteoid that is produced is normal in quality and pattern but abnormal in quantity and position, the lesion is a hamartoma. Of these there are two examples in the osteogenic series, the osteoma and the osteochondroma. If the osteoid is normal in quality but abnormal in pattern, the lesion is a reactive process. Examples of these are osteoid osteoma and osteoblastoma. There are two true neoplasms of osteoblastic origin, the osteosarcoma and the parosteal sarcoma. The former, as previously stated, is of an embryonic cell type that grows rapidly, is highly destructive and metastasizes early. The latter is a paradox because it forms collagen, chondroid and osteoid, yet the tumor is slow growing and late of metastasis. The explanation here is that the parosteal sarcoma is in reality a combination of relatively mature cell types, each type producing its special intercellular material. In the sense of Stout's mesenchymoma of soft tissues the parosteal sarcoma is a mesenchymoma of bone.

One other tumor type must be mentioned in this category, the osteoclastoma, giant cell tumor of bone. Actually its cytogenesis is unknown though the giant cells are probably vaguely related to osteoclasts and the stromal cells to fibroblasts from which osteoblasts and thence osteoclasts arise. Therefore, though osteoclastoma could be considered an osteoblastic tumor, it is more reasonable to think of it as a type of fibrosarcoma. Because any disposition of this complex neoplasm is apt to engender controversy we shall treat it under a separate heading of its own.

OSTEOSARCOMA

The osteosarcoma is a malignant neoplasm arising from the undifferentiated, multipotential, fibroblastic cells of bone. It is more generally called osteogenic sarcoma. Ewing used the term "osteogenic" to indicate that the tumor is of osseous genesis but other writers use it to mean that it forms bone tissue. Because the cells of osteosarcoma may be less mature than the bone-forming osteoblast and because they may or may not form osteoid, the present writers prefer to use the noncommittal term "osteosarcoma."

Until relatively recently the term "osteogenic sarcoma" was used to include all primary malignant tumors of bone with the exception of malignant giant cell tumors and those arising from marrow elements. Thus, osteosarcomas, chondrosarcomas and fibrosarcomas of bone were all grouped together. Because these three tumors have quite different age and site incidence, radiologic and cytologic features and mortality statistics, this unfortunate situation has led to confusion and quite inaccurate reporting. Recently a more definitive classification has led to clearer concepts and more trustworthy prognostication.

Once the importance of the primary malignant bone tumors as entities is established, further classification becomes largely a matter of opinion. Osteosarcoma has been subdivided into many categories, the most generally used being sclerosing, osteolytic, subperiosteal, medullary and telangiectatic. We hold that any classification of a disease that is not concerned with the manner and extent to which the patient is affected is tedious pedantry. The previously mentioned classification may be of some use to the radiologist but because it

in no way indicates the behavior of the tumor type, its general usage should be abandoned. We recognize two subtypes of osteosarcoma whose radiologic and microscopic features are sufficiently different from the usual osteosarcoma to merit special comment, the sclerosing osteosarcoma and the primitive bone sarcoma.

With the exception of plasma cell myeloma, osteosarcoma is the most commonly occurring primary malignant tumor of bone. It is encountered nearly twice as often as chondrosarcoma and, excluding the special type in the jaw, about three times as often as fibrosarcoma. In almost all reported series its incidence in males is greater than in females and in some, twice as great. The age incidence of osteosarcoma is most interesting. If one analyzes the various available series one finds that there is a preponderance in the age group under 30 years, but a rather bountiful scattering throughout the ages over 30. However, if one considers the type of bone involved, one sees a more distinct separation of two types of osteosarcoma. In our series of 185 cases, 157 were in large cylindrical bones and of these, 80 per cent were in patients under the age of 30. Of the 28 cases occurring in flat bones, 85 per cent were in patients over the age of 30. Thus, it appears that osteosarcoma is more frequent in those under 30 and usually occurs in cylindrical bones. A second and smaller rise occurs in the age incidence curve after 50 and these tumors are almost always found in flat bones. In this latter group there is a very high percentage of associated Paget's disease (see Fig. 16–4); in our total series there were only 12 cases, but if calculated on the basis of osteosarcoma over 50 years of age there was slightly over 50 per cent.

The most common bone to be involved in all series is the femur; in fact, nearly 50 per cent of all osteosarcomas occur in this bone. The humerus and tibia are next most commonly involved, and because the usual area is distal femur and proximal tibia about 75 per cent of all osteosarcomas in the juvenile-cylindrical bone group occur in the region of the knee. The upper end of the humerus is much more commonly involved than the lower end. It will be noted that these are the sites of principal growth in these bones. Of the flat bones the ilium is most often involved but the sacrum, sternum, ribs and skull are not invulnerable. Osteosarcoma rarely affects the small bones of the hands and feet. There are only four in our material and not more than a dozen in the entire literature. The tumor has been reported recently in the phalanges following irradiation; these are presumably secondary tumors. A number of lesions commonly occurring in these short cylindrical bones may mimic osteosarcoma and it is well to remember that this diagnosis in these bones is almost certain to be wrong.

In cases in which osteosarcoma affects the cylindrical bones, it usually is the metaphysis that is involved. The tumor arises very near the epiphyseal line, practically always within 5 cm. of it. Only six long bone osteosarcomas in our material have occurred outside the metaphysis (Fig. 16–1). Osteosarcoma probably does not arise in or on the cortex, although because they are massively destructive, the site of origin is not always determinable. A bone-forming tumor does arise in the perios-

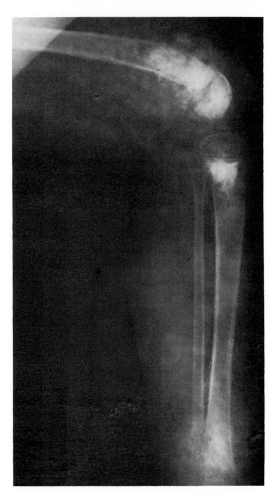

Figure 16–2 Multiple sclerosing osteosarcoma. Note areas of radiopacity in the distal femur and proximal and distal tibia. These tumors are usually found in multiple cylindrical bones, in young children. The epiphyseal center of the femur is involved.

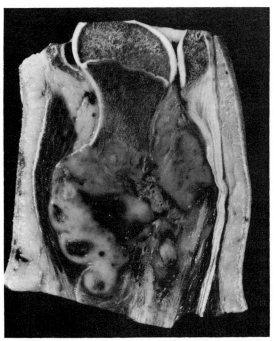

Figure 16–1 This is an unusual site for an osteosarcoma. The tumor apparently started several centimeters shaftward from the metaphysis.

teum—the parosteal sarcoma—but it has quite distinctive clinical, radiologic and pathologic features. Of course, osteosarcomas secondary to Paget's disease or irradiation may occur in any portion of any bone. The literature contains numerous instances of primary osteosarcoma of the diaphysis and the validity of these reports will not be denied, but it is worthy of mention that any lesion in a long bone involving other than the metaphyses should be very carefully considered before a diagnosis of osteosarcoma is made.

A peculiar and rare type of multiple osteosarcoma involves many sites simultaneously (Fig. 16–2). Both cylindrical and

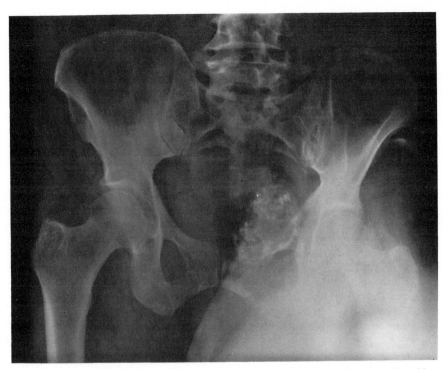

Figure 16-3   Extraosseous osteosarcoma. This tumor arose in the gluteal muscles. It produced large amounts of radiopaque bone and metastasized to the lungs.

flat bones are involved and the reported cases have usually been in patients under 15 years of age.[1] These osteosarcomas usually are of the sclerosing type producing irregular areas of dense radiopacity. It is unknown, of course, whether the tumor is multicentric or whether the many lesions represent bone metastases. Bone metastasis is unusual in osteosarcoma, lending credence to the former idea.

Extraosseous osteosarcoma is a rare tumor. Fine and Stout[2] collected 12 cases and reviewed those in the literature. Seven of 46 cases apparently began in myositis ossificans. The preponderance of the tumors occurred in the muscles of the extremities, most frequently in the legs (Fig. 16-3). They behaved very much in the same manner as do osteosarcomas of bone. Most of them ran a rather rapid course and metastasized to the lungs. There was only an 8.8 per cent five-year cure rate among the cases on which there was sufficient data for analysis. These authors urge caution in diagnosis of a group that they term "pseudomalignant," stating

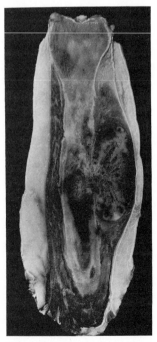

Figure 16-4   Osteosarcoma superimposed on a Paget's lesion. In this instance the tumor may be found in any part of the bone rather than in the usual site, the metaphysis.

that this lesion is a type of myositis ossificans.

Osteosarcoma, chondrosarcoma and fibrosarcoma may be superimposed on Paget's disease (Fig. 16–4). In the series of Thomson and Turner-Warwick,[3] of 32 cases of osteosarcoma, 5 were associated with Paget's disease. In our material there were 23 osteosarcomas in patients over the age of 50. Putting it another way, of the combined series there were 40 patients over the age of 50 with osteosarcoma. Twenty-three or slightly more than half of these had Paget's disease. Paget's disease is common, and if one estimates the percentage of associated osteosarcoma the figure must be very low. Indeed, an authority on Paget's disease has stated that no case of Paget's which he has followed has ever developed osteosarcoma. However, osteosarcoma in patients over the age of 50 is quite uncommon and the figure of 50 per cent is probably not far wrong in expressing an association, especially if occult monostotic Paget's disease is considered.

Osteochondroma predisposes to sarcoma. It is impossible to give an accurate estimate of the number of osteochondromas that eventually develop into malignant tumors, but the figure has been variously stated as 5 to 15 per cent. If a careful study is made of these tumors it will be found that most or even all of them are parosteal sarcomas.

Recently, it has been shown that osteosarcoma may evolve at a site affected with fibrous dysplasia. A paper[4] reviews the literature on four cases and reports a fifth. We have studied two such cases. The osteosarcoma, which may be multicentric, runs the usual rapid course with death in about 18 months.

Massive irradiation of bone tissue appears to increase the incidence of bone sarcomas. Osteosarcomas, chondrosarcomas and fibrosarcomas have been reported following x-ray therapy for other lesions in bone or contiguous soft tissue. Hatcher reviewed the literature[5] and found 24 cases, 15 of which were osteosarcoma. One osteosarcoma of the ilium in our material followed irradiation therapy for a genital carcinoma. In most cases, though not in all, excessive doses have been administered. The sarcoma has usually appeared in the area of bone most heavily irradiated rather than in the customarily involved sites. Its course is like that of primary osteosarcoma. There is some evidence that not only is the dosage important but also divided doses administered over an extended period, such as a year, are more apt to be cancerogenic. The interval between therapy and the advent of symptoms of sarcoma has averaged about 11 years. It has been stated that in cases in which sarcoma appears within three years of irradiation, the latter probably has no etiologic relation. Martland studied the cases of 800 girls[6] who had worked in a luminous dial factory and who had ingested significant amounts of zinc sulfide combined with radium and mesothorium. Several of these girls developed osteosarcomas. He found the lethal dose to be approximately 10 to 180 μg. These cases are reminiscent of the lung cancers that were reported in the Schneeberg cobalt and Joachimsthal pitchblende miners.

X-ray, radium, mesothorium and the radioactive isotope of calcium have been used to induce osteosarcoma in experimental animals. Typical osteosarcomas can also be induced in rabbits with intravenous injections of zinc beryllium silicate.[7] Beryllium causes a rather extravagant cellular proliferation of any body tissue in which it becomes lodged. Apparently the bones have a greater affinity for beryllium than do other tissues and when a certain concentration is reached, a neoplastic proliferation of osteogenic tissue results. It is not suggested here that either radiant energy or beryllium is an important causative agent of osteosarcoma in humans but the possibility of causing a bone sarcoma by giving irradiation for any reason is sufficiently real to make this type of therapy inadvisable, especially in children, except as a last resort.

Finkel et al.[8] have reported that hamsters given injections of extracts of human osteosarcoma developed osteosarcoma, suggesting a virus as an etiologic factor. Morton and Malmgren[9] found antibodies to tumor tissue in the serum of four patients with osteosarcoma.

Pain is the only consistent symptom of osteosarcoma. It is often insidious in onset and at first there may be remissions. Later, the pain becomes severe, deep, boring and constant. Osteosarcoma is a destructive tumor. It infiltrates and causes lysis of the overlying cortex and then lifts the periosteum. It is probably the latter that causes much of the pain. Soon a palpable tumor mass develops (Fig. 16–5). Because osteosarcomas of long bones are near a joint the pain may be referred into this area. Soon there is limitation of motion and disability. A pathologic fracture is apt to occur because of the cortical destruction. The tumor mass often becomes erythematous, hot and exquisitely tender, suggesting acute inflammation. The superficial veins in relation to it may become dilated and prominent. Eventually there is apt to be fever, malaise, weight loss, anemia and progressive debilitation. The systemic signs and symptoms of osteosarcoma probably arise because of the destruction of normal tissue and the degeneration within the tumor itself. It is a rapidly growing tumor and though it is usually highly vascular it is probable that large fields become necrotic because of loss of adequate blood supply.

The serum alkaline phosphatase level depends, among other things, upon osteoblastic activity. It has been shown that tumor osteoblasts may contain and probably secrete phosphatase. Serum phosphatase levels are usually elevated in osteosarcoma[10] and a level of 20 Bodansky units is not infrequently noted. It should be remembered, however, that the amount of phosphatase depends upon the number of osteoblasts that produce it. The number in an early and small tumor may be inadequate to elevate the level above normal or an osteosarcoma of immature cells may produce no osteoid and no phosphatase. An elevated level in suspected osteosarcoma is highly significant; a normal level is without meaning. The level often falls following the ablation of a large, osteoid-forming tumor. Periodic serum analysis has been used to guide the prognosis when pulmonary metastases are to be expected. The level may or may not rise with metastasis depending upon the degree of maturity and function of the tumor cells.

The diagnosis of osteosarcoma may be considered all but certain because of clinical and radiologic findings but it must be certified by biopsy before therapy may be undertaken. This rule is absolutely infallible because numerous benign and innocuous lesions precisely mimic the clinical and roentgenographic characteristics of osteosarcoma. The treatment of osteosarcoma, whatever it is, must always be radical, and overdiagnosis and overtreatment of an innocuous lesion without a biopsy is inexcusable and indefensible. It has been stated by a prominent authority that biopsy delays the advent of therapy, increases the growth rate, predisposes to pulmonary metastasis and hastens the death of the patient; therefore, treatment should be administered without it. It would be difficult

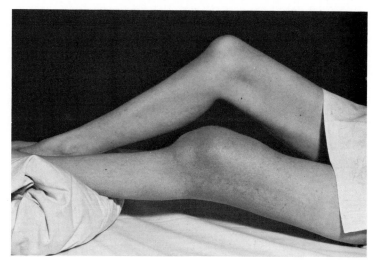

Figure 16–5 Osteosarcoma in the most common site, the lower end of the femur. After penetrating the cortex it produced a bulky soft tissue tumor.

to argue the veracity of most of the premises of the first part of this statement. Biopsy often delays the advent of therapy, though if properly done the delay need not be more than 24 hours. It is questionable whether it increases the rate of growth though such might be argued. Almost certainly, the cutting through viable tumor tissue, lymphatic and blood channels increases the probability of metastasis and hastens the death of the patient. But the most important point has been ignored. The mortality of osteosarcoma, no matter how it is treated, is probably somewhere around 95 per cent. The patient with osteosarcoma has only 1 chance in 20, at best 1 in 10, of surviving his disease. To amputate the extremity of a patient with an innocuous lesion that was thought to be a sarcoma is certainly less defensible than failing to amputate an osteosarcoma that would almost certainly have caused death no matter what the treatment.

The biopsy of choice is a frozen section taken with two tourniquets applied. Should the lesion prove to be an osteosarcoma, amputation at a line between the tourniquets may be accomplished, the proximal tourniquet theoretically preventing dislodged cancer cells pervading the general circulation by way of the return venous flow. The presence of bone may make it impossible to section biopsy tissue without demineralization, i.e., frozen section. And just as often, the nuclear detail upon which the pathologist depends so greatly in making the diagnosis of osteosarcoma may be impossible to retain with the frozen technique, though the modern cryostat has greatly improved this situation. Frozen section should be attempted but in many cases it is necessary to withhold the diagnosis until paraffin-embedded tissue may be examined.

The taking of the biopsy is exceedingly important. If cut from the superficial portion of what grossly appears to be tumor, nothing more than bone reaction may be obtained. If such material consisting of actively proliferating young osteogenic tissue is obtained from an innocent lesion suspected of being sarcomatous, the pathologist may be misled into the diagnosis of malignant neoplasm. If a deep biopsy is obtained the material may be so necrotic

that cellular clarity has been destroyed. It is better to take at least two samples of tissue and best four from different levels of the tumor. And the pathologist should remember that if a definite opinion cannot be given on frozen section, the patient is probably better off waiting for paraffin technique than taking the gamble that is necessary without cytologic guidance.

Roentgenographic Manifestations. The roentgenographic manifestations of osteosarcoma are those of bone destruction alone or in combination with the formation of new bone, neoplastic or reactive. The tumor usually begins in the metaphyseal end of a bone and results in irregular, ill-defined radiolucent defects as a result of destruction of trabeculae of bone. Periosteal new bone formation may be the first manifestation of cortical involvement and may be apparent before there is recognizable destruction of the cortex and in some instances before macroscopic evidence of the destruction of trabeculae. Codman's triangle and the "sunburst" appearance are manifestations of periosteal elevation and as such are not specific for this neoplasm. The former refers to the triangular-shaped area in which the elevated periosteum rejoins the cortex; the "sunburst" appearance results from the formation of reactive and neoplastic new bone, which is laid down perpendicular to the shaft along vessels passing from the periosteum to the cortex. In time, the periosteum is ruptured and a soft tissue mass becomes apparent that may be associated with interruption of the periosteal new bone. The presence of a soft tissue mass in association with bone destruction and new bone formation is significant in the diagnosis of a malignant tumor of bone. As a result of increased vascularity secondary to the presence of this vascular tumor, the bone may be more lucent than is normal; in fact, the lucency may be so localized as to suggest a vascular neoplasm.

If the neoplastic cells do not produce osteoid or bone in any appreciable amount, the radiographic appearance is primarily the result of bone destruction (radiolucency), and sclerosis within the neoplasm is not a feature. Radiographically, it may not be possible to differentiate this appearance from that of Ewing's tumor. Even in

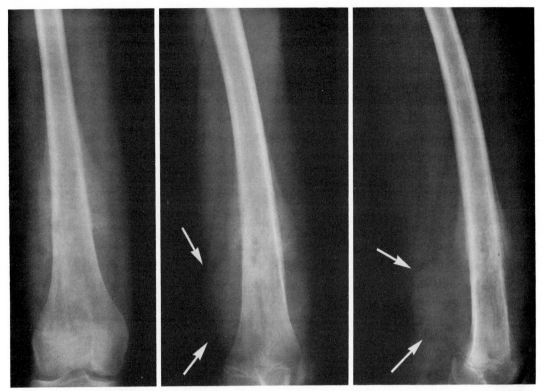

Figure 16–6 Osteosarcoma. Mottled destruction of the distal metaphysis of the femur is associated with laminated periosteal new bone, a "sunburst" of bone and Codman's triangle. A large soft tissue mass, somewhat lobulated, is most evident posteriorly (arrows), and periosteal new bone is interrupted at this site.

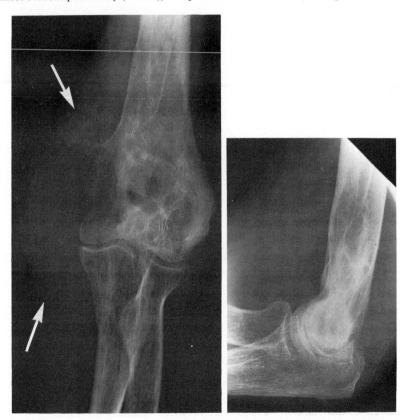

Figure 16–7 Osteosarcoma. This lesion is arising from an area of Paget's disease in the distal humerus. Destruction of bone and a soft tissue mass (arrows) are evident medially.

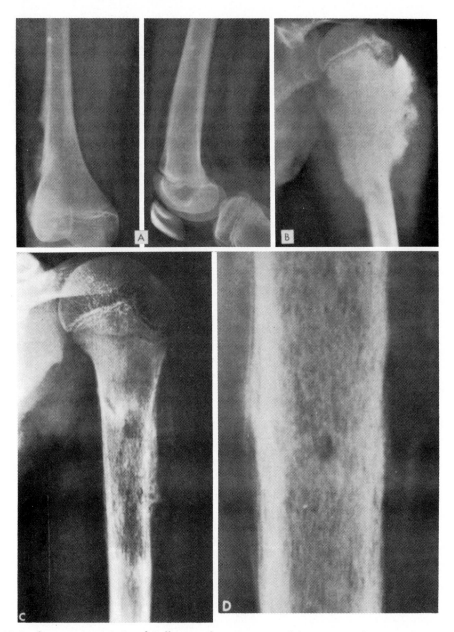

Figure 16–8   Osteosarcoma. *A, B* and *C* illustrate the appearance of this tumor in three patients. In *A* there is minimal visible involvement of medullary trabeculae. Bone production is marked in *B*. There is marked destruction of spongy and compact bone in *C* with areas of sclerosis (new bone). *D* represents a portion of the involved shaft of *C* enlarged to show the tiny areas of destruction and the nature of the periosteal new bone.

these neoplasms, however, reactive periosteal new bone may be formed. The most common type of osteosarcoma (Class I) both forms and destroys bone, so that bone destruction and periosteal and neoplastic new bone formation are apparent. The radiographic appearance of the mass of neoplastic tissue extending into the soft tissues is dependent upon the ability of the neoplastic cells to form bone. Accordingly, this mass may be of the density of soft tissue or it may be irregularly opaque as the result of the presence of multiple masses of neoplastic bone. If there is a significant cartilaginous component, calcification may be apparent within the tumor.

In those instances in which multiple bones are involved, sclerosis or the formation of new bone is a prominent feature. The epiphyses are not always spared,[11, 12] particularly in those patients in whom multiple bones are involved.

   Gross Pathology.   In most cases, osteosarcoma has destroyed a portion of the cortex and involves both intracortical and extracortical tissues by the time an anatomic examination can be made. A few bone-forming tumors are encountered that appear to be arising from the periosteum and growing outward into the soft tissues with little or no cortical destruction. In our experience the microscopy of these latter tumors has been different from that of true osteosarcoma and, moreover, from the available data it appears that they behave somewhat differently. Some writers, including us, place these in a separate category variously called juxtacortical sarcoma, periosteal osteosarcoma or parosteal sarcoma. Some writers have concluded that all true osteosarcomas arise in intracortical tissues. It is impossible to support this

statement with unequivocal evidence at this time but to us it appears that it is probably true.

   Because osteosarcoma grows rapidly it has almost always reached a considerable size by the time it is examined. In long bones, primary osteosarcoma almost always begins in the metaphysis. It usually replaces the metaphyseal cancellous tissue before it destroys the cortex. Because in long bones, it usually occurs in adolescents, the growth plate is often still unossified. Apparently cartilage is less readily invaded by osteosarcoma than cortical bone because it often remains intact until quite late (Fig. 16–10). If the growth plate is violated, the tumor grows through the ossified nucleus of the epiphysis to the articular plate, which usually restrains the neoplastic process. Osteosarcoma permeates the haversian canals of the cortex and interferes with the blood supply. Soon the cortex gives way and great portions of it simply disappear. As the tumor reaches the outer surface the periosteum is stretched over it but for some time it re-

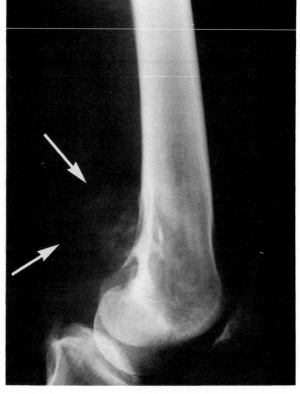

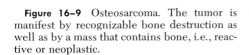

Figure 16–9 Osteosarcoma. The tumor is manifest by recognizable bone destruction as well as by a mass that contains bone, i.e., reactive or neoplastic.

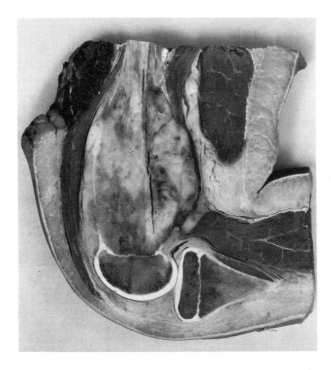

Figure 16–10 Osteosarcoma in the distal end of the femur. It began in the metaphysis and destroyed the compacta on both sides. It elevated the periosteum, which remains intact. Note that it has not violated the enchondral plate.

mains intact (Fig. 16–11). In pulling away from the cortical surface the periosteum drags along the small vessels that pass from it into the cortex and these take a vertical direction to the cortical surface. About these vascular channels columns of new bone are laid down, perhaps because of the abundant blood supply. These trabeculae of bone account for the sunburst effect, which is so often seen in the roentgenogram. Most of the bone so formed is reactive and non-neoplastic, or so it appears through the microscope. Moreover, other non–bone-forming

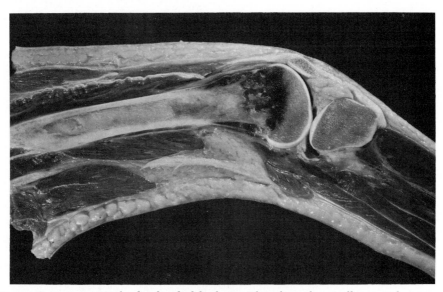

Figure 16–11 Osteosarcoma in the distal end of the femur. Though a rather small tumor it has caused marked destruction of the overlying bone. The elevated periosteum is still intact.

tumors such as carcinoma and even non-neoplastic processes may produce this identical picture. At a point near where the periosteum rejoins the cortex, the bone that it lays down is annealed to the cortical surface, causing a localized area of thickening. This produces the Codman triangle which, though it characterizes tumor elevation of the periosteum, particularly by osteosarcoma, is itself not a neoplastic proliferation. Though the periosteum may be greatly distended over the tumor before it gives way, eventually it is penetrated and the tumor infiltrates widely through the soft tissue structures.

Most osteosarcomas are highly vascular. Thus, the gross appearance is that of a frankly hemorrhagic tumor. About half of them produce considerable amounts of osteoid, which soon becomes mineralized. In the more sclerotic lesions it may be necessary to chisel out a block for section. Others produce only enough bone to give a gritty consistency and in still others there is no palpable evidence of bone. Necrosis is usual and often extensive. This involves not only the tumor but the tissue that it destroys.

The classification of osteosarcoma into medullary and subperiosteal types has already been commented upon. Separating this tumor into sclerosing and osteolytic varieties is often quite futile on an anatomic basis. One frequently finds sclerotic and lytic areas in the same tumor, the former being inside and outside the cortex and the latter in the area in which the process has broken through the compacta. In the typical sclerotic variety, large masses of dense, primitive bone characterize the tumor both radiologically and microscopically. Indeed, sections of these lesions may disclose so much bone and so few tumor cells that it may be difficult for the microscopist to be certain he is dealing with a neoplasm.

Microscopic Pathology. Though the diagnosis of osteosarcoma on the basis of microscopy is usually a fairly simple matter because of the malignant characteristics of the cells, in some instances it can be exceedingly difficult. In bone reaction in which there is very active osteogenesis it may be necessary to evaluate carefully the possibility of malignant growth. This is because an occasional osteosarcoma is composed of relatively mature bone-forming cells, and also because all too frequently the biopsy material actually submitted for osteosarcoma may consist not of tumor tissue but of bone reaction about it. Thus, the microscopist has a difficult time in establishing his criteria for osteosarcoma.

In analyzing a group of primary bone tumors we were struck by the variation in cellular pattern. A cytologic classification was made with the hope that the recognition of at least some varieties might help in the planning of therapy and in prognosis. A series of 20 cases was selected in which there were a reasonably good clinical record and a five-year follow-up, adequate roentgenograms and ample histologic material. The clinical and radiologic data were analyzed by a participating worker and the coded slides were examined by us. By microscopy the cases fell quite naturally into five fairly distinct groups. There was some overlapping between classes in some cases and a few showed transition from one class to another in which biopsy and autopsy samples were both available, but in general there were five dominant cytologic pictures.

When the clinical data were considered in relation to the histologic types it became apparent that no correlation could be made. Regardless of whether the tumor was bone-forming, cartilage-forming or was too immature to form either, there was no relation to the rate of growth, the advent of metastasis or the length of the survival period. It was deemed impossible to predict the behavior of osteosarcoma on the basis of histology alone.

The grouping of the tumors into the five cytologic classes became largely an academic exercise, useful only to the pathologist in recognizing the lesion and in recording its characteristics. To serve the latter purpose it will be used in the following discussion.

Class I osteosarcoma: In this group the tumor matrix cells are spindled or less frequently pleomorphic. They align themselves along irregular masses of crude bone and are obviously active in the production of osteoid. Tumor giant cells are usually rare. Sometimes the tumor cells orient themselves in relation to spicules of normal bone and form tumor osteoid around it. When this happens it is not always possible to be sure which is neoplastic and which is normal bone tissue. This is particularly true in the region of the subperiosteal, perpendicular rays in which both reactive and neoplastic bone formation occur simultaneously. There is a considerable degree of variation in maturation of the tumor cells and in the architecture of the osteoid they produce. Usually the nuclei are obviously of malignant character though in some, one has to consider the possibility of fibrous dysplasia and even ossifying fibroma.

A subtype of the Class I, osteoid-producing variety is the so-called sclerosing osteosarcoma, which presents characteristic radiologic and microscopic features. Its bone site and age incidence are the same

as in the common variety but the roentgenogram presents a diffuse radiopacity throughout the tumor (Fig. 16–12). It may be necessary to chisel out a block from the tumor for a biopsy sample. The sections disclose large amounts of osteoid as might be expected. Usually this is laid down in a network of irregular, vermiform microspicules (Fig. 16–13). The interspicular tumor cells may present all the features of malignant tumor but more often they are sparse, spindled and show very little evidence of nuclear irregularity. The inexperienced microscopist usually diagnoses these as benign osteoblastomas. In some instances it is necessary to consider all facets of the case in order to reach a firm diagnosis.

Tumors of the Class I group (Fig. 16–14) have all the characteristics of the classic concept of osteosarcoma. Osteoid tissue is formed by tumor osteoblasts directly and

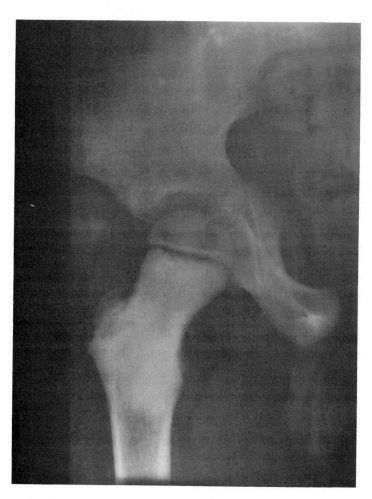

Figure 16–12 Sclerosing osteosarcoma. The proximal end of the femur, from the trochanteric area to the epiphyseal line, is almost uniform in its opacity. There is a tiny area of periosteal new bone or neoplastic bone adjacent to the medial aspect of the femoral neck.

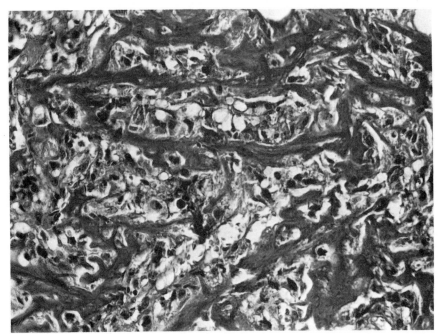

Figure 16-13   Sclerosing osteosarcoma. Large amounts of tumor osteoid are produced. The cells in this section are neoplastic but in many cases they have an innocuous appearance. (× 330.)

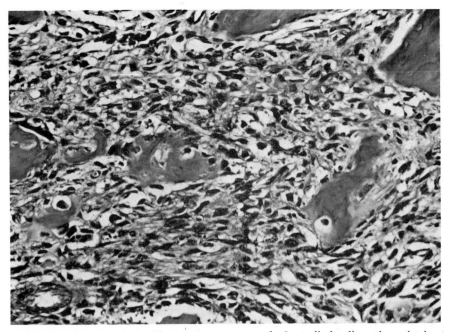

Figure 16-14   Class I osteosarcoma. The matrix is composed of spindled cells with nuclei having all the characteristics of malignant neoplasm — irregularity in size, shape and chromatin content. These cells are producing crude osteoid. (× 200.)

without the intermediary of cartilage or collagen. This is the type that Thomson and Turner-Warwick[3] would call osteoblastic sarcoma. Some writers would exclude all other types from the category of osteosarcoma. Class I osteosarcoma is the most commonly occurring type. Most of the long bone lesions in adolescents fall in this group.

Class II osteosarcoma produces areas that are identical to the cytology of Class I but they are intermingled with larger and more prominent areas of tumor chondroid (Fig. 16–15). In some tumors it may be necessary to search several sections in order to find the osteoid-producing tumor cells. The chondroid is probably an intermediary product in the formation of bone but if the biopsy is limited to this material, a diagnosis of chondrosarcoma is inevitable. These conditions may account for the occasional "chondrosarcoma," which runs a rapid and fatal course, the course that one expects in osteosarcoma.

The criticism has been made that if a tumor contains any considerable amount of cartilage it should not be called an osteosarcoma, but should be classified with the chondrosarcomas or called osteochon-drosarcoma. We agree wholeheartedly with Jaffe and Lichtenstein that if a tumor contains any considerable portion of osteosarcoma it behaves like an osteosarcoma and should be called such. To make another tumor class is making things more complicated than they need be, and to classify this tumor as a chondrosarcoma is to erase the identity of the latter as a clinical entity.

Class III osteosarcoma is the least common of the five types. It appears to be incapable of forming any intercellular substance and, therefore, there is no bone or cartilage and very little collagen. The cells are usually quite pleomorphic and obviously malignant in character. The pattern is scrambled but a characteristic feature about the lesion is slitlike spaces very similar to those seen in malignant synovioma. Sections of one such tumor were submitted to several "name" pathologists about the country. More than one classified it as a synovioma. Later a hindquarter amputation was done, affording an opportunity to examine the tumor in detail. It arose in the cancellous tissue of the ilium and at no point did it extend through the cortex. No tumor was ever found outside of

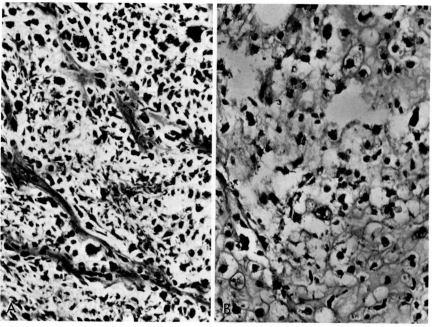

Figure 16–15 Class II osteosarcoma. A, Tumor osteoblasts forming osteoid. B, Tumor chondroblasts forming chondroid. These two photographs were made from the same section. (× 130.)

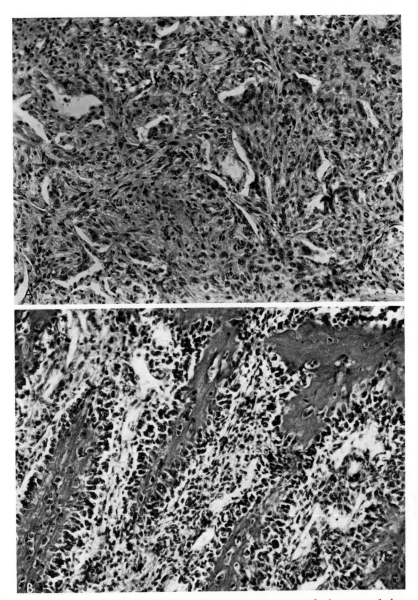

Figure 16–16   Class III osteosarcoma. *A,* The primary tumor is composed of masses of pleomorphic tumor cells with little or no chondroid, osteoid or collagen. The presence of slit spaces suggests synovioma. *B,* Section of a pulmonary metastatic deposit from the tumor illustrated in *A.* Osteoid production establishes the unequivocal diagnosis of osteosarcoma. (×130.)

bone until pulmonary metastasis and later widespread visceral metastasis occurred. The course was that of osteosarcoma. Another case almost identical in sex, age group, site and cytology metastasized to the lung. The lung metastases produced considerable amounts of well formed bone (Fig. 16–16).

Most writers contend that if a tumor forms neither osteoid nor cartilage it can-

not be classified as an osteosarcoma. They would call such a tumor an intracortical fibrosarcoma. It should be pointed out, however, that the histologic pattern of this lesion is distinct and different from that of fibrosarcoma and, more important, its behavior is that of osteosarcoma and much more malignant than fibrosarcoma of bone.

In our material there were two primary bone tumors that began in metaphyseal cancellous tissue and behaved in every way like osteosarcoma. They were destructive tumors producing no osteoid, no chondroid and almost no collagen. The morphology of the cells strongly suggested rhabdomyosarcoma. There were strap forms and even a suggestion of striations. The finding in bone tumors of cells suggesting synovia and muscle indicates that the bone mesenchyma has a greater potential in forming a greater variety of cells than is commonly supposed.

Class IV osteosarcoma: For those who like to have types and subtypes neatly segregated into classes there is some justification for making the giant cell osteosarcoma the Class IV variety. If a search is made, an occasional giant cell can be located in most types of osteosarcoma, particularly Class I. Infrequently the giant cells are so numerous and so prominent that one is tempted to diagnose the lesion osteoclastoma. But the stromal cells are more pleomorphic, irregular mitotic figures are more common and tumor osteoid more prominent. We have made the observation that these tumors arise nearer the

metaphysis than the usual osteosarcoma. In short, they appear to be an intermediary form between osteoclastoma and osteosarcoma. We hope to find eventually that their prognosis lies between that of these two tumors.

Class V osteosarcoma: Finally there is a fifth group of primary tumors of bone that may or may not produce osteoid and that describe in their behavior the course of osteosarcoma. This tumor was described by Hutter et al.[13] who called it primitive multipotential primary sarcoma of bone. They believed it to be a distinct oncologic entity. We prefer to think of it as a type of osteosarcoma which, because it arises from a very early progenitor cell, differentiates into a number of cell types. As these cases have collected in our material we have noted that the tumors, like Ewing's tumor, may arise anywhere within the bone, often involving the midshaft. We have also noted that the radiographic picture is frequently more like that of Ewing's tumor or reticulum cell sarcoma (Fig. 16–17) than of osteosarcoma. Indeed, we are inclined to believe that those tumors

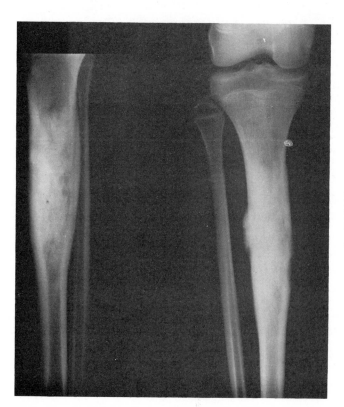

Figure 16–17   Osteosarcoma—primitive multipotential sarcoma of bone. The proximal half of the tibial diaphysis is expanded. There is thickening of the cortex in this area; there is sclerosis of medullary bone. Scattered areas of destruction are evident.

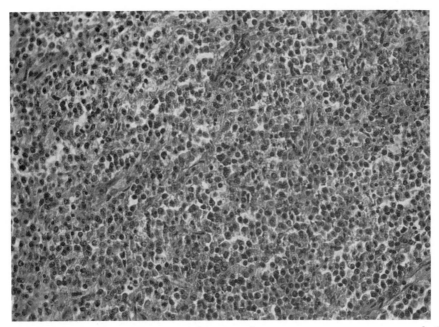

Figure 16–18 Primitive cell osteosarcoma. In this particular case many areas were composed of cells that strongly suggested a diagnosis of reticulum cell sarcoma. (× 250.)

which, in the past, we diagnosed Ewing's tumor but which produced recognizable amounts of osteoid were, in all probability, this type of osteosarcoma.

Its microscopic appearance is highly variable. It usually presents scrambled areas, some of which appear to be of bone and cartilage origin but others seem to be derived from marrow cells. In 25 cases reported by Hutter et al., the Ewing's tumor pattern dominated the sections of 10. We have encountered one in which

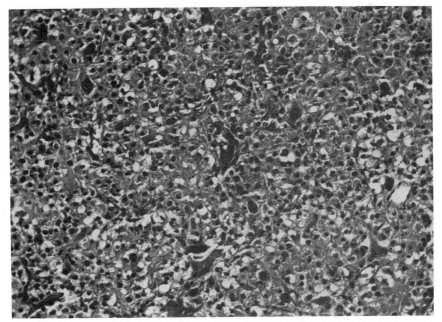

Figure 16–19 Primitive cell osteosarcoma. A variety of mesenchymal cell types may be encountered but in most cases one finds areas of primitive cells whose origins are indeterminate. (× 250.)

some areas resemble reticulum cell sarcoma (Fig. 16–18), whereas others reveal osteosarcoma. In still others the cells are so primitive that they are atypical of any recognizable type of primary bone tumor (Fig. 16–19). The original report suggested that the survival rate for primitive cell sarcoma is higher than in ordinary osteosarcoma. Behavior of the 15 tumors in our collection does not substantiate this conclusion. We have preferred to call this tumor simply "primitive" osteosarcoma.

In summary there are five recognizable cell patterns in osteosarcoma: In Class I the outstanding feature is osteoid production. This may be so dramatic that it results in what some would call "sclerosing osteosarcoma." Class II tumors form both osteoid and chondroid though the latter frequently dominates the histologic section. Class III produces neither osteoid nor chondroid and so may resemble a soft tissue neoplasm (synovioma or rhabdomyosarcoma). Class IV is the giant cell type which may be an intermediary between osteoclastoma and osteosarcoma. Finally there is a primitive osteosarcoma whose cells may resemble a primary marrow sarcoma except that small amounts of tumor osteoid and/or chondroid are found in the sections. Also its growth and behavior are more like that of osteosarcoma than of a marrow tumor. We suggest that it be designated "Class V."

A single tumor may contain more than one pattern and the pattern of the metastasis may be different from that of the primary. Whatever the pattern no inference may be made in regard to the degree of malignancy.

Price[14] attempted to classify osteosarcoma in relation to its behavior on the basis of an index of the mitotic figures seen in the sections. Most microscopists with a wide experience in the diagnosis of osteosarcoma would probably not agree that the number of mitotic figures assists in making a prognosis. At best the number of mitotic figures is but an index of the rate of growth. Too many other factors influence the effect of osteosarcoma upon the patient to make it of considerable prognostic significance.

The cytologic diagnosis of osteosarcoma is exceedingly important and not always easy. There are no special stains that are helpful. Engfeldt[15] has suggested that microradiology has reached a stage of practicability in this field. Certain, apparently characteristic patterns have been defined for osteopetrosis, osteogenesis imperfecta and Paget's disease, but the mineralization pattern in osteosarcoma is so kaleidoscopic that as yet one should hesitate to apply these patterns in cases in which an extremity may be the pawn.

Prognosis. Excluding the myelogenic tumors, osteosarcoma is the most malignant tumor of bone. The expected course is a few weeks to three months of symptoms before diagnosis is made and a postdiagnosis survival period of approximately 18 months. Death is almost always the result of pulmonary metastasis. After pulmonary metastases are demonstrable, life expectancy is not greater than six months. The reason for the grim mortality of osteosarcoma, i.e., the reason it metastasizes so consistently and so early, is not known, though it may be of significance that the osteoblast is probably derived from the capillary endothelial lining cell and one finds on careful scrutiny that sinusoids permeate the entire tumor structure. Indeed it is not unique to find areas that resemble angiomas (Fig. 16–20). This close relationship with the blood stream might help to explain the early dissemination of tumor cells. As yet there are no data to indicate that the so-called telangiectatic type metastasizes earlier than those of the less vascular group. The trauma of manipulation before and during diagnosis has been blamed, but although everyone agrees that the suspected osteosarcoma should be handled with all possible gentleness, this precaution has not seemed to prevent or delay the onset of metastasis. It is probable that most or all malignant tumors send showers of viable cells into the lymphatic and blood channels long before the cells are capable of setting up independent growth.

Green has shown by the technique of explanting tumor samples that a primary growth must exist for some time before its explant grows. It is unknown whether primary growth eventually imparts independence to its component cells or whether the primary growth affects the host organism,

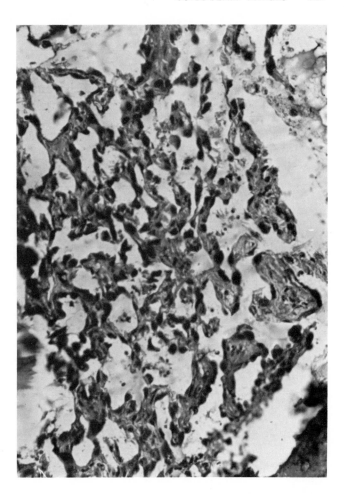

Figure 16–20 An area in a Class I osteosarcoma. These are blood sinusoids made up of tumor cells. Since these cells may be derived from endothelial cells, this relation of hemangioma and osteosarcoma may explain the early metastasis of the latter.

breaking down an early established immunity. Whatever the factor that prevents or delays independent growth at a distant site, it is of less importance in osteosarcoma than in most other tumors.

Prognosis in osteosarcoma concerning the behavior of the various types is difficult or impossible. There seems to be some evidence that the nearer the trunk the site of the primary, the higher the mortality rate and the shorter the course. Most writers agree that a 10 per cent five-year survival is as much as can be expected today. If allowance is made for tumors that are mistakenly placed in this category the figure is probably nearer 5 per cent, despite two large series in the literature in which the five-year survival approaches 20 per cent.

It is unusual for osteosarcoma to spread to the regional lymph nodes. If adequately removed, osteosarcoma rarely recurs at the primary site. Almost all osteosarcomas metastasize to the lungs first, usually within 9 to 12 months. Terminal widespread metastasis is not uncommon. Metastasis to other bones is unusual but it may occur either early or late. If multiple bone lesions should occur in a case in which one site has been diagnosed osteosarcoma, the validity of the diagnosis should be challenged.

The osteosarcoma has shown little vulnerability to irradiation therapy. Lee and Mackenzie[16] studied 160 cases of what they believed to be osteosarcoma in which they gave megavoltage radiotherapy and then waited a matter of months to see if metastases occurred. If metastases were found they did not amputate, thus sparing the patient valueless mutilation. If, after two to five months the patient failed to exhibit evidence of metastasis they undertook ablative surgery in most of the cases.

They claimed a 21.8 per cent five-year survival, a higher rate than most clinics that
practice radical surgery without delay.
The method of Lee and Mackenzie seems
valid to us since it should reduce the
number of useless amputations but we
doubt that the high rate of survival can be
attained in any series in which diagnostic
studies are as rigid as those we use.

There has been a tendency over the
past decade to increase the extent of surgery. In some clinics a hindquarter amputation is considered the proper treatment
for an osteosarcoma of the distal femur or
even the proximal tibia. Sufficient data are
not available as yet to judge whether the
salvage has been improved by this method,
but because osteosarcoma infrequently recurs and rarely spreads to regional lymph
nodes it would seem that not more surgery
but earlier surgery is what is needed. It is
probable that most osteosarcomas have already metastasized to the lungs, though
the deposits are not yet demonstrable, by
the time the diagnosis is made. A few cases
have undergone resection of a pulmonary
metastasis with cure.[17] We have two such
cases in our material. Close scrutiny of
these cases reveals that the tumors in
question, whether they were osteosarcomas or not, were not behaving like osteosarcomas at the time the lung deposit
was removed, because the interval between resection of the primary and the appearance of the metastasis was greatly prolonged. Under these circumstances
pulmonary resection is certainly justified,
but with the gamble for a good result so
great, thoracotomy for a metastasis that appeared within one year hardly seems reasonable.

Prophylactic irradiation of the lungs has
been tried at the time of treatment of the
primary tumor with the objective of killing
any pulmonary metastases that are still too
small to appear on radiographs. Early data
seemed to support the initial hope that this
technique would reduce the incidence of
pulmonary metastasis, but it should be
noted that this type of therapy is not without a considerable degree of morbidity
because of pulmonary sclerosis. Later data
failed to confirm a reduction in the number
of lung deposits.

Very recently treatment by combined
radiotherapy and chemotherapy has been
used in a few clinics. The initial data, as
yet largely unpublished, are strongly optimistic. It appears to these authors that
if our mortality figures with this vicious
cancer are to be improved, it will be
through this technique. Two or three treatment centers should be established in the
United States and all cases referred to
these clinics. In this manner treatment
could be standardized and data correlated
most efficiently and effectively.

The public must be educated to seek
counsel earlier, the clinician must maintain a higher index of osteosarcoma suspicion and insist on x-ray examination at the
outset, the pathologist must be thoroughly
acquainted with the differential diagnostic
possibilities, and once the diagnosis is
made procrastination must be abhorred by
all parties concerned. Then perhaps the
mortality figures for osteosarcoma can be
bettered, but at present the prospects appear dishearteningly grim.

PAROSTEAL SARCOMA

When one studies the radiology and histology of the osteogenic neoplasms and
carefully analyzes their clinical behavior
and mortality statistics, there emerges a
type that over the past few years has come
to be recognized as an entity separate from
central osteosarcoma. It has been called
parosteal osteoma, parosteal osteogenic
sarcoma, periosteal chondrosarcoma, juxtacortical sarcoma and desmoid of bone.
Geschickter and Copeland[18] used the term
parosteal osteoma in a paper in which they
reported what they considered to be 16
cases of this lesion in 1951. In 1954, Dwinell, Dahlin and Ghormley[19] reported a
series of 15 cases, 14 of which they believed fulfilled all the criteria for the lesion. The following year Lichtenstein,[20] in
criticizing the validity of such an entity as
described in the previous two reports, described under the heading of periosteal
chondrosarcoma one case that, judging
from the illustrations of the roentgenograms and the microscopy, is classic parosteal sarcoma. In reviewing our own material we find 32 cases that are unequivocally
parosteal sarcoma, 3 others that probably

fall in this group and 4 cases that, except that they involve the mandible where it has not yet been reported, cannot be excluded.

We prefer the term parosteal sarcoma to the other names that have been used. By using the word parosteal instead of periosteal we avoid confusion with periosteal fibrosarcoma and, if there be such an entity, true periosteal osteosarcoma. The word sarcoma is preferred to osteogenic sarcoma and chondrosarcoma because often one can find in sections of this tumor components of all three mesenchymal tissue types—collagenous tissue, cartilage and bone. In a sense it is a periosteal mesenchymoma and because the same thing can be said of some osteosarcomas, the parosteal sarcoma is considered in this section.

Parosteal sarcoma is considerably less common than osteosarcoma, chondrosarcoma and even fibrosarcoma of bone. It apparently affects females about as frequently as males. There appears to be an age predilection for those between 15 and 35 years. In the very limited material available this tumor has been reported involving only the large cylindrical bones of the extremities. In our material of 36 cases there are four lesions arising from the periosteum of the mandible, which show a remarkable similarity in both the roentgenograms and sections. The lower end of the femur appears to be the commonest site of involvement, this being the affected area in 25 of 41 reported cases. The tibia and the humerus claim most of the remainder. In our material, 28 of 42 cases in long bones were in either the distal femur or proximal tibia. The other two common sites were the humerus and ulna.

The usual clinical sign of parosteal sarcoma is a firm, smooth mass protruding from the outer cortical surface near the end of a long, cylindrical bone. The patient often has been cognizant of the mass for several months. Pain may or may not be present and usually is late in onset. Because there is little or no destruction of the host bone, fracture does not occur.

Roentgenographic Manifestations. The parosteal sarcoma has a radiographic appearance suggestive of a benign neoplasm, healing soft tissue trauma or an irregular osteochondroma. The tumor grows into the soft tissues adjacent to the periosteum and usually does not involve the underlying cortex; in some instances, however, the cortex may be eroded on its external surface. Early, a radiolucent line may be visible between the opaque tumor and the underlying cortex. Because there is no differentiation of the neoplastic bone within the tumor into recognizable trabeculae, it tends to be uniformly dense and opaque, although scattered foci of opacity throughout the mass may be present (Fig. 16–21). The non-ossifying portion of the neoplasm, which may be extensive in amount, is responsible for a mass that has the density of soft tissue (Fig. 16–22). The surgeon is frequently surprised to find extension of the tumor farther than anticipated and visible on the radiographs.

Morphology. Parosteal sarcoma appears to arise in periosteal tissue (Fig. 16–23). Most cases to date have involved the metaphyseal region. The posterior cortical surface of the lower end of the femur, the floor of the popliteal space, is the usual site of involvement. The tumor may grow from a broad base or a relatively narrow pedicle. In cases in which the base is small the tumor may produce a mushroom head, which expands laterally beyond the pedicle, sometimes resting lightly upon the surrounding cortex. The surface is fairly smooth and tends to be lobulated. About half the tumors appear grossly to have a dense fibrous capsule. The parosteal sarcoma is attached to the underlying compacta of the host bone by means of the periosteum. It has been possible to dissect the tumor away without greatly disturbing the cortex in some cases. In others there has been erosion of the cortex from without and in a few cases there appears to have been some infiltration and cortical destruction.

The parosteal sarcoma grows outward from a central pedicle or core which is usually firm and may be quite hard, depending upon the amount of mineralized osteoid present. The base and central portions of the tumor often have a bony appearance and consistency whereas a zone over the convex surface is usually frankly cartilaginous. Eventually, there is usually invasion of the contiguous soft tissues;

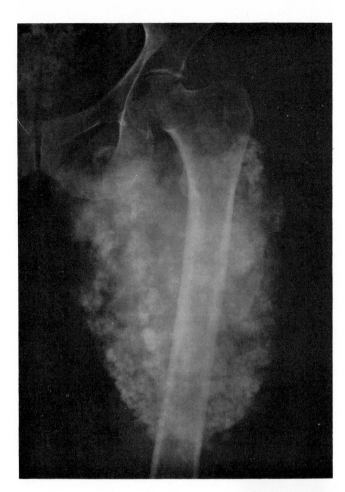

Figure 16–21 Parosteal sarcoma. The mass of the tumor is huge; its opacity is less homogeneous than is usual.

Figure 16–22 Parosteal sarcoma. A soft tissue mass (arrows) within which there is almost homogeneous opaque material is evident adjacent to the posterior aspect of the distal end of the femur. There is no apparent bone destruction.

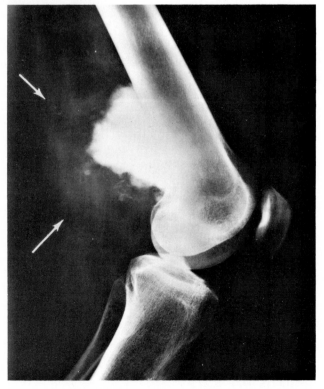

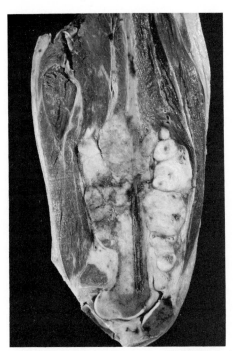

Figure 16-23 Parosteal sarcoma. Sagittal section of a tumor that arose from the posterior cortical surface of the distal end of the femur. Gradually it encircled this portion of the shaft and destroyed the cortex by involvement of its blood supply.

thus muscle bands may disappear into the substance of the tumor. Though the superficial portions or the growing frontier may be soft, to cut blocks from the tumor core it may be necessary to use a chisel.

From this description one might conclude that parosteal sarcoma is the malignant analogue of osteochondroma. We believe this to be true though there are some very important differences between the two lesions. The parosteal sarcoma does not develop a cylinder of mature bone coextensive with the cortex; it has no intracortical cancellous tissue. Though there may be a zone of cartilage overlying its convex surface, this is neoplastic cartilage and there is little or no attempt at the formation of an epiphyseal line such as is seen at the junction of the pedicle and cartilaginous cap of the osteochondroma. But the similarities are such that one can hardly escape the conclusion that they are related, one a congenital hamartoma, the other a true tumor involving the same tissues. Whether the osteochondroma always precedes the parosteal sarcoma is un-

known. Evidence of this is notable for its lack. The parosteal sarcoma may arise de novo. Such seems the most probable explanation at present for many of these tumors. However, in our material there are two cases of clearly defined osteochondroma that after trauma were activated to become parosteal sarcomas (Fig. 16-25).

The microscopic sections of parosteal sarcoma are more apt to lead to confusion than to clarification of the diagnosis unless the pathologist has samples of various levels of the tumor. It is usual to find fields of fibrosarcoma, others of chondrosarcoma and still others of osteosarcoma all in the same lesion. Or, in some cases, the characteristics of aggressiveness are so minimal that the pathologist concludes that he is dealing with a benign or even a nonneoplastic process, an osteochondroma that has failed to organize its tissue components. Lichtenstein[20] has stated that many of the lesions described as parosteal sarcoma are in fact no more than examples of heterotopic ossification such as that seen in myositis ossificans. He decries the acceptance of lesions without the microscopic criteria of malignant neoplasia in the category of aggressive tumors. His position is understandable because the adoption and casual application of such a policy would inevitably lead to unnecessary amputation. However, every experienced microscopist must eventually admit that there are tumors of malignant behavior that lack the microscopic criteria. The cellular criteria of malignancy were laid down long ago and the pathologist is apt to put his faith and stake his reputation on them. He expresses dismay and disenchantment when a tumor, whose cells appear quite mature and innocent, shows aggressive behavior. Just as one cannot always identify the criminal by his physiognomy, so one cannot always predict the activity of a cell by the appearance of its nucleus. The cells of some parosteal sarcomas may have an appearance as innocent as those of a desmoid or keloid, yet the tumor is invasive and may eventually metastasize.

In the fields of fibrous proliferation there may be sufficient collagenization to suggest scar or callus formation (Fig. 16-26). In other fields neoplastic proliferation

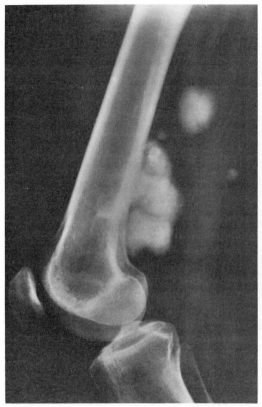
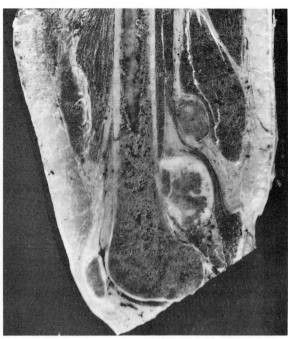

Figure 16–24 Parosteal sarcoma. Sagittal section and roentgenogram of the recurrence of the tumor illustrated in Figure 16–22. Note that the recurrent tumor has a bony core (dark central area) and is surrounded by a thick layer of cartilage. The bone is quite mature and non-neoplastic in appearance. The cartilage is composed of tumor cells. The spheroid mass above the recurrence is also tumor, probably a nodule seeded at the initial surgery.

may be obvious. In material obtained from recurrent lesions, the sections may resemble those of the most pleomorphic fibrosarcomas. Some sections are apt to show fibrocartilaginous metaplasia and it may be assumed that the cartilage constituents of parosteal sarcoma are of fibroblastic genesis. Here again, the cartilage may appear quite innocent or one may encounter the typical microscopy of chondrosarcoma (Fig. 16–27). Irregular trabeculae of cartilage are usually seen at the periphery of the fields of osteoid and it is apparent that much of the latter is formed by chondro-osseous metaplasia. Other fields show fibro-osseous metaplasia and in still others there may be osteoblastic osteogenesis (Fig. 16–28). The appearance of the bone may be quite respectable and innocent and one may be misled into the opinion that one is

dealing with material from a callus or fibrositis ossificans.

The first two cases studied by us were thought to be benign processes. Both recurred and in both the microscopic appearance of the cells of the recurrence was quite obviously malignant. The same experience has been reported by Dwinell et al.

If future reported descriptions of parosteal sarcoma are consistent with the lesion as previously described, the diagnosis to one who knows he is dealing with an extracortical lesion need not necessarily be difficult. The cytologic pattern of osteochondroma is orderly and the cells mature. Periosteal fibrosarcoma usually has a characteristic cell pattern (see p. 568), and the finding of neoplastic cartilage in some sections would make this diagnosis untena-

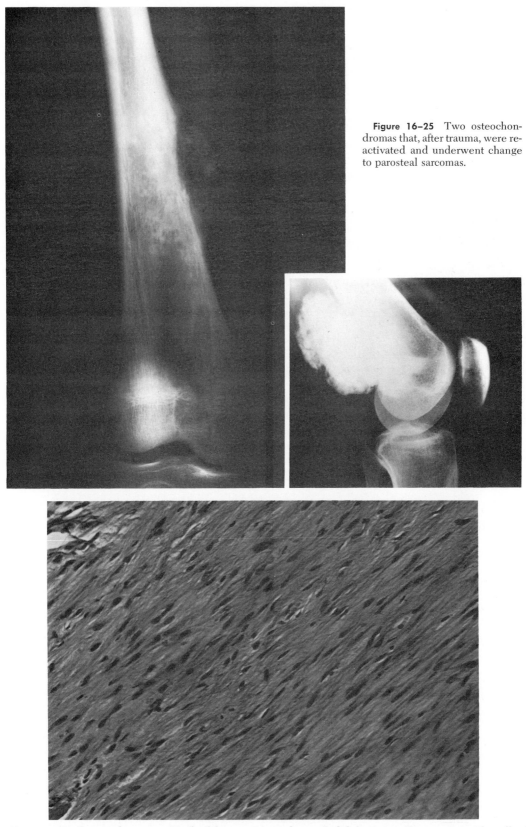

Figure 16–25 Two osteochon-dromas that, after trauma, were re-activated and underwent change to parosteal sarcomas.

Figure 16–26 Parosteal sarcoma. Much of the tumor is made up of adult bone in a fibrous matrix. The cells of the latter are quite orderly in arrangement, and their nuclei are fairly mature. In other cases the collagenoblastic cells may be extremely pleomorphic and obviously of malignant character. (× 120.)

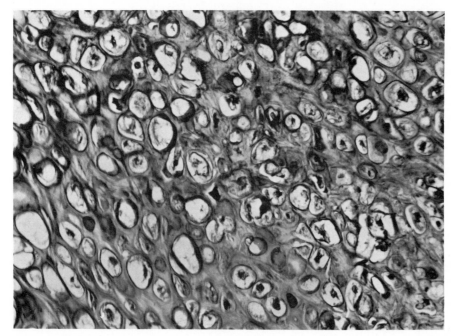

Figure 16–27 Parosteal sarcoma. Islands of cartilage are almost always present. Close examination reveals the cellular evidence of malignancy. (× 200.)

ble. One may find it necessary to differentiate central osteosarcoma on the basis of the roentgenogram.

Prognosis. Parosteal sarcoma should be held distinct from central osteosarcoma, if for no other reason than on the basis of its behavior. In most cases it is a slowly growing tumor although one case thought

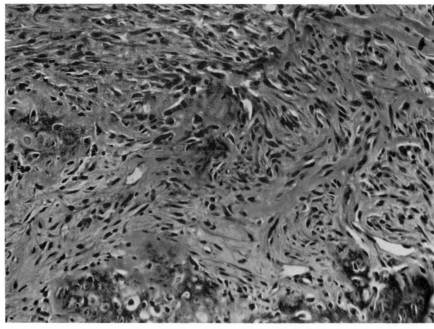

Figure 16–28 Parosteal sarcoma. Here and there one can often find fields that appear to be fibrosarcoma and elsewhere osteosarcoma. Or, as in this field, they appear to be mixed. (× 200.)

to be parosteal sarcoma in our material metastasized to the lungs and killed the patient in 13 months. This particular tumor might better have been called periosteal osteosarcoma but if there be such a tumor we are unable to distinguish it except by its behavior. Evidence of the presence of parosteal sarcoma for many years before its diagnosis has been recorded. If the diagnosis is made reasonably early and the proper treatment carried out, one can expect a cure in most cases. The proper treatment is not yet clearly apparent. One is tempted on the basis of the initial biopsy material to treat the lesion conservatively. The incidence of recurrence after local resection (nine out of ten in the series of Dwinell et al.) makes it appear that conservative measures are not enough. The change in the microscopy as shown by the recurrence following surgical intervention may be due to the manipulation or it may represent the natural behavior of the lesion.

It appears that these tumors should be treated somewhat more radically than they have been in the past. We have advised amputation in several cases in which the surgeon felt that he could not be certain of totally eradicating the lesion by regional resection. Our opinion has been conditioned by a small number of patients who had pulmonary metastases because of inadequate initial surgery. Like chondrosarcomas, these tumors frequently seed in the operative wound.

In the tumors that have recurred there is a fairly high incidence of pulmonary metastasis. Unlike osteosarcoma, however, these metastases may occur several years after ablation of the recurrent tumor, and some of them have grown much more slowly than one would expect of the osteosarcoma secondary. Only the accumulation of data on large numbers of these cases will serve to enlighten us as to how the parosteal sarcoma may be expected to behave and therefrom how it should be treated.

References

OSTEOSARCOMA

1. Moseley, J. E. and Bass, M. H.: Radiology, 66:41, 1956.
2. Fine, G., and Stout, A. P.: Cancer, 9:1027, 1956.
3. Thomson, A. D., and Turner-Warwick, R. T.: J. Bone Joint Surg., 37B:266, 1955.
4. Perkinson, N. G. and Higginbotham, N. L.: Cancer, 8:396, 1955.
5. Hatcher, C. H.: J. Bone Joint Surg., 27:179, 1945.
6. Martland, H. S.: Am. J. Cancer, 15:2435, 1931.
7. Janes, J. M., Higgens, G. M. and Herrick, J. F.: J. Bone Joint Surg., 38A:809, 1956.
8. Finkel, M., Beshes, B. and Farrell, C.: Proc. Nat. Acad. Sci. U.S.A., 60:1223, 1968.
9. Morton, D. and Malmgren, R.: Science, 162:1279, 1968.
10. Woodward, H. Q. and Higginbotham, N. L.: Am. J. Cancer, 13:221, 1937.
11. Morse, D. J., Reed, J. O. and Bernstein, J.: Am. J. Roentgenol., 88:491, 1962.
12. Singleton, E. B., Rosenberg, H. S., Dodd, G. D. and Dolan, P. A.: Am. J. Roentgenol., 88:483, 1962.
13. Hutter, R., Foote, F., Francis, K. and Sherman, R.: Cancer, 19:1, 1966.
14. Price, C. H. G.: J. Faculty Radiologists (London), 7:237, 1956.
15. Engfeldt, B.: Cancer, 7:815, 1954.
16. Lee, E. and Mackenzie, O.: Br. J. Surg., 51:252, 1964.
17. Goldenberg, R. R.: Bull. Hosp. Joint Dis., 15:67, 1954.

PAROSTEAL SARCOMA

18. Geschickter, C. F., and Copeland, M. M.: Ann. Surg., 133:790, 1951.
19. Dwinell, L. A., Dahlin, D. C. and Ghormley, R. K.: J. Bone Joint Surg., 36A:732, 1954.
20. Lichtenstein, L.: Cancer, 8:1060, 1955.

Chapter 17

CHONDROGENIC TUMORS

The classic example of the true neoplasm arising from the cartilage cells is the chondrosarcoma. The cells of this tumor may produce chondroid only, or mixtures of chondroid and collagen, but they never produce osteoid. If osteoid is found in a predominantly cartilaginous tumor it is probably the product of normal osteoblasts that are reacting to the deleterious presence of the tumor. If it can be shown that the osteoid is being produced by tumor cells, the tumor must be an osteosarcoma with a prominent cartilaginous component (osteosarcoma Class II).

There are two other lesions in the chondroid-producing category. These are chondroblastoma and chondromyxoid fibroma. Both have been identified relatively recently and as yet an adequate number of cases have not been followed long enough for us to be completely sure of their ultimate nature and behavior.

Both chondroblastoma and chondromyxoid fibroma were originally defined as benign tumors. Since their definition, a number of these lesions have shown recurrence and aggressive behavior, which makes this categorization dubious. More long-term follow-up studies must be done before unequivocal statements can be made concerning the nature of these processes.

The reader of this text will find no mention of the lesion called "chondroma" in our classification of bone tumors. Yet if one consults most clinicians and many pathologists he will be told that the chondroma is a common benign neoplasm of the skeleton. Referring to our files we found that we had not made the diagnosis of chondroma in the past 12 years, and analysis of the 15

cases diagnosed in the preceding two decades revealed that 6 had eventually developed features of malignant behavior, 3 were instances of synovial chondrometaplasia, 6 were lost to follow-up but critical review of slides and records made the diagnosis of chondroma difficult to defend. If one consults the four modern American monographs on bone tumors,[1, 2, 3, 4] eliminating hamartomatous enchondroma and such lesions as "para-articular chondroma" (synovial chondrometaplasia) and "juxtacortical chondroma" (parosteal sarcoma and periosteal chondrometaplasia) one finds no description of a benign primary bone tumor of cartilaginous origin such as is described in the older texts as chondroma. One must conclude that the chondroma does not exist. Thus, the controversy over the histologic criteria that differentiate the chondrosarcoma from the chondroma is little more than dignified double talk.

With the enchondroma and the osteochondroma, the chondroblastoma and chondromyxoid fibroma constitute an interesting group of slowly growing cartilaginous lesions that may persist for many years and then take on the attributes of chondrosarcoma. Such behavior suggests that they are hamartomas or, in the cases of the osteochondroma and chondromyxoid fibroma, choristomas, which in some instances are converted to sarcomas. The chondroblastoma develops within the epiphysis and only rarely takes on aggressive features. The enchondroma develops within the metaphysis. In cases in which it involves the large cylindrical bones, particularly the proximal humerus and proximal femur, it is quite apt to be converted to chondrosarcoma. In cases in which it penetrates the cortex it may take on the growth features of osteochondroma. The osteochondroma is a cartilaginous hamartoma growing outside bone. Perhaps as many as 15 per cent of these develop malignant features and then are known as parosteal sarcomas. Finally the chondromyxoid fibroma appears to be a heterotopic deposit of chondroid tissue in bone, which retains its capacity for growth and which apparently can develop sarcomatous growth capacity. One such chondromyxoid fibroma in our material metastasized. One might consider the hypothesis that these lesions vary in morphology and behavior only because of environmental influences and that all are subject to neoplastic alteration sometime in their existence.

The malignant cartilaginous tumor, the chondrosarcoma, most certainly must be differentiated from a number of nonneoplastic cartilaginous lesions of bone including enchondroma, synovial and periosteal chondrometaplasia and even reparative callus, and the microscopy of the lesion is frequently a most helpful adjunct. But it is time that the microscopist takes a realistic attitude concerning the cellular morphology of cartilaginous lesions. Except for a relatively small percentage of chondrosarcomas in which the sections reveal such flagrant evidence of malignant character that there can be no doubt concerning the nature of the lesion, the microscopy of all cartilaginous lesions should be interpreted in terms of the clinical and radiologic features of the case.

The chondroblasts of a rapidly developing reactive proliferation can show lacunae with one or more large, round or irregular hyperchromatic nuclei with large nucleoli and even mitotic figures, features that are widely accepted by microscopists as dependable evidence of malignant neoplasm. On the other hand, a slowly growing chondrosarcoma may show fields of cells with such innocuous morphology that the possibility of malignant behavior would appear to be untenable. Pathologists have long been in agreement that certain highly malignant carcinomas such as those of prostate and thyroid may at times reveal none of the usual cellular features of malignancy. These same pathologists repeatedly diagnose cartilage tumors as "chondromas" and express the greatest surprise when they later reveal the aggressive behavior of sarcomas. If a cartilaginous lesion occurs in a large cylindrical bone or a flat bone of a patient older than 25, if it is larger than 3 cm. in diameter or if it penetrates the cortex, it is probably a chondrosarcoma irrespective of its microscopy. In the majority of these instances the roentgenogram is of the greatest assistance in reaching a decision. But in a certain proportion, only time and behavior settle the issue. Fortunately most chondrosarcomas grow slowly enough to allow this conservative approach to diagnosis.

CHONDROBLASTOMA

The chondroblastoma is a lesion of chondroblastic cytogenesis occurring predominantly in the epiphyses of adolescents with a somewhat greater frequency in males.

Because the lesion has a predilection for the ends of large, long bones and because giant cells often appear rather prominently in its cytology, it was classified as a calcifying giant cell tumor[5] and as a chondromatous giant cell tumor[6] until the paper of Jaffe and Lichtenstein in 1942.[7] These writers described the lesion as a distinct entity, stated that it was chondroblastic in origin and gave it the name of "benign chondroblastoma." Because it may not always behave in a benign fashion, we suggest that this portion of its title be deleted.

Chondroblastoma is rather rare. To date, less than 60 cases have been reported, the largest series being 16.[8] Because of its peculiar microscopy it unquestionably has been misdiagnosed chondrosarcoma, osteosarcoma and giant cell tumor with therapeutic tragedy as a consequence. Though it is an uncommon lesion all clinicians, radiologists and pathologists must be cognizant of its features in order that overtreatment may be avoided.

Until recently, the chondroblastoma was always reported arising in relation to the enchondral plate of a large cylindrical bone of an extremity, with the exception of one lesion in the talus.[9] In Codman's early series of 9 cases, all the lesions were in the proximal epiphysis of the humerus in patients between the ages of 12 and 24. In the early series of Jaffe and Lichtenstein there were 9 patients, all in the age group 12 to 24; in the later series by Lichtenstein and Kaplan there were 6 patients, all between the ages of 10 and 20; in the series of Valls et al. there were 8 patients, 13 to 18; and in that of Hatcher and Campbell, 6 patients, 13 to 19. In the 1956 series of Kunkel et al. there were 16 patients. In 10 of these, all 21 or younger, the chondroblastoma apparently arose in relation to the enchondral plate of a large long bone; in 6 others a flat bone was involved. It is interesting that 5 of these 6 were patients over the age of 20 years. Our material consists

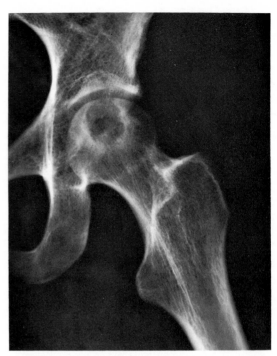

Figure 17–2 Chondroblastoma. The area of destruction in the head of the femur is rather well demarcated by a zone of sclerosis.

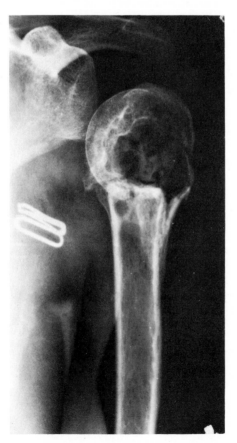

Figure 17–1 Chondroblastoma in a patient aged 44. The patient fell and suffered a fracture through the lesion, which had probably been present and asymptomatic since adolescence.

of 47 cases, 39 of these were under the age of 20.

It is obvious that the available material on chondroblastoma at present is insufficient on which to base final conclusions. Nevertheless, we must recognize it as a distinct entity of chondroblastic origin different from all other known tumors with the possible exception of chondromyxoid fibroma. It is most apt to affect adolescents. Indeed, it is probable that it always develops during adolescence though in rare instances its development may be asymptomatic and it may remain latent until its discovery years later in adult life. Wright and Sherman[10] reported a chondroblastoma in a female age 73 that was known to be present since adolescence. It had recently begun to grow. We have one such case in our material (Fig. 17–1). Certainly it is likely to involve the epiphysis in most cases and in a few there is secondary invasion of the metaphysis. These features, if they hold true in the future, set the chondroblastoma apart from all other bone tumors.

The only characteristic symptom of chondroblastoma is pain. Because the lesion is apt to be in the epiphysis, the pain is usually referred to a joint and therefore misinterpreted as a type of monarticular arthritis. The pain is insidious in onset and usually not severe at first. It may be of considerable duration, often two years or longer, suggesting that the lesion grows very slowly. A firm enlargement may be palpated in perhaps one third of the cases. There may be muscle stiffness and wasting secondary to interference with function.

Roentgenographic Manifestations. The cartilaginous nature of the chondroblastoma is responsible for a radiolucent defect. Because the lesion arises from young chondroblasts in the enchondral plate, it is located within the center of ossification, the epiphysis. The lesion subsequently may grow to involve the metaphysis and even the adjacent diaphysis. It tends to be round or ovoid and fairly well demarcated by a zone of sclerotic bone,

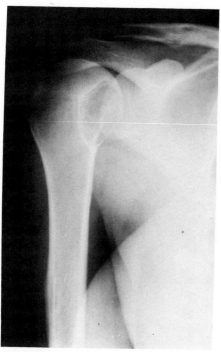

Figure 17–3 Chondroblastoma, female 28 years of age. The lesion involves the proximal humerus and obviously crosses the old epiphyseal line to lie in both the epiphysis and the metaphysis. There is a thin but well defined zone of density surrounding the area of lucency.

the result of the slow growth of the neoplasm. Tiny areas of calcification within the cartilage often produce a mottled appearance that may obscure its outline in some areas. This calcification, when present, affords a clue as to the cartilaginous nature of the neoplasm. It may be seen best by tomography. In cases in which the lesion extends into the diaphysis, erosion of the cortex results in the production of periosteal bone and widening of the involved segment of the shaft (Fig. 17–4).

The epiphyseal location of this neoplasm is quite characteristic and should strongly suggest the diagnosis, particularly in an adolescent patient.

Morbid Anatomy. It appears, from available evidence, that the benign chondroblastoma usually or always arises from the young chondroblasts in the deep portion of the enchondral plate. It almost always begins to manifest itself soon after puberty; the youngest reported patient was 8 years old. It usually invades the bony nucleus of the adolescent epiphysis to produce a mass 1 to 4 cm. in diameter. It may erode the articular plate and protrude into the joint space. Less often it progresses toward the metaphysis and in a few instances it seems to lie wholly within the metaphysis but always abutting on the epiphyseal line, suggesting an enchondral origin.

Its gross appearance is nondescript. It is usually more pale than red or brown. Areas of degeneration are common as one would expect in any cartilaginous neoplasm. Irregular deposits of calcium salts are usual and may give the tissue a gritty consistency. When it impinges on the metaphysis its slow growth allows a bony reaction in the surrounding cancellous tissue. This may produce a narrow sclerotic zone. It may erode the overlying compacta and cause the periosteum to deposit a layer of bone on the outer surface, giving the appearance of cortical expansion.

The microscopic appearance of chondroblastoma is highly characteristic but unless the pathologist is familiar with its features he is apt to misinterpret it as an undifferentiated type of bone sarcoma. The characteristic cell is the young chondroblast, somewhat larger than the normal and with a cytoplasm that is more durable

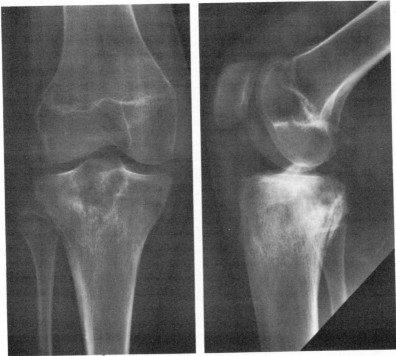

Figure 17–4 Chondroblastoma. The radiolucent lesion is evident in the proximal end of the tibia. The epiphysis is primarily involved but there is extension into the metaphysis. A line of sclerosis can be seen in relation to the tumor, particularly on its medial aspect; laterally the outline of the tumor is indistinct; posteriorly there is periosteal reaction.

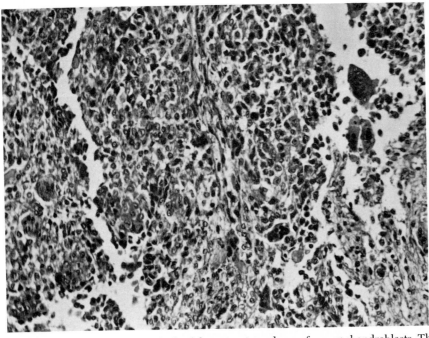

Figure 17–5 Benign chondroblastoma. Much of the tumor is made up of young chondroblasts. There is little or no chondroid production in these fields. Note the numerous giant cells. (× 200.)

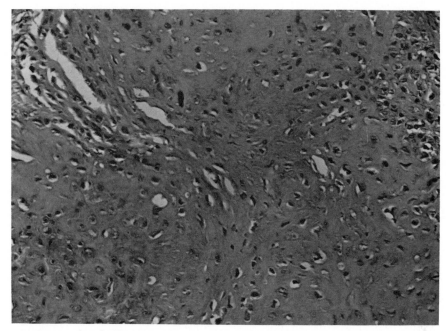

Figure 17–6   Benign chondroblastoma. In some fields the cartilage is more adult. Here a chondroid matrix is formed. (× 200.)

to the rigors of processing than the normal chondroblast (Fig. 17–5). It is spheroid, or nearly so, and its cytoplasmic membrane is usually obvious. It produces relatively little chondroid in most areas so that some fields appear very cellular. Because the morphology of these areas is quite uni-

form, this is apt to frighten the uninitiated into a diagnosis of malignant tumor. These cellular areas compose from one third to one half the tumor mass. They lie in a field of recognizable chondroid (Fig. 17–6), of myxoid material and of collagenized connective tissue. These intercellular sub-

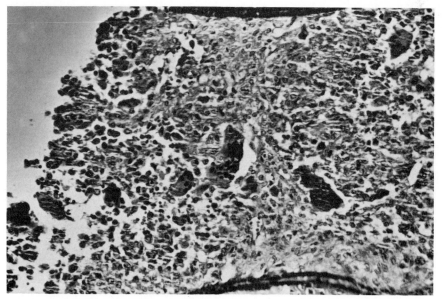

Figure 17–7   In some fields giant cells may dominate the picture. Benign chondroblastoma was originally called "cartilaginous variant of giant cell tumor." (× 200.)

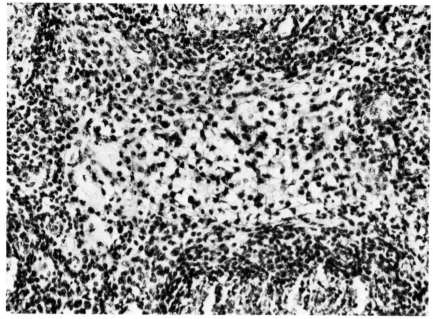

Figure 17–8   Chondroblastoma. A myxoid area resembling those seen in chondromyxoid fibroma. (× 250.)

stances almost always contain irregular masses of deeply staining calcium, much of which is in the amorphous state and, therefore, appears powdery or flocculated rather than like the crackled chips of calcified osteoid. Here and there some frag-

ments of osteoid may be recognized but it is immature and never prominent. Giant cells (Fig. 17–7) are usual but they rarely if ever dominate the picture. Because the lesion grows slowly, one expects to find mitotic figures but rarely. Areas of myxoid

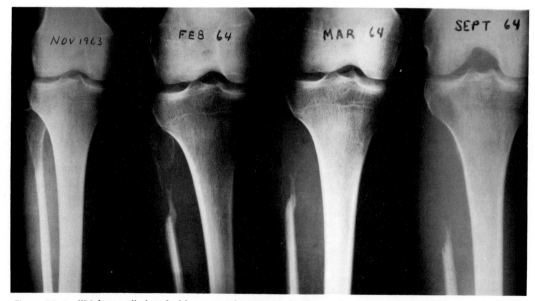

Figure 17–9   "Malignant" chondroblastoma. This series of radiographs, taken over a period of approximately one year, illustrates the aggressive nature of this lesion. Its microscopy also revealed features of malignant neoplasm. (Courtesy of Dr. Willis Hock)

change (Fig. 17–8) may be identical to those seen in chondromyxoid fibroma.

Prognosis. When Codman collected his original series from the Bone Tumor Registry he was surprised to find so many survivals with treatment that would be considered inadequate for malignant tumor. He concluded that the lesion is benign.

For a decade following its definitive description,[7] this lesion was considered a benign tumor. As our experience has broadened and our follow-ups have become more significant we have encountered recurrences and evidence of aggressiveness. Of the 47 cases in our material, five must now be classified as possible chondrosarcoma on the basis of their microscopy and behavior (see Fig. 17–9). To date we have not encountered a chondroblastoma which has produced an unmistakable metastasis. Four of our chondroblastomas have recurred. Kahn et al.[11] have reported two chondroblastomas one of which spread to contiguous soft tissues after removal and one of which metastasized to the lungs and killed the patient 15 years after original diagnosis. They review the literature and cite three other cases which behaved like malignant tumors but did not metastasize.

We must now come to one of two conclusions. Either there are two types of chondroblastoma, one that is benign and a second that is of low grade malignancy, or we must presume that all chondroblastomas (and possibly all chondromyxoid fibromas)

are actually exceedingly low grade chondrosarcomas. There is much about the latter hypothesis that makes it attractive. As our chondroblastomas collect and are treated by curettage we may be surprised by the number which recur or even metastasize many years later. The possibility is sufficiently imminent to have caused us recently to advise regional resection where feasible.

CHONDROMYXOID FIBROMA

The chondromyxoid fibroma is a slowly growing lesion of chondroblastic origin. It usually occurs in the metaphysis of cylindrical bones, most often the large, long bones of the extremities, but it has been reported in the ribs, the ilium, the metatarsals, a vertebra, and we have seen one in the clavicle, one in the patella, and one in a parietal bone (Fig. 17–10). Because the lesion is not a fibroma the name is inappropriate. If the constituents of the lesion are to be expressed in the title it would be better called a fibromyxoid chondroma.

There was no account of this entity in the literature until the paper of Jaffe and Lichtenstein[12] in 1948. They reported a series of eight cases, very clearly defining the clinical, radiologic and pathologic features and suggesting the name. Since that time Feldman et al.[13] have reviewed the world literature and reported eight cases

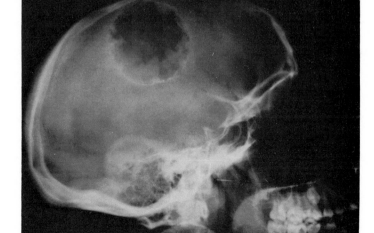

Figure 17–10 Chondromyxoid fibroma of parietal bone. (Courtesy of Dr. C. P. Schwinn)

of their own. They calculate that chondro-myxoid fibroma constitutes about 1 per cent of all primary bone tumors. In our own material we have but 17 unequivocal cases if we apply the standard criteria. In six more we could not rule out myxomatous enchondroma with absolute assurance. In 12 more cases there were areas with the microscopy typical of chondromyxoid fibroma but intermixed fields of chondrosarcoma. Of these one metastasized to the lung, one killed the patient by destroying a large portion of the spine, and five recurred from one to several times. If one accepts all of these as chondromyxoid fibromas there were 29 cases of which 12 showed evidence, behavioral or microscopic or both, of a malignant character.

In the earlier reports most of the lesions were found in patients between the ages of 12 and 30. As more cases are described it becomes apparent that any age may be afflicted, but the preponderance fall within the second and third decades.

In the large bones the chondromyxoid fibroma has always been reported in the metaphysis. In the short cylindrical bones of the hands and feet it may begin in the metaphysis but ultimately involves the entire shaft. The lesion is usually small, averaging 2 to 3 cm. in diameter, but lesions of 8 cm. have been reported. In the metaphysis of large bones it is usually eccentric, growing slowly and often producing a thin line of reactive sclerosis along the margin in contact with cancellous tissue. It may erode the compacta from within and cause the overlying periosteum to lay down a shell of bone, resulting in the appearance of cortical expansion. At times there is no reactive bone formation and then the tumor may perforate the cortex and produce a mass on the outer cortical surface, lifting the periosteum over it without invading or penetrating it. The cortex may be thinned to the point of fracture and then the resulting callus formation mixed in with the expanding cartilaginous tumor presents a most confusing picture. In the metaphysis there is usually a centimeter or more of normal spongiosa between the distal pole of the lesion and the epiphyseal line, but it may abut directly upon the epiphysis. When such is the case it becomes exceedingly difficult to be sure whether one is dealing with a chondromyxoid fibroma or a chondroblastoma. Because the histologic elements of the two lesions are so nearly the same, one might ask if a differentiation is justifiable. This has caused some, including us, to suspect that chondroblastoma and chondromyxoid fibroma are closely related processes, the peculiar features of each lesion arising from the environmental difference of its location, the one in the epiphysis and the other in the shaft.

Both lesions are chondroblastic in genesis. Both produce slowly growing, lobulated masses of embryonic cartilage cells, which may mature to the status of chondroid production and lacuna formation. Myxomatous tissue is highly characteristic of all cartilaginous tumors; it is more abundant in the chondromyxoid fibroma than in the chondroblastoma. The disparity in the age incidence is the most outstanding difference in the two lesions. The chondroblastoma probably always arises between puberty and ossification of the epiphysis, the period in which young chondroblasts are present in this region. If it occurs after epiphyseal ossification it must arise from an immature rest of chondroblasts. The chondromyxoid fibroma may occur at any age at which a group of chondroblasts, left behind in the metaphysis by the advancing epiphyseal frontier, develops the ability to proliferate. Thus the location may also explain the age incidence.

The symptoms of chondromyxoid fibroma are much like those of chondroblastoma except that the joints are not usually involved. Pain is the outstanding symptom but it is probably not very severe, because a history of a year's duration is not infrequent. If there is cortical expansion there may be a palpable mass. Tenderness is often found. In our cases, fracture occurred at least twice.

Roentgenographic Manifestations. The lobulated masses of cartilage that characterize the chondromyxoid fibroma have the density of soft tissue, as a result of which the lesion appears radiolucent in contrast with the surrounding bone. Uncommonly, spotty calcification is present reflecting calcified chondroid. Its borders tend to be scalloped and well defined by a narrow band of opaque sclerotic bone. In

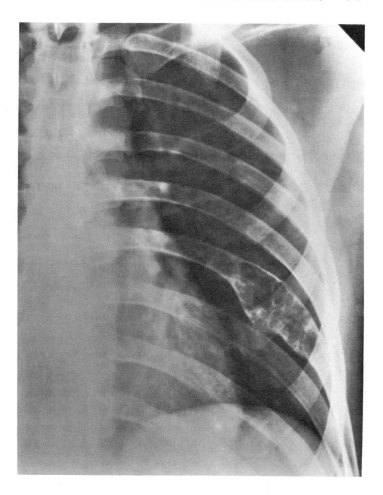

Figure 17–11 Chondromyxoid fibroma. A septate radiolucent area is seen in the rib. The lesion has caused expansion of the cortex. Chondromyxoid fibroma is more often seen in cylindrical bones.

certain instances, the amount of endosteal reactive new bone may become extensive. In the long bones this neoplasm arises eccentrically in the spongiosa of the metaphysis and erodes, thins and expands the overlying cortex as it grows. The cortex may be destroyed. The epiphyseal line is only rarely violated. Septa, often thick and relatively opaque, frequently traverse the lesion (Fig. 17–12).

In cases in which the flat bones are involved the lesion is evident as a radiolucent defect with sclerotic scalloped borders often containing trabeculations.[14]

Morphology. The chondromyxoid fibroma appears to be well circumscribed when sectioned and viewed grossly, unless it has penetrated the cortex. It is a pliable mass of soft tissue, which separates rather easily from its surrounding bony walls. It has the appearance of a rather coarse, gray fibrous tissue. There may be some gritty fragments representing calcified chondroid.

The pathologist is apt to be surprised when he examines this tissue through the microscope. The tissue that appeared fibrous grossly is largely primitive cartilage, and moreover in areas in which the tumor tissue is pressed against the bony wall it often penetrates the interspicular spaces. The myxomatous character, which may be quite dramatic on the section, usually is not appreciable on gross examination. Often the sections give the impression that the technique of preparation has been poor. This is probably because the young chondroblast is a very fragile cell and collapses under the technical stresses.

The lesion is composed essentially of lobulated masses of cartilage cells of various ages. The center of the lobule may consist of rather tightly packed immature cells, which are small, round and have a

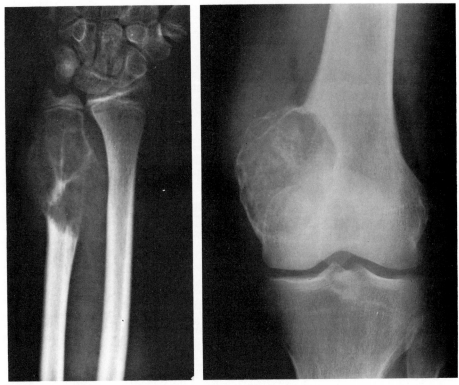

Fig. 17–12

Fig. 17–13

Figure 17–12 Chondromyxoid fibroma. The epiphyseal line is intact. The cortex is thinned medially and destroyed laterally. Thick septa are present.

Figure 17–13 Chondromyxoid fibroma. The cortex is expanded and thinned. A sclerotic border demarcates the inner aspect of the lesion.

scanty but rather intensely pink cytoplasm (Fig. 17–14). In other areas the center may have a rather amorphous, deeply pink staining character with only shadow cells to suggest its origin. About the scalloped periphery the cells are much larger and more distinct. The nuclei may be uniformly round or bizarrely folded. The cytoplasmic outlines are apt to be intact, the cytoplasm clear or pale and the configuration that of highly cellular cartilage. There may be some chondroid production between the cells. Elsewhere there should be fields of recognizable chondroid often with only sparsely scattered cells forming lacunae (Fig. 17–15). These constituents are embedded in a fibrous and myxomatous matrix. The fibrous tissue may be quite densely collagenized and this structure presumably gives the gross appearance. The myxomatous fields are made up of spindled and less often multipolar cells

loosely arranged in a pale background (Fig. 17–16). When very young chondroblasts are isolated in this matrix they are very small with a deep pink cytoplasm, vaguely suggesting plasmacytes. This material in the aspirate of one of our patients led to the first suggestion of the correct diagnosis.

In the sclerosed bony margin one may find irregular masses of large, deeply blue staining cartilage cells with considerable pleomorphism of their nuclear morphology. The nature of these cells is hard to define, whether they belong to the tumor or to the reaction consequent to infractions in its overlying cortex. These cells and groups of the younger chondroblasts at the periphery of the lobules may lead the pathologist to pronounce this lesion a chondrosarcoma. This danger becomes apparent in cases in which the biopsy is superficial.

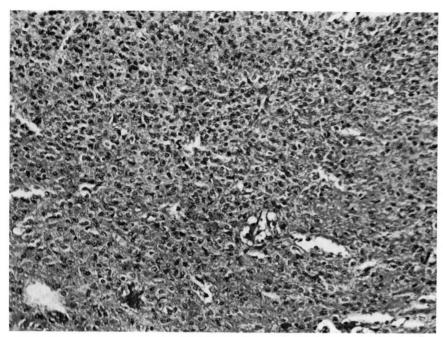

Figure 17–14 Chondromyxoid fibroma. Much of the tumor is composed of immature chondroblasts. There is little chondroid formation in these areas. Note the similarity to chondroblastoma in Figure 17–5. (× 200.)

Other constituents are less characteristic but often found. Giant cells are usual (Fig. 17–17). Their nuclei, varying from a few to more than 50, are small, deeply staining and scattered at random throughout the cytoplasm. Xanthoid cells are reported but have not appeared in our material. Pigment granules can usually be found. In the

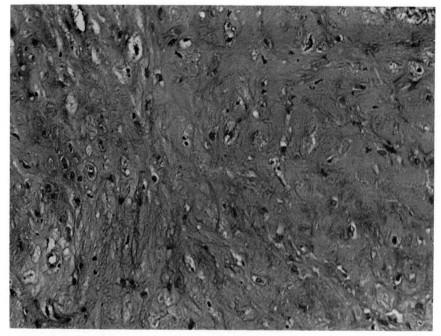

Figure 17–15 Benign chondromyxoid fibroma. In some fields the chondroblasts mature sufficiently to form recognizable chondroid. (× 200.)

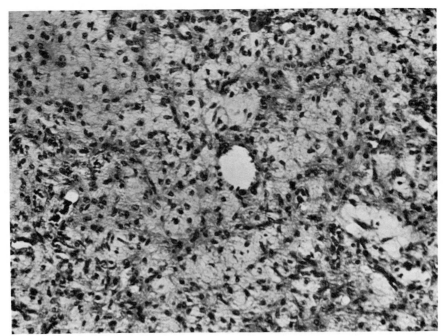

Figure 17-16 Benign chondromyxoid fibroma. The tumor is characterized by myxomatous areas made up of stellate cells in a pale mucinous matrix. (× 200.)

original series of Jaffe and Lichtenstein they mention the presence of exudative inflammatory cells. Lymphocytes and neutrophils have been more prominent in our sections than reported descriptions in other series suggest.

Prognosis. Before the definitive paper by Jaffe and Lichtenstein the chondromyx-

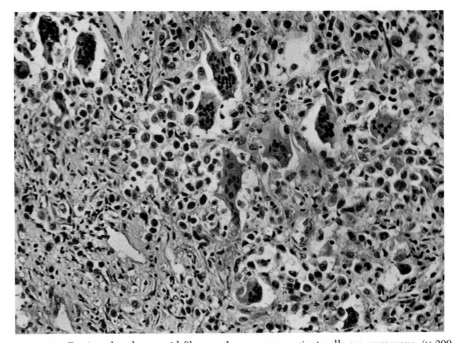

Figure 17-17 Benign chondromyxoid fibroma. In some areas giant cells are numerous. (× 200.)

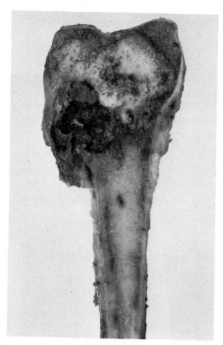

Figure 17–18 "Malignant" chondromyxoid fibroma. Ten years ago this lesion was a typical chondromyxoid fibroma both radiologically and microscopically. It was curetted. It recurred and now has many gross and microscopic features of chondrosarcoma. (Courtesy of Dr. William Campbell)

oid fibroma was considered to be a sarcoma. In that paper it was defined as a benign tumor. In the past several years more and more of these lesions have shown aggressive behavior. In the 29 cases in our collection, 12 have shown features of chondrosarcoma (Fig. 17–18). One of these has metastasized. We now believe that this tumor should be considered at least potentially malignant and treated as such.

CHONDROSARCOMA

The chondrosarcoma is the only tumor of chondrogenic origin with an expected and immediate malignant behavior. For nearly a century it was classified as a primary osteogenic neoplasm and only in the past 30 years has it been recognized as a distinct entity. In a paper by Phemister[15] in 1930, it was pointed out that the clinical behavior of chondrosarcoma is quite different from that of osteosarcoma. Since that time analysis of several series of "os-

teogenic sarcomas" has brought out differences in sites of involvement, age group, microscopy and prognosis. Though the differentiation of chondrosarcoma and osteosarcoma is often more difficult than that of osteosarcoma and myeloma, it is, nevertheless, just as important.

The osteosarcoma arises from osteoblasts and primitive fibrous tissue with the potential of forming osteoid, chondroid and collagen. It is made up of tumor cells resembling osteoblasts, chondroblasts and fibroblasts and the intercellular products of these cells. The chondrosarcoma arises from chondroblasts and collagenoblasts. It can produce only chondroid and collagen. The osteoid found in sections of the chondrosarcoma is incidental and plays no role in the tumor process. In brief, the osteosarcoma often contains neoplastic elements of all the tissue involved in normal enchondral bone formation; the chondrosarcoma is almost totally cartilaginous with only a minimal amount of supportive collagenous tissue.

Chondrosarcoma is about one half as common as osteosarcoma. It affects males somewhat more frequently than females just as do all malignant tumors with the exception of those of the genitalia, but this difference is not great enough to be helpful in diagnosis. In the largest series published to date, by Dahlin and Henderson,[16] in more than three quarters of the cases the bones of the trunk and the upper ends of the humerus and femur were affected. In a smaller group (47 cases) from our series,[17] the distribution was about the same. Excluding the myelomas, the chondrosarcoma is the most common tumor involving the bones of the trunk, shoulder and hip. Though chondrosarcoma may affect any bone, the nearer a cartilaginous tumor occurs to the trunk the more apt it is to be malignant. Chondrosarcomas of the small bones of the hands and feet are rare but they do occur. There were only four in the series of 212 cases of Dahlin and Henderson. We have seen only two.

The age incidence of primary chondrosarcoma is interesting. It is quite unusual in patients under 30. In younger patients chondrosarcoma is apt to be superimposed on other lesions; in our material six were superimposed on osteochondroma, four on

enchondroma and one on fibrous dysplasia. After 35 the incidence rises progressively and the curve is very similar to that
of carcinoma. This is in contrast to the incidence curve of osteosarcoma in which the
greater elevation is on the left. Chondrosarcoma is a very slowly growing tumor
and the question arises whether it may
begin in youth, like most other bone
tumors, but require several years to manifest itself. There are a few facts to support
this thesis and a history of symptoms of
five years' duration is not unusual.

Chondrosarcoma can be divided into
those that occur within bone and those that
arise from the outer bone and cartilage surfaces. The former is usually called central
and the latter peripheral chondrosarcoma.
Some authors have stated that most central
chondrosarcomas represent secondary
changes in enchondromas and all or most
peripheral chondrosarcomas arise in osteochondromas. In the series of Lichtenstein
and Jaffe[18] 5 of their 15 cases were peripheral and all are stated to be secondary to
osteochondromas. In the series of Dahlin
and Henderson, only 19 of their total 212
cases (they were not always able to distinguish between central and peripheral
tumors) were secondary. In our material
there was evidence that 6 were in areas in
which osteochondromas had previously
existed. Five of these were cases of hereditary multiple exostoses and one was a solitary osteochondroma. In Lichtenstein's 10
central lesions, 5 are said to have arisen in
enchondromas; in our material there were
4 in which this fact could be established.

Central chondrosarcomas in cylindrical
bones usually begin in the metaphyseal
region, but to a greater extent than osteosarcoma they may start in other portions of
the shaft. They usually replace a large
proportion of the cancellous and medullary tissue before they break through the
cortex (Fig. 17–19). The more slowly growing type erodes the compacta from within
and causes the periosteum to lay down
new bone over it. A biopsy through this
area containing new bone and neoplastic
cartilage is apt to result in a microscopist's
diagnosis of osteosarcoma. More characteristically the central chondrosarcoma infiltrates the medullary tissue and then perforates the cortex, frequently at a single

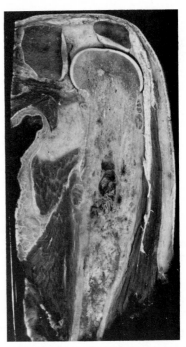

Figure 17–19 When chondrosarcoma arises in
medullary tissues it may infiltrate a considerable
proportion of the shaft before it penetrates the cortex.

small area. Then producing a large, soft-
tissue mass it develops a "collar button"
silhouette (Fig. 17–20). Thinning of the
cortex to the point of pathologic fracture is
unusual.

The peripheral chondrosarcoma grows
from the cartilaginous cap of an osteochondroma or from any area in which cartilage
normally persists. The tumors that arise
from periosteum are usually mixed, containing not only cartilage but also osteoid
and collagenous tissue. These are probably better designated "parosteal sarcomas" than periosteal chondrosarcomas.
Often surprisingly little bone erosion is
produced by the peripheral tumors, even
though they become massive as they often
do. Several reports have described peripheral chondrosarcoma penetrating the walls
of veins and producing a continuous column of tumor along the course of the
lumen (Fig. 17–21). One of these in our
collection eventually grew through the
right heart and into the pulmonary vasculature very much as hypernephromas are
apt to do. Peripheral chondrosarcoma may
be superimposed on Paget's disease of

bone. Two such instances occurred in our material.

The symptoms of chondrosarcoma depend upon the area affected and whether it is central or peripheral. Because it is slow growing, both types may be silent until a considerable tumor mass is produced. The only consistent symptom of chondrosarcoma is pain. This pain may be insidious at outset but it gradually becomes persistent and severe. In an adult any cartilaginous lesion that hurts must be considered chondrosarcoma until proved otherwise. Eventually, a palpable firm mass may be produced. Sometimes a history of osteochondroma may be obtainable. In this case, a history of trauma is probably pertinent because presumably a fracture of an osteochondroma may activate growth in the cartilaginous cap and conceivably the young chondroblasts may develop neoplastic propensities.

The expected growth rate of chondrosarcoma is much slower than that of osteosarcoma. Symptoms may persist over a period of one to ten or even more years before a

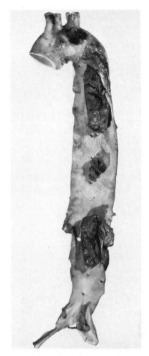

Figure 17-21 Chondrosarcoma that grew through the aortic wall to form large emboli within the lumen.

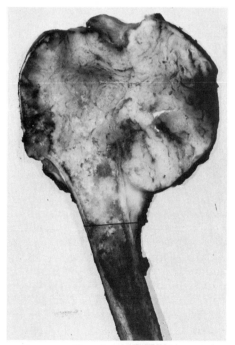

Figure 17-20 Chondrosarcoma often penetrates the cortex at a single point and then mushrooms into a soft tissue tumor to produce a "collar-button" lesion.

diagnosis is established. If treatment is inadequate, recurrence at the original site is the rule and this may not be manifest for several years after the original intervention. Surgical manipulation appears to speed up the growth process and sometimes the character of a smoldering and mildly aggressive tumor changes to that of an explosively metastasizing malignant growth. In some of these, osteoid formation is noted in the metastatic deposits and one wonders if they have not undergone metaplasia into an osteosarcoma. Chondrosarcoma has also been reported to seed itself in the soft tissues of the surgical wound. Precautions in technique should be observed in its removal.

Roentgenographic Manifestations. Chondrosarcomas, as noted on page 552, may be divided into two groups, central and peripheral. The radiographic appearance of the tumor then is dependent upon its location, whether it is within the bone or associated with its surface. In either case, the tumor presents as a lesion of soft tissue density but often containing irregular flecks and streaks of calcification. Its ef-

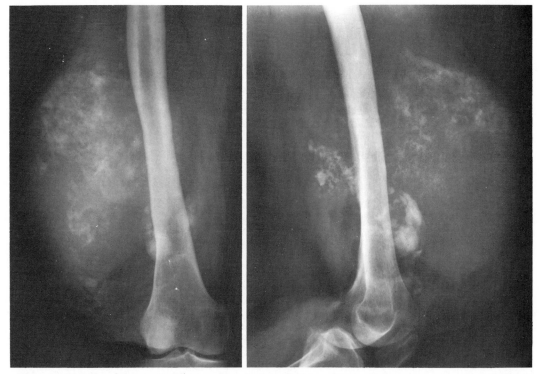

Figure 17-22 Chondrosarcoma. The neoplasm has resulted in a large soft tissue mass containing irregular patches and streaks of calcification. The cortex underlying the lesion is eroded on both its inner and outer aspects.

fect on osseous structures depends on its site of origin.

The peripheral chondrosarcoma is a bulky tumor, which presents radiographically as a mass that displaces the normal soft tissues, i.e., fatty muscle planes. Calcification is variable in its appearance but is almost always present (Figs. 17–22 and 17–23). The underlying bone may be normal or show evidence of erosion from without. The tumor may arise from osteochondromas and, if these are multiple and recognized, afford insight as to the nature of the mass.

The central chondrosarcoma usually involves the medullary portion of the diaphysis of a long bone. The tumor, whether primary or superimposed on enchondroma, for example, is apt to grow slowly. Thus expansion of the medullary canal and erosion of the inner surface of the cortex are associated with the formation of reactive periosteal new bone and irregular thinning of the cortex (Fig. 17–25). The inner aspect of the cortex may become wavy in outline as it is thickened and thinned in relation to the growth of the tumor. With the passage of time, the margins of the tumor become indistinct and when the cortex of the bone is perforated, a soft tissue mass is evident.

Pathology. The chondrosarcoma usually produces a tissue that is grossly recognizable as cartilage. A lobulated, white or bluish mass of glistening, moderately firm consistency is found (Fig. 17–27). Though malignant, it is often quite well delineated by a capsule of compressed normal tissue or a subperiosteal lamina of bone. The lobular pattern is often conspicuous and there is apt to be discoloration from degeneration and old hemorrhage. Two features are helpful. Areas of myxomatous change are usual and sometimes the major portion of the tumor may consist of a slimy mass. The second feature is calcification. Irregular areas of chalky white, never very large, may be grossly obvious. The chondrosarcoma is apt to be a large tumor (Fig. 17–28). Any

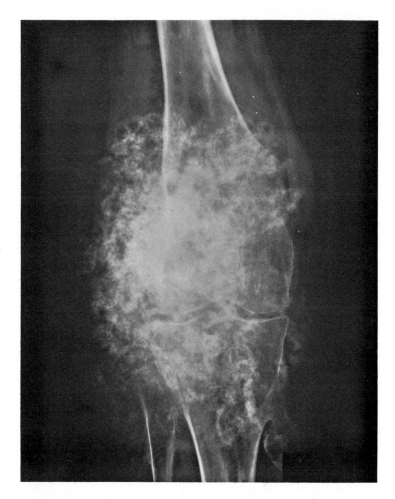

Figure 17–23 Chondrosarcoma. This lesion has arisen in association with hereditary multiple exostoses.

abnormal cartilaginous mass larger than 3 cm. in diameter should be regarded with suspicion. Destruction and perforation of bone are incriminating evidence of malignant character (Fig. 17–29).

The diagnosis of chondrosarcoma by microscopy alone is, more often than not, impossible. Lichtenstein and Jaffe[18] and Lichtenstein[2] carefully listed the features to be evaluated in making the distinction between "chondroma," chondrosarcoma and osteosarcoma. The last usually can be ruled out by the paucity of cartilage and the presence of neoplastic osteoid. These authors point out that only viable, noncalcified areas should be judged. If, here, more than a few lacunae per field contain more than one cell (Fig. 17–30) and if there are cells with more than one nucleus, the pathologist should seriously consider chondrosarcoma. If the nuclei are

large and heavily chromatized this is added evidence (Fig. 17–31). We have found irregularity in nuclear outline and the presence of prominent nucleoli helpful. Areas of calcification and myxomatous change are usual but not very valuable. Mitotic figures need not be common in chondrosarcoma, but in cases in which they are abundant they are very significant. The inadvisability of evaluating a cartilaginous lesion on the microscopic features alone has been discussed earlier in this chapter. Unless the microscopy is overwhelmingly that of malignant tumor the pathologist should refuse to commit his diagnosis until he has had an opportunity to weigh the clinical and radiologic findings.

Very clearly etched in our memories are three cases, a brief account of which may be informative to those who deal with the

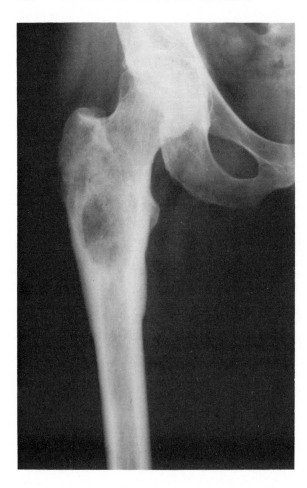

Figure 17–24 Central chondrosarcoma. The tumor is characterized by a lytic defect and overlying cortex of varying thickness. Calcification is not visualized.

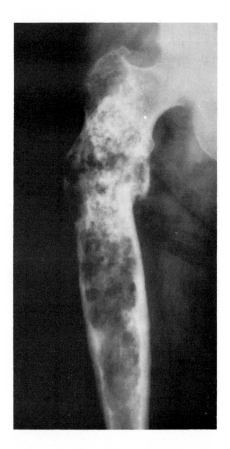

Figure 17–25 Central chondrosarcoma. The femur is expanded; irregular areas of cortical thinning are present. A pathologic fracture has occurred through the proximal end of the diaphysis at the point at which the cortex is thinnest. Calcification is present within the tumor.

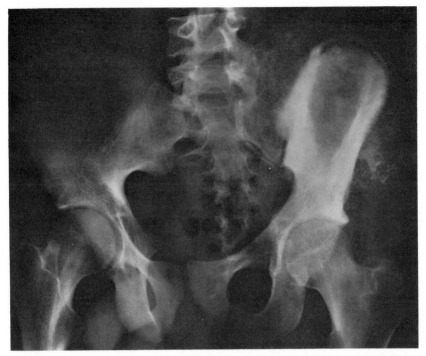

Figure 17–26   Chondrosarcoma. Destruction of the left lateral aspect of the sacrum and ilium is evident as well as a soft tissue mass within which there are irregular scattered areas of calcification.

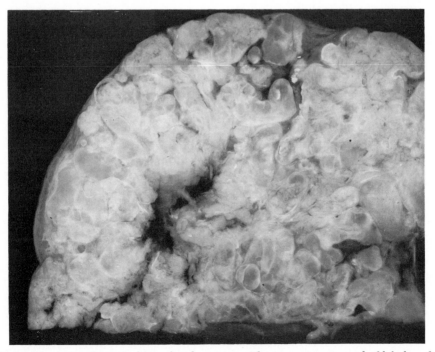

Figure 17–27   The cut surface of a large chondrosarcoma. The tumor is composed of lobules of glistening blue-white translucent tissue. Myxomatous areas are found throughout.

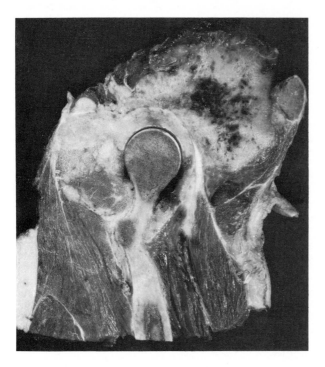

Figure 17–28 Chondrosarcoma of the ilium. The tumor has penetrated the cortex to form a huge, lobulated, extraosseous mass with hemorrhage and myxomatous change.

problem of cytologic diagnosis of chondrosarcoma. All were males whose ages were 40, 52 and 59. All had pain of long standing in the region of the hip. Two had x-ray–discernible lesions of the ilium in relation to the acetabulum, the third a lesion in the neck of the femur. On clinical and radiologic evidence the diagnoses in all were chronic inflammatory or degenerative disease. In each a series of four biopsies was done before a correct diagnosis was achieved. The earlier diagnoses were consistently "degenerating bone and cartilage with necrosis and calcification." All three patients eventually died of metastatic chondrosarcoma. In reviewing these cases it was established that a correct diagnosis might have been made at least a year earlier if all facets of the cases had been known and all features of the microscopy sections had been properly evaluated. The earlier biopsy material in all cases consisted almost entirely of myxomatous tissue, calcium deposits, necrotic cartilage and bone and other products of degenerative inflammation. But on hindsight one could find viable cartilage cells, some singly and some in small groups, some embryonic and others more mature, whose

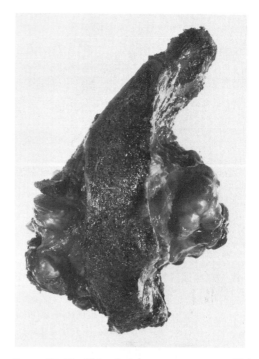

Figure 17–29 This chondrosarcoma arose within the cancellous tissue of the ilium. It penetrated both the inner and outer tables. Cartilaginous tumors of flat bones are apt to be malignant. Penetration of the cortex and the formation of a soft tissue tumor make the diagnosis of malignancy almost certain.

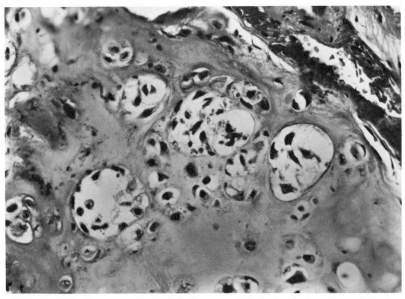

Figure 17–30   If many of the lacunae contain more than one cell, the lesion is more apt to be sarcoma. (× 300.)

presence should have been weighed more seriously. This experience has allowed us to make the diagnosis of chondrosarcoma in a fourth case, again a male, aged 64, and again in the hip region on material that casually treated is no more informative than that of the earlier three.

One of the most disconcerting features of the chondrosarcoma for the microscopist is the almost constant occurrence of myxomatous alteration. Chondroid is the normal product of the normal chondrocyte. When the metabolic routine of this cell is altered in the neoplastic cell the resulting product, a myxomatous liquid or gel, is very similar in chemical constituency but quite dissimilar in physical character. There is also a distressing tendency for the tumor cells to become spindled or stellate or rounded and chondroblastic in appearance. Two malignant cartilaginous tumors have been described and called mesenchymal chondrosarcoma[19] and chondroblastic sarcoma.[2] We have seen "typical" instances of both these tumor types and prefer to consider them simply microscopically atypical types of chondrosarcoma. It seems reasonable at the time of this writing to suggest that the neoplastic chondroblast manifests a variety of structural forms and functions which produce what

superficially appears to be a group of lesions varying from chondroblastoma through mesenchymal chondrosarcoma to classic chondrosarcoma. They all may be variations of the same lesion.

Most pathologists see too few chondrosarcomas to feel comfortable in evaluating these quantitative differences. It is a trying experience to place a tumor with such minimal evidence of malignancy in a category that will necessitate mutilating surgery. This is probably the reason chondrosarcoma, more than any other tumor, has the reputation of developing from a benign forerunner. It is probable that the primary lesion in most instances was chondrosarcoma from the start and only behavior following the initial investigation made the final diagnosis apparent. A careful evaluation of all the available criteria and comparison with sections of known lesions, both benign and malignant, will help to better the diagnostic acumen but there will still be border cases in which technique, notably poor in cartilaginous lesions, and inadequate biopsy material will give the sincerest microscopist trouble. And if the general pathologist seeks solace he may be assured that not even many years of experience are a guarantee of accurate prognosis.

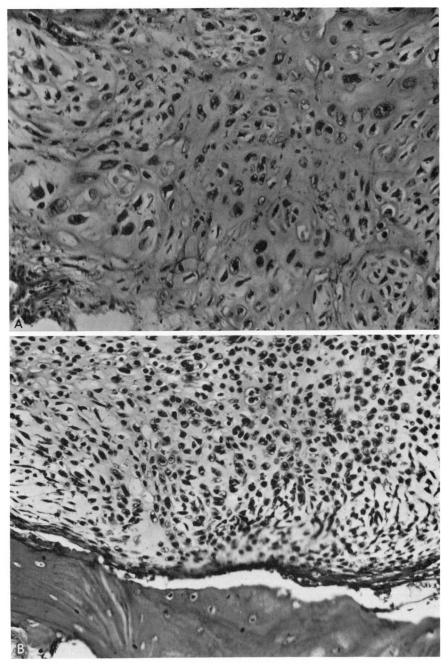

Figure 17–31   Chondrosarcoma. *A*, Variation in cell size, irregularity in nuclear borders and hyperchromatism are important features of malignancy. *B*, Sometimes the cells are rather small and uniform but one can still find more than one cell in a lacuna and there is usually hyperchromatism. (× 200.)

Prognosis. The typical chondrosarcoma grows slowly and metastasizes late. Only an occasional tumor runs a rapid and fatal course and one may suspect that these are actually osteosarcomas in which the biopsy sections failed to reveal osteoid tissue. Chondrosarcoma is much more apt to recur at the site of operation than is osteosarcoma, and even after recurrence a cure is often obtained if adequate excision is still possible. But repeated surgery may cause a change in the degree of malignancy of a chondrosarcoma. Every effort should be made to secure a firm diagnosis and once the diagnosis of chondrosarcoma is made the surgeon should proceed with the courage of his convictions. The rule is that "all neoplastic tissue must be removed widely enough to give assurance that none remains." In a large percentage of cases this means amputation through the proximal bone, because chondrosarcoma may infiltrate through the medullary tissues farther than the eye can discern. If there is recurrence, excision should be repeated. If there is metastasis, even pulmonary metastasis, excision should be considered. The value of persistent vigilance and determined surgery is nowhere so great in bone tumors as in chondrosarcoma.

In conclusion, only about half of our chondrosarcomas are primary. The other half arise on preceding lesions, most often osteochondroma and enchondroma. The primary tumors rarely occur before age 35; the secondary type often occur earlier. The primary tumor is unusual distal to the hip and shoulder areas. Secondary chondrosarcoma is more apt to be peripheral. It tends to grow slowly; a history of 10 years of symptoms is not unprecedented. It is apt to recur and to seed itself in the operation site. With adequate surgical treatment, five year survival figures should be approximately 35 per cent.

References

1. Jaffe, H.: Tumors and Tumorous Conditions of the Bones and Joints. Philadelphia, Lea & Febiger, 1958.
2. Lichtenstein, L.: Bone Tumors. Ed. 3. St. Louis, C. V. Mosby Co., 1965.
3. Dahlin, D.: Bone Tumors. Springfield, Ill., Charles C Thomas, 1957.
4. Ackerman, L. and Spjut, H.: Tumors of Bone and Cartilage. Washington, D.C., Armed Forces Institute of Pathology, 1962.

CHONDROBLASTOMA

5. Ewing, J.: Report International Conference on Cancer. Bristol, John Wright and Sons, Ltd., 1928.
6. Codman, E. A.: Surg. Gynecol. Obstet., 52:543, 1931.
7. Jaffe, H. L. and Lichtenstein, L.: Am. J. Pathol., 18:969, 1942.
8. Kunkel, M. C., Dahlin, D. C. and Young, H. H.: J. Bone Joint Surg., 38A:817, 1956.
9. Valls, J., Ottolenghi, C. E. and Schajowicz, F.: J. Bone Joint Surg., 33A:997, 1951.
10. Wright, J. and Sherman, M.: J. Bone Joint Surg., 46A:597, 1964.
11. Kahn, L., Wood, F. and Ackerman, L.: Arch. Pathol., 88:371, 1969.

CHONDROMYXOID FIBROMA

12. Jaffe, H. L. and Lichtenstein, L.: Arch. Pathol., 45:541, 1948.
13. Feldman, F., Hecht, H. and Johnston, A.: Radiology, 94:249, 1970.
14. Turcotte, B., Pugh, D. G. and Dahlin, D. C.: Am. J. Roentgenol., 87:1085, 1962.

CHONDROSARCOMA

15. Phemister, D. B.: Surg. Gynecol. Obstet., 50:216, 1930.
16. Dahlin, D. C. and Henderson, E. D.: J. Bone Joint Surg., 38A:1025, 1956.
17. Levy, W., Aegerter, E. and Kirkpatrick, J.: Radiol. Clin. North Am., 2:327, 1964.
18. Lichtenstein, L. and Jaffe, H. L.: Am. J. Pathol., 19:553, 1943.
19. Dahlin, D. and Henderson, E.: Cancer, 15:410, 1962.

Chapter 18

COLLAGENIC TUMORS

The true neoplasms included in the collagenic group are angiosarcoma and fibrosarcoma. The latter is relatively common, grows rather slowly, produces collagen but no chondroid or osteoid and metastasizes late. Because both chondrosarcoma and osteosarcoma often contain sizable fields of tumor collagenoblasts, these tumors are sometimes labeled fibrosarcoma in cases in which insufficient blocks are available. Moreover, the cells of an osteosarcoma may be so undifferentiated that they are mistaken for spindled collagenoblasts. Thus, one may encounter a series of tumors, all diagnosed fibrosarcomas, that describe great variation in behavior. It is our belief that, in such series, the very malignant behaving tumors are probably osteosarcomas.

The angiosarcoma of bone is a rare tumor. It is included in this group because the cell type may at times produce collagen though the predominant cell in the tumor may be endothelial, a cell that may derive from the collagenoblast.

Finally, the giant cell tumor of bone might be included as justifiably with this group as with the osteogenic tumors. Indeed, there is much to justify the belief by many, including the authors, that the giant cell tumor of bone is only a giant cell variation of fibrosarcoma. If there be such an entity we should not envy the microscopist who is called upon to make the distinction.

ANGIOSARCOMA OF BONE

The majority of the lesions of bone composed primarily of vascular elements are hamartomas called angiomas or hemangiomas. The great preponderance of these occur in the vertebrae or the skull. (See p. 502.) Most of them are asymptomatic. In the vertebral body they may cause lysis of enough bone to bring about weakening and collapse, producing cord pressure and impingement on nerves. Lesions of the calvarium may stimulate an eruption of bone growth on the outer cortical surface, the bony mass being intermingled with angiomatous tissue. Because the trabeculae stem from a central point and fan outward they produce a sunburst appearance on the roentgenogram.

The blood vessel is made up of three types of cells, which are transitional forms of one another. These consist of collagenoblasts that form the wall, endothelial cells that make up the lining, and perithelial cells (hemangiopericytes) in the adventitia. The malignant tumor of vessel origin may be composed more or less purely of one of the cell types (hemangioendothelioma, hemangiosarcoma or hemangiopericytoma), of a primitive vascular cell type (hemangioblastoma) or of mixtures of these cells. Though behavior appears to vary considerably, the degree of malignancy is not well correlated with the cell type. Malignant tumors of vascular tissue primary in bone are quite rare. There are only 11 in our material and we have never seen a hemangioblastoma or a hemangiopericytoma of bone. The malignant vessel tumors of bone that we have encountered have been composed predominantly of endothelial cells, which attempt to form vascular channels in a loose fibrous matrix. To simplify terminology we have called these angiosarcomas.

In surveying various published accounts

562

of this tumor[1] one can find no predilection for sex or age. Eight of our 11 cases were in males. Nor does there appear to be a preference for any particular bone of the skeleton. There is no evidence to suggest that the angiosarcoma is a malignant metaplasia of a hemangioma. In a most interesting case studied by us[2] the patient had had a bayonet stab wound at the tumor site 10 years before tumor diagnosis was made. The wound healed and was asymptomatic for five years. Pain and swelling occurred and persisted for another five years. Eventually radiologic changes occurred in the bone. The patient was dead of multiple metastases within six months after diagnostic biopsy. Because of the variety of cell types of the tumors of vessels, it is impossible to form an opinion concerning behavior from the few reports in the literature. Of our patients, four died of widespread blood-borne metastases within a few months after diagnosis.

The tumor appears to spread in a typical fashion, first to healthy areas in the same bone, then to multiple areas in nearby bones and finally widely throughout the skeleton and soft tissues.

Multiple sites of involvement are common. It is unknown whether the tumor is multicentric or whether the multiple foci represent metastases from a primary site. Multiple hamartomatous angiomas are the rule and we have seen cases with combined bone, soft tissue and visceral involvement. Our cases of angiosarcoma, however, appeared to start as a primary focus with early metastasis to other bones and to viscera.

Roentgenographic Manifestations. The roentgen manifestations of angiosarcoma are those of bone destruction as manifest by areas of radiolucency without surrounding sclerosis. Calcification is not found within the areas involved by the tumor. When the cortex has been destroyed and the periosteum elevated, periosteal new bone may be seen but is uncommon, as the growth of the tumor is rapid. Multiple areas of destruction within a bone are common, as is involvement of multiple bones.

Microscopic Features. In the cases that we have studied, though the radiograms were convincingly characteristic, diagnosis could be made only on examination of microscopic sections. The diagnoses were not always clearly obvious even

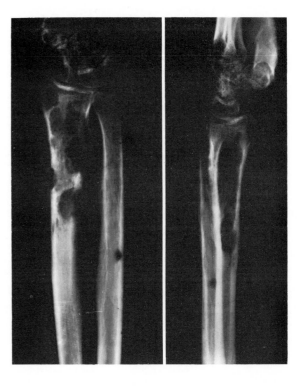

Figure 18–1 Angiosarcoma of bone. Multiple areas of destruction are apparent in the radius and ulna. There is no evidence of bone reaction around the lucent areas.

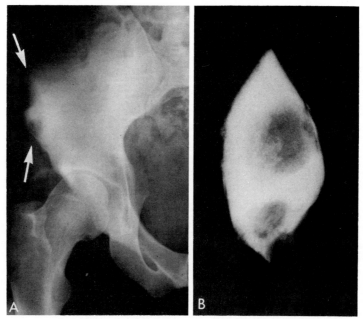

Figure 18–2 Hemangiosarcoma of the ilium. There are at least two large peripheral areas of destruction (arrows); smaller foci are visible on the radiograph of the resected specimen.

there. The proliferating endothelial channels often lay in a loose supportive stroma revealing considerable edema and inflammatory reaction. Unless the microscopist is alert he may interpret these sections as inflammatory granulation and search in vain for the agent that provoked its formation. Inadequate biopsy samples foster the making of such mistakes.

Diagnosis must be made on finding fea-

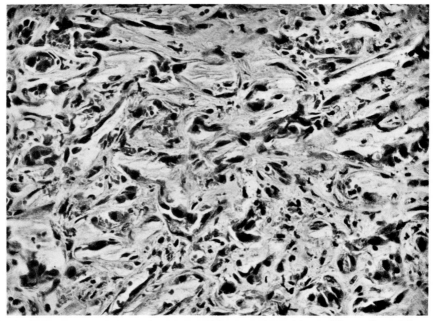

Figure 18–3 Angiosarcoma of bone. There is a proliferation of very pleomorphic cells with hyperchromatic nuclei. The growth pattern suggests an attempt to form vascular sinuses. ($\times 200$.)

tures of malignancy in cells that form vascular spaces. Often the latter is merely a suggestion of channel formation by cells that have the appearance of greatly enlarged and distorted endothelial lining cells (Fig. 18–3). The nuclei are apt to be quite pleomorphic and hyperchromatic. The channels may or may not contain red blood cells.

FIBROSARCOMA OF BONE

Fibrosarcoma of bone is one of the most poorly defined and poorly described of the primary tumors of the skeleton. Like giant cell tumor of bone it has been confused with many other lesions, some non-neoplastic, such as the reticuloendothelioses, non-osteogenic fibroma, subperiosteal cortical defect and Paget's disease, and some highly malignant, such as Class III osteosarcoma. As a result most accounts portray the fibrosarcoma of bone as a tumor of highly variable morphology and behavior.

Some authors[3] deny the existence of a primary intracortical fibrosarcoma. They believe that the lesions so diagnosed are all either osteosarcomas or chondrosarcomas that are too undifferentiated to produce their intercellular osteoid or hyalin. That many highly undifferentiated osteosarcomas are diagnosed as fibrosarcomas cannot be denied. However, to state that intracortical fibrosarcoma does not exist appears to us to be a stand that is difficult to defend. Occasionally, one encounters a tumor of the metaphyseal or medullary tissues that has the microscopic features of the fibrosarcoma of soft tissues; it grows slowly and metastasizes late if at all, just as do fibrosarcomas elsewhere in the body. Its behavior is quite different from the rapidly growing, early metastasizing, undifferentiated Class III osteosarcoma. (See p. 524.) To classify this tumor with the osteosarcomas because it grows within bone is to confuse and complicate the characteristics of both tumor types.

Fibrosarcoma is the least common of the primary malignant tumors of bone, excluding parosteal sarcoma and reticulum cell sarcoma. Batts[4] described 27 cases in 200 primary bone tumors but this proportion is much higher than reported in any other series. In some series there is a prepon-

derance in males; in others the sex incidence appears to be fairly equal. It is said that fibrosarcoma of bone has a predilection for those in the second and third decades of life. In our series of 69 cases the greatest number occurred in young adults, but there was a wide age distribution, the youngest being 11 and the oldest 61.

Bone fibrosarcoma is of two types, those arising in the metaphyseal and medullary tissues—central fibrosarcoma—and those that spring from the periosteum. The periosteal fibrosarcoma (Fig. 18–4) is said to be much less common than the type that arises within bone. In our series, of 52 cases (excluding those involving the jaws and three multicentric tumors) 26 arose within bone and 16 primarily involved the periosteum. Fibrosarcoma usually occurs eccentrically in the metaphysis of a large cylindrical bone. Classic sites are a condyle of the femur or an epicondyle of the humerus. Fibrosarcoma is not rare in flat bones, particularly if those of the jaws are included. If it occurs in the small bones of the hands and feet, this event must be rare.

There are 69 cases in our material. Twenty-two occurred in the femur, and

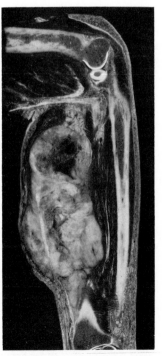

Figure 18–4 A periosteal fibrosarcoma involving the radius. It forms a bulky, firm, pale, soft tissue tumor mass, which erodes the bone from without.

eight occurred in the tibia. Fourteen occurred in the jaws, mostly the mandible. Ten involved flat bones (including vertebrae) other than the mandible. Almost half these tumors occurred between the ages of 20 and 30. The remaining half were fairly evenly scattered between the ages of 10 and 65.

Fibrosarcoma grows slowly. In Batts' series of periosteal fibrosarcomas the average duration of symptoms before diagnosis was 20 months. Pain is the principal symptom of central fibrosarcoma. It is usually not as severe or persistent as that of osteosarcoma and pathologic fracture is much less characteristic. Periosteal fibrosarcoma produces a palpable tumor mass (Fig. 18–5). It is sometimes present for years before the onset of pain causes the patient to consult his physician. The periosteal type rarely causes pathologic fracture. Though both central and periosteal fibrosarcomas are aggressive and invasive they do not metastasize until late, often not until after there has been inadequate surgical intervention. Recurrence at the site of original resection is much more common. There may be multiple recurrences before metastasis is seen.

Some writers make the distinction between periosteal desmoid and fibrosarcoma of periosteal origin. We believe that this distinction is usually impossible and sometimes unwise. The diagnosis of periosteal desmoid may give the clinician a sense of unwarranted security. If the identities of the two lesions are distinct, they appear to merge after recurrence of the latter.

Multicentric fibrosarcoma has been reported[5] and we have encountered one such case. We have seen two cases of central fibrosarcoma apparently superimposed on bone infarcts.[6] Central fibrosarcoma, when located in the ossified epiphysis, always has a prominent component of giant cells and then, of course, it is an osteoclastoma (giant cell tumor of bone). Its behavior and prognosis are not changed by its billing but it is all too commonly confused with other giant cell lesions, particularly giant cell reactions to injury.

Roentgenographic Manifestations. The roentgenographic manifestations of fibrosarcoma of bone depend upon the site of the tumor. The periosteal fibrosarcoma may present as a large soft tissue mass that is visualized radiographically only because of distortion of more radiolucent muscle planes. Although no evidence of underlying bony abnormality may be present in some instances, in others there is destruction of bone ranging from irregular cortical roughening to frank destruction of cortical bone and spongiosa (Fig. 18–6). The central fibrosarcoma is apparent when there is macroscopic destruction of trabeculae. When the tumor involves the metaphysis it is apt to be eccentric in location (Fig. 18–7). In the medullary canal it destroys trabeculae and, later erodes the inner aspect of the surrounding cortex (Fig. 18–8). As it grows, the spongiosa and later the cortex are destroyed. Because there is no bone reaction, the margins of the tumor are poorly defined (Fig. 18–9). When the cortex is destroyed, however, periosteal new bone may be evident, but this is subsequently destroyed as the tumor grows and the soft tissues are involved. Calcification within the tumor, central or peripheral, is uncommon and when seen probably is the result of necrosis of bone.

Gross Anatomy. Central fibrosarcomas usually begin in the metaphysis but in

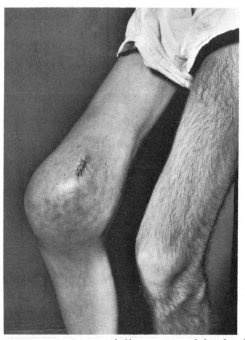

Figure 18–5 Periosteal fibrosarcoma of the distal end of the femur.

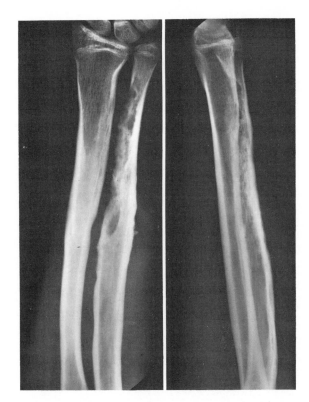

Figure 18–6 Periosteal fibrosarcoma. Irregular destruction of the cortex of the diaphysis of the ulna is evident associated with a soft tissue mass. The bone is almost encircled.

some instances they appear to start in the tissues of the medulla. They may replace the cancellous and medullary tissues of a considerable portion of the bone before cortical erosion is noted. The edges of the tumor are usually poorly delineated and are apt to extend farther than the naked eye can discern. The central type is usually more vascular than the peripheral fibrosarcoma. Eventually, it penetrates the cortex and causes extensive lysis, producing a soft tissue tumor mass whose origin is

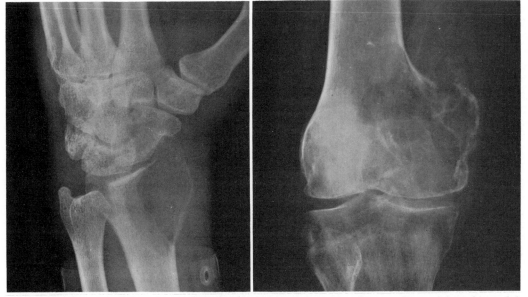

Figure 18–7 Central fibrosarcoma. The destructive areas are located in the metaphysis of the radius and the femur. The cortex has been expanded, thinned and perforated.

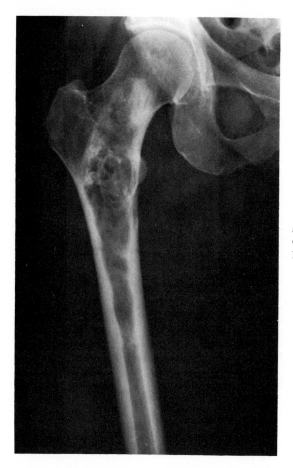

Figure 18-8 Central fibrosarcoma. An ill defined area of medullary destruction is present as well as erosion of the inner aspect of the cortex of the proximal end of the femur.

hard to determine (Fig. 18-10). The periosteal fibrosarcoma is firmly anchored to the host bone but usually can be dissected away, leaving a concavity with a roughened surface. It is unusual for the periosteal fibrosarcoma to perforate the compacta and continue its growth in the intracortical tissues but this has been observed. Usually it grows outward, sometimes completely surrounding the bone with a collar-like mass. If a tumor of this configuration contains areas of radiopacity it is probably a parosteal sarcoma. Many of the peripheral type appear to be encapsulated, but this line of delineation is usually only a zone of compressed normal tissue, which through the microscope is found to be infiltrated with advancing tumor cells. The periosteal fibrosarcoma is usually pale, sometimes white and glistening. Mineral deposits have been recorded but they are not characteristic as in chondrosarcoma.

Microscopic Anatomy. The fibrosar-

coma of bone has much the same microscopy as that of the fibrosarcoma of skin, viscera and the soft parts. The cells are fusiform or spindled. They course in fairly well organized trabeculae, which weave irregularly through the substance of the tumor (Fig. 18-11). In central fibrosarcoma there is a tendency for whorl formation, which is less frequently noted in the peripheral type. In most cases the cells are moderately mature and considerable amounts of collagen may be formed. When such is the case it may be exceedingly difficult to differentiate the fibrosarcoma from the non-osteogenic fibroma. To make the matter more difficult, when marrow and bone tissues have been destroyed there may be lipid-bearing macrophages and giant cells scattered through the sections. Prediction of the behavior of the fibrogenic lesions in general is more difficult than with any other class. Those composed of mature fibrocytes with abundant collagen production are obviously non-

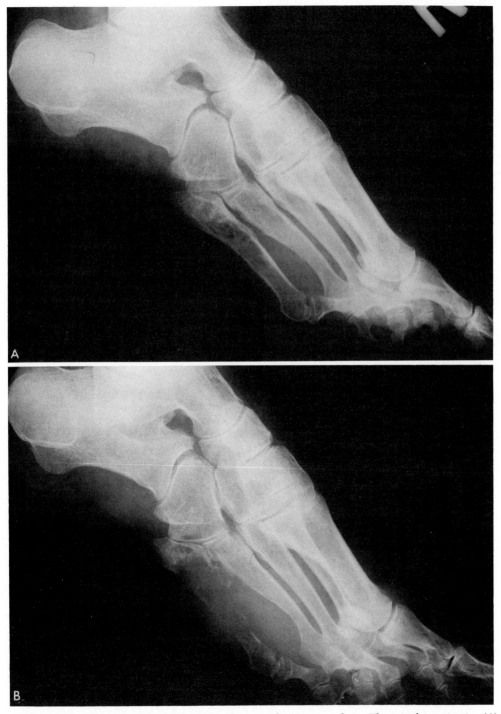

Figure 18–9   Fibrosarcoma of the fifth metatarsal in a male 29 years of age. The initial examination (A) reveals medullary destruction; 9 months later (B) the destruction is extensive and associated with a large soft tissue mass.

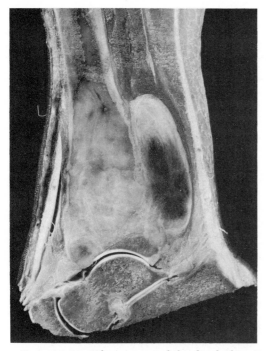

Figure 18–10 Fibrosarcoma of the distal tibia. It arose in the metaphysis, perforated the cortex and produced an extramedullary soft tissue tumor. This behavior is similar to that of intramedullary chondrosarcoma.

neoplastic and those of pleomorphic cells with numerous mitotic figures and no collagen are just as obviously neoplastic and

malignant (Fig. 18–12). But the majority fall somewhere between and the line of distinction grows thinner and thinner until, like the Cheshire cat, it may disappear altogether.

The fibromatoses throughout the body, including those of the palmar and plantar fascias and the muscle desmoids, are notable prognostic hazards. The fibrous proliferations of bone share this characteristic. Silver stains may be done to demonstrate the reticulin fibrils, which are woven about and between the cells, but they have not been of great help to us. The clinician frequently becomes impatient when the pathologist admits that he cannot distinguish between a fibrosarcoma and an innocuous, non-neoplastic fibrosing process. He should be reminded that morphology is all the microscopist has to go by, and one cannot always tell by its appearance what a cell is doing.

Prognosis. The prognosis of bone fibrosarcoma is certainly better than that of osteosarcoma and probably somewhat better than that of chondrosarcoma. Its tendency to recur rather than metastasize usually gives the surgeon a second chance. We believe that giant cell fibrosarcoma and osteoclastoma (giant cell tumor of bone) are probably one and the same. Certainly no distinction can be made on the

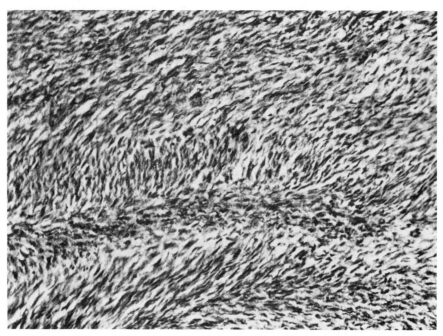

Figure 18–11 The periosteal fibrosarcoma often shows fascicles of palisaded cells. The nuclei may be quite mature in appearance. (× 200.)

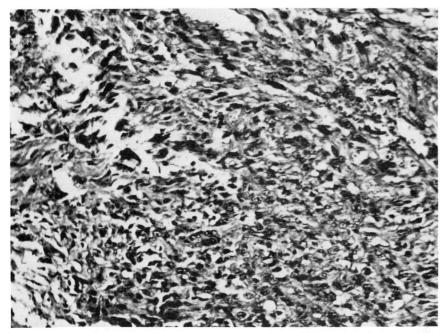

Figure 18–12   The endosteal fibrosarcoma is apt to appear more malignant than the periosteal variety; see Figure 18–11. In this section the cells are quite pleomorphic and there is no evidence of collagen. ($\times$ 200.)

basis of behavior. Fibrosarcoma, like parosteal sarcoma and chondrosarcoma, has been noted to change its cytologic characteristics toward the malignant side following surgical manipulation. Fibrosarcoma should be completely resected and often this necessitates amputation. If the diagnosis is firm and there is question whether local resection will remove all of the tumor, obviously amputation is the only course to be taken.

It has always been the dictum that fibrosarcomas do not respond well to irradiation therapy. Actually, modern irradiation methods have been tried too infrequently to justify this statement.

This prognosis holds for fibrosarcoma whether it be of soft tissue or bone, with one exception. The fibrosarcomas of the jaw appear to be more malignant than fibrosarcomas of other bones. This may be because mandibulectomy is attempted less often than limb amputation. Like the tumor elsewhere, that in the jaw usually does not metastasize but destroys locally.

Perhaps with more adequate facial surgery, the behavior of these tumors will prove to be no worse than those in other bones.

In cases in which bone fibrosarcoma eventually metastasizes it usually goes to the lungs. There is a somewhat greater incidence of lymph node metastasis than is found in osteosarcoma and chondrosarcoma.

References

ANGIOSARCOMA OF BONE

1. Carter, J., Dickerson, R. and Needy, C.: Ann. Surg., *144*:107, 1956.
2. Bundens, W. and Brighton, C.: J. Bone Joint Surg., *47A*:762, 1965.

FIBROSARCOMA OF BONE

3. Stout, A. P.: Cancer, *1*:30, 1948.
4. Batts, M.: Arch. Surg., *42*:566, 1941.
5. Steiner, P.: Am. J. Pathol., *20*:877, 1944.
6. Furey, G., Ferrer-Torells, M. and Reagan, J.: J. Bone Jont Surg., *42A*:802, 1960.

Chapter 19

MYELOGENIC TUMORS

The term "myelogenic tumors" arises from the assumption that these neoplasms are derived from marrow cells all of which come from the marrow reticulum. Four tumors are usually included in this group: the plasma cell myeloma, Ewing's tumor, the reticulum cell sarcoma and Hodgkin's disease of bone. Lymphosarcoma of bone should probably be included. These tumors occur in frequency in the order named. The marrow infiltrations, which sometimes occur in the various types of leukemia and cause bone changes, might be included in this group, but as a matter of practice they rarely are. They are dealt with in another section of this text. The four tumors named are included in the term "myelomas" because they are all considered to be of marrow origin.

Actually, the precise cytogenesis of none of the myelomas is known. Though the plasma cell myeloma is almost certainly composed of plasma cells, no one knows for certain from which primitive marrow cells plasmacytes arise. We do not know the exact types of cells that constitute the other three marrow tumors. For purposes of description and study we assume the Ewing's tumor arises from the marrow reticulum. Ewing originally thought that it was derived from capillary endothelial lining cells and there is recent evidence that suggests he may have been right. The other two marrow tumors, plasma cell myeloma and Hodgkin's disease, are almost certainly derivatives of marrow reticulum. The cytogenesis of the reticulum cell sarcoma is completely problematic. Could it be an attenuated form of Ewing's tumor?

Because the cells derived from the reticulum elaborate the serum globulins, pathologic alterations in the latter frequently are associated with some of the marrow tumors (plasma cell myeloma) and other marrow diseases.

When normal globulin is broken down it yields polypeptide chains, some of which are light (22,000) and others heavy (55,000). Rarely the plasma cells apparently are able to produce only the latter, causing a condition known as heavy chain disease. Many of the clinical features are similar to those of malignant lymphoma with which it is frequently confused. There is apt to be lymphadenopathy, hepatomegaly, splenomegaly, fever, weakness, anemia and thrombocytopenia. The course may proceed rapidly to death or be chronic and indolent. An excessive number of plasma cells are found in the bone marrow and sometimes in the lymph nodes. Because mature globulin (specific antibody) cannot be produced, the patient usually dies of infection.

In another clinical entity there is proliferation of cells that appear to be transition forms between lymphocytes and mature plasmacytes in the marrow. They apparently elaborate a heavy chain macromolecular globulin (1,000,000). The condition is called Waldenström's macroglobulinemia. It is encountered in the elderly, causing mild lymphadenopathy, hepatomegaly, lymphocytosis and anemia. The disease runs an indolent course with a diffuse deossification of the skeleton.

Myelosclerosis is an idiopathic disease in which the marrow appears incapable of maturation to form normal blood cells. As a result the patient develops a profound anemia. The marrow tissues undergo metaplasia to cartilage and osteoid, causing obliteration of the medullary architecture.

Most patients succumb to anemia or infection but some undergo proliferation of the remaining marrow cells to terminate in a leukemic phase.

PLASMA CELL MYELOMA

The plasma cell myeloma is a malignant neoplasm arising from a reticulum derivative. Because reticulum, or derived cells that under certain conditions may revert to reticulum, are found in most body tissues, the tumor may be primary in many body sites. The great preponderance of these tumors arise from hematopoietic reticulum of the bone marrow and it is to this large group that the term plasma cell myeloma is applied. In cases in which, rarely, it is primary in the viscera or soft tissues it is called extramedullary plasmacytoma.

Other names for the plasma cell myeloma are multiple myeloma and myelomatosis. Because the tumor may be solitary, at least for a period of years, or because it may exist as numerous, probably multicentric focal deposits or involve the entire marrow, these terms should be avoided except when referring to a specific type. The term solitary myeloma is permissible when referring to a type or to an early stage in which a single focus only is demonstrable, multiple myeloma when more than one focus is evident, and diffuse myeloma or myelomatosis when all hematopoietic tissue is involved. The various types are not necessarily stages of the tumor process though most or all solitary myelomas may be expected eventually to develop into the multiple myeloma type, and some of the last may eventuate as diffuse myeloma in the terminal stage. Some trustworthy observers contend that they have studied rare cases of solitary myeloma that have regressed and disappeared spontaneously. We have not encountered such a case.

Until recently there has been valid argument as to whether the term "plasma cell" should be applied to these tumors. Though the tumor cells may closely resemble plasma cells, the precise cell of origin is not known and no one has answered the question why the tumor so consistently arises in bone marrow in which the plasma cell is such an inconspicuous part of the normal cell population. Since we have learned more of the function of the plasma cell, i.e., its role in gamma globulin production, the disturbance in serum globulin levels in this neoplasm relates the cell in function as well as morphology.

Plasma cell myeloma is a tumor of the older age group, almost always occurring after the age of 40. It has been said that the chief incidence is between the ages of 40 and 60, but if one corrects the incidence with the life expectancy one finds no decline in the curve after the age of 60. The tumor is occasionally seen in the fourth decade and has been reported in adolescence[1] (see Fig. 19–8) and even in childhood, but these are medical curiosities. The disease has been reported in a female 13 years of age in whom extensive extramedullary involvement, particularly of the breasts, was the first manifestation of the disease.[2] It is somewhat more common in males than females but the difference is not great enough to be of diagnostic significance.

Multiple myeloma is the most common form of the tumor, though since the diffuse type has been more generally recognized[3] it can by no means be considered uncommon. Earlier and better clinical work-up and roentgenographic surveys are disclosing an increasing number of tumors in the solitary stage. All types included, plasma cell myeloma is the commonest primary malignant bone tumor.

In the solitary and multiple myeloma types the flat bones are the ones most commonly affected. In a series of 85 cases in our material, only nine were initially found in cylindrical bones. This is a tumor of red marrow and almost all the hematopoietic tissue in the latter half of life is located in flat bones. The fatty marrow of cylindrical bones acts as a reserve tissue, undergoing conversion to red marrow only when the normal tissue is injured or replaced. This is probably the reason cylindrical bones are involved usually only in the advanced stages of the multicentric and diffuse types.

The vertebral bodies are the most commonly involved, and after them the bones of the pelvic and shoulder girdles and the skull. Plasma cell myeloma is rather unusual in the bones distal to the elbows and knees.

Plasma cell myeloma is a neoplastic proliferation of the cells that normally produce gamma globulin. This substance and globulins which are more or less closely related to it are produced in excess quantities. These abnormal proteins are excreted through the kidney and interfere with its function. The symptoms and signs of plasma cell myeloma may, therefore, be divided into three groups: (1) those due to the presence of the tumor mass, its replacement of normal hematopoietic marrow and its lytic action upon bone; (2) those due to the excessive proteins; and finally (3) those secondary to impaired kidney function. They will be discussed in this order.

The most common symptom related to the skeleton is pain. Depending upon the site of the lesion it may begin as back pain, pain in the thoracic cage or in the pelvic bones. Pain often precedes recognizable roentgenographic changes. In the early stages it may be intermittent or occur only on motion but eventually it may be intense, deep and constant. The symptom of back pain is so common in patients over 40 that it alone is of little diagnostic value.

Most plasma cell myelomas begin insidiously, the duration of skeletal symptoms before diagnosis is made averaging about nine months. The cells of this tumor apparently have a lytic action upon bone. Cancellous bone is melted away and eventually the cortex is eroded from within. The areas of deossification are usually quite sharply delineated. In thin flat bones such as those of the calvarium, the tumor may perforate both inner and outer tables to invade the contiguous soft tissues. Often the apparent metastatic deposits in the orbit, scalp, epidural and retroperitoneal regions are actually extensions of a tumor arising in medullary tissue. Thinning of cortical bone causes weakening and eventual pathologic fracture is common (Fig. 19–1). At times the tumor may be silent until this event. Compression fracture of a vertebra may injure nerve roots and give rise to a wide range of symptoms of neurogenous origin. Sciatica is a common chief and sometimes initial complaint. It has been estimated that 40 per cent of

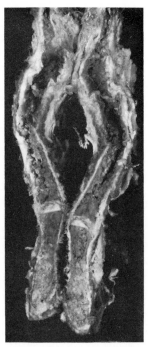

Figure 19–1 Sagittal section through a sternum, the site of plasma cell myeloma. The cortices are thinned and expanded. The normal medullary tissues have been replaced by a mushy, reddish brown material representing the tumor. Fracture has occurred because of cortical thinning.

presenting cases of myeloma have neurologic symptoms.

Four cases of plasma cell myeloma, in which the tumors caused appositional bone formation over them so that the cortex appeared expanded, have come to our attention. One of these cases, contributed by Warner Bundens, is illustrated in Figure 19–12. It appears that though bone lysis is the rule in plasma cell myeloma, bone production to cause cortical expansion does not rule out this diagnosis. We make the suggestion that the appearance of cortical expansion superimposed on plasma cell myeloma may represent the advent of aneurysmal bone cyst complication.

In cases in which the tumor is multiple or diffuse, almost all the bones of the skeleton excluding those of the distal portions of the extremities are involved. Huge amounts of calcium salts are freed; the level of serum calcium rises and it spills out into the urine. The serum calcium level depends upon the extent of skeletal involvement. It is elevated at the time the diagnosis is made in about one half the cases of plasma cell myeloma. Prolonged serum calcium levels above 12 mg. constitute a hazard because of metastatic calcification. The kidneys are most often affected and this insult compounds that caused by the excessive proteins. Pure nephrocalcinosis is rarely found as a serious complication of plasma cell myeloma.

In cases of myelomatosis the marrow may be so extensively replaced by tumor that a serious anemia may result. Some degree of anemia is present in more than one half the patients with myeloma at the time of diagnosis, regardless of the extent of roentgenographically demonstrable lesions. This is because the marrow is more extensively involved than can be grossly appreciated. This fact makes marrow aspiration a very valuable diagnostic procedure. Tumor cells often may be found in sternal marrow even though there is no radiographic evidence of a tumor mass or of bone destruction (Fig. 19–2). The anemia may be enhanced by the bleeding that is such a common occurrence in plasma cell myeloma. This bleeding may be the result of a thrombocytopenia due to widespread destruction of megakaryocytes, but another factor appears to play a part. The disturbance in protein formation apparently interferes with normal fibrinogen action though the exact mechanism is not known. The bleeding phenomenon is sometimes manifested by patients with normal platelet levels. Clot retraction time is often prolonged or retraction is sometimes completely lacking. Epistaxis is the commonest form of hemorrhage but melena and bleeding of the gums are also seen.

The total serum protein may rise to 10 gm. or higher. The excessive protein is in the globulin range and usually the albumin level is lowered. The curve obtained by the electrophoretic method is illustrated in Figure 19–3. Though the contour of the curve varies considerably in different cases, the elevations are within a range that is highly diagnostic for plasma cell myeloma. The albumin curve is usually smaller than normal, the alpha$_1$ and alpha$_2$ waves are usually not altered, the beta wave may or may not be elevated and the gamma wave is usually many

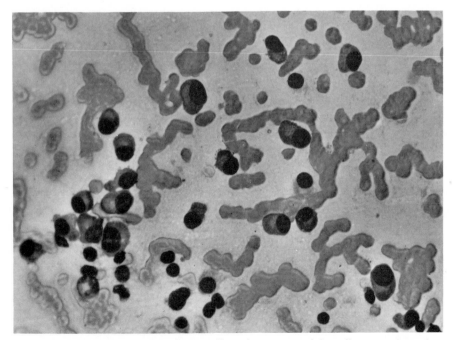

Figure 19–2   Marrow aspiration smear in plasma cell myeloma. Most of the cells pictured are obvious tumor plasma cells. These cells are often found in areas that give no evidence of bone involvement. Sternal or ilial aspiration should be done in all cases of suspected plasma cell myeloma. (× 440.)

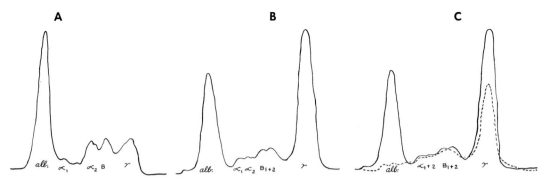

Figure 19–3   Electrophoretic tracing in plasma cell myeloma. *A*, Tracing of normal serum proteins. Note the relation of the curve representing albumin to those of alpha$_1$, alpha$_2$, beta and gamma globulins. *B*, Tracing in a case of multiple myeloma. The gamma globulin is greatly elevated. *C*, An extract of the tumor was made in the case represented in *B*. The tracing made with this extract is represented by the broken line showing that the tumor cells contain the protein which is elevated in the serum.

times its normal height. Protein diffraction has taught us that the kinds of globulin produced in plasma cell myeloma vary considerably from case to case. Some of these globulins are chemically but not biologically normal. For example, though the gamma globulin level may be high, specific antibody formation may be seriously impaired. But new and abnormal globulin curves may appear in the diffraction pattern. A common variation is a peak between the beta and the gamma elevations, which has been called the M (for myeloma) wave. The curves are usually broader than normal curves indicating a lack of specificity of the proteins that produce them. The M fraction globulins have been divided into gamma A and gamma B types. These are produced by neoplastic cells and are usually mixed with some light chain fractions. About 65 per cent of the cases of plasma cell myeloma demonstrate an excess of gamma globulin. A considerably smaller proportion reveal an abnormal quantity of beta globulin. Though a few cases of myeloma with increased alpha globulin have been reported, some observers question the existence of a specific alpha globulin myeloma. Some cases of plasma cell myeloma manifest no abnormal alterations in the serum proteins. To date there is no trustworthy correlation between the type of protein alteration and the behavior of the tumor.

That a variety of globulins are present should not surprise us. This material is produced by tumor cells whose metabolic activities have been greatly altered by the neoplastic process. Their function is no more normal than their shape and often considerably less so. The failure of normal antibody production makes the patient vulnerable to infection and this may be the important factor in causing death. The excessive and abnormal serum proteins may cause the erythrocytes to adhere so that rouleau formation is common. Clumping of red cells speeds the sedimentation rate. Abnormal serum proteins may also cause bizarre serologic reactions. The viscosity of the blood may be increased sufficiently to cause pulmonary and perhaps kidney embarrassment.

Cryoglobulins are a group of proteins that precipitate when the serum is cooled. The presence of cryoglobulins in the serum is simply another manifestation of deranged protein synthesis in plasma cell myeloma.[5]

Henry Bence Jones in 1850 described a curious protein in the urine of patients with plasma cell myeloma. This protein was found to form a white precipitate when the urine was heated to a temperature around 50° C., and cleared when the temperature reached approximately 100° C. This protein acquired the name of its discoverer and today is considered a highly characteristic sign of plasma cell myeloma. Bence Jones protein occurs in the urine in probably less than one half the patients with this tumor. In these cases it is usually intermittent and several analyses may be necessary to detect its presence. It is a light chain globulin and because its molecular size (37,000) is about half that of albumin it passes the glomerular filter. Only rarely can it be found in the serum by ordinary methods but a precipitin test has been described that is said to be helpful in the early diagnosis of the lesion.[6] The protein has been extracted from the tumor cells. Bence Jones proteinuria is not pathognomonic for plasma cell myeloma because it has been found in carcinoma with extensive bone metastases and in certain types of leukemia. Liberal amounts of protein other than the Bence Jones type are almost constantly found in the urine in myeloma. Indeed, this finding has been the first indication of the tumor in some cases. A simple test has been reported by Kyle and McGuckin[7] in which crystalline urethane is added to serum, which then forms a gel. The test does not distinguish myeloma and macroglobulinemia.

Excessive amounts of uric acid may sometimes be demonstrated in the serum. This is probably produced by the breakdown of nucleic acids, which come from the degenerating tumor and normal marrow cells.

Amyloid may be demonstrated in the tissues of about one quarter of the patients dying of plasma cell myeloma (Fig. 19–4). Careful microscopic search must be made for it and rarely does it occur in sufficient amounts to be of diagnostic value. Amyloid is a sugar-linked protein that appears to be formed by the leakage of abnormal proteins out of the vascular channels. As it permeates the collagenous tissues it is transformed to a substance that is foreign to normal tissue economy. Amyloidosis is usually divided into two types according to its distribution. In the primary or idiopathic type it is found predominantly in the skeletal, visceral (gastrointestinal) and cardiac muscles, lying in the supportive tissues between the muscle fibers. In the secondary type that usually follows longstanding infections, the amyloid is found among the parenchymal cells of the viscera. A number of stains may be used to demonstrate amyloid, but because its chemical components are not constant its staining reaction is variable and sometimes it takes none of the usual stains. The distribution of the amyloid in plasma cell

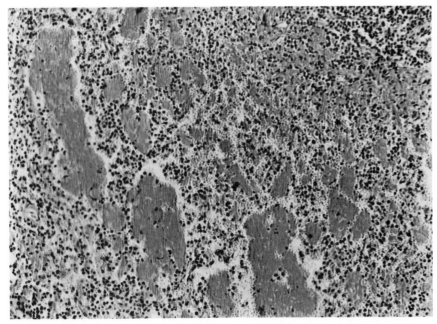

Figure 19–4 Deposits of amyloid in a lymph node of a patient with plasma cell myeloma. The amyloid appears as islands of homogeneous, acellular material. One of the amyloid stains may be helpful in demonstrating it because it stains much like collagen with hematoxylin and eosin stain. (× 130.)

myeloma is characteristic of neither of the classic types, though in general it is more apt to be like that of idiopathic amyloidosis. It is seen best in the tumor and medullary tissues, occasionally in muscles and sometimes it may be demonstrated in the viscera. Quite often it fails to take the amyloid stain. One must assume that the abnormal globulins formed by the tumor cells make up the protein moiety of the amyloid substance.

Evidence of kidney insufficiency occurs in about two thirds of the cases of plasma cell myeloma. The type of kidney disease is peculiar inasmuch as it is not associated with hypertension, and alterations in kidney function are different from both diffuse glomerular nephritis and lipoid nephrosis.[8] The morbid physiology of the kidney disease is not understood. Some authors believe that the Bence Jones protein acts as a toxic agent to the glomerular filter, others[9] contend that the Bence Jones and other proteins form casts in the distal tubules (Fig. 19–5), which obstruct the urine flow to cause what Ehrich has called

an "internal hydronephrosis." This mechanism may play a role but not all cases demonstrate a decreased urinary output, which would of necessity be the outcome of massive tubule obstruction. Because some patients have developed severe renal damage in the absence of Bence Jones proteinuria, it has been postulated that the kidney disease may be due to nephroischemia secondary to the increased viscosity of the blood because of excessive amounts of a number of proteins in the serum.

The typical "myeloma kidney" results from deposits of Bence Jones protein within the tubules and, in one reported case,[10] the glomeruli (Fig. 19–6). The protein here obviously acts as an irritant causing a striking giant cell foreign body reaction. A few cases of hypophosphatemic–vitamin D refractive rickets have been reported with myeloma kidney. It is assumed that the crystals of Bence Jones protein may inhibit phosphorus reabsorption from the glomerular filtrate. In any event nephritis is a serious

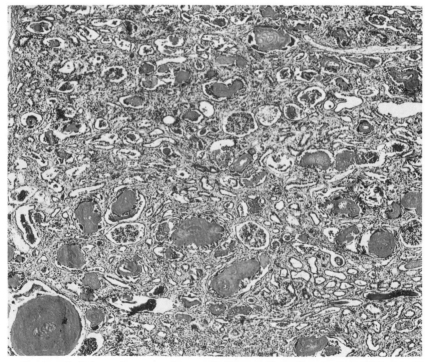

Figure 19–5 Section of a kidney of a patient dying with plasma cell myeloma. Many tubules are filled and distended with protein. In this case it is protein that gives a negative Bence Jones test. Bence Jones protein stimulates a foreign body inflammatory reaction in kidney tissue. (See Fig. 19–6.) (× 30.)

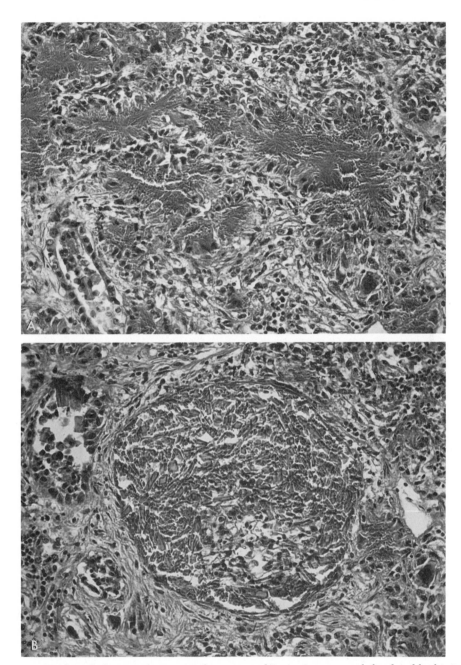

Figure 19–6   Myeloma kidney. *A* shows irregular masses of Bence Jones crystals bordered by histiocytes in epithelioid pattern and foreign body giant cells. *B* shows a glomerular structure, which is now almost completely replaced by masses of Bence Jones protein. (× 440.)

complication and many patients die in uremia. Nephrocalcinosis secondary to the high serum calcium levels may contribute to the kidney inefficiency.

Some authors have attempted to establish the concept of solitary myeloma as a separate entity. It has been stated that early diagnosis and radical therapy in this type result in a much better prognosis than that of multiple or diffuse myeloma.[11, 12] Others[13, 14] are of the opinion that the solitary myeloma is merely an early stage of the multicentric form and that the patient with a single lesion eventually develops the full-blown disease regardless of his treatment. The weight of evidence is with the latter group. Even in the solitary form one can sometimes find tumor cells scattered through the marrow in areas remote from the primary lesion.

The incidence of plasma cell myeloma in families is probably somewhat greater than is the average in the population at large. The tumor has been reported in a father, son and daughter[15] and we have seen two brothers affected with the disease.

Roentgenographic Manifestations. The roentgenographic manifestations of plasma cell myeloma vary considerably and in approximately 25 per cent of patients there are none. As with many bone lesions, one speaks of the classic picture, but variations are common. Flat bones, because they contain hematopoietic elements, are involved first. The process is a medullary destructive one and the radiographic appearance is dependent on the degree of local marrow involvement and the extent of the process.

Classically, there are multiple areas of bone destruction, sharply defined areas of intermediate density involving the skull, vertebrae, pelvis and shoulder girdle. This is often associated with a generalized decrease in bone density. There is no associated sclerosis. The cortex may be quite thin over a lesion and may bulge, and when the cortex is completely destroyed, a soft tissue mass is associated with the bony lesions. In the spine, collapse of vertebral bodies occurs, often associated with a soft tissue mass; the pedicles are involved late in the course of the disease. Rarely, involvement of the cortex may stimulate considerable new bone formation (Fig. 19–12). These destructive foci are manifestations of local proliferation of neoplastic cells within the medullary tissues. In some instances, a single osteolytic lesion may be present, solitary myeloma.

The process may present radiographically as a less well defined destructive process with mottled areas in the bones. A type of myeloma in which all or most of the marrow tissue is involved to produce a diffuse deossification of the skeleton without localized destruction may be recog-

nized. Here, trabeculae are fine and sparse and the cortices thin, and pathologic fracture of the ribs or vertebrae is not uncommon.

The radiographic manifestations then are secondary to proliferation of neoplastic cells within the medullary spaces. Marked local proliferation causes focal bone destruction and perhaps expansion, whereas diffuse involvement destroys the trabeculae and cortices uniformly to produce an osteoporosis-like appearance. When the process is seen early in its course, there may be no macroscopic evidence of its presence. One must be aware of the less classic manifestations of the disease to be suspicious of it radiographically.

Morbid Anatomy. The plasma cell myeloma usually has a red-gray color, often with the appearance and consistency of raspberry custard. This soft creamy mass oozes from the medullary area when the involved bone is opened. The tumor is often surrounded by a thin layer of cortical bone that may show multiple infractions. When the tumor perforates bone and forms a soft tissue mass it is frequently surrounded by a capsule of compressed fibrous connective tissue or muscle. The spleen is sometimes moderately enlarged,[16] and less often the liver and lymph nodes.

As a rule the diagnosis of plasma cell myeloma by microscopy is an easy matter. In most instances the tumor cells resemble plasma cells sufficiently to leave little doubt in the mind of the pathologist. Only rarely is the similarity so close that one may be concerned about whether the lesion is a chronic inflammatory reaction or a neoplasm. In the former, one may expect to find other exudative inflammatory cells scattered among the plasmacytes. Also in the inflammatory reaction there is usually a more prominent fibroblastic reaction. In rare instances in which the mature type of myeloma has perforated bone and been involved in a secondary inflammatory reaction, the distinction on sections alone may be quite difficult.

As a rule the tumor cells are round or ovoid (Fig. 19–13). The nucleus is often eccentrically placed just as it is in the normal plasmacyte. The cell membrane or at least its outline is usually discernible. The

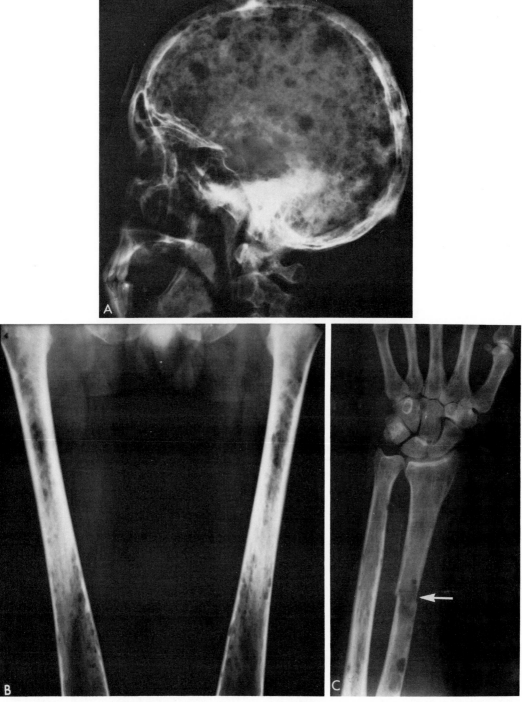

Figure 19-7   Plasma cell myeloma. Distinct areas of bone destruction are evident. There is no bone reaction to this diffuse process. A pathologic fracture of the left radius is present (arrow, *C*).

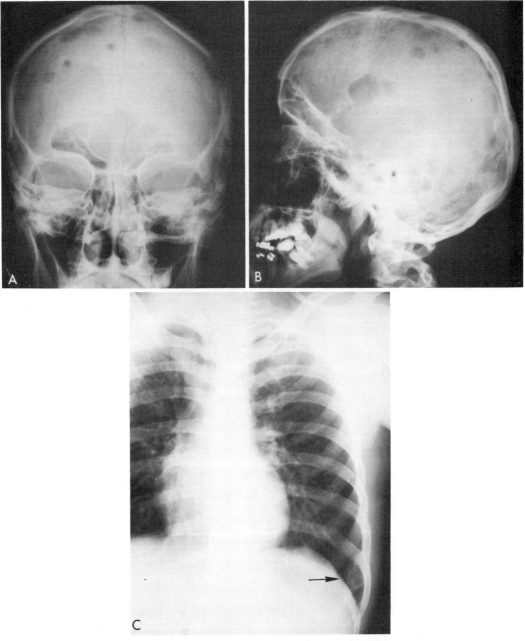

Figure 19–8   Multiple myeloma, male 17 years of age. While quite uncommon at this age, the roentgen findings are as expected, i.e., well defined lucent defects without surrounding reaction. The lesion in the eighth rib on the left has caused expansion of the bone (arrow).

cytoplasm has much the same intense red-blue quality that is seen in the normal plasmacyte with hematoxylin-eosin technique. The nuclear chromatin is sometimes broken and clumped beneath the nuclear membrane in a peripheral distri-bution but more often this "clock-face" arrangement is lacking. Usually, but not always, there is considerable disparity in nuclear size, shape and staining reaction and the cells are obviously neoplastic in character. There is great variation in the

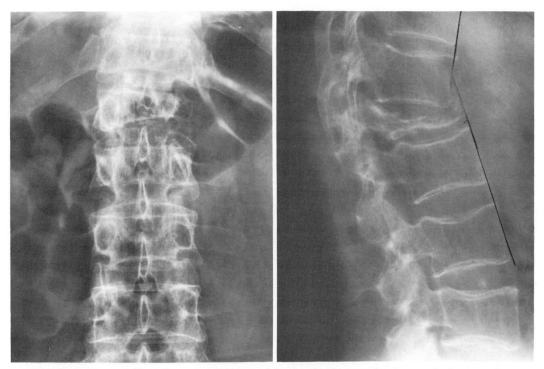

Figure 19-9 Plasma cell myeloma. Involvement of the first lumbar vertebra has resulted in its collapse.

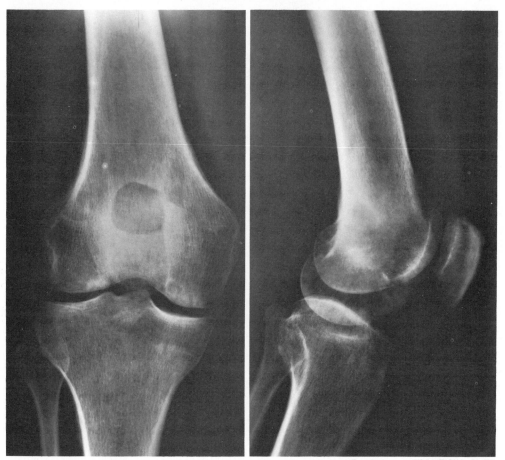

Figure 19-10 Plasma cell myeloma. A solitary lesion is present in the distal femur. It is discrete with no surrounding sclerosis.

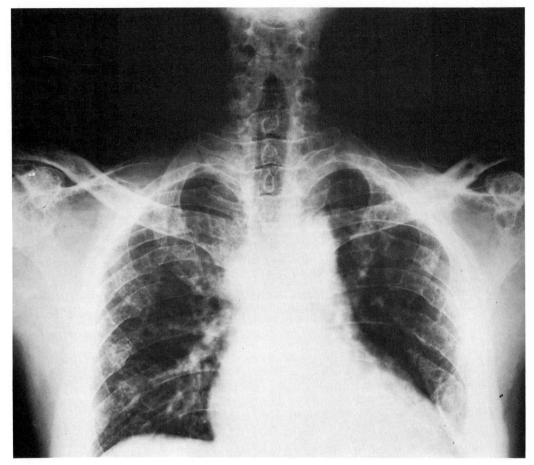

Figure 19-11 Multiple myeloma. There is extensive involvement of the skeleton; expanding lesions are noted in many ribs.

morphologic types, from those that are almost identical to plasma cells to those in which the resemblance is completely lacking (Fig. 19–14). In the latter the cells are larger, more irregular in outline and often contain two or more nuclei. At this end of the scale these cells may be difficult or impossible to distinguish from those of Ewing's tumor or reticulum cell sarcoma.

In a very small percentage of cases tumor plasma cells may be found in the peripheral blood. Usually these are few in number but in rare instances they may dominate the blood smears. In cases in which this occurs it is usually encountered in the last few months of the disease and becomes in all respects a plasma cell leukemia.

In about 50 per cent of the autopsied cases one may find plasma cells infiltrating the spleen, liver, lymph nodes and less frequently the other viscera.[17] This aspect of myeloma leads to the concept that this is a systemic disease of the body reticulum. If such is the case, radical surgery (i.e., amputation) could not be conscientiously recommended for the solitary lesion. On the other hand, cures for as long as 16 years have been reported following this method of treatment. Johnson and Meador[18] have described a lesion that they call "benign myeloma of bone." They claim that this may be mistaken for myeloma because it is a reticulum cell reaction and may be multiple. They believe it to be a type of inflammation that should be differentiated from myeloma by careful analysis of the microscopy.

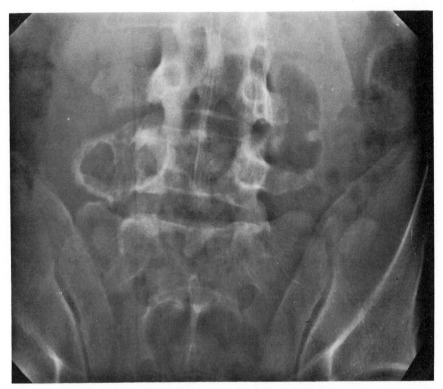

Figure 19–12   Plasma cell myeloma. The lesion has involved the pedicle and a portion of the body of the fifth lumbar vertebra. Appositional new bone marks the extent of this expanding tumor.

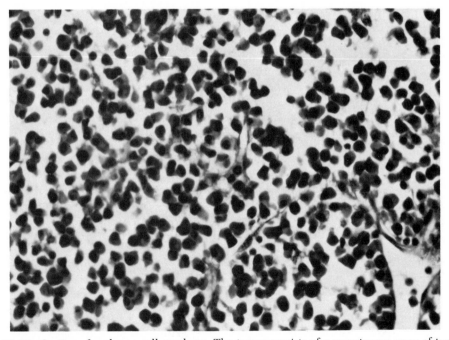

Figure 19–13   Section of a plasma cell myeloma. The tumor consists of a monotonous array of tumor cells resembling plasmacytes. The nuclei usually vary enough in size, shape and staining reaction to establish the diagnosis of tumor. ($\times$ 440.)

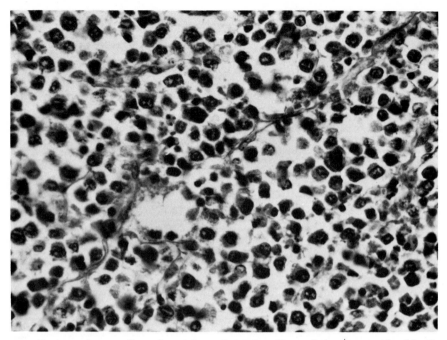

Figure 19–14   In some plasma cell myelomas the variation in cell morphology is considerable. Some typical tumor plasmacytes are found but other cells show little resemblance to the plasma cell. (× 440.)

The variation in cell morphology has led to an attempt to classify the plasma cell myelomas on this basis. They have been divided into four types: plasma cell myeloma, myelocytoma, erythroblastoma and lymphocytoma of bone. Because these types cannot be correlated with a characteristic clinical behavior and because all types almost certainly came from the same stem cell, such classification becomes an academic exercise of no practical importance. In recent years there has been an attempt to correlate the cell type with the kind of globulin found in the serum. Myeloma cells produce a mixture of globulin types, some of which are light chain globulins. These have been divided into lambda and kappa fractions. Whereas the normal plasma cell produces both fractions the tumor cell can produce only one or the other leading to the expressions "lambda" or "kappa myelomas." Such association might prove to be of value if it is found to be related to prognosis. As yet our knowledge of the types of globulins involved is too superficial to construct such a classification. The protein chemistry of plasma cell myeloma needs much more extensive investigation.

The plasma cell tumors of soft tissues, extramedullary plasmacytomas, are still a mystifying group. About half of these occur in the upper respiratory passages, the nasal and oral pharynges, the larynx and the paranasal sinuses. Another quarter are encountered in the conjunctivae. The remainder involve the mucosal linings of the various body tracts and the soft tissues of the neck. Hellwig[19] reviewed 127 cases from the literature in 1943. In many of these cases accompanying myelomas are found in the bones; others go on to develop the picture of skeletal myelomatosis. Many of these cases, however, run a completely benign course. The microscopic appearance in these is apparently the same as that of plasma cell myeloma, yet one cannot help but feel that these are curious plasma cell inflammatory reactions that have been misdiagnosed as tumors.

Prognosis. Plasma cell myeloma is a fatal disease. A few cases of cures have been reported following radical therapy of the solitary type, but one must always suspect the possibility of incorrect diagnoses in these cases. The average survival time after the diagnosis of multiple myeloma is made is about two years. In a small percentage of cases, the process appears to advance much more slowly. The possibility of confusion with macroglobulinemia, however, must always be borne in mind. The use of urethane is believed by many to prolong life for a year or longer.

In general, plasma cell myeloma must be regarded as a tumor with a prognosis similar to that of leukemia. Some patients die in a few months, the average survive about two years, and an occasional case runs a course comparable to that of chronic lymphocytic leukemia in the older age group.

EWING'S TUMOR

Ewing's tumor is a malignant neoplasm that always arises in medullary tissue. It has several clinical characteristics that set it apart from other primary bone tumors. It almost always involves the bones of patients under the age of 30. It has a tendency to perforate the overlying cortex and form a soft tissue mass, which is often larger than the intracortical lesion. It is usually accompanied by the systemic manifestations of fever and leukocytosis. It quite often metastasizes to other bones.

Ewing's tumor is the third most common malignant primary bone tumor, being surpassed in incidence only by plasma cell myeloma and osteosarcoma. It is surprising, therefore, that it was not delineated as an entity until 1921.[20] It was described in several earlier papers but was always grouped with other tumor entities and was usually thought of as a type of endothelioma. It was perhaps this precedent that caused James Ewing to consider it a tumor arising from the lining cells of the medullary blood or lymphatic channels. It was largely because of Ewing's three published discussions of the lesion that it was known as "endothelial sarcoma of bone." Oberling first published the opinion that this neoplasm came from the marrow stem cell, the reticulum, in 1928, and Stout,[21] Lichtenstein and Jaffe,[22] and McCormack, Dockerty and Ghormley[23] eventually subscribed to this theory of genesis. Since, in truth, the endothelial vessel lining cell is itself a derivative of the marrow reticulum, Ewing's original thesis was not entirely incorrect but the term "endothelial sarcoma of bone" was abandoned when Ewing himself recanted his original thesis, and now to avoid cytogenic implication the term "Ewing's tumor" is widely used.

Because the hematopoietic cells of the marrow are derived from the reticulum it seems logical to classify the plasma cell tumor, Ewing's tumor and the reticulum cell sarcoma together as tumors of marrow or myelomas. It seems odd to us that Lichtenstein categorizes Ewing's tumor separately as a neoplasm of "medullary fibrous connective tissue," but the occasional presence of primitive osteoid among the tumor cells has fathered the idea that these cells may represent the earliest types of osteoblasts. Because osteoblasts may stem from capillary endothelial lining cells one is led to wonder if Ewing's original concept may not have been correct. It is in no sense a fibrosarcoma, and though it forms no recognizable blood cells there is as much reason to place its progenitive cells among the myelogenous or lymphogenous series as there is for plasma cell myeloma and reticulum cell sarcoma.

It is usually stated that Ewing's tumor is more common in the male. In our material there are 132 cases and the sexes are about equally divided. The age incidence is diagnostically more helpful. It is usually stated that the chief incidence is in the age group of 10 to 25 years. Actually, if one extends the age limit to 30 years and includes the numerous cases in those younger than 10, one rarely encounters a Ewing's tumor outside this group. In our material consisting of 132 cases there were only four patients over 30, the youngest was 18 months and there were 40 patients under 10. Ewing's tumor does occur over the age of 30, but rarely. When this diagnosis is contemplated in older patients the possibility of reticulum cell sarcoma, histiocytosis, metastatic carcinoma or atypical plasma cell myeloma should always seriously be considered.

The skeletal location of Ewing's tumor is not as precise as with most other bone tumors An epiphyseal primary location is quite unusual but other than that it may occur in almost any part of any bone. About two thirds of the cases begin in cylindrical bones and the younger the patient the more apt this is to be true. In our material, of those cases in patients under 20 years, 61 began in cylindrical bones and 44 in flat bones. Of the 25 cases in patients 20 or over, a flat bone was the primary site of involvement in all but 10. This is another way of saying that the Ewing's tumor arises in hematopoietic tissue and after the age of skeletal maturity most of the red marrow is found in the cancellous tissue of flat bones. Most of the primary bone tumors that affect the shaft characteristically begin in the metaphysis. In contrast, Ewing's tumor may begin anywhere in cylindrical bones. For this reason a malignant tumor involving the middle third of the diaphysis of a cylindrical bone in a patient under 30 years of age is very apt to be Ewing's. When it occurs in the metaphysis the anatomic position is of little diagnostic aid.

Just as with most other bone tumors the femur is the most common bone affected and the tibia is second. The small bones of the feet, especially the os calcis, are

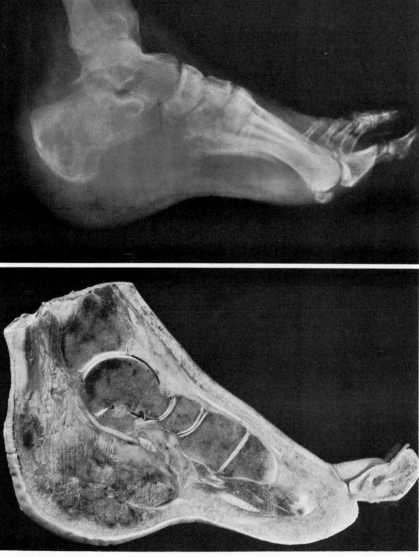

Figure 19–15 Ewing's tumor of os calcis. Above, roentgenogram showing destruction within calcaneus and large soft tissue mass. Below, sagittal section of amputated foot.

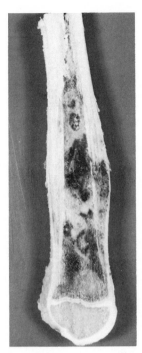

Figure 19–16 Ewing's tumor. The tumor arose within the shaft, penetrated the cortex without wholly destroying it and elevated the periosteum. This behavior accounts for the pain and also the "onion skin" appearance of the roentgenogram.

frequently affected (Fig. 19–15). Of the flat bones, those of the pelvic girdle are most commonly involved, but primary sites in the ribs and vertebrae are common.

The outstanding symptom of Ewing's tumor is pain. At first it may be vague and transient with quite long periods of remission. Eventually, it persists and becomes severe. As in most bone lesions the pain is often worse at night. More so than in most bone tumors, tenderness over the involved area may develop early. The explanation for the pain and tenderness is obvious when one examines a series of amputated specimens. Ewing's tumor has a strong propensity for the invasion and penetration of bone without destroying its contours. Very early it grows through the fine nutrient canals of the cortex to reach the extraosseous soft tissues including the nerves (Fig. 19–16). This character accounts for the considerable mass of extraosseous tumor before the underlying cortex gives roentgenographic evidence of

permeation. We have seen a 16 cm. soft tissue tumor mass growing out from the medulla of the calcaneus without any roentgenographic evidence of bone involvement. Eventually the nutrient vessels are closed by the pressure of the finger-like processes of growing tumor tissue, and then the bone begins to show change. In areas in which there is partial closure the bone becomes sclerotic; in areas in which closure is nearly complete there is rapid bone necrosis. This behavior is responsible for the generally accepted idea that Ewing's tumor is highly lytic in nature. Actually, the process is very similar to that of infection with the inevitable thrombosis and formation of granulation that occur. The roentgenograms of the two conditions may be strikingly similar.

Two other characteristic features of Ewing's tumor, fever and leukocytosis, can be explained on the basis of the gross appearance and cytologic nature of the lesion. For some reason this tumor characteristically outgrows its blood supply, or perhaps it would be more accurate to say that the blood supply that sustains its growth does not remain to keep it viable. As a result large areas of the tumor degenerate; indeed it may be necessary to take samples from several levels in order to find one in which the cells have retained their morphologic character sufficiently for recognition. This fact probably accounts for the wide variation in morphology that is encountered by the microscopist. The nature of the degenerating cells, i.e., their marrow origin, probably explains the fever and leukocytosis. These cells are closely related to pus cells and it is understandable that they should give rise to the same symptoms that one finds in suppurative infection. Indeed, it has been noted more than once that completely degenerated tumor tissue takes on the exact gross appearance of suppurative exudate.

Abnormal temperatures range around 100 to 101° F. early in the disease. Later the fever may rise to 105°. The leukocytosis is usually moderate, often remaining under 20,000. Occasionally it may rise as high as 40,000. The sedimentation time is usually shortened.

Roentgenographic Manifestations. The most striking roentgenographic manifestation of Ewing's tumor is bone destruction. Classically, this first involves the medullary canal and then the cortex. Finally, the neoplasm elevates and penetrates the periosteum to produce a large soft tissue mass. The medullary destruction appears as mottled areas of intermediate density replacing the bony trabeculae. As cortical destruction occurs, the continuity of the cortex is interrupted or with less extensive destruction its outlines become indistinct. The elevation of the periosteum results in the production of one or more layers of new bone (onion skin appearance), and the extremes of the periosteal elevation form an angle with the cortex (Codman's triangle). This periosteal new bone is a response to the elevation of the periosteum. It is not neoplastic bone and is not specific

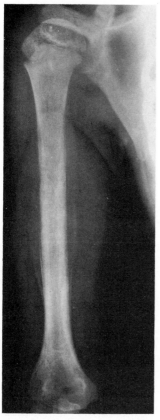

Figure 19–17 Ewing's tumor. The shaft is the site of the neoplasm. Irregular areas of bone destruction are evident as well as layers of periosteal new bone. Soft tissue swelling and local tenderness are present. The fat between muscle groups is displaced but not obliterated as would be expected in osteomyelitis.

for Ewing's tumor. Irregular patches of sclerosis or opacity may be seen within the area involved by the tumor that reflect vascular impairment and bone reaction.

It has been reported that approximately 25 per cent of Ewing's tumors present the classic appearance, i.e., a lesion in the medullary zone of the midshaft with cortical destruction and multiple layers of new periosteal bone.[24] As might be expected, this radiographic appearance may be entirely compatible with osteomyelitis except for its location in the midportion of the shaft. The metaphysis is frequently involved and the lesion may even arise in the epiphysis. Ewing's tumor may involve the cortex primarily and mimic an extraosseous lesion with secondary involvement of bone. At times, a large soft tissue mass is evident with only minimal bony changes or associated with thick periosteal new bone at the edges of the soft tissue extension of the tumor (Fig. 19–18). The soft tissue mass of a Ewing's tumor may be evident on properly exposed films by virtue of displacement of more radiolucent muscle planes. Massive calcification within this mass is not common but spotty ossification, presumably of periosteal origin, may be seen.

Involvement of flat bones and the small bones of the feet follows the same pattern of destruction with or without associated sclerosis (Fig. 9–15). Sclerosis may produce a streaky appearance of the involved portion of the bone, which is accentuated by contrast with areas of radiolucency produced by osseous destruction.

It now appears to be probable that in the past those tumors of both flat and cylindrical bones that exhibited considerable amounts of osteoid production (sclerosis) were, in fact, primitive osteosarcomas (Hutter's primitive multipotential, primary sarcoma). This type of tumor has much the same clinical appearance as Ewing's tumor and indeed could be considered a more primitive subvariety of the same group.

Radiographically, this neoplasm produces a response that is primarily that of a destructive process. The pattern produced by this destructive process is modified by the extent of involvement, the location of the lesion, the degree of vascular involve-

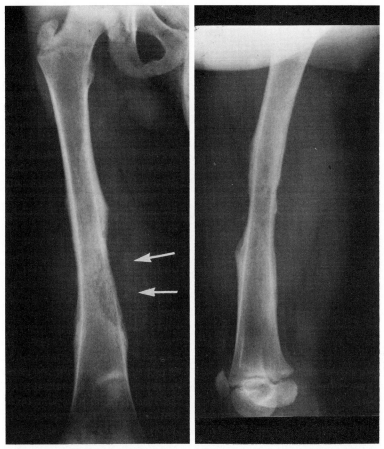

Figure 19–18 Ewing's tumor. The lesion has destroyed the cortex medially and practically envelops the shaft. Calcification (arrows) is evident within the accompanying soft tissue mass. Involvement of the spongy bone of the medullary canal is not marked radiographically.

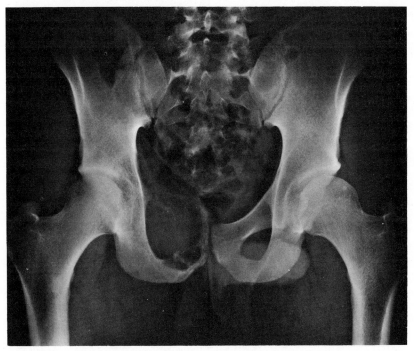

Figure 19–19 Ewing's tumor. The neoplasm has expanded and destroyed the right pubic bone and a portion of the ischium. A large soft tissue mass is present.

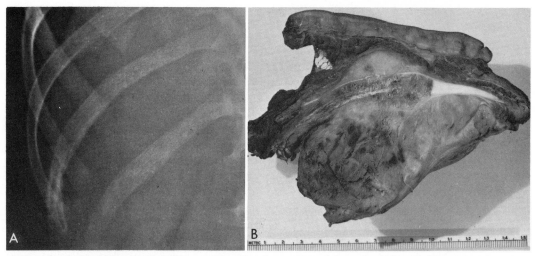

Figure 19–20   Ewing's tumor. *A*, There is irregular destruction of the trabeculae and cortex of the eleventh rib. The huge soft tissue component is best seen in *B*, the pathological specimen. Tumors of ribs may be first manifested by pleural effusion.

ment and the nature of associated bone reaction. Microscopic involvement is universally greater than are the macroscopic changes. The radiographic diagnosis, which can only be suggested rather than positively established, is dependent upon an understanding of the basic pathologic process coupled with a high index of suspicion. The differential diagnosis is commonly concerned with osteomyelitis, eosinophilic granuloma, osteosarcoma and reticulum cell sarcoma.

Gross Pathology. Ewing's tumor is a soft, pultaceous mass of cells with a pale color. Areas of degeneration mottle the white to gray color with patches of yellow or greenish brown. Hemorrhage is not usual but in the areas of degeneration there may be sufficient hemosiderin to give a dark red or brown color. Because the tumor causes thrombosis of and pressure on blood vessels it alters the blood supply of the involved bone and soft tissue. Reactive bone formation and collagen production are usual. As the periosteum is dissected away from the diaphysis (Figs. 19–16 and 19–22) it often produces a thin layer of mineralized bone along its inner layer. This is soon penetrated by the tumor and the periosteum is again lifted and again it forms a shell of bone. This may be repeated several times before the perios-

teum is destroyed and the tumor advances beyond its limiting influence. This mechanism accounts for the thickening of the cortex and the laminated "onion skin" appearance that often appears in the roentgenogram. If the periosteum is elevated by a rapidly growing tumor, the reactive bone may be laid down in strands about nutrient vessels, which are perpendicular to the cortical surface. Thus the sunburst appearance, which is so characteristic of osteosarcoma, may also appear on the roentgenograms of Ewing's tumor.

When the nutrition of the affected bone falls below the level of viability, bone lysis occurs. The cortex becomes necrotic and fragmented. This appearance has given Ewing's tumor the reputation of being a bone-lysing neoplasm. Tumor tissue replaces the destroyed bone and advances out into the soft tissue. In turn its vessels are choked off and large areas of degeneration occur. These areas often become cystic and they may be filled with liquid debris that grossly resembles pus. This appearance sometimes convinces the surgeon that he is dealing with an infectious process.

Microscopic Pathology. Ewing described the morphology of the cells of this tumor as "monotonously uniform" and most text authors have borrowed this term in their accounts of it. If one carefully eval-

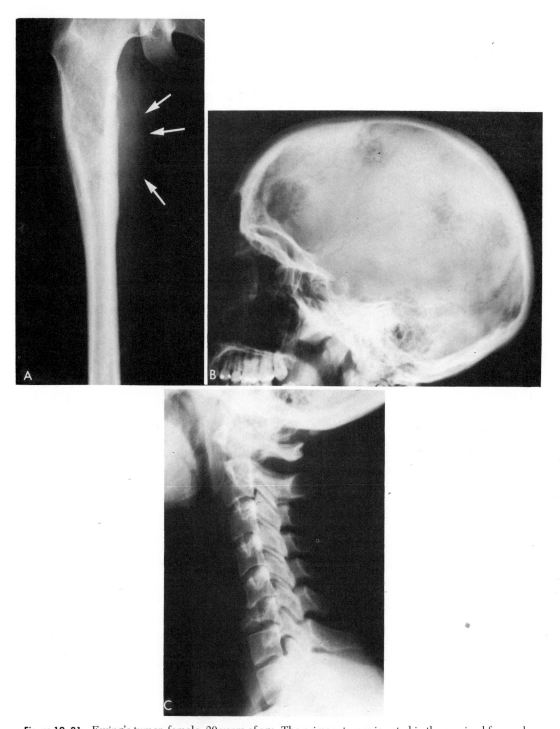

Figure 19–21   Ewing's tumor, female, 20 years of age. The primary tumor is noted in the proximal femur characterized by tiny areas of destruction, abundant periosteal new bone and a soft tissue mass (arrows, *A*). Metastatic foci involve the skull and the body of the sixth cervical vertebra.

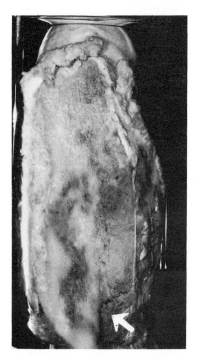

Figure 19–22 Ewing's tumor in the upper end of the femur. It arose in the shaft proximal to the metaphysis, infiltrated the cortex without destroying it and elevated the periosteum, which laid down a thin shell of bone.

uates these cells on the basis of their microscopic appearance, "monotonous" does not seem to be a very apt term. This tumor is very cellular, the cells usually are quite undifferentiated and there is little apparent supportive tissue, but if one examines the highly magnified fields one notes considerable variation between tumors and between areas of the same tumor.

Large areas of degeneration are as characteristic of Ewing's tumor as they are in Hodgkin's disease of lymph nodes. If the biopsy is small one may have difficulty in finding enough intact cells on which to base an opinion. A second characteristic that has been inadequately emphasized is the considerable amount of bone and fibrous tissue that is found in the sections. The bone is largely reactive in type and one must be careful on frozen section not to conclude that it is being formed by the tumor cells, thus suggesting a diagnosis of osteosarcoma.[25] But if one searches many sections one can almost always find microspicules of poorly formed osteoid, which certainly appear to be formed by the tumor cells (Fig. 19–23). It is difficult to explain this curious metaplasia of apparent reticu-

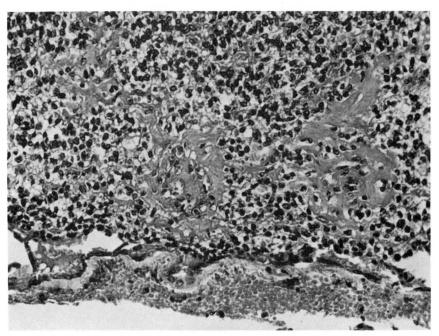

Figure 19–23 Ewing's tumor. Microspicules of poorly formed osteoid are produced apparently by the tumor cells. (× 250.)

lum derivatives into osteoblasts unless one remembers that all cellular elements of bone arise from a common stem cell. One finds Ewing tumor cells and reticulum cell sarcoma elements mixed with osteoid-forming cells in the primitive cell osteosarcoma (primitive multipotential primary sarcoma of bone). Indeed, it now seems probable that there is a transition group lying between this tumor and the classic one of Ewing. They scarcely deserve a class of their own and probably should be placed with one or the other on either side depending upon the amount of osteoid production.

The fields may be irregularly divided by bands of fibrous connective tissue of varying width. Some of this is doubtless invaded tissue but much of it appears indigenous to the tumor growth.

The appearance of the tumor cells themselves is also variable (Fig. 19–24). The nucleus ranges in size from one half again to three times the size of the normal erythrocyte. The amount of chromatin is variable but it is almost always finely divided and diffusely dispersed. Mitotic figures in most tumors are inconspicuous but rarely they may be abundant. In most lesions the nucleoli are small or lacking; in

others they may be prominent. The nucleus is usually ovoid, sometimes round, and though there may be variation in size the outline is rarely irregular. This may be an important differential point in distinguishing Ewing's tumor from reticulum cell sarcoma. The nuclear membrane is usually distinct.

The cell size is two to three times that of the nucleus. The cytoplasm is usually clear with whatever stain is used, but at times it takes eosin and appears very similar to the cytoplasm of the macrophage. In either case the cell membrane usually remains intact, describing a fine tracery through the matrix. Sometimes no cytoplasm is demonstrable and the nuclei appear naked.

Eosinophilic granules are usually apparent in the cytoplasm when P.A.S. stain is used. This feature is not pathognomonic for Ewing's tumor (the granules are found in other tumors) nor is their absence significant. However, when present they probably rule out lymphoma and neuroblastoma.

The appearance of the tumor cells apparently depends greatly upon the technique used in processing the sections. These cells probably contain a higher

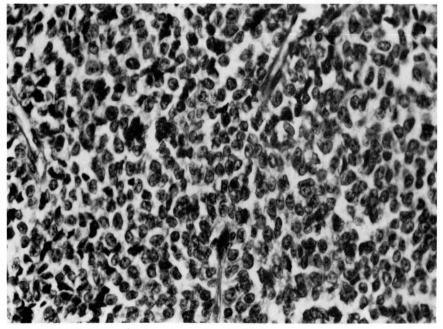

Figure 19–24 Section from a Ewing's tumor. In good preparations the nuclei vary somewhat in size and chromatin distribution. The cytoplasm stains poorly. (× 440.)

water content than most and often the dehydrating agents cause the cytoplasm to shrink to nothing and the nuclei to appear heavily chromated and pyknotic. This may account for the description that Ewing gave, one which seems so at variance with what we now consider the typical Ewing's tumor

If one examines this tumor closely, a fine meshwork of stromal fibers often can be seen forming a netlike support for the tumor cells. These fibrils stain like collagen and one can often demonstrate spindled fibrocytes, which apparently form them. In other areas no fibrocytes can be demonstrated and the grouping of the tumor cells suggests that they have a genetic relation to the intercellular substance. One must consider the possibility of shrunken reticulum elements. Silver stains are of no help because fine collagen fibers and reticulin fibrils, if there be a difference, are both argentophilic (Fig. 19-25).

The microscopic diagnosis on carefully prepared viable tissue should give the microscopist little difficulty except in excluding reticulum cell sarcoma, the rare neuroblastoma and the still rarer lymphosarcoma of bone. It is probable that metastatic neuroblastoma and Ewing's tumor cannot be differentiated by microscopy alone in many instances. In cases in which the rosettes of neuroblastoma are present they are most helpful because though the cells of Ewing's tumor frequently form circles, these cells are usually arranged around blood vessels, or nidi of degenerating cells. The fact that these two tumors may have an identical microscopy does not constitute proof that they are the same tumor or that one or the other does not exist, a hypothesis that has been offered by a few distraught writers who have had difficulty in making the distinction. If primary lymphosarcoma of bone occurs, it is a close relative of Ewing's tumor. We know of few differentiating features as long as bone alone is involved. If one can be sure that his staining technique is reliable, the nucleus of the tumor lymphoblast is a bit smaller, is more compact with a greater amount of chromatin obscuring the nucleolus and there is relatively less cytoplasm which, of course, should contain no eosinophilic staining granules. The most

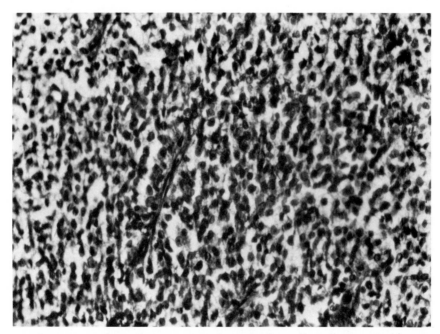

Figure 19-25 Counterstained reticulin preparation of a section from a Ewing's tumor. In this case no reticulin fibrils are seen. They may be present, however, and the reticulin stain cannot be used as a dependable guide in differentiating Ewing's tumor from reticulum cell sarcoma. (× 300.)

obvious and helpful feature, when present, is a tendency for the cells of lymphosarcoma to group themselves in imperfect follicles.

The variability of the microscopic morphology of the cells of Ewing's tumor has led some microscopists, principally in Great Britain, to the conclusion that no such entity exists, a disturbing contention that has caused us many hours of serious consideration. Whatever the opinion of the microscopist, the clinician finds he must deal with a large number of primary bone tumors in young patients that have remarkably similar radiographic pictures and clinical behavior. We are unable to explain the structural variability satisfactorily though doubtless the tendency for necrosis and the cell fragility to handling during processing are important factors. We have wondered if the cell genesis may have a wider range than most tumors, limited only by the multiple cell types derived from marrow reticulum. In short, we may be using the term "Ewing's tumor" to cover not only the tumors of myelogenous series origin but also the several types of lymphomas that arise in bone marrow. The constant clinical features of these types are sufficient reason to retain the classification of Ewing's tumor as long as we admit that, as the English have long contended, there is no such specific, microscopic entity, only a closely related group with much the same clinical behavior.

Prognosis. Ewing's tumor is highly malignant because of its propensity to metastasize. Secondary deposits soon occur in the lungs and in other bones. Less frequently the lymph nodes, viscera and even the skin may be involved. The duration of symptoms before diagnosis ranges from three to nine months. Metastasis after diagnosis usually occurs within six months.

Multiple bone involvement has caused some to conclude that Ewing's tumor, like plasma cell myeloma, is multicentric. There is very little other evidence in support of this hypothesis. In most cases a single focus is present for some time before other bone lesions appear. About one half the cases do not develop multiple bone lesions. Examination of the marrow removed from a site remote from the tumor has not revealed the presence of tumor cells, and to our knowledge no case of Ewing's tumor has ever eventuated in leukemia. Pulmonary metastases are not as constant in Ewing's tumor as in osteosarcoma, but death is caused in the majority of cases by this complication.

The over-all mortality rate of Ewing's tumor is exceedingly high. Some writers place it at 95 per cent even with early diagnosis and proper treatment. There is some evidence that the younger patient has a more rapid course and less hopeful outlook. This may be because reticulum cell sarcoma has a wider age range and better prognosis, and some pathologists still refuse to make the distinction between Ewing's tumor and reticulum cell sarcoma.

At the present, the treatment considered most definitive is radical radiation therapy to the primary tumor combined with intensive chemotherapy. The latter serves to destroy or delay the growth of metastatic deposits. Although the results are encouraging, more time and data will be necessary for evaluation of this form of therapy.[26]

RETICULUM CELL SARCOMA

In 1939, Parker and Jackson[27] reported 17 cases of what they called reticulum cell sarcoma of bone. The tumor occurred in all age groups, in both cylindrical and flat bones, caused extensive bone destruction and soft tissue growth, and though often diagnosed late had a very much better survival rate than Ewing's tumor. This was the first reported account of this tumor as an entity in which the comparatively good response to therapy was associated with a specific tumor cell morphology. In 1928, Oberling published a paper in which he stated that the Ewing "group" of tumors arose not from endothelium but from the marrow reticulum. Since 1940, several series of 25 or more cases[28, 29, 30, 31] have been published and in 1957, Schwingen[32] reviewed the world literature and found 154 cases published under the name of reticulum cell sarcoma of bone. Despite this publicity there still are authors of eminence who state that they are unable to distinguish this lesion from other marrow tumors, particularly Ewing's tumor, and who thereby cast some doubt on the authenticity of the lesion as a separate entity. Today, though there are cases in which the microscopy appears to lie somewhere between the two classic concepts of Ewing's tumor and reticulum cell sarcoma, we believe that, in the majority, the two lesions can be distinguished on the basis of cellular characteristics. The two tumors certainly describe quite different clinical courses.

Why the reticulum cell sarcoma of bone is quite a different tumor in behavior from the reticulum cell sarcoma primary in lymph nodes and other soft tissue is a question that we cannot at present answer, but these two tumors are apparently unrelated. Though the cells of the two tumor types may be similar, the clinical courses are very different. Reticulum cell sarcoma of lymph nodes occurs about equally in both sexes. It usually affects patients over 40 years old. It is a fatal disease that metastasizes to the reticulum-bearing structures of soft tissue — lymph nodes, spleen and liver — and much less commonly to bones. Its response to irradiation is transient and its course is rapid. It is associated with a variety of forms — follicular lymphoma, lymphocytic lymphosarcoma, lymphatic leukemia and Hodgkin's disease. The behavior of reticulum cell sarcoma of bone as reviewed here will be seen to be quite different from that of the non-osseous reticulum cell sarcoma, suggesting that the two tumors are not the same despite their nomenclature.

The following account of reticulum cell sarcoma is drawn largely from the literature on the published cases. A review of the accounts produces much contradictory data and many inconsistent statements, but today the records are sufficient to settle the controversy concerning its existence and to give us a fairly good concept of the behavior and morphology of this neoplasm.

Reticulum cell sarcoma of bone is probably less than half as common as Ewing's tumor. Most series stress the male predominance, usually calculated at about two to one. Whereas all but a very few patients with Ewing's tumor are under 30 years of age at the time of onset of their tumor, reticulum cell sarcoma is quite evenly scattered throughout the life span. Thus the age incidence of reticulum cell sarcoma of bone differs from that of both Ewing's tumor in the young age group and reticulum cell sarcoma of soft tissues in the older age group. There is a fairly widespread impression that reticulum cell sarcoma of bone is a tumor most often occurring after the age of 40. This is not supported by an analysis of the available case reports and probably is due to the frequently heard statement that reticulum cell sarcoma occurs in an older age group than does Ewing's tumor; this is true, but it also occurs in the Ewing's age group.

The skeletal distribution is apparently about the same for reticulum cell sarcoma as for Ewing's tumor and like the latter it may occur anywhere in the shaft rather than predominantly in the metaphysis. According to Ivins and Dahlin, reviewing a series of 49 cases, about one half occur in the lower extremities, one quarter in the shoulder and upper extremities and the remaining quarter in the bones of the head and the vertebrae. There is probably less tendency for the tumor to occur in the small bones of the hands and feet than there is in Ewing's tumor.

In our material there are 48 reticulum cell sarcomas. Of these 33 occur in patients over 30 years of age, the oldest 83. There are but four patients under the age of 20, 11 under 30. Of those patients available for follow-up, 33 per cent were alive five years after treatment.

The symptoms of reticulum cell sarcoma of bone are minimal. In their original paper Parker and Jackson state "In no other bone tumor is the contrast between the comparative well-being of the patient and the size of the tumor so marked." Pain and, in about one half the patients, a palpable tumor are the outstanding clinical features. Neither of these helps to differentiate the lesion from Ewing's tumor though the pain is apparently less severe than in the latter. Fever and leukocytosis have been lacking in most tumors though an increase in sedimentation rate has been reported in some. Characteristic alterations in the serum chemistry in relation to calcium, phosphorus, alkaline phosphatase, albumin and globulin have not been found.

Reticulum   cell   sarcoma   apparently

evolves more slowly than Ewing's tumor. If one averages the time from the reports in which this data is given, the duration of symptoms is usually between 15 months and two years. In some cases it has been reported as 10 years or longer.

Though this tumor grows quite slowly it eventually produces the same considerable bone destruction as does Ewing's tumor. Apparently because the process is more insidious, pathologic fracture is more common. It is said to occur in one quarter to one third of cases. Some reactive bone formation occurs in reticulum cell sarcoma. This may be sufficient to produce the picture of cortical expansion.

This tumor metastasizes much later than Ewing's tumor and its pattern of metastasis is somewhat different. Whereas approximately one half of the Ewing's tumors eventually affect other bone sites and only occasional lymph node deposits are found, this pattern is reversed in reticulum cell sarcoma of bone. About 20 per cent have metastasized to lymph nodes and only occasionally are tumor deposits encountered in other bones. Both tumors kill by eventual metastasis to the lungs.

Roentgenographic Manifestations. Reticulum cell sarcoma is manifested radiographically by small, irregular foci of destruction often accompanied by patchy opacification resulting from the formation of reactive new bone. The neoplasm arises from reticulum elements and hence first involves the medullary canal. Trabeculae of bone are destroyed and replaced by tumor tissue. Small areas of normal bone isolated by the tumor and areas of reactive new bone contribute to the mottled appearance of the involved bone noted radiographically (Fig. 19–27). Reactive bone is a reflection of the slow growth of the tumor.

As the medullary neoplasm grows, the cortex is eroded and thinned, usually in a most irregular pattern so that the islands of normal cortex remain. The edges of the tumor are poorly defined. Periosteal new bone is usually not a prominent feature of

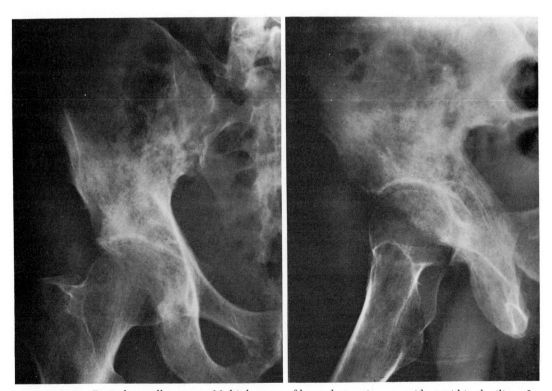

Figure 19–26 Reticulum cell sarcoma. Multiple areas of bone destruction are evident within the ilium. Interspersed opacity reflects reactive bone formation.

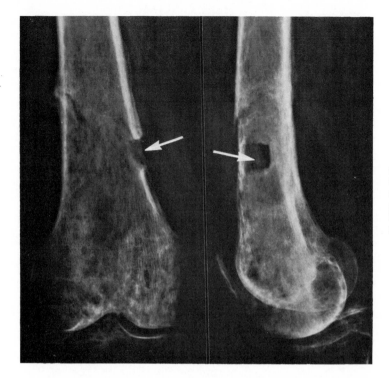

Figure 19–27 Reticulum cell sarcoma. Patchy areas of destruction involving the trabeculae and cortex are evident with little periosteal new bone. A pathologic fracture is evident. An arrow marks the site of a biopsy.

reticulum cell sarcoma early; it is evident as the cortex is penetrated and the periosteum elevated, however. The latter is particularly true in metaphyseal lesions.

Soft tissue extension of the tumor is not common early, but in tumors present for a long period of time and in cases in which flat bones are involved, the soft tissue mass may be quite large and be the presenting physical finding. Calcification within the soft tissue mass is not to be expected.

Pathologic fracture through the involved area is not uncommon and, too, may be an early clinical manifestation of this tumor.

Morbid Anatomy. Reticulum cell sarcoma of bone usually has a pink or a pinkish gray color. It always begins in the medullary tissues and erodes bone from within. Sometimes the erosion is slow enough to permit the periosteum to lay down a shell of bone over it, causing cortical expansion. Pathologic fracture is reported more frequently and there is said to be less necrosis in reticulum cell sarcoma than in Ewing's tumor.

However slender the evidence for a difference in clinical behavior of these two tumors, the microscopic details of the cells concerned are sufficiently different in some cases at least to warrant separation. It will be remembered that the cells of Ewing's tumor are moderate in size, the nuclei are about half the mass of the cell, ovoid or round, and have a distinct, regular contour. The cells of reticulum cell sarcoma of bone are usually larger than those of Ewing's tumor (Fig. 19–28). The cell membrane is usually not demonstrable and in cases in which it is, it is irregular with processes that have been likened to pseudopods. The cytoplasm is smooth or moderately granular. Cytoplasmic volume in relation to nuclear volume is greater than that of Ewing's tumor, in which it is approximately one to one or at most one to two. In some sections the cytoplasm appears more basophilic than most tissue cells.

The character of the nucleus is the most outstanding feature of the lesion. In the more mature forms it is large and reniform; in the younger cells it is frankly lobulated. In some the lobulation is so pronounced that the appearance is that of a cluster of small spheroid nuclei. Actually some cells are binuclear or even trinuclear. The nuclei are usually quite irregular in outline. As in the cells of Ewing's tumor the nuclear chromatin is sometimes finely divided and evenly dispersed, but more often it is coarsely clumped and quite irregular. Mitotic figures are much more common in reticulum cell sarcoma of bone than in Ewing's tumor. The nucleoli are apt to be quite prominent. Thus, one gets the impression of quite marked cellular pleomorphism in reticulum cell sarcoma whereas in Ewing's tumor the cells are more uniform. Mixed in with the obvious tumor cells there is often a scattering of similar round cells with scant cytoplasm, which have the appearance of lymphocytes (Fig. 19–29). Some authors believe that these are an indigenous part of the tumor and represent the more mature components of reticulum differentiation.

It has been reported that the cells of Ewing's tumor contain glycogen in their cytoplasm, whereas those of reticulum cell sarcoma do not and that a glycogen stain makes the distinction. To date we have been unable to evaluate this test on a sufficient number of cases to formulate a conclusion.

The pattern and the supportive stroma of reticulum cell sarcoma are not of great differential help. There is probably less necrosis than in Ewing's tumor. Some sections show the tumor cells aligned along syncytial bands that are purported to be primitive reticulum. Actually, if these sections are carefully examined these bands may be seen to contain mature fibrocytes and at least some collagen. They appear to be a network of supporting fibers and the cellular arrangement is an artifact, a shrinking of the cells toward their scaffolding thus producing a reticulum pattern.

Special silver stains have been used to differentiate reticulum cell sarcoma from Ewing's tumor (Fig. 19–30). In our hands, and admittedly in a very limited number of cases, this has been a futile exercise. In terms of the differentiation of these particular two tumors, argentophilia is a property not of the cell but of the physical state of the intercellular substance. The intercellular material of many of the mesenchymal derivatives takes the silver stain to some extent. Broad bands of collagen stain a pale reddish brown; narrower bands stain more deeply. If the collagen fibrils

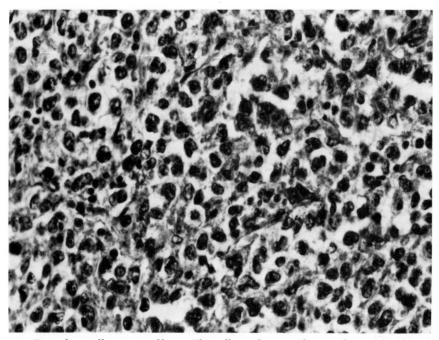

Figure 19–28   Reticulum cell sarcoma of bone. The cells are larger and more pleomorphic than those of Ewing's tumor (Fig. 19–24). The nuclear outlines are reniform or frankly irregular. Sometimes the nucleus is lobulated or there may be more than one nucleus. (× 440.)

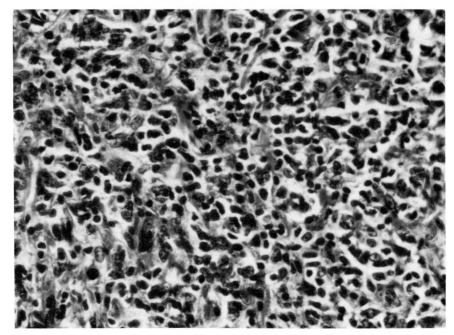

Figure 19–29   In some sections of reticulum cell sarcoma one can find small round nuclei resembling those of lymphocytes. Here they are quite densely infiltrating the reticulum cell elements. (× 440.)

are very fine they take an intense black stain similar to the neurofibrils in the central nervous system. The fine reticulin fibrils supposedly produced by the reticu-lum cells give the same staining reaction. If the cells of the reticulum cell sarcoma of bone produce reticulin fibrils they have not been helpful in distinguishing this

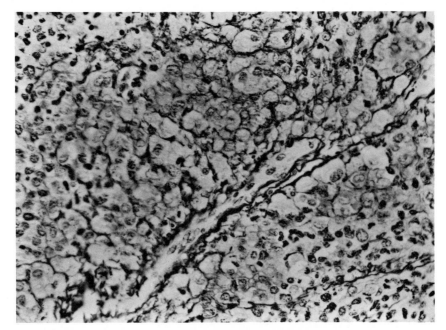

Figure 19–30   Reticulum stain of a section of reticulum cell sarcoma. The fine, black reticulin fibers are woven between the tumor cells. They are not always present in this tumor. (× 300.)

tumor for us. Indeed, the fine collagen fibrils of Ewing's tumor have been more prominent in some cases.

Some clinicians are under the impression that the reticulum stain has a special affinity for the reticulum cells, which it has not. Because it stains collagen fibrils as well as reticulin fibrils, a differentiation must be made on the basis of whether the fibrils surround single cells or groups of cells. To date there is lack of agreement on the character and arrangement of the intercellular fibrils of reticulum cell sarcoma of bone. Not until the properly prepared sections of large numbers of cases, proved by clinical behavior as well as by microscopy to be reticulum cell sarcoma of bone, have been studied and compared with those of Ewing's tumor can the virtue of reticulin staining be factually evaluated. Until then we must rely almost entirely upon the nuclear morphology to make the distinction between these two tumors. It is obvious that in cases with atypical morphology, mistakes in diagnosis will almost certainly occur.

Prognosis. It is the definitely more cheerful outlook that makes the differentiation of reticulum cell sarcoma of bone from Ewing's tumor so important. Approximately 30 per cent of reticulum cell sarcomas of bone can be cured by adequate irradiation therapy if the correct diagnosis is made reasonably early. Excellent results have been reported even after lymph node metastasis has occurred. It is becoming apparent that reticulum cell sarcoma grows more slowly, metastasizes later and is more vulnerable to x-irradiation than are the other marrow tumors. It is now believed by those who have had the greatest experience with this tumor that x-ray therapy is as efficient as surgical ablation. It is often the only available means of treatment in cases in which the vertebral and pelvic bones are involved.

The mortality statistics of reticulum cell sarcoma of bone must be carefully evaluated in terms of years of survival. Recurrences and metastases have been reported as late as 10 years after the original treatment. All cases of plasma cell myeloma and Ewing's tumor with five-year survival should be reevaluated with the possibility that they might represent reticulum cell sarcoma of bone with atypical microscopy. Therapeutic perseverance, even in the face of multiple site involvement, is probably warranted.

HODGKIN'S DISEASE OF BONE

Hodgkin's disease, malignant granuloma, is a disease of lymphoid reticulum. In the United States it is quite generally considered a malignant neoplasm, one of the lymphomas. Other tumors in the lymphoma group are lymphosarcoma, reticulum cell sarcoma, follicular lymphoma and lymphatic leukemia. These cancers arise from the lymphoid reticulum throughout the body, the lymph nodes, the spleen, the intestinal follicles, the liver, the skin and the thymus in approximately that order of incidence. Presumably, any one of these lymphomas may involve the bone marrow reticulum as a part of a more generalized neoplastic process or even develop as the primary lesion at this site. Actually lymphatic leukemia usually infiltrates the marrow and occasionally it produces bone changes, which are described in another section of this text. Focal deposits of lymphosarcoma have been reported within the bone marrow. If we have ever seen an instance of this, we have been unable to distinguish it from one or the other of the myelomas on the basis of its microscopy alone. Follicular lymphoma, to the best of our knowledge, has never been encountered in bone marrow, and it is our opinion that the reticulum cell sarcoma of bone marrow is not the same tumor as that affecting extraskeletal tissues, because though they may be morphologically identical their behavior is quite dissimilar. Hodgkin's disease commonly affects bones as a part of a generalized body involvement. It has been demonstrated in marrow most often by autopsy examination and obviously in the terminal phase of the disease. Rarely has it been discovered by biopsying a roentgenographic bone lesion and is thus thought to be the initial lesion of the process. There are only nine such in our material of 17 cases of Hodgkin's disease of bone.

Hodgkin's disease is more common in the male. It is rarely encountered in patients under the age of 15 and though it is sometimes seen in older patients, the common age incidence is between 20 and 30.

The lesion of Hodgkin's disease of bone is no different from that of soft tissue or viscera. The disease recently has been divided into six histologic types by Lukes et al. Types one and two have an average survival of 8 to 16 years. Types five and six have an average survival of one to eight years. Types three and four fall somewhere between these types. An analysis of our cases confirms these figures. The older classification of Hodgkin's disease into paragranulomatous, granulomatous and sarcomatous types should probably be discontinued.

Roentgenographic Manifestations. The osseous lesion of Hodgkin's disease may present as a fairly well circumscribed area of radiolucency within a bone. If, as may be the case when a vertebral body is involved, destruction of trabeculae has weakened the bone but not to a degree that is apparent radiographically, a pathologic

fracture may be the first manifestation of osseous abnormality. As in any expanding and destructive medullary tumor, when the cortex is destroyed and the periosteum elevated, periosteal new bone may be evident but is uncommon. Infrequently an area of intense opacity may be evident, the result of an osteoblastic reaction to the neoplasm or there may be a mixed blastic and lytic reaction. At times, one may see fine, diffuse areas of destruction, poorly defined as to extent within a bone, that resemble reticulum cell sarcoma.

The distribution of the osseous lesions parallels the location of active marrow, so that the vertebral bodies, the pelvis, the ribs and the femurs are most often the sites of radiographic abnormality.

Pathology. The common lesion of this condition is called granulomatous Hodgkin's disease. It is a complex of a variety of cells most of which are of inflammatory nature, and for this reason in Europe the disease is still widely regarded as an inflammatory process. In all six types of

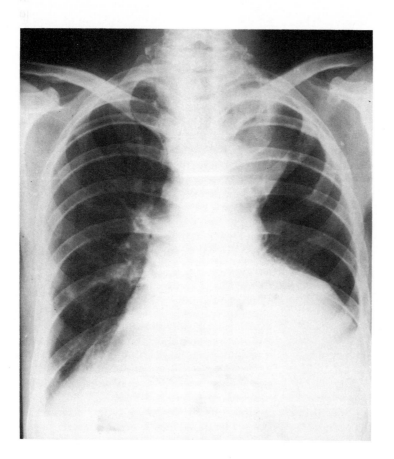

Figure 19–31 Hodgkin's disease. Destructive areas are apparent in the first, second and third ribs on the left.

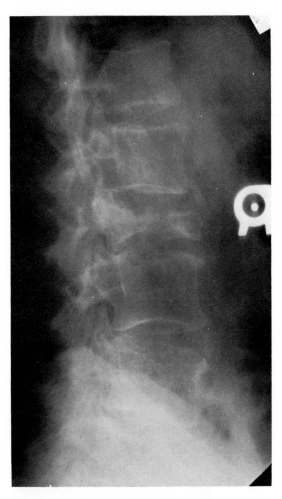

Figure 19–32 Hodgkin's disease. Involvement of the body of the second lumbar vertebra has resulted in its collapse.

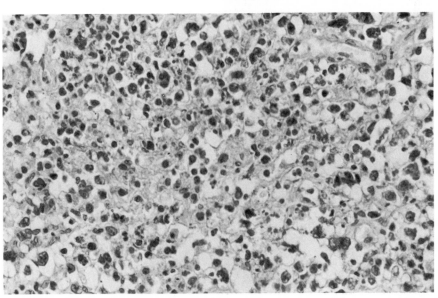

Figure 19–33 Granulomatous Hodgkin's disease of bone. This section reveals numerous irregular Reed-Sternberg cells with histiocytes and cells of inflammatory origin. ($\times$ 250.)

Hodgkin's disease there is always a hyperplasia of reticulum elements. This may appear as large numbers of epithelioid cells, of histiocytes, of young lymphocytes, of the more primitive reticulum cells or of the pathognomonic Reed-Sternberg giant cells. The last are large cells, usually multinucleated. The chromatin is often condensed along the nuclear membrane giving a penciled delineation. The nucleolus is usually very large and pink staining. When more than one nucleus is present they usually overlap or are arranged in a cross-stick pattern, usually in the central area of the cell. In granulomatous Hodgkin's disease (Fig. 19–33) the Reed-Sternberg cells are usually accompanied by scattered eosinophilic granulocytes, sometimes in abundance, plasmacytes and lymphocytes. There may be extensive fibrosis with collagen formation. Rarely the lesion may be converted to a mass of scar tissue. More commonly there is necrosis, which is often caseous.

Prognosis. Hodgkin's disease runs a varied and unpredictable course to a fatal termination. At one time it was quite generally believed that the disease was multicentric so that eradication of a single site was futile. Because there is often an astonishingly good initial response to irradiation, many clinics used to treat with the minimal amount of irradiation that would control symptoms and repeat therapy as indicated until maximal dosage had been administered. Today, an increasing number of observers believe that Hodgkin's disease is unicentric and metastasizes like other such neoplasms. With this concept it is reasonable to make the diagnosis at the earliest possible moment and to treat the lesions with surgery or cancericidal dosage of x-ray with the objective of achieving a cure. Whatever method of therapy is used the mortality rate is high in types five and six, though duration may vary from a few months to a decade. In types one and two the survival period is considerably longer and the survival rate is higher.

References

PLASMA CELL MYELOMA

1. Wood, H., Quinlan, J. W. and Merrill, E. F.: Am. J. Roentgenol., 53:466, 1945.

2. Maeda, K., Abesamis, C. M., Kuhn, M. and Hyun, B. H.: Am. J. Clin. Pathol. 60:552, 1973.
3. Aegerter, E. E. and Robbins, R.: Am. J. Med. Sci., 213:282, 1947.
4. Craver, L. and Miller, D.: CA, 16:142, 1966.
5. Waldenström, J.: In Dock, W. and Snapper, I., Eds.: Advances in Internal Medicine, vol. 5. Chicago, Year Book Publishers, 1952.
6. Collier, F. C. and Jackson, P.: N. Engl. J. Med., 248:409, 1953.
7. Kyle, R. and McGuckin, W.: Am. J. Clin. Pathol., 43:157, 1965.
8. Bell, E. T.: Am. J. Pathol., 9:393, 1933.
9. Blackman, S. S., Barker, W. H., Buell, M. V. and Davis, B. D.: J. Clin. Invest., 23:163, 1944.
10. Sickel, G.: Am. J. Med., 27:354, 1959.
11. Esposito, J. J.: Radiology, 40:195, 1943.
12. Toth, B. J., and Wintermantl, J. A.: Radiology, 41:472, 1943.
13. King, B. B.: J.A.M.A., 115:36, 1940.
14. Paul, L. W. and Pohle, E. A.: Radiology, 35:651, 1940.
15. Nadeau, L. A., Magalini, S. I. and Stefanini, M.: Arch. Pathol., 61:101, 1956.
16. Lowenhaupt, E.: Am. J. Pathol., 21:171, 1945.
17. Schindler, J. A.: Ann. Intern. Med., 19:140, 1943.
18. Johnson, L. and Meador, G.: Bull. Hosp. Joint Dis., 12:298, 1951.
19. Hellwig, C. A.: Arch. Pathol., 36:95, 1943.

EWING'S TUMOR

20. Ewing, J.: Proc. N.Y. Pathol. Soc., 21:17, 1921.
21. Stout, A. P.: Am. J. Roentgenol., 50:334, 1943.
22. Lichtenstein, L. and Jaffe, H. L.: Am. J. Pathol., 23:43, 1947.
23. McCormack, L., Dockerty, M. and Ghormley, R.: Cancer, 5:85, 1952.
24. Sherman, R. S. and Soong, K. Y.: Radiology, 66:529, 1956.
25. Garber, C. Z.: Cancer, 4:839, 1951.
26. Sutow, W. W., Vietti, T. J. and Lernbach, D. J.: Clinical Pediatric Oncology. St. Louis, C. V. Mosby Co., 1973.

RETICULUM CELL SARCOMA

27. Parker, F. and Jackson, H.: Surg. Gynecol. Obstet., 68:45, 1939.
28. Shuman, R. S. and Snyder, R. E.: Am. J. Roentgenol., 58:291, 1947.
29. Jackson, H., Jr., and Parker, F., Jr.: Hodgkin's Disease and Allied Disorders. New York, Oxford University Press, 1947.
30. Ivins, J. C. and Dahlin, D. C.: J. Bone Joint Surg., 35A:835, 1953.
31. Wilson, T. W. and Pugh, D. G.: Radiology, 65:343, 1955.
32. Schwingen, R. S.: Am. J. Surg., 93:41, 1957.
33. Fucilla, I. S. and Hamann, A.: Radiology, 77:53, 1961.

Chapter 20

OSTEOCLASTOMA

In the first edition of this text (1958) we gave the standard, world-accepted description of giant cell tumor of bone faithfully copied from standard, world-accepted texts. We did so because we had so little proof of the implausibility of this description that we felt it unwise publicly to attack it. In the second edition (1963) the proof was still tenuous but the conviction that the general concept was erroneous was so strong that we refused to propagate it by inclusion. We simply ignored the existence of giant cell tumor. In this, the fourth edition, we have gathered together the shreds of evidence painfully collected over 30 years of experience with giant cell lesions of bone and boldly record our conclusions with the prayer that eventually they will be proved correct.

Kolliker described and named the osteoclast nearly a century ago. The term "giant cell tumor of bone" began to appear in the literature shortly thereafter. Papers concerned with this lesion have continued to flow from the pens of pathologists, radiologists and clinicians ever since, until a vast literature, certainly more massive than that of any other bone neoplasm, has accrued. Most authors have offered new hypotheses for the nature or pathogenesis of this enigmatic tumor and respecting precedent, this account will be no exception. In the usual course of medical progress the more recent theories most closely approximate the truth. We can hope the trend will not be reversed in this writing.

In 1947 we published a paper on giant cell tumor of bone and thereby unwittingly became a reluctant consultant on the subject. Since that time hundreds of samples of giant cell lesions of bone have been submitted for our scrutiny from all parts of the country. Most of these have been accompanied by radiographs and at least a thumbnail sketch of the clinical features. In admittedly a small proportion we have been able to obtain follow-up data. An analysis of this material serves as the source of this account. It is our opinion that a review of the literature can provide the reader nothing better than a sense of frustration. If such is his intention, he may direct his efforts thence but we shall remain aloof from this objective by providing only the most salient references.

Much of the difficulty that has obscured an understanding of this tumor has been our ignorance concerning the giant cell itself. We are still uncertain of its origin, its function and its disposition. We cannot be unequivocal concerning whether it is an osteoclast or a foreign body giant cell or whether it causes bone lysis, is the product of bone lysis or an innocent bystander, related only because it is the product of a common cause. To formulate a thesis of the giant cell tumor of bone one must first determine some working concept of its giant cell component.

It is now widely accepted that osteoclasts are derived from osteoblasts and possibly osteocytes by the merging of these mononuclear cells. Some evidence has been presented to suggest that osteoclasts may divide and reestablish themselves as osteoblasts [1] but we hold grave doubts concerning this eventuality in human bone tissue. The origin of the osteoblast is also controversial. Johnson,[2] Trueta,[3] and others have suggested recently that they may arise from the endothelial lining cells of sprouting capillaries. Our experience supports this view to a measure. When

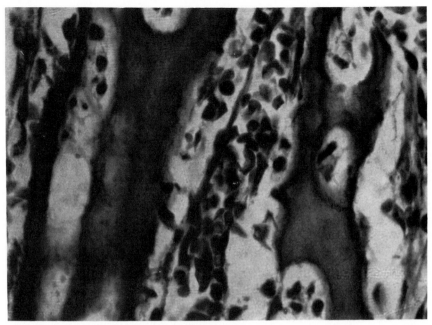

Figure 20–1 Subepiphyseal zone, growing bone. Three bars of darkly staining, mineralized chondroid cross the field vertically. Between the two heavier of these one can see a blood-filled arteriole, which courses toward the epiphyseal line just off the field above. The vessel's endothelial lining cells appear to form osteoblasts, which are pressed against the surfaces of the chondroid bars. (× 700.)

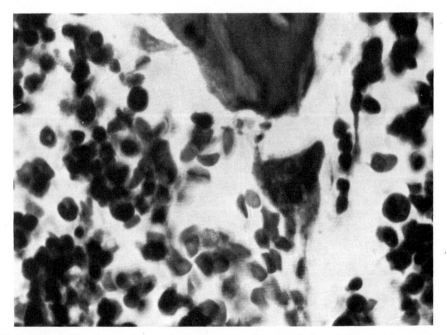

Figure 20–2 Subepiphyseal area of normal growing bone. The tip of a bar of chondroid protrudes onto the field from above. Below it is an osteoclast. One can barely discern the wall of a sinusoid of which the osteoclast is a part. The osteoclasts appear to arise from the vessel lining cells and to spearhead the sinusoid, perhaps breaking down the walls of the mature cartilage cells, which the sinusoid is destined to replace. (× 950.)

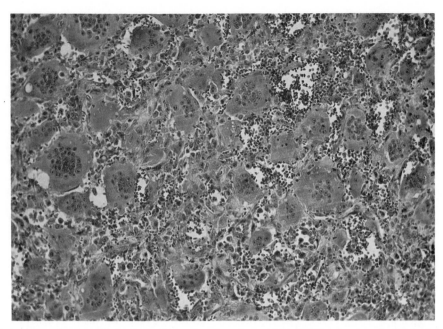

Figure 20–3   Osteoclastoma. The giant cells are found within endothelial lined sinusoids. Often these are not discernible but in cases in which the tumor is congested, as in this illustration, the spaces are distended with red blood cells. (× 110.)

cellular activity at the epiphyseal line is studied in tissue sections it appears that, in the zone of interdigitation, osteoblasts are formed from the capillary lining cells or from intermediate cells of the same origin (Fig. 20–1). Heading the capillary column one can usually find an osteoclast that appears to have the same genesis (Fig. 20–2). A number of accounts[4] have suggested that the osteoblast, chondroblast, collagenoblast and histiocyte are all variations of the same cell type. Thus the inclusion of the capillary endothelial cell is less heretical than it may seem on first consideration. When sections of both giant cell tumors and giant cell reactions in bone are carefully studied one finds that most of the multinucleated cells lie within the lumina or walls of endothelial lined blood channels. This is particularly obvious in cases in which the lesion has been congested so that these channels are dilated (Fig. 20–3).

Most American writers have considered the giant cells of giant cell tumor as nonspecific cells of different type from osteoclasts. British authors, on the other hand, who call the giant cell tumor an osteoclastoma, have generally supposed the multi-

nucleated cell of the tumor to be a neoplastic form of the osteoclast. We have made a study of the matter and cast our vote on the side of the British. If the tumor cell is not a form of the osteoclast, the distinction cannot be made by any technique known to us at this time.

Thus inherent implication is made in the previous discussion that both giant cell tumor and giant cell reactions in bone are variations, neoplastic and reactive, of proliferating granulation tissue and are therefore of vascular origin. It is inferred that a proliferation of capillary buds is intrinsic to the production of large numbers of cells which, depending upon as yet unknown local factors, may develop into osteoblasts, chondroblasts, collagenoblasts or histiocytes. We infer that osteoblasts, again as the result of some unknown local or systemic (parathormone?) stimulus, merge to form osteoclasts and that osteoclasts, though perhaps not the sole agents of osteolysis, do play a role in bone resorption. If we can accept this concept of the origin and function of its cellular components, the giant cell tumor or, as we prefer to call it, the osteoclastoma may be conceived as a neoplasm with pathogenesis and behavior in accord with other oncologic entities.

Most of the misunderstanding associated with this tumor can be accredited to three facts stemming from certain peculiarities intrinsic to the healing and neoplastic proliferation of bone tissue. An understanding of these facts is essential for a correct concept of the tumor.

1. Whenever there is an injury to bone, particularly in the epiphyseal or adjacent metaphyseal areas of long bones, there is apt to be a florid, proliferative, reactive process. The matrix cells are spindled fibroblasts that are capable of maturing to collagenoblasts, chondroblasts or osteoblasts and they form giant cells which are identical in every morphologic feature with osteoclasts. The presence of the giant cells, whatever their exact nature and function, has given rise to the descriptive title of this lesion, benign giant cell tumor of bone. It is no more a neoplasm than is reparative callus an osteosarcoma, yet in both instances distinction may be difficult on the basis of microscopic appearance.

2. The principal cells of both osteosarcoma and chondrosarcoma, particularly when they affect the metaphyses of cylindrical bones are prone to form giant cells which again may be difficult to differentiate from the non-neoplastic variety on a morphologic basis. This type of osteosarcoma is highly malignant; we call it giant cell osteosarcoma. The chondrosarcoma is of very low grade malignant potential; we call it malignant chondroblastoma. Though both are neoplastic, neither can be regarded as osteoclastoma, though in the past they have been so classified.

3. Finally an elusive but none-the-less precise lesion of bone, aneurysmal bone cyst, which has very similar clinical, radiologic and microscopic features, has emerged over the past decade. Until recently it was generally confused with giant cell tumor. To make the matter infinitely more complex, the two lesions are often associated at the same site.

As a result of the above facts, giant cell reactions to bone injury, giant cell osteosarcomas and chondrosarcomas and aneurysmal bone cysts have all been, from time to time and in certain reports, mixed together in the classification of giant cell tumor of bone. It is little wonder that it now becomes impossible to evaluate the literature since the data refer to varying lesions whose behavior differs from healing reaction to highly lethal neoplasms.

We found it advisable to disregard all previous concepts and start anew, formulating our conclusions on contemporary cases as they have accumulated in our files. In doing so the lesion that emerges bears little resemblance to that shadowy enigma described in earlier reports. It is emphatically not a tumor that may be benign or malignant, that may involve any part of any bone in any age group. When giant cell lesions of bone are analyzed with the most painstaking care there emerges a tumor that rarely if ever involves other than the metaphyseal area of cylindrical bones within the first decade after fusion of the epiphysis, that is slowly growing but destructive and has a penchant for recurrence, that is always of low grade malignancy and that, if allowed to progress over a considerable period of time, is often, perhaps usually, superimposed by aneurysmal bone cyst. In the latter instance the behavior of the giant cell lesion changes to a much more rapidly destructive character, with pathologic fracture and extension into soft tissues.

We have suggested that the name of this lesion be limited to "osteoclastoma" thus attempting to dissociate it from the numerous other giant cell lesions with which it has been so regularly confused. The English have used this term almost from the outset and recent evidence indicating that the giant cell components of this tumor (if not osteoclasts) have the same progenitor cells, makes this an accurately descriptive name.

Finally, if the above observations are valid, then an inescapable conclusion becomes apparent. There is no such pathologic entity as giant cell tumor of bone. There are only a variety of giant cell reactions to a variety of bone injuries by hemorrhage, ischemia, infection or neoplasm. Osteoclasts normally arise from osteoblasts and they are normally present in great numbers in the growing bone in the metaphyses of cylindrical bones (the ring of Ranvier), where they are responsible for modeling. However, the progenitor cells remain and when an injury occurs at this site, giant cells are formed in the reaction. If the injury is related to normal collagenoblasts, chondroblasts or osteoblasts, the giant cells behave in physiologic fashion, carrying out their appointed duties. If the involved cells are neoplastic in nature, then so are the giant cells and the product is a giant cell osteosarcoma, a giant cell chondrosarcoma (chondroblastoma or chondromyxoid fibroma) or a giant cell collagenoblastoma. This last, or better yet a tumor with a slightly earlier cell progenitor (the fibroblast), is identical with osteoclastoma. More accurately it could be called giant cell fibrosarcoma. All clinical, radiologic and microscopic evidence, properly interpreted, leads to this conclusion.

The clinical aspects of fibrosarcoma (whether of bone or soft tissue) and of osteoclastoma are identical. They affect the same age group, they grow slowly but are infiltrative and destructive, they frequently recur and they metastasize late, usually to the lungs. The microscopic aspects are highly convincing. When neoplastic giant cells are added to the section of fibrosarcoma one has osteoclastoma. Indeed, if one searches through numerous sections of typical osteoclastoma, one is almost sure to find a few sections in which there is an absence of giant cells, presenting the precise histologic picture of fibrosarcoma. There is no report of the classic, textbook fibrosarcoma arising in the metaphysis of a cylindrical bone. If it did occur there, and we know of no reason why it should not, then it would probably give the radiographic picture of osteoclastoma.

We choose to believe that the osteoclastoma is nothing more than a fibrosarcoma which, because it arises in the metaphysis of a cylindrical bone, displays large numbers of tumor giant cells in its spindle cell matrix. If this be true then there would be little purpose in retaining the name "osteoclastoma." However, to attempt to eradicate the term from the minds of clinicians, radiologists and pathologists would be as futile as disclaiming the existence of flying saucers and the Loch Ness monster. We must content ourselves with the continued use of the name and pray that the outworn ideas of its origin and nature will be replaced by a concept nearer the truth.

The concept of osteoclastoma has been changing over the course of a century. For the first half of this period it was considered to be a benign tumor and descriptions of this lesion embraced such widely varying conditions as what we now recognize as chondroblastoma, brown tumor of hyperparathyroidism, solitary cyst and even reaction to hemorrhage. Ewing recognized a malignant form of the tumor but it was not until the definitive paper of Jaffe, Lichtenstein and Portis[5] that the concept was refined to exclude the lesions of hyperparathyroidism, bone reactions and bone cysts. These authors discovered on restudy of the cases in their files diagnosed as giant cell tumor that only about half were indeed giant cell tumors. The remainder, though presenting giant cells in their tissue sections, could not be included in the giant cell tumor category. During this same period we were reviewing our own material and arrived at the identical conclusions. We published our findings some years later.[6]

In the course of the ensuing several years seven new and distinct bone lesion entities were defined: non-osteogenic fibroma (1942),[7] solitary cyst (1942),[8] chondroblastoma (1942),[9] chondromyxoid fibroma (1948),[10] aneurysmal bone cyst (1950),[11] intraosseous villonodular synovitis (1954)[12] and osteoblastoma (1954).[13] Large numbers of giant cells may be found in the sections of all these lesions. It seems reasonable to presume that before definition of these entities, many instances of these conditions, particularly those with extravagant giant cell populations, were diagnosed giant cell tumors.

Because of this and because the concept as presented by Jaffe and Lichtenstein, i.e., a completely benign tumor (their class I), a malignant tumor (their Class III) or a tumor of intermediate type (their Class II) composed of two cell type components, seemed unrealistic in the general terms of oncology, and particularly because an attempt to prognose the behavior of giant cell tumors on the basis of the cell criteria[14] that they gave usually resulted in failure, we came to the inevitable conclusion that the giant cell tumor as a distinct clinicopathologic entity probably does not exist. We reasoned that the Class I lesions were all giant cell reactions to some type of bone injury, that the Class III tumors were all osteosarcomas, chondrosarcomas or fibrosarcomas with giant cell reactions and that the Class II category was a twilight zone, containing bone reactions with extraordinarily brisk cell proliferation and sarcomas with unusually slow cell division.

However, there is a clinical entity which must be dealt with. We can call it what we like, giant cell tumor of bone, osteoclastoma or a giant cell variant of fibrosarcoma. Whatever its definition we must recognize its features in order to diagnose it correctly; we must know how it will behave in order to treat it correctly. The following is an account of this specific lesion.

Clinical Aspects. Osteoclastoma most frequently occurs in young adults within 10 to 20 years after fusion of the epiphysis of the site involved. It is infrequently encountered after the age of 40; it rarely, if ever, involves the area of an unclosed epiphysis. Like most primary neoplasms it most commonly involves the distal end of the femur and the proximal end of the

tibia, the knee region, but more than any other true bone tumor it is apt to affect the distal end of the radius and the cylindrical bones of the hands and feet. Here its differentiation from enchondroma and aneurysmal bone cyst must always be considered, though the latter may occur concurrently with it. There are numerous accounts of osteoclastomas arising in the bones of the skull, particularly the jaws and the vertebrae. Bhaskar et al.[15] reviewed 104 giant cell lesions of the jaws without encountering a single case of true osteoclastoma. Jaffe[16] designated most giant cell lesions of the jaws as reparative granulomas. It is apparent that hemorrhage within the cancellous tissue of the jaws or related to their periodontal membranes or periosteum is often associated with a striking giant cell response. This lesion has been called central or peripheral giant cell epulis. These, despite their microscopic similarities, must not be confused with true osteoclastoma. We have never (with one possible exception) encountered an unequivocal osteoclastoma of a flat bone of the head or trunk including the jaws and vertebrae.

Though diagnosable osteoclastoma is

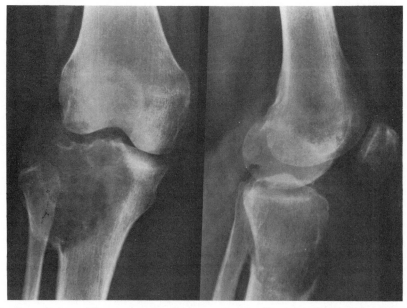

Figure 20–4   Osteoclastoma. The tumor in the tibia is eccentric and has expanded the bone laterally; however, a very thin shell of bone is evident around the periphery of the lesion. Fine trabeculae of bone traverse the area of destruction. No reactive bone is evident medially.

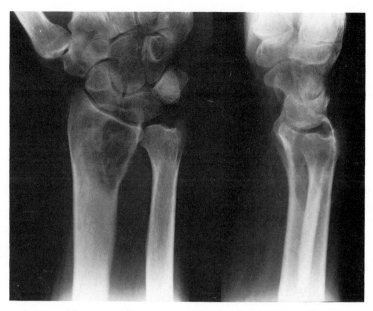

Figure 20–5 Osteoclastoma. The area of destruction in the distal end of the radius is eccentric. Its border is not distinct from surrounding cancellous bone of the metaphysis and shaft. The tumor abuts the subchondral bone.

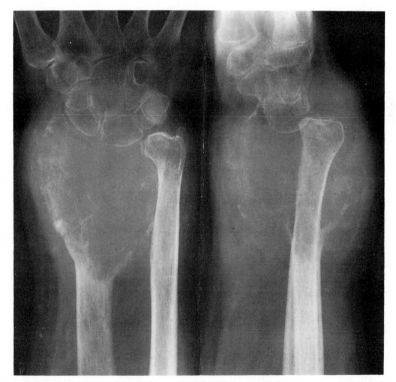

Figure 20–6 Osteoclastoma. This radiograph was exposed two years after the one illustrated in Figure 20–5. The area of destruction is huge and the distal end of the radius expanded. Only fragments of the expanded cortex are visible around the lesion. Extension distally has resulted in dislocation of the wrist. An aneurysmal bone cyst was found to be superimposed.

rarely seen until the involved growth center is closed, it almost certainly began at the site of the zone of interdigitation. Because this zone is effaced by fusion it is interesting to speculate if the tumor began at or about the time of the closure but grew so slowly that it could not be appreciated until years later. It begins within cancellous tissue and progresses to involve what was the epiphysis and somewhat less obviously the metaphysis. Though it must progress through the epiphyseal cancellous bone toward the articular plate, in its early stages we have found it risky to make a diagnosis on the basis of the radiograph until the full epiphyseal depth is involved (Fig. 20–4).

Characteristically the lesion is eccentric. It erodes the overlying cortex from within, at the same time stimulating the periosteum to lay down concentric layers of bone over its advancing peripheral margin. Thus, it is one of the few true bone neoplasms that causes cortical expansion. In some instances the progress is slow, in a few well documented cases, over a period of years. Sometimes, it is explosively rapid. This disparity in behavior suggests either that there are two types of osteoclastomas or that a second lesion is overlaid upon it. We believe that the latter is probably true and that the secondary lesion is aneurysmal bone cyst. More will be said about this in the section on differential diagnosis but the larger, the more destructive and the more rapid the growth, the more apt is the lesion to be a combined one (Fig. 20–6). In cases in which it is combined with aneurysmal bone cyst the osteoclastoma is exceedingly bloody. In cases in which it is uncombined it is more apt to be brown, resembling the brown tumor of hyperparathyroidism. In either event its vascular component is usually obvious. The complication with aneurysmal bone cyst explains cases in which the lesions are rapid in growth and wildly destructive. We have seen this combination of lesions completely destroy the head and proximal one third of the femur of a young adult male in six weeks.

Roentgenographic Manifestations. The primary radiographic manifestation of the osteoclastoma is bone destruction. Presumably related to the rate of its growth is the absence of reactive bone around its advancing margin. However, as the cortex is thinned and expanded, the periosteum attempts to cover the tumor with a shell of new bone. Incomplete septa are often evident within the substance of the tumor; these are remnants of trabeculae and are not newly formed bone (Fig. 20–5).

The osteoclastoma is most apt to involve the epiphysis of long bones, particularly the ends at which growth is most rapid. It is eccentric initially, but grows to involve the width of the bone. While it extends to the articular plate, it uncommonly destroys it. Aneurysmal bone cysts may be superimposed and result in extremely rapid growth, extensive destruction and a soft tissue component (Fig. 20–6).

Microscopy. Because the osteoclastoma, we believe, arises from cells that have the potential of becoming collagenoblasts, osteoblasts, chondroblasts or histiocytes we should expect to find vestiges of the products of these cells in this tumor. Collagen is the most commonly encountered intercellular substance. Some fields may be composed entirely of spindled cells elaborating large amounts of collagen and it may be impossible in those areas without giant cells to distinguish the lesion from fibrosarcoma. Tiny, irregular microspicules of osteoid are exceedingly common in sections of osteoclastoma (Fig. 20–7). We agree with the dictum that if considerable amounts of osteoid are found in these sections, the correct diagnosis is more apt to be giant cell osteosarcoma, but in cases in which the osteoid content is restricted to minute curved or curled spicules, the correct diagnosis is usually osteoclastoma. Small islands of chondroid, apparently elaborated by the matrix cells, are rare but their presence does not rule out the diagnosis (Fig. 20–8). Small aggregates of lipid-bearing histiocytes are not uncommon in osteoclastoma.

Some writers have counseled the microscopist to ignore the giant cells when evaluating the osteoclastoma. Occasionally we have found these cells offering the decisive evidence for a diagnosis. Usually they are closely ensheathed by the endothelial lining of the sinusoid of which they are a part. If the tissue was congested at the time the block was taken, the giant cell

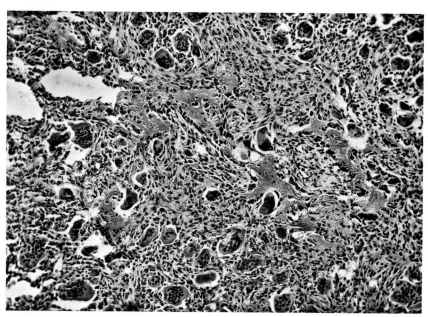

Figure 20–7   Osteoclastoma. It is usual to find small spicules of osteoid in this tumor. Because stromal cells are probably neoplastic osteoblasts, this finding should not surprise us. (× 110.)

appears to lie within the lumen of a blood filled sinusoid or it forms a portion of its wall. Because they may not arise directly from endothelial cells[2] but from intermediate cells of the same source, the sinusoidal architecture may not be apparent. Their nuclei in the visualized plane may number a few to more than 30 (Fig. 20–9). Chromatin is apt to be rather sparse. Mitotic figures are rare in most cases, but we have seen more than one instance in which they were common. We feel very sure that the giant cells are made up of merged matrix cells. In the reactive process the giant cells often show the sinusoidal relationship; they are large, discrete and their nuclei are apt to be numerous and regular. In the osteoclastoma the sinusoidal pattern is usually discernible if sought; the giant cells are often smaller, the nuclei fewer and their profiles less regular. Often the cells are less discrete, appearing partially merged with the surrounding matrix cells (Fig. 20–10).

We agree that the most important diagnostic evidence is provided by the cells of the stroma. But just as the cells of a youthful and florid fibromatosis may have all the morphologic features of a fibrosarcoma and a slowly growing example of the latter may

give the appearance of the more innocuous lesion, so it may be impossible to distinguish the giant cell reaction from the osteoclastoma on the basis of its cell constituents alone. Though we have spent many hours in deliberation over these sections we have been compelled to accept the previous statement as fact. Histochemical techniques have as yet provided no help. A careful analysis of the clinical and radiologic features often gives most rewarding assistance.

The differential features in the stromal cells are simply those of fibrosarcoma and as in fibrosarcoma, they are not always present. Occasionally the diagnosis is easy. Unbalanced mitotic figures appear in every field, collagen is scant and osteoid and chondroid are lacking (Fig. 20–11). Giant cells are small and indiscrete. Their nuclei are few and pleomorphic. One needs nothing more than the sections to make a firm diagnosis. In most cases the diagnosis is not so easy and in a few it is impossible. When such slides are encountered the final conclusion should lean heavily upon the clinical and radiologic features and the diagnosis of osteoclastoma made only after every other reasonable possibility has been ruled out. The

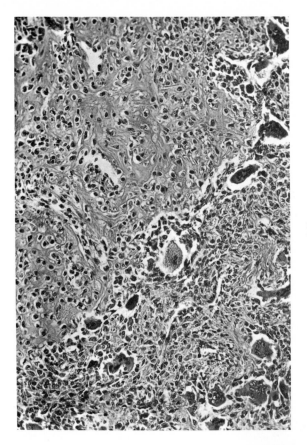

Figure 20–8 Osteoclastoma. Rarely one may find small, irregular islands of chondroid in this tumor. (× 110.)

Figure 20–9 Osteoclastoma. Giant cells should always be evaluated in osteoclastoma. Frequently they show features of the more malignant appearing stromal cells. (× 400.)

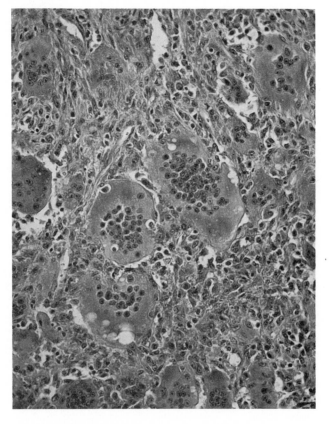

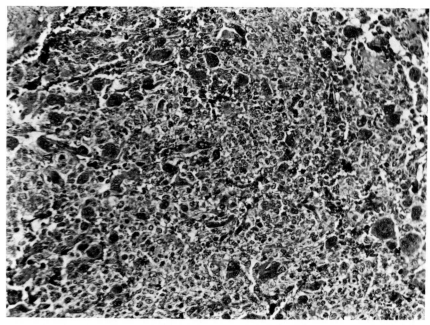

Figure 20–10   Osteoclastoma. The giant cells of this tumor are frequently smaller and contain fewer nuclei than those found in giant cell reactive processes. Sometimes they appear to merge with the stromal cells. (× 95.)

lesions that are most commonly diagnosed osteoclastoma on the basis of sections alone are aneurysmal bone cyst, intraosseous villonodular synovitis, brown tumor of hyperparathyroidism and giant cell reaction in response to hemorrhage of various causes within cancellous tissue. These conditions constitute the differential diagnosis of osteoclastoma.

Differential   Diagnosis.   Aneurysmal

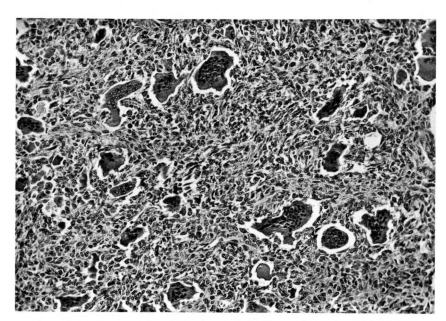

Figure 20–11   Osteoclastoma, a typical section. The stromal cells are obviously neoplastic. Because they produce neither osteoid nor chondroid, they more closely resemble the cells of fibrosarcoma. (× 110.)

bone cyst (see p. 507) is the curious response of bone tissue to the presence of multiple large fibrous walled channels, which are probably arteriovenous fistulas. The extreme vascularization of these lesions probably predisposes to hemorrhage, which in turn appears to provoke the production of large numbers of giant cells. In one report[17] six of seven aneurysmal bone cysts were diagnosed giant cell tumors.

In pure aneurysmal bone cyst the vascular channels should always be found, the giant cells are not usually so profuse, there is more evidence of hemorrhage and old blood pigment and, of course, the stromal cells should have an innocuous appearance. In recent years, however, we have been forced to the conclusion that aneurysmal bone cyst frequently is superimposed on osteoclastoma. Thus, some fields may present the classic features of tumor, whereas others show reactive tissue. Now a clear distinction is impossible.

We believe the unique pathogenesis of osteoclastoma, its origin from vessel-forming cells and its rich sinusoidal content make it peculiarly liable to aneurysmal bone cyst complication. There is much clinical and radiologic evidence as well that supports this hypothesis (Fig. 20–6). It explains the sudden growth spurt encountered in some osteoclastomas and the massive destruction that sometimes occurs. There can be little doubt now that aneurysmal bone cyst is usually engrafted on a preemptive lesion though the mechanism is still obscure. We believe that osteoclastoma is a common precursor of the aneurysmal bone cyst.

To make the distinction between aneurysmal bone cyst and osteoclastoma on microscopic sections alone is often easy; in other cases it is impossible. The diagnosis of the former should probably never be made without the obvious presence of the fibrous walled channels. The giant cell reaction is often spotty throughout the lesion and in the giant cell fields, these cells are not as numerous. There is apt to be more hemosiderin pigment and osteoid production. But the decisive quality of the lesion is the structure of its stromal cells. The stromal cells of the osteoclastoma are those of a true neoplasm. There are degrees of pleomorphism, hyperchromatism and mi-

toses that are usually not reached by the stromal cells of aneurysmal bone cyst. Unfortunately in some cases these differences are not great enough to permit distinction by methods available today.

Villonodular synovitis apparently occasionally involves subarticular cancellous bone tissue as well as joint and tendon sheath synovia. The pathogenesis of this curious lesion is still unknown but it is assumed that usually it begins within the joint and then penetrates, or creeps around the periphery of the articular plate. Because it is composed of a matrix of collagen-forming spindled cells with giant cells, on the basis of sections alone, it is usually most difficult to differentiate from osteoclastoma. Indeed, we believe that it is safe to presume that most of these lesions have been in the past and still are being misdiagnosed osteoclastomas. There are certain differences that should appear in the sections. The giant cells of villonodular synovitis are morphologically identical to those of osteoclastoma but they arise from cells that would normally produce synovial lining rather than vessel lining. Thus the spaces in which these cells lie should never contain blood cells except as artifacts. The difficulty arises in that both types of giant cells may arise from intermediate cells and thus spaces may be found in neither. Again, the red cells may have been drained or hemolysed from the spaces of the osteoclastoma. In many instances of villonodular synovitis the lining cells are apt to be more plump, resembling synovial lining cells rather than the flat, vascular sinusoid lining cells of osteoclastoma. One may get some help in making the differentiation from the radiographs. Evidence of intra-articular villonodular synovitis may accompany the intraosseous lesion and sometimes both bones on either side of the joint are involved. This is overwhelming evidence of villonodular synovitis.

We have little idea of the incidence of intraosseous villonodular synovitis. It is probably rather unusual because we encounter so few cases of the intra-articular type. But tenosynovitis is exceedingly common and no one has proved that the intraosseous lesion cannot arise as a result of metaplasia of the tissues native of the area, thus making it unnecessary to have the intraosseous type preceded by involvement of the joint synovia.

Brown tumor of hyperparathyroidism may be identical in some fields to the microscopic features of osteoclastoma. However, any microscopist who hands down the diagnosis of osteoclastoma without knowing the serum calcium and phosphorus levels is practicing a degree of abandon that will inevitably bring him the reputation he deserves. We usually refuse to make a firm diagnosis of hyperparathyroidism when the serum calcium level is below 12 mg. and one should be most reticent in making a diagnosis of osteoclastoma when the level is higher. The phosphorus level in hyperparathyroidism, of course, should be low but it varies considerably and is much less dependable. A multiplicity of lesions is presumptive evidence that they are not osteoclastomas. Though the giant cells of brown tumor, we believe, are frequently identical to those of osteoclastoma, the stroma should be less cellular, more hemorrhagic and less uniform. Though hyperparathyroidism is definitely unusual, the microscopist should never encounter a giant cell lesion without thinking of it. Failure to do so inevitably leads to an embarrassing oversight. The brown tumor is quite probably nothing more than a delineated area in which hemorrhage has occurred because of weakening and infraction of a bone in a stress area in hyperparathyroidism. Thus the lesion is quite similar to that of ordinary intraosseous hematoma except that the high parathormone level may predispose to a more florid giant cell reaction.

Giant cell reaction to intraosseous extravasation of blood has been only scantly noted in the American and English literature. This subject was reviewed by Cottier.[18] He noted that as early as 1912 the German pathologists Lubarsch[19] and Looser[20] recognized and described this entity. He produced giant cell reactions, cysts and areas of fibrous scarring by injecting autolysed and acidified blood into rabbit bones.

We have frequently seen extravagant giant cell reactions of bone following trauma and apparently more often following vascular damage due to other mechanisms. Because this reaction is rarely encountered in tissue removed from fracture sites its existence is denied by American pathologists and surgeons, though the giant cell "tumors" that occur in relation to the jaw in response to central or subperiosteal hemorrhage have been recognized for a long time. Why it occurs only occasionally following trauma and apparently more often following vascular damage without loss of integrity of the overlying cortical bone, we are not prepared to say. Elsewhere (see p. 324) we have described the post-traumatic rib cyst, which now appears to be a definite entity. Giant cell reactions play a more or less prominent part in the formation of these lesions. Because this process is not generally recognized among American pathologists it is reasonable to presume that most of these cases end up in giant cell tumor files.

In cases in which the preceding four conditions have been ruled out the chances are that the lesion is an osteoclastoma. One still must bear in mind that giant cell reactions may be caused by other mechanisms. Thus, we may find them the result of bone injury due to primary or metastatic bone tumor. If only the bone reaction is sampled by the surgeon a diagnosis of giant cell tumor is made. When the original tumor explodes in metastatic growth the process is called an innocuous giant cell tumor that has developed a remarkably malignant quality. Giant cell reactions may be found in solitary cysts, non-osteogenic fibromas, osteoblastomas, chondroblastomas, chondromyxoid fibromas, fibrosarcomas and osteosarcomas.

In cases in which the pathologist encounters a host of giant cells in the sections, he should attempt to diagnose the lesion as something other than osteoclastoma. Failing this, he should carefully analyze the clinical and radiologic features of the case. Only when all of the criteria are in favor of osteoclastoma should the firm diagnosis be made.

Treatment. If the previously discussed concept of osteoclastoma is accepted, i.e., a uniformly malignant tumor with a propensity for recurrence but late of metastasis, frequently overlaid by aneurysmal bone cyst, the treatment becomes immeasurably simpler than it has been in the

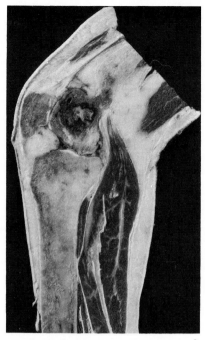

Figure 20–12　Osteosarcoma superimposed on an irradiated osteoclastoma.

cellent results. In the case of the large destructive tumors, particularly those with complicating aneurysmal bone cyst, it may be necessary to resort to amputation. At present it appears that if an osteoclastoma recurs, the patient has only about a 50 per cent chance of ultimate cure. This probably means that nearly all *correctly diagnosed* osteoclastomas which recur are lethal. Thus the initial treatment should be sufficiently radical to assure all concerned that the tumor is completely ablated, and there must be no doubt that the diagnosis is correct before therapy is undertaken. Only when a conservative attitude is coupled with the teamwork of able and informed orthopedists, radiologists and pathologists will the chaos that characterizes present day concepts of this unique tumor be dispelled. Then we may be able to collect and analyze our cases on the basis of valid statistics.

past. Until some such realistic concept is accepted, the orthopedist finds little solace in the pathologist's verdict that the tumor is benign, malignant or something in between. In the past his classification of this tumor into Class I, II or III has provided little more specific information on which to base therapy. X-ray therapy should probably never be used. Many lesions so treated have been converted to highly malignant osteosarcoma (Fig. 20–12). The lesion must be completely eradicated as conservatively as is compatible with the surgeon's best judgment. It is obvious that in some cases, curettage is sufficient but we have had to learn by experience that the number of these cases is in the minority. Worse, it is impossible to say in which cases this treatment is adequate. A safer procedure is block resection. Often, particularly in the non-weight-bearing limbs, a bone graft or prosthesis may be substituted for the resected bone with surprisingly ex-

References

1. Bloom, W., Bloom, M. and McLean, F.: Anat. Rec., *91*:443, 1945.
2. Johnson, W.: Arch. Pathol., *10*:197, 1930.
3. Trueta, J.: Scot. Med. J., *11*:33, 1966.
4. Bassett, A.: J. Bone Joint Dis., *44A*:1217, 1962.
5. Jaffe, H., Lichtenstein, L. and Portis, R.: Arch. Pathol., *30*:993, 1940.
6. Aegerter, E.: Am. J. Pathol., *23*:283, 1947.
7. Jaffe, H. and Lichtenstein, L.: Am. J. Pathol., *18*:205, 1942.
8. Jaffe, H. and Lichtenstein, L.: Arch. Surg., *44*:1004, 1942.
9. Jaffe, H. and Lichtenstein, L.: Am. J. Pathol., *18*:969, 1942.
10. Jaffe, H. and Lichtenstein, L.: Arch. Pathol., *45*:541, 1948.
11. Lichtenstein, L.: Cancer, *3*:279, 1950.
12. Carr, C., Berley, F. and Davis, W.: J. Bone Joint Surg., *36A*:1007, 1954.
13. Dahlin, D. and Johnson, E.: J. Bone Joint Surg., *36A*:559, 1954.
14. Goldenberg, R., Campbell, C. and Bonfiglio, M.: J. Bone Joint Surg., *52A*:619, 1970.
15. Bhaskar, J., Bernier, J. and Godby, F.: J. Oral Surg., Anesth. & Hosp. Dent. Ser., *17*:30, 1959.
16. Jaffe, H.: Oral Surg., *6*:159, 1953.
17. Beeler, J., Helman, C. and Campbell, J.: J.A.M.A., *163*:914, 1957.
18. Cottier, H.: Schweiz. Z. allg. Path., *15*:46, 1952.
19. Lubarsch, O.: Med. Klin., *41*:1651, 1912.
20. Looser, E.: Dtsch. Z. Chir., *189*:113, 1924.

DISEASES OF JOINTS AND MUSCLES; SOFT PART TUMORS

Chapter 21

ARTHRITIS

Pathologic alterations in structure and function of the tissues of the joints constitute the most important group of crippling diseases, from the standpoint of incidence and economic loss, in the world today. It has been estimated that more than 10 million people in America suffer from some type of arthritis and, of these, nearly a quarter of a million are completely disabled.

Because there are a considerable number of types of arthritis and some of these types are exceedingly complex with poorly understood pathogenesis, a detailed discussion of the subject would be far too lengthy for the limitations of this volume. The subject is included in this book because it has been our observation that too many clinicians regard the subject of arthritis as impossibly complex and it is obvious that they have never had a concept of a classification. A classification has been devised and is offered here with the hope that it may simplify the matter for those who feel they cannot master the complete texts, such as the excellent volume edited by Hollander.[1]

Because this book is concerned principally with pathogenesis and roentgenographic aspects of orthopedic diseases, our classification is based on the pathologic alterations that characterize the various processes. This simplifies the matter considerably inasmuch as joint tissues can express disease processes in only a limited variety of alterations. Because symptoms and physical findings in the joint diseases present a much wider and more subtle spectrum of variation, classifications based on clinical aspects are usually much more complex. The one used here is a modification of that suggested by the American Rheumatism Association with some regrouping, additions and change in order to facilitate the discussion from the standpoint of the pathologic alterations.

THE PATHOGENESIS OF ARTHRITIS

I. Secondary arthritis
Gout and pseudogout
Alkaptonuric arthritis
Hemophilic joint disease
Psoriatic arthritis
II. Degenerative joint disease
Osteoarthritis and arthritis of chronic trauma
Chondromalacia
Neurogenic arthropathy and congenital indifference to pain
Cortisone arthropathy
III. Villonodular synovitis
IV. Infectious arthritis
Suppurative arthritis
Nonsuppurative arthritis
V. Hypersensitivity (collagen disease) arthritides
Rheumatoid arthritis
Arthritis of the collagen diseases
VI. Miscellaneous types of arthritis
Intermittent hydrarthrosis
Palindromic rheumatism
Arthritis mutilans
Cysts of the menisci
Baker's cyst
VII. Diseases of periarticular tissues
Fibrositis
Bursitis
Ganglia
Synovial chondrometaplasia

623

Anatomists have divided the joints into three types. When two bones are connected by collagenous tissue such as that in the sutures of the infant calvarium the joint is called fibrous. Cartilaginous joints are those in which two bones are connected by a mass of cartilage, which acts as their growth center. Joints in which a fibrous capsule connects two bone members and defines a space between them that is lined with a synovial membrane are known as synovial joints. These joints are involved in arthritis. Before describing the disease alterations of these structures a review of the anatomy and physiology of synovial joints is important.

THE SYNOVIAL JOINTS

All the tissues of the joint structure — the fibrous capsule, the cartilage articular plates, the synovial lining and the collagenous and osteoid supportive structures — are mesenchymal in origin. They are apt to suffer, therefore, in diseases that result from perversion of mesenchymal tissue function, e.g., the hypersensitivity diseases, and those that are caused by collagen degradation, the collagen diseases, more properly termed mesenchymal diseases. They most often suffer from long continued traumatizing overuse, especially when inadequately nourished.

When a joint of the adult skeleton is sagittally sectioned one finds the end of each bone covered by a disc of hyalin cartilage, the articular plate (Fig. 21–1). This is the remnant of the cartilage mass that formed the epiphysis of the growing bone. This cartilage is supported at the periphery by a ring of very thin compacta and centrally by a network of arches of cancellous bone tissue. The capsule appears as a continuation of the periosteum as the latter approaches the periphery of the articular plate. Like the periosteum it is composed of heavy collagenous bands but it is thicker, and replacing the cambium there is a highly vascular layer, which is the synovial membrane. In the hinge-type joints the capsule is reflected backward from its attachment to form a fold over the portion of the ossified epiphysis that supports the articular plate. This fold allows

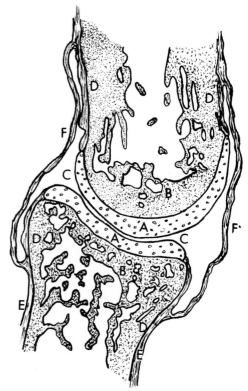

Figure 21–1   Drawing of a synovial joint. The articular plates, *A*, are supported by arches of cancellous bone, *B*, which rest upon the compacta, *D*, of the shaft. The capsule, *F*, is folded on itself to attach at the periphery of the articular plate enclosing the joint space, *C*. At the point at which it is reflected it merges with the periosteum, *E*.

movement of the two bones concerned in relation to each other without exerting excessive tension on the capsule. The synovial membrane is also attached at the periphery of the articular cartilage. The weight-bearing surfaces of the latter are naked. In areas in which the capsule is folded the synovia is thrown into finger-like villous processes. Elsewhere it consists of a layer of rounded, rather plump mesothelial cells resting on a loose fibrous connective tissue (Fig. 4–39, page 73), which contains an extraordinary number of small vessels. The joint ligaments merge with and support the capsule. Ligamentous tissue is less cellular, more densely collagenous and less vascular than capsule tissue.

It should be noted that the arteries that supply the joint tissues arise from the same source as those that supply the contiguous end of the adjacent bone. They branch within the capsule and form a capillary network within the synovia. The veins from the synovia merge with those from the metaphysis. There is also a rich communication of lymphatic channels between the synovia and the metaphysis and the importance of this becomes apparent in discussing the infectious diseases of either area.

A consideration of the physiology of these tissues is pertinent to an understanding of the pathogenesis of the diseases that affect them. The articular plate is composed of laminae of chondroid, which consists of a feltwork of collagen fibers in a gel ground substance, largely chondroitin sulfate. Because the refractive indices of the fibers and ground substance are about the same, the fibers are not visible by transmitted light. Thus the substance has a glassy appearance and, therefore, is called hyalin cartilage.

Though the chondrocyte is admirably adapted to living at low oxygen tension it must receive some oxygen and nutrition. The adult articular plate usually has no vessels. This means that nutrient materials must reach the cells by seeping along the submicroscopic planes between the laminae to reach the cells from other sources. These sources are the plexuses of vessels in the subchondral cancellous tissue and those of the joint capsule in the region of attachment for the deeper two thirds of the chondroid and for the superfi-

cial layers of the articular plate, i.e., those that bound the joint cavity, from the synovial fluid. Truetta believes that the alternate compression of exercise is an important factor in "pumping" nutrient-bearing fluid through the chondroid to the cells and that without exercise the cells eventually atrophy, the lacunae enlarge and merge to form cysts, the surface integrity is lost and the plate disintegrates, causing degenerative joint disease. Whether this be true or not it is obvious that the synovial fluid plays an important role in the nutrition and health of the articular plate. This fact is too little stressed by those interested in joint disease. A discussion of this matter helps to explain the pathogenesis of several types of arthritis.

Synovial fluid is a dialysate of blood plasma plus mucin. It contains essentially the same electrolytes and antibodies as those found in plasma. In addition, it contains large quantities of hyaluronic acid loosely bound to protein. It is obvious that the fluid elements of synovial fluid are dialyzed through the synovial membrane from its plexus of vessels. It is supposed that the mucinous portion, the hyaluronic acid, is secreted directly into the synovial fluid by the surface synovial cells. When the synovia and its vessels are healthy the dialyzing function is extremely efficient in maintaining a normal and delicate balance between the synovial fluid and blood plasma. Permeating fluids injected into the blood appear in the synovial fluid in min-

TABLE 21-1   CHARACTERISTIC FEATURES OF ARTHRITIS FOR USE IN ANALYSIS OF SYNOVIAL FLUID

| Type | Gross Appearance | | Viscosity | Acetic Acid Clot | Cells | | Urate Crystals | Cartilage Debris | Bacteria in Smear or Culture |
	Color	Clarity			WBC	RBC			
Normal	Clear straw	Clear	Viscid (high)	Good	200± 25% N.	0	0	0	0
Traumatic	Amber to bloody	Hazy to bloody	High	Good	1,500± 40% N.	Few to many	0	+	0
Degenerative joint disease	Yellow to straw	Clear to sl. hazy	High	Good	800± 20% N.	Rare	0	Many fragments and fibrils	0
Gout	Yellow to milky	Cloudy to turbid	Fairly low	Fair to poor	15,000± 75% N.	Rare	Many	0	0
Rheumatoid arthritis	Yellow to greenish	Cloudy to turbid	Decreased to low	Fair to poor	20,000± 75% N.	Rare	0	0	0
Infectious arthritis	Grayish creamy to bloody	Turbid	Low	Poor	50,000± 90% N.	Few to many	0	0	Few to many

utes and they have been shown to travel in the opposite direction in a somewhat longer interval. Substances of small molecular size are removed from the joint directly by means of the capillaries in the synovia. Particulate matter is removed by macrophages through the lymphatics. Normal synovial fluid contains about 200 cells per cubic millimeter. The cells are the same and in about the same proportions as those found in tissue fluids, i.e., lymphocytes, plasma cells, macrophages, red cells and granulocytes. The last should not exceed 25 per cent in a normal cell population.

Analysis of the synovial fluid of the involved joint is a most helpful aid in diagnosing and differentiating the various types of arthritis. In our hospital we maintain a special rheumatology laboratory in which this procedure is carried out. Table 21–1 is a chart of the features that characterize the five most commonly encountered types of arthritis.

The functions of the synovial fluid are twofold: lubrication and nourishment of the articular cartilage. Failure of either results in a deleterious effect upon the plate. The viscous (lubricating) quality of the fluid may be altered by impairment of the secretory capacity of the synovial cells, by dilution in effusion, or alteration by mixing with exudate or by depolymerization by chemicals, bacteria or enzymes. The nutrient-supplying capacity of the fluid may be impaired by alterations of the blood supply in the synovia (thrombosis, inflammation, sclerosis, etc.), by changes in the quality of the fluid (hemorrhage, exudates) or by barriers set up at the cartilage level such as a pannus of fibrin or granulation tissue.

If one is cognizant of the importance in maintaining a normal synovial fluid it is easier to appreciate the pathogenesis of many diseases that beset joint tissues.

SECONDARY ARTHRITIS

Several types of arthritis are merely the joint manifestation of a more generalized disease. Such is the case, of course, of the rheumatoid group, but because these will be discussed together in a special section, the more varied types are grouped together for consideration here.

Gout

Gout is a congenital disturbance in uric acid metabolism probably caused by an excessive formation of uric acid, which is deposited in various mesenchymal tissues as monosodium urate crystals which provoke an inflammatory reaction in the involved tissues. The exact mechanism of the production of this inflammatory response is of course unknown but an attractive hypothesis suggests that the urate crystals are adsorbed to or phagocytized by the granulocytes. The latter are known to degranularize. It is assumed that the salt crystals break down the lysosome capsules freeing cathepsin into the tissue. The latter hydrolyzes the ground substance of collagen, cartilage and bone. When sufficient amounts of tissue are involved there may be a systemic reaction of fever and anorexia. In the late stages of progressive gout, joints are destroyed, kidney function may be impaired and deposits in the collagen structures of the heart may lead to cardiac insufficiency.

Primary gout is inherited by an autosomal dominant gene with low penetrance in the female. More than 90 per cent of cases are in males. In females the deposition of urates apparently does not usually begin until menopause whereas in males deposition probably begins at puberty. Probably all patients with primary gout have increased serum uric acid levels some time during the course of the disease, and if the families of these patients are examined, hyperuricemia is found in about 25 per cent. The earlier the disease is manifested, the more severe it is apt to be.

The disease in its classic form consists of repeated attacks of arthritis involving one or more joints, the first metatarsophalangeal joint being the most common. The onset of each attack is apt to be dramatically sudden and is characterized by angry flushing of the skin, swelling, pain and exquisite tenderness. There may be effusion. It is obvious that the joint and periarticular tissues are involved in an acute inflammatory reaction. Each attack may last a few days to two weeks or even longer; then the symptoms spontaneously subside, and until deposits of urates have caused joint destruction, joint function returns to normal.

A few patients suffer only one acute attack, without recurrence. In most victims of the disease the attacks are repeated, the intervals becoming shorter and shorter, more and more joints being involved and greater and greater destruction resulting as the urate salts accumulate. In the very severe cases these collections of urates, called tophi, in nonarticular tissues lead to

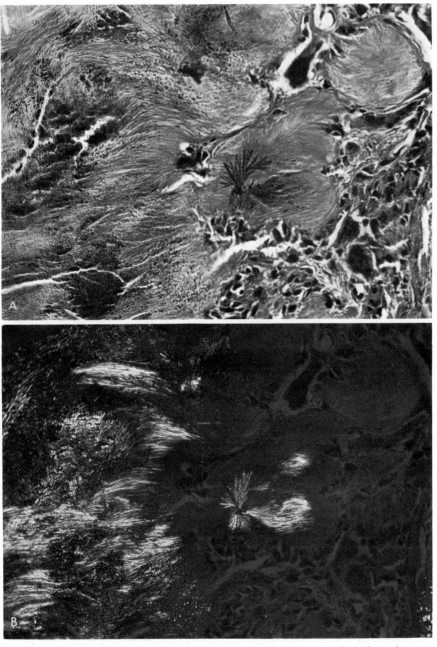

Figure 21–2 Gouty tophus. *A*, The urate crystals, dark linear bodies, are seen throughout the section. In the central area they are arranged in a sheaf. In the lower right one sees the giant cell foreign body reaction of the tissues. *B*, The same field taken with polarizing lenses. (× 330.)

serious systemic disease, which may terminate in uremia or cardiac failure.

Urate salts are deposited in sheaves of sharp pointed crystals in the affected tissues, and either their mechanical or their chemical properties, or both, cause an inflammatory reaction with the production of granulation and a giant cell foreign body reaction (Figs. 21–2 and 21–3). It appears that the increased blood flow of active inflammation plays a role along with the release of lysosomal cathepsin in causing the dissolution of cartilage and bone and the healing process promotes the growth

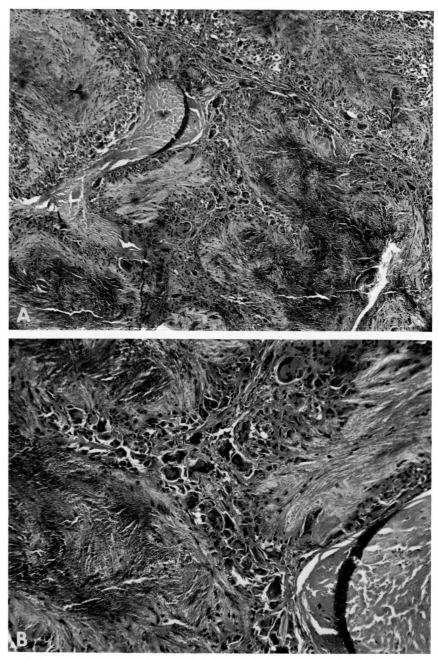

Figure 21–3   Gouty tophus. *A*, Numerous focal areas of sodium urate deposits with surrounding foreign body tissue reaction. (× 40.) *B*, A higher magnification of the tissue reaction between the nodules of crystals. (× 150.)

of a thick collagenous capsule. The tophi measure a few millimeters to several centimeters in diameter (Fig. 21–4). When near the surface they may ulcerate to discharge a white pasty mass of sodium urate. They are often first apparent when they involve the cartilage of the ear, usually the helix.

Because joint structures are composed entirely of cartilage, collagen or bone it is not surprising that these tissues are most commonly involved. Crystals are deposited in the synovia to which the urate salts are brought by the blood. From here they get out into the synovial fluid and then are deposited on the articular surfaces. The inflammatory reaction that they stimulate causes a pannus of granulation to form. In areas in which this comes in contact with the cartilage, the latter undergoes resorption perhaps because of the action of urate-released lysosomal hydrolases or the increased oxygen tension, which appears to act in the same manner. The cavity is eventually filled in with precipitated urates, inflammatory exudate including giant cells and collagen-producing fibroblasts. There may be effusion. The lesion increases in size to cause bone resorption and x-ray alteration. Tophi occur not only in synovia, articular cartilage and its supportive bone but also in the capsule, ligaments, subchondral marrow and even muscles. Extensive joint involvement may fill the cavity with fibrous pannus, which may calcify and later ossify, causing a stiff, useless joint.

In the kidneys, crystals of sodium urate are found in the capillary tuft of the glomerulus and in the lining cells particularly of the collecting tubules. Inflammatory reaction here leads to vascular sclerosis and eventually arteriolonephrosclerosis. The collagen structures of the heart may be the site of tophus formation and these may lead to valvular disease or muscle destruction. After the large toe the intertarsal joints and those of the fingers, ankles and wrists are most likely to be involved.

Secondary gout may occur because of excessive breakdown of nucleoproteins in such diseases as polycythemia, leukemia, multiple myeloma and sickle-cell anemia. The lesions produced are identical to those of primary gout.

The pathogenesis of the acute attack is unknown. Though probably all patients with primary gout have hyperuricemia, the high serum levels are not related to the attacks. The chronic arthritis and joint destruction are of course due to the presence of tophi and the inflammatory reaction they induce.

A number of laboratory tests are helpful in cases in which the diagnosis of gout is suspected. The serum urate level should always be determined. Though a normal level does not rule out gout, in the absence of treatment it makes this diagnosis unlikely. If there is joint effusion the fluid may be aspirated and searched for crystals of sodium urate. These are needle shaped, usually with pointed ends (Fig. 21–2). They exhibit negative birefringence with polarized light subjected to a mica retardation plate.[2] They are digested with uricase. In the early phases of the disease they are usually found within the granulocytes. Later they are found free in the fluid. The finding of crystals is one of the most helpful and certain procedures in making the diagnosis. Tophi may be aspirated and examined through the microscope. Tissue biopsy by needle aspiration has been reported successful in a small series of cases.[3]

Roentgenographic Manifestations. The earliest radiographic evidence of gout is swelling of the soft tissues around the affected joint, a reflection of effusion into the joint and inflammation of the overlying tissues. The swelling tends to involve the more superficial soft tissues and to be sym-

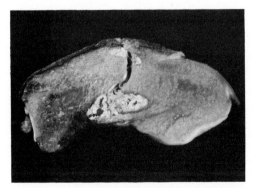

Figure 21–4 Gout. A large toe was sagittally sectioned to reveal a tophus of the anterior portion of the metatarsophalangeal joint. The nail is at upper right. The tophus has eroded the articular plates and bones and ulcerated the overlying skin surface.

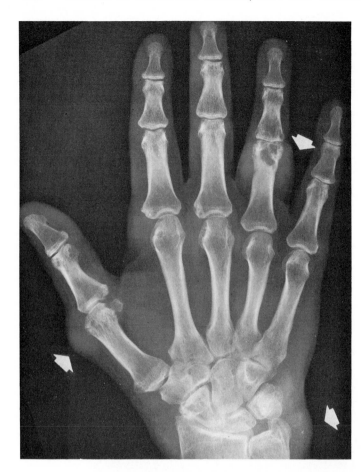

Figure 21–5 Gout. There are multiple areas of involvement in the hand and wrist (arrows). There is soft tissue swelling, a tophus, in relation to the distal end of the first metacarpal in which there are small foci of destruction. More extensive osseous and soft tissue alterations are present in the fourth digit.

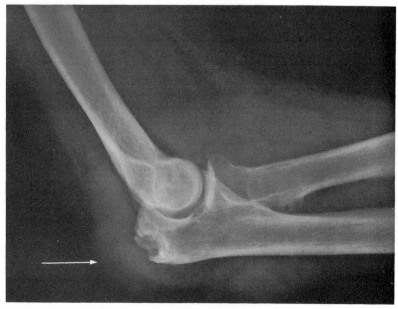

Figure 21–6 Gout. Localized swelling, a tophus, is evident in relation to an area of destruction in the olecranon process. There is bone reaction around the osseous defect as well as an overhanging lip extending outward from the lower margin of the defect.

metric about the joint except in the localized area of the tophus. The latter is nonopaque but may calcify as the disease progresses. It may be intracapsular or may occur in the subcutaneous tissues.

The destruction of bone in relation to a tophus is characterized by a defect with sclerotic margins and an overhanging edge, manifestations of bone reaction to the process (Fig. 21–6). There may be extensive osseous destruction and soft tissue alterations in a joint with preservation of the joint space.[4] However, such involvement of a joint may result eventually in osseous ankylosis.[5]

Treatment. It has long been known that gout is a disturbance of purine metabolism and the limiting of purine-rich foods as a part of the therapy regimen is traditional. Better comprehension of the routes of purine metabolism recently charted makes it seem doubtful if this restriction has accomplished anything because apparently most uric acid in man is synthesized from simpler chemical components. Today a number of drugs are available that induce increased uric acid elimination through the kidney with reduction of serum urate levels. These are known as uricosuric agents. They include salicylates in large doses, colchicine, probenecid, phenylbutazone and adrenal cortical and corticotropic hormones. If the acute attack is treated with colchicine or phenylbutazone immediately upon onset and probenecid given in the intervals as a prophylactic, and if the patient is taught to avoid such precipitating events as bouts of alcoholism, exposure, exhaustion and trauma, the patient with primary gout may live a life of normal duration with but a minimum of pain and inconvenience.

Pseudogout (Chondrocalcinosis)

In the past several years a number of reports have appeared describing cases of a peculiar calcification of the articular plate in one or more joints (Fig. 21–7). Some of these cases have been associated with joint disease resembling rheumatoid arthritis. The disease appears to have a familial incidence. Dr. Warner Bundens has allowed us to examine the sections

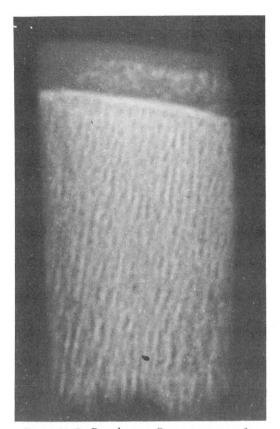

Figure 21–7 Pseudogout. Roentgenogram of resected proximal fibula showing flecks and striations of opaque calcium salts in the articular plate. (Courtesy of Dr. Warner Bundens.)

from such a case. This condition is best described in the American literature by McCarty et al.[6] under the title of "pseudogout." The disease has been described in the European literature as chondrocalcinosis.

This arthritis closely simulates gout clinically though there are certain rather constant differences. The condition is more apt to affect the knee rather than the first metatarsophalangeal joint though it has been noted in almost every joint in the body including the sternoclavicular joint. The onset may be sudden or insidious, causing pain, tenderness, swelling, heat and redness. The attacks last one to several days with remissions of months. Most patients are in the latter half of life. Like gout the disease is seen more often in patients who have hypertension or diabetes mellitus. Attacks may be initiated by exposure,

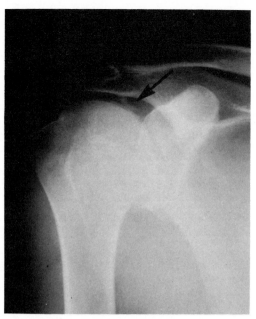

Figure 21–8   Pseudogout. Calcification of cartilage of the head of the humerus is present (arrow).

Roentgenographic Manifestations.
The radiographic manifestations of pseudogout are those of swelling of the joint and calcification of cartilage, particularly in relation to joints. In the acute episode only effusion into the joint may be seen; in cases in which the disease is chronic, calcification and degenerative alterations may be evident. Calcification of cartilage in sites other than the articular plates has been reported,[6] e.g., the ear. Calcification of the menisci of the knee has been seen as well as calcification in the bursa of the knee. Localized areas of destruction of the subchondral bone have been noted that are quite similar to those associated with gout.

There may be roentgen findings in joints that are not associated with symptoms. It is to be noted that such calcification of cartilage may occur in hyperparathyroidism and diabetes as well as in other arthritides, such as gout and rheumatoid arthritis. The condition in this country is sometimes referred to as chondrocalcinosis, whereas the symptomatic form is called pseudogout.

Alkaptonuric Arthritis

Alkaptonuria is a hereditary inability to oxidize homogentisic acid. This substance, an intermediary metabolite of phenylalanine and tyrosine, accumulates in the body fluids and spills over into the urine. The inability to oxidize homogentisic acid is apparently due to the congenital absence of its oxidizing enzyme in the liver cells.[7] The defect is transmitted by a single recessive autosomal gene. As homogentisic acid is oxidized it forms a dark brown to black pigment. Freshly voided urine appears normal but as it stands and becomes alkaline the color develops. Homogentisic acid is a reducing agent and, with Benedict's reagent, used for testing for the presence of sugars in urine, it forms a yellow precipitate. This should not be mistaken for the positive sugar reaction because in alkaptonuria the supernatant urine reveals the characteristic darkening. Homogentisic acid reduces other substances as well, and the reduction of silver on photographic film and of molybdate in urine serves as empiric tests for this substance.

trauma, surgery or injections of mercurial diuretics. Several cases have been associated with pernicious anemia. The disease is apparently hereditary and familial. Patients may have had symptoms for 20 to 40 years before a correct diagnosis is made. The serum chemistry, including calcium, phosphorus, alkaline phosphatase, uric acid and homogentisic acid levels, remains normal.

The diagnosis is made by eliciting a pertinent history, by noting characteristic roentgenograms, and most important by finding the crystals of a calcium salt rather than urate crystals in the synovial fluid. These crystals are said to be the hydrated calcium salt of a complex phosphate closely resembling pyrophosphate.[6] They are produced in rodlike and rhombic forms. In the acute stage they are found within the granulocytes; in the chronic phase they are apt to be free in the fluid. Injection of these crystals into the joint of a human and into dogs causes an acute synovitis. The crystals are not digested by uricase and they are birefringent by polarized light.[2] The diagnosis has been made by use of needle biopsy.[3]

The symptoms in a few cases apparently have been relieved by treatment with colchicine.

If the homogentisic acid accumulates in sufficient amounts over a long enough period, usually by the thirtieth yeãr, a granular brown to black pigment is deposited in numerous tissues of mesenchymal origin. Apparently these tissues have an affinity for this pigment just as they do for sodium urate in gout. When sufficient amounts are eventually collected by the collagen in the cutaneous tissues, the sclerae[8] and the cartilage of the ear and nose, which lie close to the epidermis, the dark color appears through the overlying tissue and this condition is known as ochronosis (Fig. 21–9). Cartilage apparently has a special affinity for homogentisic pigment and when sufficient amounts are aggregated within the articular plates there is death of the chondrocytes and calcification of chondroid. This occurs in probably less than one third of patients

with ochronosis so that arthritis is a rather exotic entity occurring in only a small percentage of patients with alkaptonuria.

The most common site of arthritic involvement is the spine. Alkaptonuric spondylitis is more common in males in whom it occurs at a younger age than it does in females. The intervertebral plate becomes blackened, then it atrophies and eventually calcifies, being ultimately replaced by a craggy mass of coal black mineral. The normal spinal curves are effaced and movement of one vertebra on the next is lost. A poker spine similar to that of ankylosing spondylitis is the eventual result. A lumbar and dorsal kyphosis develops. There is loss of stature because of reduction in the height of the discs. In severe cases the peripheral joints may be affected. There is pigmentation and degeneration of the articular plates and an ac-

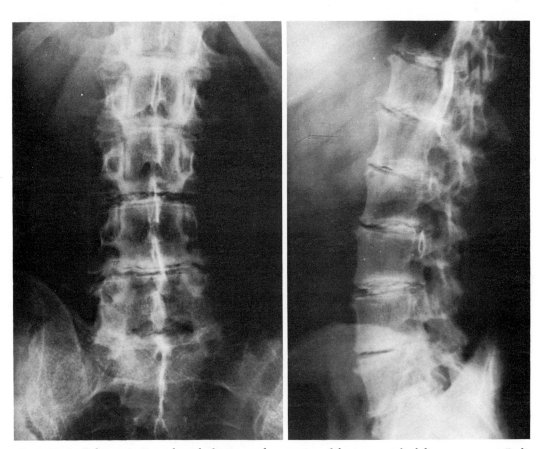

Figure 21–9 Ochronosis. Irregular calcification and narrowing of the intervertebral discs are present. Radiolucent streaks, evident anteriorly between the vertebral bodies, are not uncommon. There is only minimal lipping of the vertebral bodies. (Courtesy of Dr. Samuel Fisher.)

companing inflammatory reaction may cause effusion. This arthritis may result in pain, tenderness and limitation of motion. The commonest sites of involvement are the knees, shoulders and hips. The cartilage becomes brittle and eventually may fragment.

A curious complication of alkaptonuric arthritis is the stimulation of the synovial cells lining tendon sheaths to form cartilaginous bodies in the periarticular tissues. These may calcify and then ossify, producing the roentgenographic picture of periarticular tenosynovial chondrometaplasia. (See p. 682.)

Other tissues that may be involved in alkaptonuria are the trachea, the walls of vessels, the tympanic membrane (sometimes causing loss of hearing), the valve cusps of the left side of the heart (sometimes producing murmurs), and the prostate, in which pigment calculi may cause prostatic enlargement. Renal calculi may form and necessitate surgical intervention.[9]

Hemophilic Joint Disease

Hemophilia is the generic term for a group of diseases characterized by a defect in the clotting mechanism. These diseases have been divided into eight types depending upon the plasma protein deficiency responsible for the defect.[10] Most cases of hemophilia fall into two groups and these deficiencies are transmitted by a sex-linked dominant gene. Hemorrhage results from trauma, often so trivial that the patient himself is unaware that it has occurred.

More than three quarters of patients with hemophilia suffer episodes of acute hemarthrosis. When these episodes are repeated, eventual damage to the joint occurs, the failure to return to normal function being more apparent with each episode. Eventually deformity and ankylosis may be complete. The pathogenesis of the arthritis is actually unknown but we believe that repeated bleeding into the joint cavity disturbs the blood-synovial fluid balance and interferes with nutrition of the cartilage plate. The surface becomes pitted, often in a geographic pattern. Deposi-

tion of huge amounts of hemosiderin, residuum of hemolyzed red cells, within the synovia probably leads to fibrin production with thickening of the membrane and sclerosis of the vessels. In this stage the membrane resembles that of pigmented villonodular synovitis. Further impairment of nutrition of the cartilage follows and the pits deepen and extend into the subchondral bone. Peripheral cartilage hyperplasia may occur but this is never marked.

Several theories have been offered to explain the cartilage destruction that occurs in repeated hemarthroses. Experimentally, plasmin, a fibrinolysin, has been shown to cause lysis of cartilage to some extent. It has been proposed that this is the

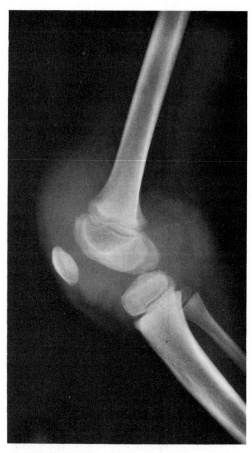

Figure 21–10 Hemophilia. There is massive distention of the knee joint as a result of hemorrhage into it. There is irregular synovial thickening present as well as blood. Osseous alterations are minimal.

mechanism that pertains in hemophilic arthritis.[11]

Three complications of hemophilic arthritis are worthy of mention. There may be accelerated maturation of the epiphysis adjacent to the affected joint. The reason for this has not been satisfactorily defined. There also may be massive subperiosteal hemorrhage about the end of the shaft of a long bone in hemophilia. The appearance may then closely simulate severe scurvy. Intraosseous hemorrhage into the cancellous tissue produces the large tumor-like mass known as pseudotumor of hemophilia. Because of the giant cell reaction to hemorrhage this has been mistaken for osteoclastoma. Often there is dramatic expansion of the cortex over the hematoma. These have much the same appearance in the radiograph as aneurysmal bone cyst and indeed, the pathogenesis is almost certainly the same.

The hemarthroses always begin early in childhood and become less frequent as the patient ages. They may cease entirely after puberty.

Treatment consists of supplying the lacking serum protein that is responsible for the clotting defect. The patient must be carefully studied to determine which factor this is. Transfusion with fresh blood or freshly frozen blood supplies the deficient protein in most cases.

Roentgenographic   Manifestations. The radiographic manifestations of hemophilic arthritis result from bleeding into the joint. A single episode is marked only by swelling of the joint. Soft tissue swelling, irregular synovial thickening, is associated with repeated hemorrhages. Repeated episodes result in the destruction of cartilage, eburnation of the subchondral bone, the erosion of subchondral bone, eventual narrowing of the joint and, in the adult, degenerative spurring in areas of weight bearing. The subchondral erosions are cystic and tend to be multiple. The bones of the joint may in time enlarge. In the child, the deformity of epiphyses may be marked as a result of irregular overgrowth. Particularly is this seen at the ankle where there may be slanting of the tibiotalar joint. Ir-

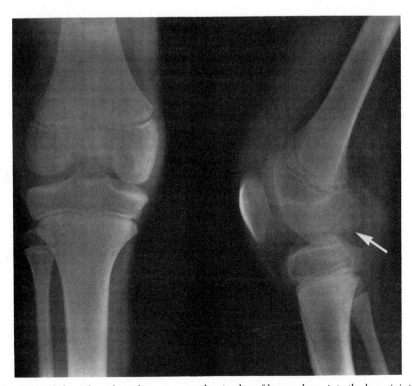

Figure 21–11   Hemophilia. There have been repeated episodes of hemorrhage into the knee joint. The suprapatellar pouch is slightly distended. The intercondylar notch is wide and irregular in outline. Subchondral cystic areas (arrow) are present in the femoral condyle.

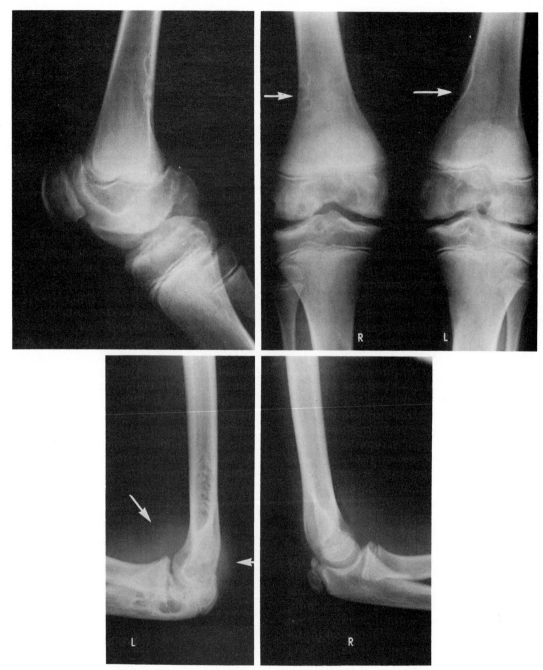

Figure 21–12   Hemophilia. There are multiple cystic lesions on the bones of the knee and the left elbow as a result of intraosseous hemorrhages. The inferior aspect of the patella is straight. Incidental benign cortical defects are present in both femurs (arrows). The elbow joint is distended by blood and thickened synovium (arrows).

regular and premature closure of epiphyses may occur as well, adding to the deformity. Localized hemorrhage into a bone at times causes an area of destruction and evokes new bone formation that may mimic a malignant neoplasm.

Other Diseases Associated with Arthritis

Certain other diseases may be accompanied by manifestations of joint disease. In these the joint disturbance resembles a prodromal stage or a mild form of rheumatoid arthritis in most instances. At present there is no satisfactory explanation for the arthritic components in these diseases.

Patients with *psoriasis* not infrequently (probably less than 10 per cent) manifest symptoms of joint disease. Though the latter most closely resembles rheumatoid arthritis, only rarely does it progress to cause the extreme joint destruction and loss of function that characterize that condition. Recurrences appear suddenly and are apt to be more complete. Because rheumatoid arthritis and psoriasis are common diseases in the same age group it is inevitable that they coexist in a percentage of patients, thus accounting for some of these cases. But the inflammatory reaction of psoriasis, which usually affects the skin, may affect the synovia, presenting a pathologic picture that cannot be differentiated from rheumatoid arthritis. It is notable that the arthritic symptoms of these patients usually improve with treatment for the skin manifestations. Psoriasis is most frequently associated with ankylosing spondylitis.

Perhaps one quarter of patients who suffer from *agammaglobulinemia* also have arthritis (Fig. 21–14). In this instance, both clinical and pathologic aspects of the joint disease are those of a mild rheumatoid arthritis. The episodes of inflammation are transient and regress rapidly without residua of joint tissue destruction. The association of these two conditions raises some interesting questions concerning the pathogenesis of each. Because gamma globulin is the seat of antibody, the arthritis of agammaglobulinemia can hardly be said to be the result of antigen-antibody reaction.

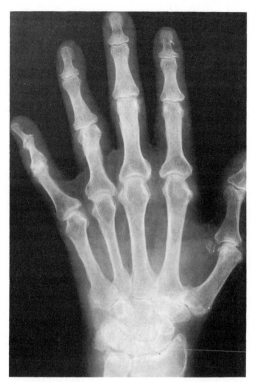

Figure 21–13 Psoriatic arthritis. There is involvement of the distal interphalangeal joint of the fourth and fifth digits. Flexion deformity of the fifth digit is evident with considerable destruction and narrowing of the distal interphalangeal joint. Deossification is not present. Ankylosis of involved joints may occur.

In these cases there obviously is no rheumatoid factor. This fact suggests that the rheumatoid factor is only a byproduct and not an etiologic factor in the disease. The association of agammaglobulinemia and rheumatoid arthritis does not, however, necessarily preclude the possibility that the latter may be the result of a perversion of function of the cells that normally supply antibody and related tissues of the same cell genesis.[12] It is almost certainly more than coincidence that in all the collagen diseases, including rheumatoid arthritis, alterations of one kind or another in the immune mechanism play an important role.

It has been noted that there is an increased incidence of arthritis in patients with *ulcerative colitis*. The joint symptoms are usually relatively mild and clear with little or no residual damage to joint tissues. In rare instances it may become chronic

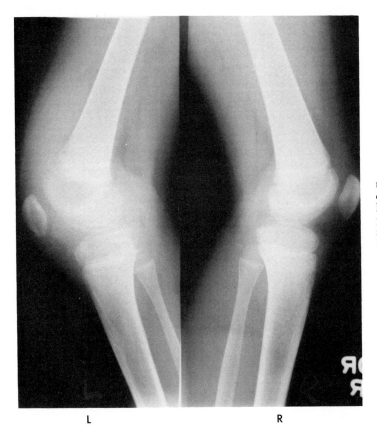

Figure 21–14 Agammaglobuline-mia, male, 11 years of age. There is extensive synovial reaction on the left; no osseous alterations are apparent except deossification. Left x-ray is left leg; right x-ray is right leg.

L   R

and destroy articular cartilage. Structural changes have been inadequately investigated but apparently show nothing to distinguish this condition from rheumatoid arthritis. The rheumatoid factor has been isolated only from patients with the unusual, severe form of the disease. Both peripheral arthritis and spondylitis have been reported. The prognosis for the latter is much poorer than for the former. The arthritis is reported to have cleared following radical surgery for the ulcerative disease in the bowel.

DEGENERATIVE JOINT DISEASE

Occasionally, a single episode of gross, acute trauma may produce joint changes that may be classified as arthritis. Most such trauma causes bone fracture within the joint or strain or sprain of ligaments outside the joint and these are usually not included under the heading of arthritis. Repeated minor trauma, often occupational, results in what is today best called degenerative joint disease, not implied in the term traumatic arthritis. If trauma breaches the integrity of the surface of the articular plate, or causes a shifting of the stress-bearing surfaces out of alignment, or produces a gross hemarthrosis, the reparative process or the residuum of the damage may be accompanied by pain, swelling and effusion. This reaction may persist over a period of months and thus justify the term arthritis. In most instances the trauma causes a disturbance in the normal physiology of the joint structure either by scarring the articular plate or by interfering with the circulation in the synovial vasculature. Roentgenographic changes occur related to the structural changes induced by the trauma.

The most common type of arthritis is what is usually called today "degenerative joint disease." This term, suggesting as it does the pathogenesis of the process, has evolved after many decades of conflicting theories concerning its cause and nature. The numerous names with which it has been identified in the past, osteoarthritis,

arthritis deformans and hypertrophic arthritis to name a few, testify to the lack of agreement concerning the morbid physiology of this disease.

About 50 per cent of all persons 50 years or older who for some reason have a complete skeletal survey reveal some alterations of their vertebral or peripheral joint structures that are characteristic of degenerative joint disease (osteoarthritis). Less than half of these, however, give a clear history of arthritis. Likewise, at least a few patients may recite the typical symptomatology of the disease and reveal no structural changes on the roentgenogram. Thus, though degenerative joint disease is the commonest of all joint ailments, it is not always easy to diagnose because we know less about it than about many less common types. The variation in clinical, radiologic and pathologic expression has led some authors to suggest that a variety of entities have been grouped together under this heading. If such is the case, there is too little evidence at present to make a distinction between the types. The consensus is that degenerative joint disease is what its name implies, a progressive structural and functional deterioration of the joint with

an attempt at repair by lateral proliferation. The causes for the degeneration are apparently numerous and varied but the commonest type of the disease is the result of a continued demand for excessive function in the face of a decreasing efficiency of blood supply.

Thus the disease is one of the middle-aged and the elderly. In most series the incidence is higher in males; in others there is no sex difference. The disease usually first manifests itself in a single joint, most often a large weight-bearing joint; however, it is unusual for it to remain confined to one joint. When it is polyarticular at the outset the distal phalangeal joints of the fingers are most commonly involved. Degenerative joint disease is not a systemic illness like rheumatoid arthritis and, therefore, there are no clinical or laboratory findings other than those referable to the joints.

Symptoms are pain and stiffness. The patient is rarely disabled unless the hip joints are involved. The pain is worse after inactivity and tends to decrease as the joint is "warmed up" by activity. It is increased by continued use and fatigue and is improved with rest. The amount and type of

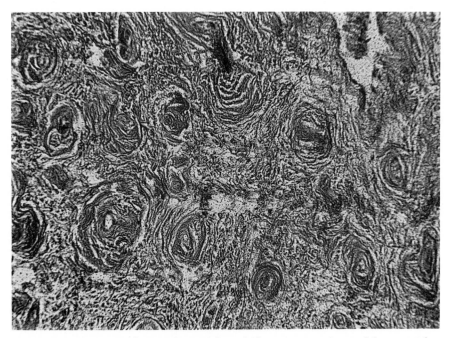

Figure 21–15 Degenerative joint disease. Section through the supportive tissue of the synovial membrane. The arterioles show proliferation of their fibrous walls and diminution of their lumina. (× 165.)

deformity depend upon the joint involved but deformity is less apt to be as severe as in rheumatoid arthritis.

Pathology. Because degenerative joint disease does not cause death or severe disability and because in the active phase it is not helped by surgery, it has taken over a century to collect sufficient material to provide data concerning the structural changes in the various aspects of the disease. By combining numerous reports such as the very complete and informative studies of Bennett et al.[13] and by carefully collecting the surgical material from patients with degenerative joint disease who have been operated upon for other reasons, we have been able to arrive at an appreciation of the chronologic changes that take place in the joint tissues.

The earliest changes that we believe are associated with degenerative joint disease are collagenization of the synovial membrane and sclerosis of its fine vascular network (Fig. 21–15). We are aware of reports that have failed to find evidence of correlation between the degree of sclerosis and joint degeneration. This does not necessarily mean that failing blood supply is not a cause, even a very important cause of the disease. It only means that there are reasons other than failing blood supply for articular cartilage degeneration.

The next changes are found in the articular plate, near the joint surface. With ordinary staining methods the chondroid about the young cartilage cells of this area takes up more hematoxylin and therefore stains a deeper blue than normal chondroid.[14] Next one may note changes within the nucleus of the cartilage cell; it may swell and rupture or become exceedingly pyknotic. This is followed by death of the chondrocyte and lysis of the surrounding chondroid to accomodate an excess of fluid, which collects within the lacuna. Thus a microcyst is formed (Fig. 21–16). These changes occur in groups of cells giving the impression that the cells are clumped. As the microcysts enlarge they agglomerate to form larger cysts and eventually there is rupture through the surface laminae. Now if the articular plate is examined with a hand lens, numerous irregular pits are seen to interrupt the integrity of the surface. In the early stages, while they are shallow, they involve only the superficial laminae, which are almost horizontal to the joint surface, but as they deepen into the laminae that are more vertical in arrangement they progress more rapidly,

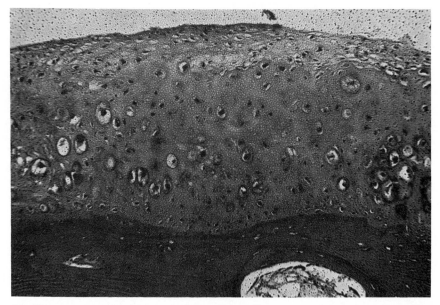

Figure 21–16 Degenerative joint disease. Articular plate with supportive arch of bone at bottom and joint space at top. Microcysts have formed with clumping of lacunae and degeneration of chondrocytes. (× 165.)

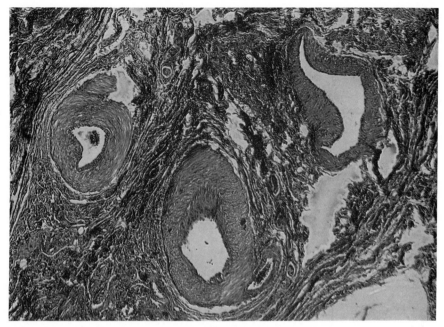

Figure 21–17   Degenerative joint disease. Section through joint capsule. Medium-sized vessels show sclerosis, thickening of subintimal tissues and decrease in lumen diameter. (× 60.)

producing irregular crevices and fissures. About these injury zones, which develop in the stress-bearing areas, the chondroid atrophies and disappears. Thus the surface becomes more and more irregular and the thickness of the plate diminishes. By this time the capsule usually has become thickened and fibrotic and even the larger vessels show thickening of their walls and diminution of their luminal diameter (Fig. 21–17).

In areas in which articular plates have undergone change in contour there must be shifting of stress trajectories. Whether because of its capacity for reaction to injury, stimulation by new stress lines or simply regeneration at the site at which the blood supply still allows it, the cartilage at the margins of the plate grows outward to produce spurs, osteophytes or exostoses. In the early phase this is best described as marginal lipping. This cartilage forms a plate of its own, which in turn forms a semblance of an epiphyseal line and a chondroid scaffolding. The sequence of normal bone growth is precisely duplicated, even to metaplasia of cells to osteoblasts, which now lay down bone. Thus

we have enchondral bone growth that is normal in everything except direction. These spurs are the basis for the usual roentgen diagnosis of hypertrophic arthritis.

In the distal interphalangeal joints of the fingers the spurs protrude on the extensor surface within the joint, pushing the capsule outward. These hard protrusions are called "Heberden's nodes." In the spine, the lipping may interfere with normal motion and with the course of spinal nerves. In the hip it interferes with motion.

As the articular plate is thinned its shock absorber function is diminished. The arches of bone that support the plate become heavier. When the cartilage plate eventually disappears completely there is left a smooth rounded surface of eburnated bone with irregular bony spurs springing from its periphery. The synovia and supportive capsule are now a fused mass of collagen scar tissue. Effusion is not usual but may come and go with periods of increased activity. The joint may be grossly deformed by deviation or subluxation. Ankylosis does not occur. Unlike the joint destroyed by rheumatoid arthritis, that in degenerative joint disease remains functional and painful.

Before the subchondral cancellous bone becomes eburnated, cysts may appear in this area. The cysts may be small (0.1 to 1 cm.) and multiple, in which case they are usually located superficially near the joint surface; in the femoral head they may agglomerate to form a single cyst of greater than 3 cm. in diameter. Landells[15] believes that these cysts are formed by the hydraulic action of synovial fluid forced by pressure from the joint space through a degenerated area of the articular plate into the subchondral cancellous tissue. He bases this opinion on finding openings between the cyst cavity and the joint space, and structures he interprets as synovial cells and synovial mucopolysaccharides within the cysts. Eventually the fluid or gel content of these cysts may be replaced by collagenous tissue. The lesion is now no longer cystic though it remains radiolucent. The surrounding bone often forms a sclerotic zone measuring as much as 0.5 cm. in thickness.

These cysts are quite different in pathogenesis from those found in rheumatoid arthritis though the end products may appear identical both radiologically and on section. In rheumatoid arthritis the subchondral inflammatory pannus unites with that of the joint space. In the active phase of the disease the "cyst" is filled with granulation, which later becomes converted to scar tissue. However, the cysts of degenerative arthritis are identical with the so-called subchondral or ganglion cysts. In these latter, however, the overlying articular plate is breached by some mechanism other than degenerative joint disease.

Roentgenographic Manifestations. Radiographically, the earliest manifestation of osteoarthritis is narrowing of the joint, which means a thinning of the articular plates. This is followed by sclerosis of the subchondral bone (Fig. 21–18). These alterations are the result of atrophy of the chondroid. At the margins of the articular plates the growing masses of cartilage ossify and form marginal osteophytes or hooklike projections (Fig. 21–19). Osteophytes are commonly found in the vertebral column, the hips and the knees. In

the bone near the joint, cysts may be evident and are seen as rounded radiolucent areas (Fig. 21–20).

The distal interphalangeal joints of the hands are commonly involved. The marginal lipping here is responsible for Heberden's nodes (Fig. 21–21).

Any involved joint may be deformed but the articular cortex will remain distinct. Periarticular demineralization is not a feature of osteoarthritis.

Pathogenesis. As has been stated in preceding paragraphs, the pathogenesis of degenerative joint disease is not known with certainty. It is generally believed that this is a degenerative process, a part of the general aging phenomena, hastened by excessive functional demand and a decreasing efficiency of blood supply. We have emphasized that the delicate balance between blood and joint fluid must be maintained if the articular plate is to be properly nourished. Truetta has stated that the intermittent compression and expansion of the articular plate produced by activity acts as a pumping mechanism, which promotes circulation of the synovial fluid into the cartilage and around the cells. This is doubtless true but leads to the conclusion that lack of activity causes degenerative joint disease. He states that in England this ailment is a disease of desk workers and not of gardeners. His observations seem to differ from those of authors in this country who find the incidence higher, the onset earlier and the joint damage greater in those who use their joints excessively. It might be observed also that an obese person of relatively sedentary habits might inflict more damages to his joints than a much more active, though lithe, athlete or laborer.

It is certain that excess stress and nutritional deficiencies are not responsible for all cases of degenerative joint disease. This ailment is almost sure to follow any situation that results in alteration of the weight-bearing contours, such as epiphyseal ischemic necrosis (Perthe's disease), slipped epiphysis (epiphysiolysis), infarction within the epiphysis and other types of arthritis. We have suggested that damage to the vascular apparatus of the synovium or alteration of synovial fluid, by impairing interchange of oxygen, nutrients

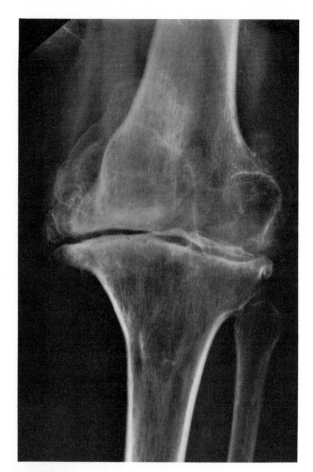

Figure 21–18 Osteoarthritis. The knee joint is narrow, the subchondral bone is sclerotic and marginal lipping is present.

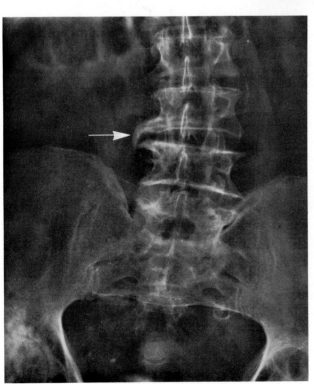

Figure 21–19 Osteoarthritis. The bodies of the lumbar vertebrae, particularly the fourth and fifth, are involved. Lipping is prominent on the right (arrow).

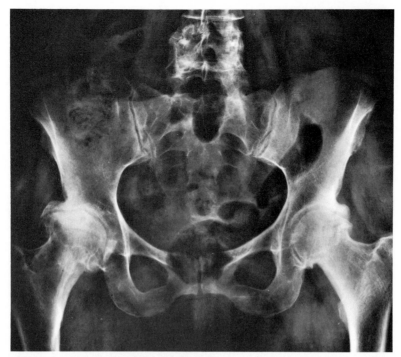

Figure 21–20 Osteoarthritis. Sclerosis of the articular cortex is evident on the left side. On the right side, the hip joint is narrow, osteophytes are present and cysts are evident in the head of the femur and in the acetabulum.

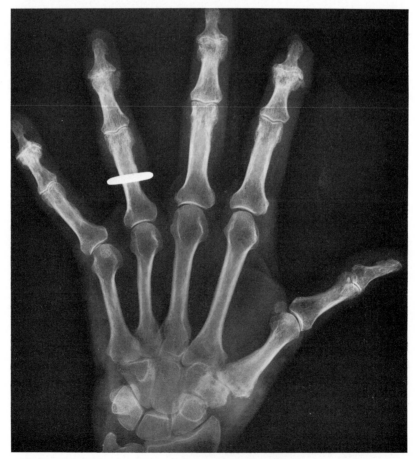

Figure 21–21 Osteoarthritis. The distal interphalangeal joints are affected and marginal lipping is prominent. A similar change is present in the wrist, particularly at the base of the first metacarpal.

and metabolic products across the joint space from articular plate chondrocytes to synovial blood, is a very important cause of degenerative joint disease. Thus it becomes obvious that some degree of osteoarthritis is seen wherever this impairment applies and must be prominent in rheumatoid arthritis. It is difficult for the writers of this book to imagine an instance of rheumatoid arthritis severe enough to cause structural damage without a considerable overlap of osteoarthritis. Thus associated disease processes may present a picture that is difficult to analyze. It has been stated repeatedly that stress is unimportant in this disease because of its incidence in the interphalangeal joints. It should be noted that degenerative joint disease occurs most frequently in those who use their hands a great deal. Excessive stress does not necessarily imply excessive weight bearing.

The treatment for degenerative joint disease is prophylactic by rest, supportive by analgesics, massage, heat and regulated exercise, and later, corrective by arthroplasty. Once alterations have occurred they are permanent because the articular plate has little capacity for repair. Though pain and stiffness may limit function the joint remains movable. Reassurance and relief of pain are the objectives of therapy.

Chondromalacia

The term "chondromalacia" usually refers to the patella though occasionally other articular cartilage plates are involved.

The undersurface of the patella loses its smooth, glistening surface but appears to be softened and fibrillated. The pathogenesis is unknown but it almost always is associated with trauma, either a single episode or less often chronic and repeated. It is classically elicited by joint tenderness, sometimes called the Fouchet sign. The trauma probably causes changes in the intercellular chondroid that interfere with the normal dispersion of the synovial fluid that is responsible for nutritional maintenance of the cartilage layer on the posterior surface of the patella. Thus the lesion

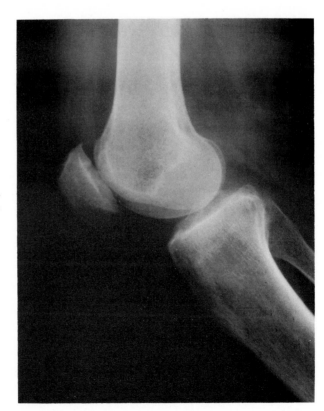

Figure 21–22 Chondromalacia. The inner aspect of the patella is roughened and irregular in outline.

is almost certainly a metabolic or degenerative process caused in all or most cases by chondroid alterations secondary to trauma.

Neurogenic Arthropathy

In this condition there is massive destruction of the stress-bearing portion of the joint and dramatic hypertrophic changes at the periphery. The disease has been known generally as Charcot's joint since Charcot's recognition and description of the pathogenesis in 1868.

In adults this type of joint disease is seldom seen under the age of 40 though rarely a neurogenic arthropathy may occur in children. In most instances a single joint is affected, but two or more large joints may be involved in this extensive degenerative change, or rarely a segmental group of small joints. Though both structural and functional changes in the involved joint may be dramatic, there is almost always a disproportionate paucity of symptoms. The lesion has been described as a painless bag of bones.

The pathogenesis and end result of neurogenic arthropathy is that of a greatly exaggerated and fulminant degenerative joint disease (osteoarthritis). The onset is insidious but the pace of the degenerative process, particularly if the patient remains active, is much more rapid than that of osteoarthritis. At the outset it is assumed that the degenerative changes in the articular plate are identical to those of degenerative joint disease. Soon, however, the stress-bearing portions of the joint cartilage undergo fibrillation and eventual fragmentation. These irregular fragments may become the nidi of joint bodies. One of the most important early features of the disease, and one that is more often than not overlooked, is loss of stability of the joint. This is probably due to early decrease in tendon and ligament tone. With destruction of the joint cartilage, this loss of stability is more obvious. The involved tissues attempt to compensate for this loss by a remarkable peripheral growth of cartilage, which matures to form bone. Thus long struts and bizarre craggy masses of bone are produced in the joint space, the joint

capsule about the joint and extending far beyond the joint along muscle planes, sometimes to attach to the adjoining bone member (Figs. 21–23 and 21–24).

Just as in degenerative joint disease with more or less complete destruction of the articular plate, there is a grinding down and eburnation of the end of the shaft. Destruction of normal weight-bearing surfaces results in a subluxation and even dislocation. Continued activity under these conditions causes fractures, within the joint, through the joint and in the contiguous bone outside the joint. Mechanical injury to the synovia is probably the most important cause of the effusion that plays such an important role in the Charcot joint. This effusion is less painful than one might expect it to be and it may continue to be the most prominent and most complained of feature for many months of the early phase of the disease. Eventually destruction of all joint structures becomes so complete that all usefulness vanishes. Then the structure resembles a swollen, de-

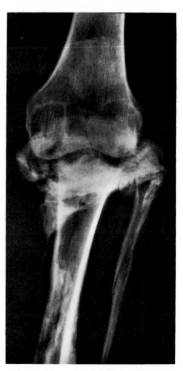

Figure 21–23 Neurogenic arthropathy. The tibia and fibula are primarily involved. There are obvious distortion and destruction of the knee joint.

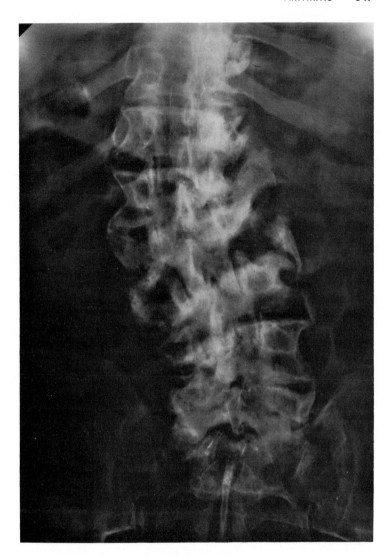

Figure 21–24 Charcot spine. There are sclerosis and destruction of the lumbar vertebrae with lateral osteophytic projections of new bone.

formed and shapeless mass with loss of all architectural normalcy and with complete disability (Figs. 21–25 and 21–26).

Since the recognition of neurogenic arthropathy as an entity, its pathogenesis has been a matter for discussion and argument among those interested. Today there is little proof that any one of the proposed theories is the correct one but an overwhelming amount of circumstantial evidence has accumulated to show that the cause lies not within the joint but in the nervous system. The disease may stem from degenerative or inflammatory alteration of the proprioceptive and sensory cells of the brain or cord or of the pathways that conduct their impulses. Why abolition of the proprioceptive or sensory (or more probably both) impulses from joint tissues results in massive deterioration of those tissues is unknown. Some have thought that the joint vasculature was affected but there seems little or no evidence of this. One may presume that, with loss of tone in the structures that stabilize the joint, stress lines are changed and the joint tissues are exposed to unusual trauma. If sensory appreciation is also lacking, continued activity prolongs the insult beyond tolerance and joint tissues give way as a result of accumulated trauma. But because the blood supply is not deficient, new bone forms in areas in which stress does not inhibit it and therefore the astonishing exophytic growth occurs. Mechanical irritation causes excessive fluid formation and effusion, and eventually tearing of synovial vessels may cause hemarthrosis.

The joints most apt to be affected are those most exposed to stress insults. Thus the weight-bearing joints—the knees, the hips, the ankles and the lower spine—are involved in that order of frequency. This is particularly true when tabes, the most common cause of the disease, is responsible. In diabetic neurogenic arthropathy the joints of the feet are most often involved. In a case studied by us there was demyelinization of the peripheral nerves of the lower extremity (Fig. 21–27). In syringomyelia the joints of the shoulders and upper extremities are more often involved than those of the lower extremities. This is presumably because the neurogenic arthropathy is apt to occur after the patient is confined and the joints of the lower extremities are put at rest. Myelomeningocele is the most common cause of Charcot's joint in childhood. Neurogenic arthropathy may occur in any nervous sys-

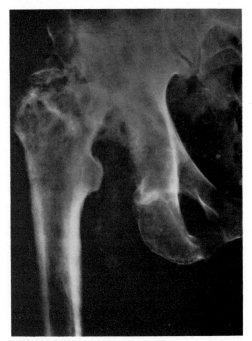

Figure 21–25 Neurogenic arthropathy. Destruction, but with minimal new bone being formed, is common in instances in which the hip is involved.

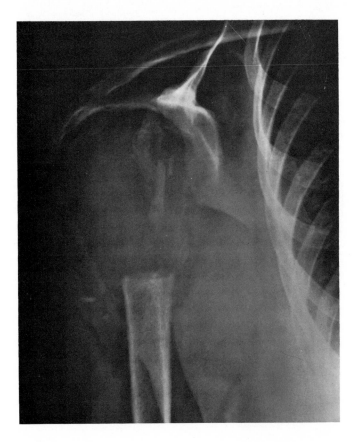

Figure 21–26 Neurogenic arthropathy. There are massive joint effusion at the shoulder and destruction of the humerus in this patient with syringomyelia.

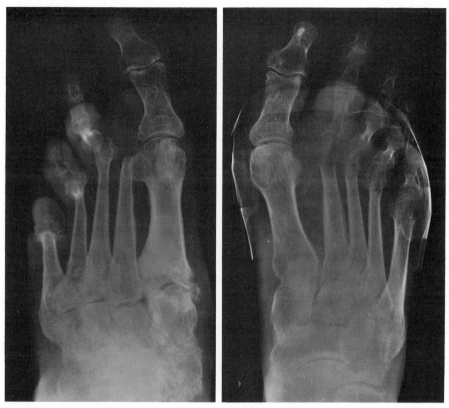

Figure 21–27 Neurogenic arthropathy. Periarticular demineralization and articular destruction in a patient with diabetes mellitus.

tem disease that abolishes sensory appreciation of proprioceptive tone. These include leprosy, spinal cord injury or compression, pernicious anemia and peripheral nerve section.

The only therapy that benefits the patient is complete protection of the joint from stress and injury and even then the advance of the process may be only slowed. Early diagnosis is seldom made for obvious reasons but must be attempted because protection at this stage probably encourages recovery. When destructive changes are advanced, the involved tissues are long since past their capacity for repair. Surgical reconstruction offers little because of the poor healing potential.

The destructive changes in joints that are rarely seen following cortisone therapy demonstrate all the radiologic features of neurogenic arthropathy. Because of the florid proliferation of cartilage at the joint peripheries, if this area is sampled, the pathologist may be misled into a diagnosis of chondrosarcoma.

Congenital Indifference to Pain

This unusual disturbance is the result of an intrauterine degeneration or a congenital absence of sensory ganglion cells of the trigeminal ganglion and those distal to it. It is familial and is more common in Jewish children. They cry without tears and the insensitivity is usually accompanied by mental retardation of moderate to severe degree. These patients frequently die of mediastinitis. The pathogenesis of the multiple and symmetric Charcot's joints, which develop in this condition, is apparently the same as that of other types of neurogenic arthropathy discussed previously.[16] (See p. 245.)

Cortisone Arthropathy

For the past decade there have been numerous reports of Charcot's joints occurring in patients on cortisone therapy.[17] Degenerative changes have followed single or multiple injections of this agent directly into the joint and in patients taking the drug orally. In the latter group, it is most often seen after 9 to 18 months of therapy with 50 to 100 mg. daily. The pathogenesis of the dramatic alterations in cartilage and bone that characterize the lesions is poorly understood. Because cortisone stabilizes the lipid lysosome membrane, it may interfere with normal hydrolase release and thus affect ground substance of mesenchymal tissues. It has been shown that steroids induce a fatty liver and probably produce abnormal levels of the serum lipids. Fisher et al.[18] report one case in which fat emboli were found in sections of the head of the femur.

VILLONODULAR SYNOVITIS

The term "villonodular synovitis" has a number of synonyms. In English, these are xanthoma, xanthogranuloma, giant cell tumor of tendon sheath, xanthomatous giant cell tumor, giant cell fibroangioma and benign synovioma. Lesions that are histologically identical are seen most frequently in relation to tendons, less commonly within joints, rarely in bursas and recently they have been described within the cancellous tissue of bone.

These lesions were first described by Broca in 1861, later in the French literature by Heurtaux in 1891, and finally the three types were definitively described and associated by Jaffe, Lichtenstein and Sutro[19] under the name of villonodular pigmented synovitis in 1941. This term is probably preferable to the others because it designates the lesion as a non-neoplastic one. However, it implies that it is an inflammatory reaction, which it may or may not be, and it is descriptive only inasmuch as it is applicable to the first phase of the process.

We have collected 144 of these cases. Twenty-four were within the joint, in all cases the knee joint. Eighty-four were in the soft tissues near a joint, five the wrist, eight the ankle, four the toes, two the knee and 72 involved the periarticular joint tissues of the hand, half of them the thumb and index fingers. There was a 3 to 1 preponderance in females. In 25 cases the lesions were located within a bone, most often but not always in an ossified epiphysis near a joint afflicted with the same process. Two lesions were located in bursas.

There is at present a general belief that all these processes, though varying in location, are the same pathologic entity, though the symptoms and x-ray appearance are quite dissimilar because of variation in site involvement. We share this belief only because the microscopy of the various lesions is the same and we have no evidence to indicate that they are different. We admit, however, that synovial tissue has only a limited capacity for reaction and the microscopic picture that we see in villonodular synovitis may represent the change caused by any of a number of agents.

Microscopy. In the early stages of villonodular pigmented synovitis one finds a nonspecific inflammatory reaction (Fig. 21–28). The synovia is thickened by edema and an infiltration with lymphocytes. In some cases large amounts of hemosiderin darken the tissue to a red-brown color. There may be considerable fibroblastic reaction which, if it enlarges the villous processes, gives the lesion a shaggy or bearded appearance. As the proliferative reaction becomes more dominant, nodules of solid tissue are produced. Eventually the composition is one of fibroblastic and synovial cell hyperplasia (Fig. 21–29). Spaces and clefts are formed, many of which are lined with synovial cells. Within the spaces are found giant cells, which appear to have arisen from the contiguous lining cells. Small groups of lipid-bearing macrophages, xanthoid cells, are usually found scattered through the fibrous stroma. The stromal cells may be so immature that they suggest undifferentiated mesenchymal tumor cells. When the stroma is young and active this lesion may quite easily be mistaken for a giant cell tumor and it is probable that at least a few of the "benign giant cell tumors" of the past were, in reality, examples of this con-

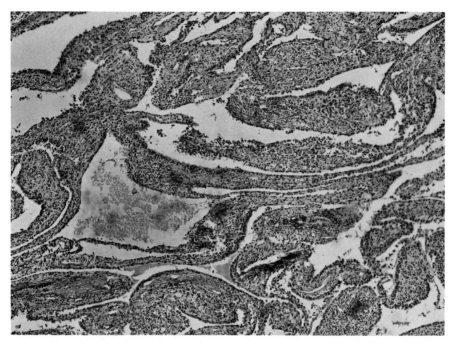

Figure 21–28 Section showing the enlarged inflamed villous processes of the synovia in early villonodular pigmented synovitis. (× 40.)

dition. When the lesion is composed of sheets of rather undifferentiated synovial cells in which giant cells have failed to appear, there is a temptation to consider this a malignant tumor.

The term "benign synovioma" is an unfortunate one because it implies that the lesion is a true tumor and moreover related to a neoplasm with a high mortality rate. In all probability this condition is a type of

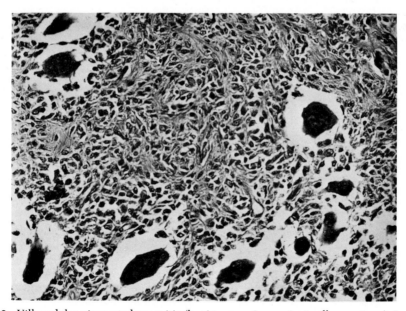

Figure 21–29 Villonodular pigmented synovitis (benign synovioma, giant cell synovioma). In the terminal stage the proliferation of synovial cells predominates in the section, producing a tumorlike mass. Irregular sinuses are formed in which lie giant cells. (× 170.)

chronic proliferative inflammatory reaction. The tendon lesions are apt to erode bone from without and they may recur after surgical removal. One such lesion in the ankle region involved most of the soft tissues about the tarsal bones but eventually these proliferating cells matured and the lesion became static, still allowing function. To our knowledge no such lesion has ever metastasized.

The pathogenesis of villonodular synovitis is unknown. Because of large amounts of hemosiderin pigment and lipid that are phagocytized by the synovial covering cells it was long presumed that this process was a reaction to hemorrhage within the tendon sheath, joint or bursa. It still seems probable that hemorrhage is a factor in the development of this lesion, though apparently not the only factor in the development of this lesion, and perhaps not the important one. Though there is some disagreement in results, villonodular synovitis cannot be produced consistently by injecting blood or mixtures of blood and lipids into the joint cavity. It should also be noted that the incidence of villonodular synovitis has not yet been reported to be higher in the patient with hemophilia who frequently bleeds into his joints than in the normal population.

Some recent work suggests that the culprit in the pathogenesis of villonodular synovitis is the residuum of the hemosiderin which has been broken down by the phagocytizing synovial cells and perhaps histiocytes. These products may become antigenic, initiating a proliferative hypersensitivity reaction.

Intraosseous Villonodular Synovitis

In 1944, Smith-Petersen[20] reported a case of villonodular synovitis of the hip joint with an erosion of the articular plates. The latter he interpreted as due to accompanying, but unassociated, degenerative joint disease. Seven years later Clark[21] reported a similar case in which the prolif-

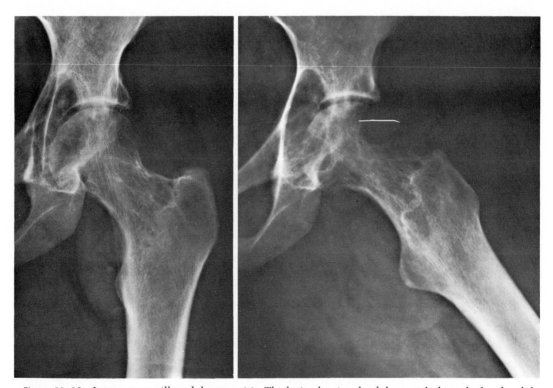

Figure 21–30   Intraosseous villonodular synovitis. The lesion has involved the acetabulum, the head and the neck of the femur. The mass of proliferating synovia is evident adjacent to the medial aspect of the neck of the femur; there are no calcifications within it.

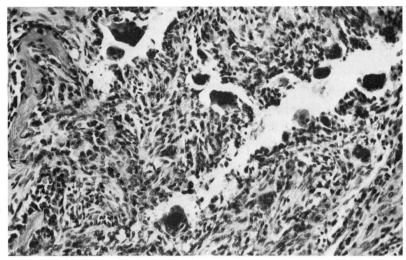

Figure 21–31   Section from the metaphysis of a patient with villonodular pigmented synovitis in the hip joint. Compare this section with one of typical synovitis within a joint seen in Figure 21–29. (× 170.)

erating joint synovia had penetrated into and replaced much of the cancellous tissue of the femoral head. In 1954, Carr, Berly and Davis[22] reported an instance of villonodular synovitis of the left hip joint in which the proliferating synovial tissue had penetrated through the acetabular roof to produce a soft tissue mass in the retroperitoneal area of the pelvic cavity. It had also penetrated the articular plate of the femoral head and invaded the intraosseous substance of the head and neck. Shortly thereafter Deakins, Wohl and Pietroluongo, at a meeting of radiologists and orthopedists in Philadelphia, reported two similar cases, one in a hip joint and the other in the shaft of a fractured humerus at the site of a delayed union.

In the past 10 years we have been able to collect 25 additional cases of villonodular synovitis involving bone structures in relation to joints. To distinguish this from the usual manifestation of the process we have called the condition intraosseous villonodular synovitis.

In most of these cases there have been obvious disease within the joint and an irregular area of radiolucency in the adjacent subchondral bone, often of both bones (Fig. 21–30). Villonodular synovitis should be thought of in all triple sited

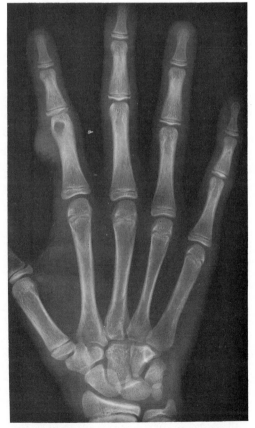

Figure 21–32   Intraosseous villonodular synovitis. There is prominence of the soft tissues proximal to the first interphalangeal joint of the second digit. The distal end of the proximal phalanx is widened and a circular radiolucent defect is evident within the bone. Osteopenia is not present.

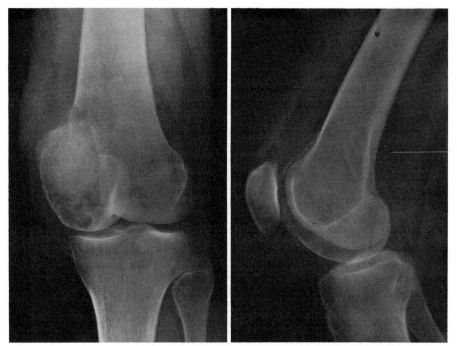

Figure 21–33 Intraosseous villonodular synovitis. Cystlike lesions with slightly sclerotic borders are present in the medial condyle of the femur. There is an associated soft tissue mass.

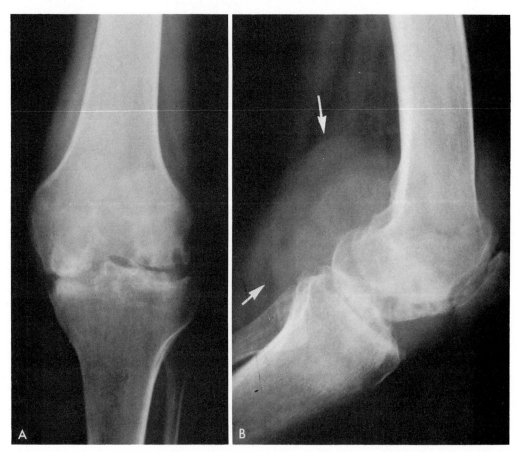

Figure 21–34 Pigmented villonodular synovitis. There is a large mass of synovial tissue that distends the knee joint (arrows, *B*). Destructive changes with associated sclerosis are present on both sides of the joint (*A*).

lesions of this type. In all of our cases, surgical biopsy of the lesion within bone was done[12] and samples of synovial tissue showing the alterations of villonodular synovitis were obtained. It is assumed in these cases that the proliferating synovia (Fig. 21–31) brings an increased blood supply into contiguity with the articular plate or the thin cortical collar that supports it. The cartilage or the bone is resorbed and the synovial tissue penetrates into the underlying cancellous tissue and continues to proliferate there.

In two cases of our series the lesion was found deep within the shaft. In both instances a villonodular synovitis of a nearby bursa had extended beyond the walls of the latter and presumably invaded the bone.

In one case of our series the radiolucent bone lesion was located within the greater trochanter of the femur at some distance from any normally existing synovial tissue. This case provoked the question, "Can cancellous mesenchymal tissue undergo metaplasia to form synovia?" The question cannot be answered, but because cancellous tissue can produce bone, cartilage or collagen it would not seem too extraordinary to find it producing synovia. If such is the case, it would not be necessary to find channels between the joint space and lesions within bone to explain the presence of synovial tissue in the latter.

INFECTIOUS ARTHRITIS

Following is a working classification of the inflammatory diseases of the joints considered to be of infectious origin:

A. Suppurative
  1. Bacterial infections
  2. Reiter's syndrome
B. Nonsuppurative
  1. Tuberculosis
  2. Fungal infections
  3. Viral infections
  4. Syphilitic arthritis

Suppurative Arthritis

BACTERIAL INFECTION

Most bacterial infections of the joints have a sudden onset and develop rapidly into an acute suppurative arthritis. There are pain and limitation of motion. Swelling, redness, heat and tenderness soon develop. Joint effusion is common to most of the infections. The patient usually manifests fever and there is often a leukocytosis. Examination of the joint aspirate usually discloses an increased number of leukocytes, from 1000 to 100,000, depending upon the type of organism, the duration and the severity of the infection. The synovial fluid sugar is usually reduced in amount. In most joint infections, the disease is monarticular and a large joint is much more apt to be involved than a small one. Notable exceptions are gonococcal arthritis and Reiter's syndrome in which involvement of more than one joint is the rule.

Suppurative arthritis with the exception of gonococcal arthritis and Reiter's syndrome is seen most often in children, in the debilitated and aged and in those taking steroid hormones. Though almost all pathogenic bacteria have been incriminated in joint infections the ones that most commonly attack these tissues are the staphylococcus, the gonococcus, the pneumococcus, the hemolytic streptococcus and the meningococcus. Less common offenders are the influenza bacillus, the typhoid bacillus and *Salmonella choleraesuis*. Infectious arthritis may develop in the more generalized cases of brucellosis and shigellosis.

The infecting organisms usually reach the joint tissues by means of the blood, as the result of a primary septicemia such as subacute bacterial endocarditis or a secondary septicemia of such diseases as lobar pneumonia or meningitis. Occasionally the organisms are apparently disseminated from a focal infection such as a furuncle, an otitis media or a sinusitis. Sometimes the infection extends into the joint from a nearby focus of osteomyelitis (Fig. 21–35).

The infection in joint tissues manifests itself in the same manner as infections elsewhere in soft tissue. There is hyperemia with swelling and later edema of the synovial membrane. This is followed by an infiltration with inflammatory cells, principally granulocytes. Small vessels may rupture to produce petechial hemorrhages and focal areas of necrosis may develop.

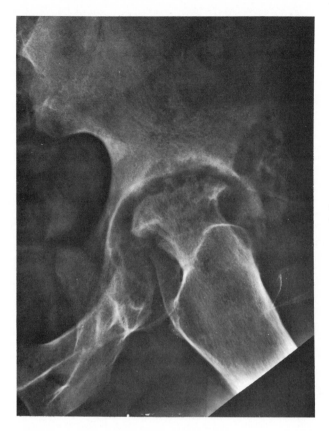

Figure 21–35 Suppurative arthritis. Gross destruction of the acetabulum and head of the femur has resulted from infection of the joint.

There is usually an outpouring of fluid into the joint. This has a high protein and a low sugar content. Granulocytes are shed into the synovial fluid to produce pus cells. When these cells are broken down they release lysosomal cathepsin and other enzymes that destroy cartilage. Such destruction is often found in the central portions of the articular plate where weight-bearing has ground the cells into the plate. Replacement of the normal synovial fluid with effusion and suppuration doubtless interferes with nutrient and cell waste transport making the cartilage more vulnerable to injury, inducing a superimposed degenerative joint disease. When the healing reaction is initiated a pannus of granulation forms from the fibrin covering the synovial surface. It is composed of myriads of new vessels, which when spread over the articular plate further cause its lysis.

Even before this stage of infection within the joint, exudative inflammatory cells may be demonstrated in the subchondral cancellous tissue. It is our belief that this is general and due to the association of the two sites by a common lymphatic system. If the articular plate barrier is penetrated there follows a frank suppurative osteomyelitis of the end of the shaft.

Today, because of the development of specific antibiotic agents, the complete course of suppurative osteomyelitis is rarely seen. This is fortunate indeed because the articular plate has little or no capacity for regenerative healing. With loss of the articular plates there is usually an extension of granulation from one subchondral area to the other across the joint space. As the granulation ages it forms collagen scar tissue, a fibrous ankylosis. The collagen often calcifies as it condenses and this is usually followed by ossification — bony ankylosis. In short, if the joint infection proceeds to destruction of the articular plate, joint destruction and permanent crippling are almost inevitable. It behooves the modern clinician to make the diagnosis early so that the infection can be curbed before irreversible joint damage takes place.

Examination of synovial fluid is probably the most valuable single means of making the correct diagnosis. By the time x-ray alterations have occurred, other than enlargement of the joint space because of effusion, irreparable damage may have been done.

REITER'S SYNDROME

This disease is a curious association of inflammatory reactions within the urethra, the conjunctiva and synovial membrane. It is preceded by a mucositis in the bowel in some series in up to one third of the cases. It sometimes is accompanied by a rash of

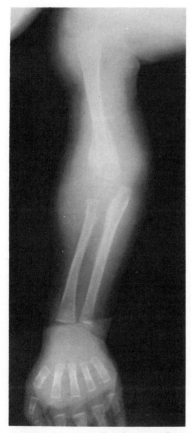

Figure 21–36 Gonococcal arthritis and osteomyelitis, male, 6 weeks of age. There is marked distention of the elbow joint associated with deep soft tissue swelling. Destruction is present in the distal end of the humerus and there is thick solid periosteal new bone about the distal humerus and proximal end of the ulna.

the palms and soles, which most closely resembles pustular psoriasis.

The cause of Reiter's syndrome is unknown. Because the inflammation of the mucous membranes is usually suppurative it has long been thought to be bacterial in origin, but no organism has been consistently isolated. There has been much discussion on the pleuropneumonia-like organisms that undergo morphologic alteration with therapy but there is no universal agreement concerning this matter.

The condition usually affects young adults, most often males. Characteristically, it begins as a suppurative inflammation of the urethra. Then the conjunctivae become inflamed and they too may develop a suppurative exudate. Pain is noted in the joints and this aspect of the disease predominates symptomatically. The inflammatory reaction has all the gross and microscopic features of a suppurative bacterial arthritis except that an organism cannot be recovered consistently. The course differs from ordinary suppurative arthritis inasmuch as it is less apt to destroy the joint structure leaving residual crippling and it is apt to recur, sometimes several times over a period of years.

Multiple joints are usually involved. In a few instances the cartilages have been thinned and fibrosis has distorted the joint structure. The course is usually run in a few months but sometimes it is prolonged over a period of years. In some recent series, cardiac complications have been reported. The signs suggest endocardial involvement.

Nonsuppurative Arthritis

TUBERCULOSIS

Like most other infections, the incidence of tuberculous arthritis has greatly diminished in the past two decades. As elsewhere in the body, tuberculosis is a chronic infection characterized by an insidious but progressive extension of a necrotizing process that eventuates in massive tissue destruction. One of the interesting features of tuberculous arthritis is that it is usually, perhaps always, accompanied by a similar infection in the adjacent subchondral cancellous tissue. Some authors believe that it always starts in bone and spreads to the joints; others think that the route of spread is in the opposite direction. The organism must always reach the joint or bone tissue by the blood from a primary infection elsewhere, today almost always from the lungs, in the past more often from infections in the gut.

The tubercle bacillus characteristically causes tissues to react in such a manner that granulomas are formed. (See p. 268.) There is central necrosis surrounded by a zone of histiocytes intermingled with giant cells and lymphocytes that in turn are encircled by fibroblasts. The granuloma of tuberculosis is relatively avascular. It is in essence the foreign body and hypersensitivity inflammatory reaction as expressed by the reticuloendothelial derivatives. The accompanying inflammatory reaction usually causes the formation of granulation tissue in which the granulomas are embedded (Fig. 21–37).

Except in the spine, tuberculous arthritis is usually monarthritic. Any joint may be involved but the spine is very much the most common and the hip second (Fig. 9–20, p. 269).

The infection is more insidious in onset and more chronic in course than suppurative infections in joints. Unless diagnosed early and treated properly it progresses over a period of months, gradually destroying all the tissues of the joint structure. Granulomas are formed within the synovia. The latter becomes thickened and fibrotic. A granulation pannus forms on its surface and grows to spread over the articular plates, slowly eroding them as it does so. Focal areas of necrosis in the capsule agglomerate to form channels that rupture outside the joint to form chronic sinuses. The same process goes on simultaneously within the subchondral bone. The sinuses may extend long distances in the soft tissues to produce masses near a tissue surface—cold abscesses. Secondary infection of this necrotic mass may now cause a suppurative reaction. Joint effusion in the absence of secondary infection is uncommon. Because of the necrosis and relative avascularity there is less fibrous proliferation than in other types of arthritis and, therefore, less tendency for fibrous ankylosis. The same reason is probably valid in explaining the lack of spur formation at the periphery.

Most tuberculosis of the spine occurs before the age of 15. In the peripheral

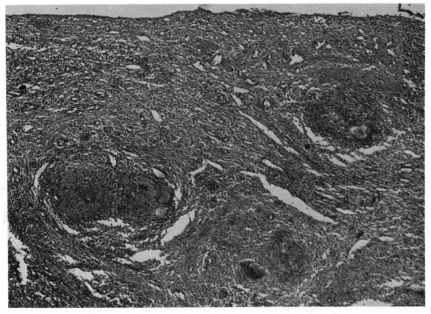

Figure 21–37   Tuberculous arthritis. A matrix of granulation tissue contains three granulomas showing the characteristic arrangement of cells including multinucleated giant cells. (× 65.)

FUNGAL INFECTIONS

Rarely a fungus may reach the joint tissues and establish an infection there. The commonest of these is blastomycosis. Most fungi cause a granulomatous type of inflammatory reaction that may be indistinguishable from the granulomas of tuberculosis. In most instances, however, suppuration is much more prominent and caseation necrosis is lacking. Such is the case with blastomycotic arthritis. The incidence of blastomycotic infections is highest in the southeastern section of the United States. The infection may be polyarticular and is apt to be stubbornly persistent. In one case studied by us a systemic infection led to death with huge abscesses scattered everywhere throughout the body (Fig. 21–39).

The ray fungus may produce joint infection and like actinomycosis of other sites it produces massive necrosis and distortion of the affected tissues. It too is a persistent infection that is difficult to eradicate. Other types of fungal infection in joints include cryptococcosis, coccidioidomycosis and histoplasmosis.

VIRAL INFECTION OF JOINTS

Joint pain and sometimes swelling are not uncommonly encountered in certain systemic viral diseases. This association is particularly likely to occur in influenza, rubella, viral hepatitis and lymphopathia venereum. The pathogenesis of the joint disease is not clear. Because it is usually transient and of short duration it is thought by some to represent a hypersensitivity reaction though there is little evidence to substantiate this idea.

SYPHILITIC ARTHRITIS

Today the incidence of luetic infection of joint tissues is exceedingly low. The Charcot joint, a neurogenic arthropathy due to tabes dorsalis, has been described. (See p. 646.) Both secondary and tertiary types of syphilitic inflammatory reaction may rarely occur in joint tissues as well as elsewhere in the body. The process may

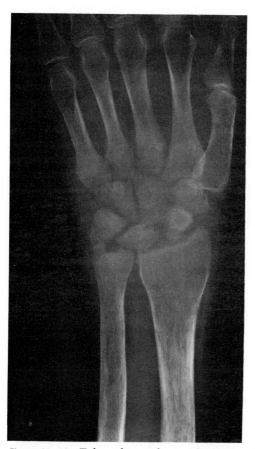

Figure 21–38 Tuberculous arthritis. The bones of the wrist are undermineralized and their margins indistinct. The joints are only slightly narrowed. Swelling of the soft tissues is evident.

joints the infection may occur in an older group. Tuberculosis of the spine, Pott's disease, is practically always a combination of osteomyelitis and joint infection. (See p. 265.) Cold abscesses may point in the neck, in the loin or in the groin depending upon the site of the bone and joint infection.

Treatment of tuberculous arthritis is based on putting the affected part at rest by immobilization on a frame or in a cast and chemotherapy with combinations of streptomycin, isonicotinic acid and para-aminosalicylic acid. With early diagnosis and proper treatment the prognosis today is excellent though many months are necessary before the joint structures can be put to normal use again.

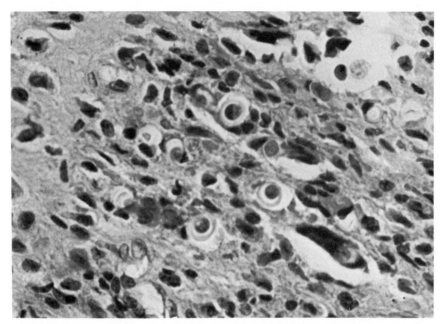

Figure 21-39   Blastomycotic arthritis. A group of blastomyces with characteristic double contours are seen in the central field. H and E stain. (× 660.)

simulate rheumatoid arthritis and the clinician should be alerted to the possibility of mistaking a rheumatoid arthritis precipitated by syphilis (with a positive Wassermann reaction) for luetic joint disease.

The types of joint disease of congenital syphilis are now only names to most of us. Clutton's joint was a type of painless hydrarthrosis seen in children and adolescents with congenital syphilis. Parrot's syphilitic osteochondritis was a more destructive and serious type of infection seen in young infants in which there was massive necrosis of the epiphysis.

ARTHRITIS OF THE HYPERSENSITIVITY GROUP

Grouped under this heading are several types of joint disease or possibly a single disease of joint tissue with considerable variation in clinical expression. The pathologist finds the microscopy of these conditions so similar that he is unable to make a clear distinction between them. He is, therefore, inclined to think of them as a group, admitting that a variety of etiologic factors may produce the structural alterations that characterize the disease.

The predominant member of this group and by all odds the most important is rheumatoid arthritis. Two subvarieties of this condition are spondylitis ankylosans and juvenile rheumatoid arthritis (Still's disease). In rheumatoid arthritis, normal healthy joints are attacked and run the gamut of the disease, from an acute inflammatory reaction with effusion to complete joint destruction and finally an attempt at repair that results in bony ankylosis.

Joint disease is frequently an important facet of several of the so-called collagen diseases. Though the arthritis attacks healthy joints it rarely runs the complete course of rheumatoid arthritis and in most instances the joints heal without residual loss of function. The microscopy is that of a mild type of rheumatoid arthritis, usually without articular plate destruction. Occasionally, however, the arthritis in a collagen disease may run a course similar in every way to that of severe rheumatoid arthritis.

In a third group of diseases, which includes rheumatic fever, the joints are affected with an inflammatory process that has all the features of the earliest stage of rheumatoid arthritis but that produces no lesions beyond this point. In this group the articular plate is never damaged and there is no gross scarring of the synovia. Though the bouts of inflammation may be recurrent they always heal completely leaving a normal joint.

Rheumatoid Arthritis

Rheumatoid arthritis (sometimes called proliferative arthritis) is a systemic disease of mesenchymal tissues. The connective tissues throughout the body are affected but because the joint is constituted entirely of mesenchymal tissues and because disease of the joints gives rise to pain and disability, the patient's chief complaint is that of arthritis.

In most series the incidence of rheumatoid arthritis is two to three times greater in females. It often begins during adolescence, more often during the third decade, and sometimes after 50. Rarely there may be but a single episode lasting a few weeks to one or two years. The usual course is one of exacerbations and remissions. Complete cure is rarely seen following more than two to three years of persistent activity. The onset is often sudden, just as often insidious. Usually a single joint is first affected with spread to other joints as the disease progresses. Early manifestations may be polyarticular; often there is symmetric involvement of the proximal interphalangeal joints of the fingers. Other joints of the hands and feet are commonly affected early and no joint, including those of the spine and jaw, is invulnerable.

Rheumatoid arthritis is a disease of the temperate zone. Attacks are more common in the spring. Joint pains are usually introduced by bouts of malaise and fatigue. One or more joints become painful, swollen, red, hot and tender. The inflammatory reaction in and about the joint presents a fusiform or spindled appearance. After inactivity the pain is more intense on motion and accompanied by stiffness. The attack may clear leaving an undamaged joint but recurrence is probable. Eventually the joint tissues are destroyed by the inflammatory process ending in flexion contractures, subluxation and ankyloses. The arthritis may be accompanied by a mild fever and tachycardia. As the disease progresses there may be marked weight loss and muscle atrophy. The extremities are cold but moist. The skin over the involved joints becomes atrophic, tight and shiny. In about 20 per cent of patients subcutaneous nodules develop at pressure points, often where the skin is in close approximation to bone, as over the olecranon process. During the attacks one often finds generalized lymphadenopathy and less often splenomegaly.

The most consistent laboratory finding is an increased sedimentation rate. There may be a mild leukocytosis and in longstanding cases there is usually a normocytic, normochromic anemia. The serum globulin level is often increased at the expense of the serum albumin level. The globulin elevation is in the $alpha_2$ and gamma fractions. Investigation of the rheumatoid factor has stimulated much interest and controversy in the past several years. This factor is found in about 75 per cent of all patients who have had severe rheumatoid arthritis for one year or longer. Unfortunately it is rarely found in the early stages of mild arthritis when diagnostic aids are most needed. It is sometimes found in patients with lupus erythematosus (about 15 per cent) and less often with polyarteritis nodosa and dermatomyositis so that it cannot be considered specific for rheumatoid arthritis. It is found in the sera of relatives of rheumatoid arthritis patients oftener than in a normal population. The factor is a gamma globulin (IgM) with a large molecular weight (19S) which has the capacity to react with gamma globulins in the smaller molecular weight range (7S) or particulate matter such as latex particles or tanned sheep cells coated with this globulin.

The rheumatoid factor (Rh factor, IgM) is now generally considered to be an antibody; its antigen is probably the specific immune gamma globulin (IgG, 7S) elaborated by lymphocytes. Why this substance becomes antigenic is not completely understood. It may be abnormally split in the rheumatoid patient or perhaps it remains normal and the fault lies in the metabolic choreography of the plasma cells which apparently are stimulated by it to elaborate the abnormal IgM or Rh factor. The Rh factor now apparently complexes with its antigen IgG and the agglutinated product together with complement is phagocytized by granulocytes on the synovial surface and in its supportive tissues. This complex destroys the lysosome capsules, releasing stored enzymes that have the capacity for lysing collagen and chondroid. This activity sets up an inflammatory reaction which attracts more lymphocytes and plasma cells to the area and thus a vicious cycle is established which operates until either the abnormal antigenic action is righted or the joint structure is destroyed. Of the two widely used laboratory tests for Rh factor, the latex agglutination test is more sensitive but less specific than the sensitized sheep cell agglutination test. Both tests should be done in establishing a firm diagnosis.

L.E. cells are found in perhaps 15 per cent of patients with established rheumatoid arthritis.

Examination of the aspirated synovial fluid may be helpful in reaching a diagnosis of rheumatoid arthritis though no changes are specific for the disease. The leukocyte count is moderately increased during activity. Counts of more than 200 per mm. are significant, particularly if 25 per cent or greater are granulocytes. Counts of 100,000 or more are apt to be of septic origin. Granulocytes usually contain inclusion bodies within their cytoplasm, probably complexed antigen-antibody. These cells have been called ragocytes. They are present in most types of inflammatory arthritis and so are not specific for rheumatoid arthritis. Joint fluid also has increased turbidity and decreased viscosity (see Table 21–1).

Measurement of urinary hydroxyproline and of urinary mucopolysaccharides helps to determine the rate of collagen metabolism and turnover, the former for collagen fibers, the latter for ground substance. These are quite nonspecific tests and are positive in a wide variety of diseases affecting connective tissues.

Pathology. Rheumatoid arthritis is a disease that is characterized by chemical and physical alterations in the fibers and ground substance of collagen, cartilage, osteoid and possibly the cytoplasm of striated muscle cells. All of these tissues are derivatives of mesenchyme and there-

fore, in a sense, belong to a system of support and locomotion. It is of interest that another mesenchymal derivative, the reticulum and its offspring cells which elaborate the protective proteins, gamma globulins, are probably involved in rheumatoid arthritis. At least gamma globulins are increased in amount and tend to lose their antibody specificity. The rheumatoid factor itself is an abnormal gamma globulin.

One may summarize the pathologic alterations of rheumatoid arthritis by stating that there are a variety of changes in the supportive tissues of the body that begin as an acute inflammation, pass through a stage of necrosis and terminate in masses of scar tissue. The changes are most characteristically seen in the tissues of the joint and in the rheumatoid nodule but they have been reported in almost every tissue of the body including the brain and its meninges.

Within the joint the disease first manifests itself as a thickening of the synovia with edema. Histiocytic proliferation with fibrinoid alteration is usually prominent at this time (Fig. 21–40). Within a short time there is an infiltration of lymphocytes, sometimes with a few neutrophilic and eosinophilic granulocytes into the synovia. The synovia becomes thickened by a chronic exudative inflammatory reaction (Fig. 21–41). The lymphocytes tend to aggregate in follicles and at times the synovia may be studded with nodules of densely clustered lymphocytes (Fig. 21–42). In the stroma between the follicles one usually finds a scattering of plasma cells. In cases in which we had the opportunity of examining subchondral cancellous tissue the same pathologic alterations were found routinely (Fig. 21–43). It is our belief, without proof from a large amount of material, that the exudative inflammatory stage of rheumatoid arthritis begins in the synovia and the subchondral bone tissue concomitantly.

With progression of the disease there is hyperplasia of the covering synovial cells to form several layers of irregular thickness (Fig. 21–44). The synovial membrane now appears more vascular than normal but this is probably because of congestive filling of otherwise inconspicuous vessels rather than the formation of new

(*Text continued on page 666.*)

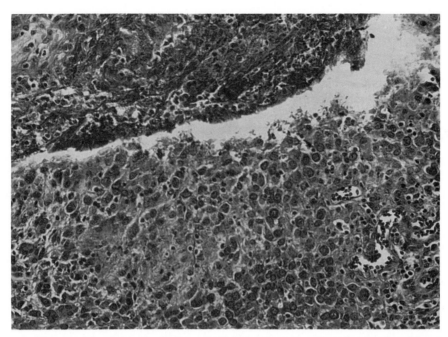

Figure 21–40   Rheumatoid arthritis. In the lower half of the illustration there is a florid proliferation of histiocytic cells. The material above stained deeply with eosin. The linear structures in this area represent fibrinoid alteration. (× 250.)

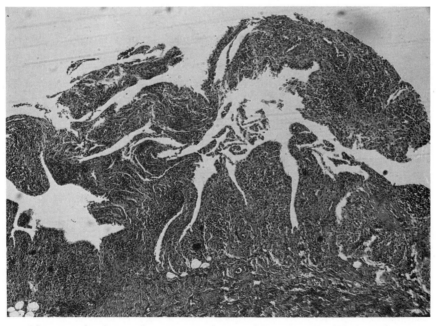

Figure 21–41   Rheumatoid arthritis. The synovia is thickened by a chronic exudative inflammatory reaction. Most of the black dots in the illustration are nuclei of lymphocytes. There are areas of necrosis with some edema and fibrosis. (× 50.)

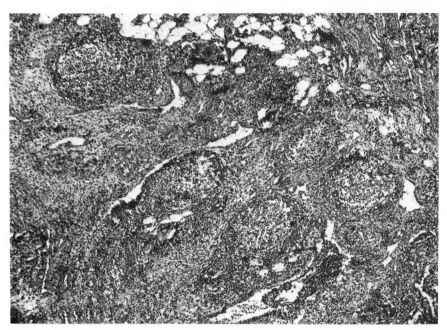

Figure 21–42 Rheumatoid arthritis. Section through thickened synovial membrane at very low magnification to show the follicles of lymphocytes. Five nodules can be seen here though delineation is poor. The germinal centers of the follicles are pale. A vague rim of condensed lymphocytes surrounds each center. (× 50.)

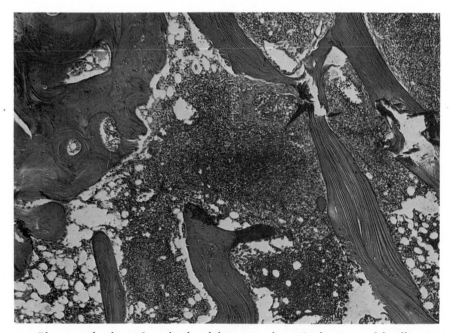

Figure 21–43 Rheumatoid arthritis. Lymphoid nodule in metaphysis. In the center of the illustration there is a dense aggregate of cells in which there are no fat cells. On higher magnification these cells are found to be uniform lymphocytes. (× 65.)

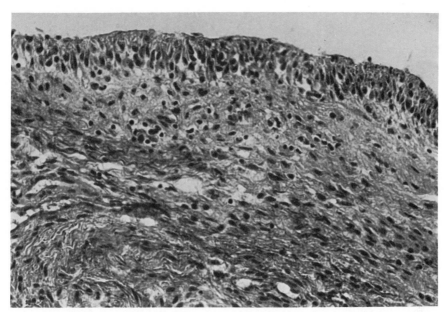

Figure 21–44   Rheumatoid arthritis. Section through synovial membrane. Normally there is only a single layer of synovial cells. Early in the disease they undergo hyperplasia to form several layers of cells such as those seen along the upper edge of the tissue in the illustration. (× 300.)

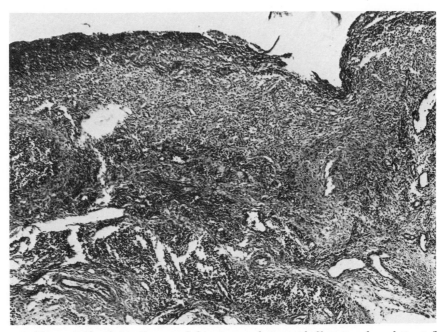

Figure 21–45   Rheumatoid arthritis. Pannus of chronic granulation with fibrosis and exudative inflammatory reaction. The dark zone along the upper edge of the tissue is deeply eosinophilic in the section. It is precipitated fibrin. (× 60.)

channels. There is escape of edema fluid into the joint space to cause effusion and then precipitation of a layer of fibrin over the synovial and articular surfaces (Fig. 21–45). This fibrin layer becomes organized by a growth of collagenoblasts and vessels grow into it from the synovia. This membrane of granulation tissue is known as a pannus. It is highly vascular, and as it spreads over the surface of the articular plate, releasing lytic enzymes from its infiltration of inflammatory cells, the cartilage undergoes lysis and the pits that are formed fill up with a newly formed granulation that continues and extends the lytic process. The same sequence of events goes on beneath the articular plate by the inflammatory reaction in the subchondral epiphysis (Fig. 21–43). Thus the articular plate is attacked from both sides (Fig. 21–46). Weight-bearing surfaces are soon altered so that subluxation occurs. There is extension of the inflammatory reaction into the joint capsule and periarticular ligaments and tendons. Muscle contractures, usually of the stronger flexor muscles, occur. Eventually the joint space is filled with thickened nodular synovia and granular pannus. The articular plate is destroyed

and the joint distorted. There follows a proliferation of collagenous tissue in an attempt to heal the lesion. Fibrous adhesions grow from one subchondral area to the opposite, producing fibrous ankylosis. The dense collagen of these adhesions undergoes calcification and then goes on to ossification – bony ankylosis. The capsule and the synovia are merged into a thick mass of dense scar tissue, which extends beyond the joint to encase ligaments and tendons. The distorted joint is now stiff and functionless.

The rheumatoid nodule develops in about 20 per cent of all cases of rheumatoid arthritis. It is usually found in the subcutaneous tissue at points of pressure, the commonest site being the olecranon area. Nodules may occur in joint capsules and ligaments and rarely in a wide variety of tissues far removed from the joint structure. It is probably this nodule that when it occurs in the sclera causes scleromalacia perforans.

In the early stages the nodule of rheumatoid arthritis is indistinguishable from that of rheumatic fever. Later it may be indistinguishable from the tuberculoma. It is essentially a reactive process manifested

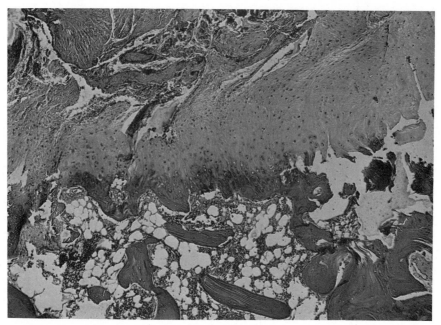

Figure 21–46 Rheumatoid arthritis. The articular plate is attacked from above and below. Areas of lysis produce pits in the cartilage that fill with granulation, which causes further lysis. The plate becomes thinned, split and eventually penetrated. (× 50.)

by the reticuloendothelial system. It begins apparently as an aggregate of histiocytes similar to the Aschoff nodule. Instead of stopping in this stage with necrosis and fibrous scar formation, as is characteristic of the lesion in rheumatic fever, it continues to enlarge to 2 cm. or more in diameter. The central portion becomes necrotic and often caseous (Fig. 21–47 A). Occasionally it may liquefy and then an inflammatory cyst is formed. These nodules, often with cavitation, are occasionally found in the lungs[23] and then must be differentiated from pulmonary tubercu-

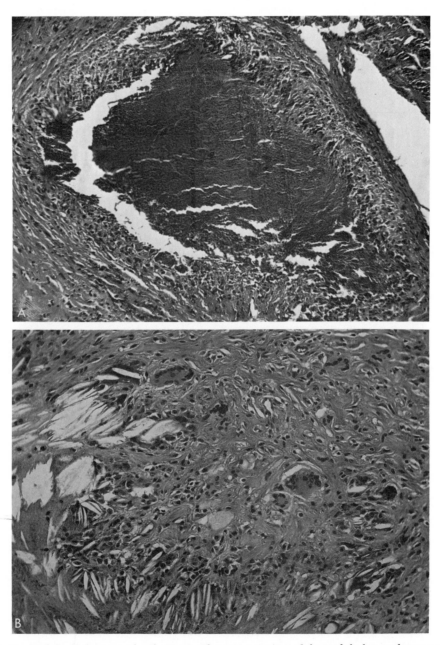

Figure 21–47 Nodule of rheumatoid arthritis. *A*, The major portion of the nodule has undergone necrosis. This dark central area is surrounded by a zone of palisaded inflammatory cells better appreciated in the higher magnification. Outside this zone there is a fibrous capsule. (× 150.) *B*, Reaction at margin of rheumatoid nodule. Clefts are formed by crystals of cholesterol due to caseous necrosis. Giant cells are foreign body type. (× 185.)

losis. About the caseous area there is a zone of histiocytes, which tend to describe a palisade pattern—epithelioid cells. Giant cells are frequently formed (Fig. 21–47 B). If the histiocyte is not expended in the battle to restore normalcy it becomes a collagenoblast, so that these spindled forms are found scattered through this zone. Lymphocytes are also intermixed and tend to aggregate more densely at the periphery, and about this the collagenoblasts form a fibrous capsule. As one surveys the rheumatoid nodule one cannot help but note the similarities to the tissue reaction in tuberculosis, a reaction that is largely composed of what among allergists is known as the delayed immunity response.

Pseudo-rheumatoid nodules may occur in adults without other evidence of rheumatoid arthritis.[24] These nodules are identical to those appearing in the typical disease. They may be followed by symptomatic joint disease and thus be the earliest manifestation of rheumatoid arthritis. When occurring in children they are never followed by rheumatoid arthritis and rarely by rheumatic fever.

Skeletal muscles undergo such rapid atrophy in this disease that it is held by most that the loss in muscle mass is more than can be accounted for on the basis of inactivity because of pain. Because the muscle syncytium is a close relative of the collagen-producing cell, this atrophy may represent a degenerative process akin to that within collagen. Follicles of lymphocytes similar to those found in the synovia are found scattered through skeletal muscle with apparently no geographic relation to involved joints. The same type of exudative inflammatory reaction occasionally may be encountered in lupus erythematosus, rheumatic fever and dermatomyositis.

Follicles similar to those seen in muscle have been reported in the supportive tissue of peripheral nerves. These are apparently common enough to account for the neuritic symptoms, pain, paresthesias, sweating and Raynaud's phenomena that are seen in rheumatoid arthritis. Nerve nodules are also encountered in lupus erythematosus, rheumatic fever and dermatomyositis.

An iridocyclitis sometimes develops in this disease, more frequently in ankylosing spondylitis and somewhat less often in juvenile rheumatoid arthritis. It is usually not severe but occasionally progresses to blindness.

Spontaneous rupture of tendons has been reported in rheumatoid arthritis.[25]

Occasionally rheumatoid arthritis in the adult is associated with splenomegaly and severe hypersplenism with pancytopenia. This is known as Felty's syndrome. Abnormalities of the blood disappear with splenectomy.

Occasionally rheumatoid arthritis may affect children. This is known as juvenile rheumatoid arthritis or Still's disease. Clinical and pathologic features are much the same as those in the adult form but the systemic aspects are apt to be more severe. The juvenile form may be exceedingly difficult or impossible to differentiate from rheumatic fever until joint destruction takes place. The rheumatoid factor is less commonly found in the juvenile form. The inflammatory reaction within the osseous epiphyseal nucleus may destroy the enchondral growth plate, with subsequent replacement by bone, thus arresting longitudinal growth.

RHEUMATOID SPONDYLITIS. One type of arthritis selects exclusively or predominantly the joints of the spine. Except for the differences related to site, the pathologic changes are identical to those of rheumatoid arthritis. This disease is best called ankylosing spondylitis but is variously known as spondylitis rhizomélique, Marie-Strumpell disease and von Bechterew's spondylitis. The age incidence is about the same as for rheumatoid arthritis but it is about 10 times more prevalent in males. The disease has the same tendency for exacerbations and remissions, and when it runs its full course, usually 10 to 15 years though it may describe a fulminant and steadily active course of perhaps three years, it causes bony ankylosis of all the vertebral joints—the poker spine or bamboo spine (Fig. 21–48).

There is said to be a greater incidence of cardiac involvement in spondylitis than in ordinary rheumatoid arthritis. Moreover this complication is apt to involve the aor-

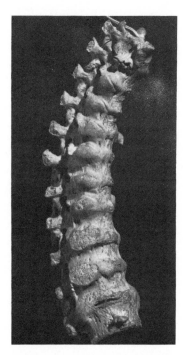

Figure 21–48 Rheumatoid spondylitis. There is bony ankylosis of the entire spine. The anterior longitudinal ligaments are accentuated as bony struts. There is lipping of the vertebral margins.

tic valve, its ring and the ascending aortic segment. Rheumatoid nodules rarely are formed and Rh factor can be found in only about 15 per cent of cases. Reiter's syndrome is sometimes associated. Clinically ankylosing spondylitis and typical rheumatoid arthritis are quite dissimilar. For this reason many writers prefer to consider spondylitis a separate entity. There can be no doubt, however, that the pathogenesis of the two diseases is the same.

The hereditary features of spondylitis are more obvious than in rheumatoid arthritis. The disease most commonly begins in the sacroiliac joints and extends cephalad. In cases in which the spine alone is involved the rheumatoid factor is rarely present in the serum. Peripheral joints are involved in about one fifth of the cases. The incidence of ankylosing spondylitis is perhaps one fifth that of rheumatoid arthritis.

Roentgenographic Manifestations. The earliest roentgenographic manifestation of rheumatoid arthritis is related to the involvement of synovia, with synovial thickening and fluid within the joint. Periarticu-

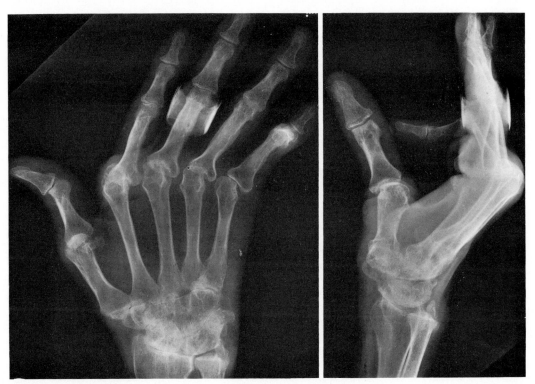

Figure 21–49 Rheumatoid arthritis. There is narrowing of the proximal interphalangeal joints, the metacarpophalangeal joints and the wrist. Ulnar deviation of the fingers is evident.

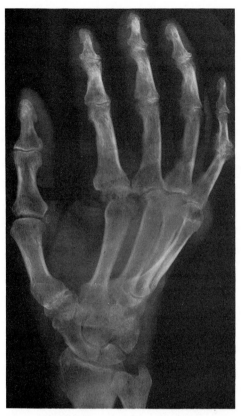

Figure 21–50 Rheumatoid arthritis. Destructive areas are evident in the distal ends of the second, third and fifth metacarpals. In the second, they are most conspicuous at the margins of the articular plate.

lar deossification is commonly present early, but later involves the entire bone. Periosteal reaction in relation to the joint is frequently encountered in juvenile rheumatoid arthritis, but may also be noted in the adult. As the pannus of granulation tissue spreads over the articular surfaces, the joint narrows. Erosion of the cortex indicates destruction of cartilage and these are first manifest as loss of subchondral bone, usually of the proximal end of the first phalanx of a finger or the radial aspect of the distal end of the second and third metacarpals.[26] Irregular circumscribed radiolucent areas appear in the cancellous bone beneath the articular plate as the pannus invades the bone. Later in the course of the disease there will be marked destruction of joints and bones in relation to joints (e.g., the distal end of the clavicle) as well as such subluxations as muscle atrophy and contractures. Ossification of the pannus results in bony ankylosis.

Involvement of the odontoid process is not uncommon. This is characterized by erosion of the odontoid, but just as important, by laxity of its ligamentous support and subluxation of the atlantoaxial joint.[28] The latter is demonstrable on film studies made during flexion, i.e., the posterior dis-

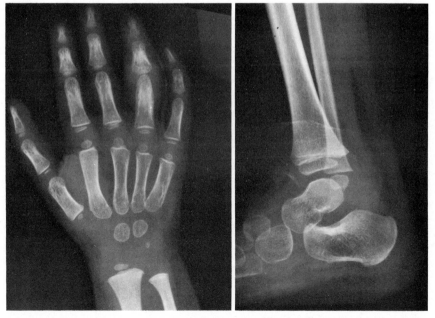

Figure 21–51 Rheumatoid arthritis in a white female 3 years of age. Periarticular swelling and osteopenia are present at the proximal interphalangeal joint of the fourth digit. Periosteal reaction surrounds the proximal phalanx. An effusion into the right ankle joint is evident.

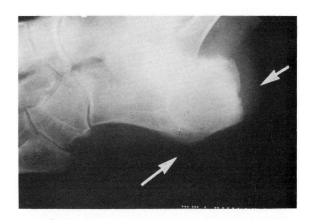

Figure 21–52 Rheumatoid arthritis. There is sclerosis of the os calcis with roughening of the surface at the attachment of the Achilles tendon and the plantar fascia (arrows). Soft tissue swelling is present at the former site. Similar alterations may be seen in Reiter's syndrome and psoriasis.

placement of the odontoid in relation to the anterior arch of the first cervicle vertebra. Atlantoaxial subluxation is also observed in rheumatoid spondylitis and juvenile rheumatoid arthritis.

The manifestations of *juvenile rheumatoid arthritis* are different from those in the adult[29] because of the characteristics of

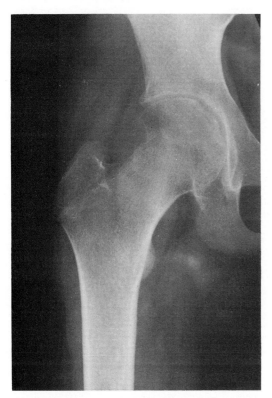

Figure 21–53 Rheumatoid arthritis. The hip joint is narrow. There are small, irregular areas of subchondral destruction with more marked alterations in relation to the lateral aspect of the femoral head.

the growing skeleton, i.e., the large amount of epiphyseal cartilage and the affect of hyperemia and disuse on growth. There will be fluid in joints, deossification and the effects of pannus formation. However, because of the amount of cartilage present, narrowing of joints and bone erosion may be appreciated later. Enlargement of epiphyses is common, but so is accelerated maturation and premature closure of the epiphyseal line. Thus cylindrical bones will be either longer or shorter, depending on the stage of epiphyseal involvement. The diameter of the diaphyses may be decreased. Periosteal new bone is often present in the vicinity of an involved joint (Fig. 21–51). Atlantoaxial subluxation may be apparent. The cervical spine may be further affected as manifest by apophyseal ankylosis and narrowed intervertebral discs.

In *ankylosing spondylitis*, the sacroiliac joints and the lumbar segments of the spine tend to be involved first, particularly the sacroiliac joints. The hip joints and shoulders are involved as well in the majority of patients. The sacroiliac joint becomes indistinct in outline and wider than is normal; marginal sclerosis, particularly of the iliac aspect of the joint, appears and in time ankylosis occurs with disappearance of sclerosis. Involvement tends to be bilateral. In the spine, the anterior aspect of the vertebral bodies becomes squared off followed by calcification and ossification of the soft tissues anterior to the spine and finally of the anterior longitudinal ligament. The result is the bamboo spine (Figs. 21–48 and 21–55). Involvement of the odontoid process with subluxation of

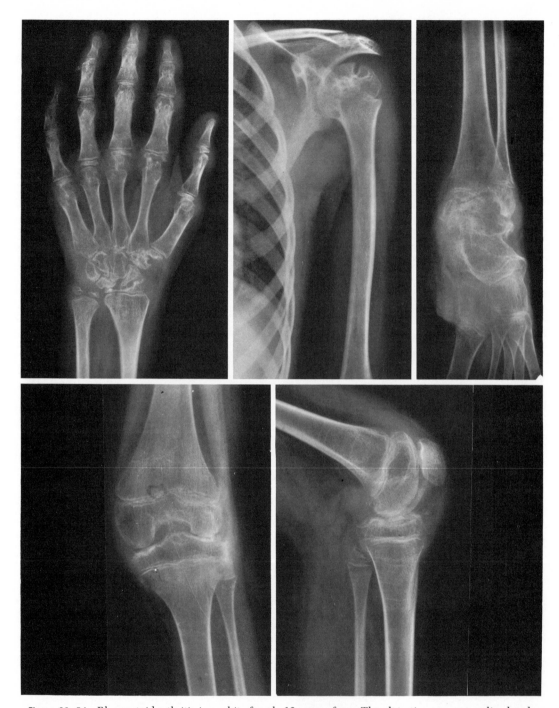

Figure 21–54 Rheumatoid arthritis in a white female 12 years of age. The alterations are generalized and severe. Periarticular osteopenia is marked. There are deformities of the epiphyses, a flexion deformity of the knee and a diminution in size of the muscle bundles.

the cervical spine at the level of the first and second cervical segments may occur.[28] Abnormalities of the remainder of the vertebral bodies in the cervical region are to be expected, characterized by a squared off appearance and often reactive sclerosis. The alterations in the hips and shoulders are those associated with rheumatoid ar-

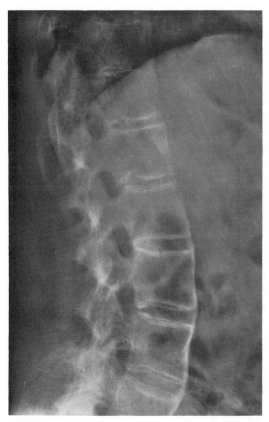

Figure 21–55 Rheumatoid spondylitis. The anterior longitudinal ligament has ossified. The anterior borders of the vertebrae tend to be straight.

thritis. They are characterized by synovial reaction and the effect of pannus formation.

Arthritis of the Collagen Diseases

Joint disease frequently constitutes an important aspect of several of the collagen diseases. This is most often the case in *disseminated lupus erythematosus,* in about 90 per cent of the cases of which there is evidence of joint involvement. The arthritis is apt to run a milder course than in uncomplicated rheumatoid arthritis, but occasionally joint deformity with ankyloses and contractures is the end result of the disease. In the mild or early stage the microscopic aspects of the joint tissues usually are identical to those of rheumatoid arthritis. The rheumatoid factor may be present, though in a smaller percentage than in rheumatoid arthritis.

Serum sickness is usually associated with joint symptoms. Microscopic examination of tissue has been possible in a few cases in which death took place from unrelated diseases during the active phase of a bout of serum sickness. The tissue changes are identical to those of rheumatic fever or presumably the earliest phase of rheuma-

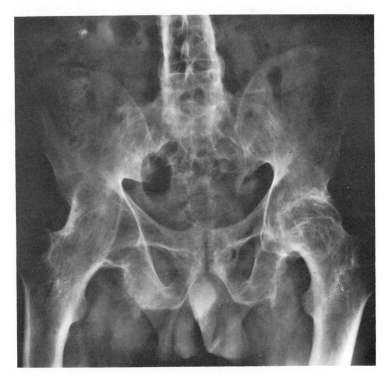

Figure 21–56 Rheumatoid spondylitis. Ankylosis of the sacroiliac and hip joints has occurred. Ossification of the vertebral ligaments is evident.

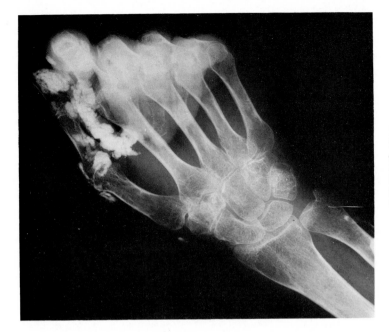

Figure 21–57 Scleroderma. There are flexion deformities of the fingers and considerable calcification of soft tissue, particularly in relation to joints. The bones are undermineralized and the interphalangeal joints are narrowed.

toid arthritis. The lesions never progress to tissue destruction and scar formation.

In perhaps half the cases of *dermatomyositis* the joints are involved in what usually proves to be a mild rheumatoid arthritis. The joint disease may continue into the destructive phase. The rheumatoid factor has been identified in a few of these cases.

In *erythema nodosa*, transient joint disease commonly develops. The signs and symptoms are those of early rheumatoid arthritis that does not progress to tissue destruction.

In a small percentage of cases of *scleroderma* and *polyarteritis* the symptoms of rheumatoid arthritis complicate the picture. We have studied one case in which there were tissue changes characteristic of lupus erythematosus, rheumatoid arthritis and polyarteritis nodosa. The terminal phase of the disease in this patient most nearly resembled polyarteritis and tissues at autopsy revealed the classic arterial lesions.

RHEUMATIC FEVER

Rheumatic fever is a systemic disease; the outstanding feature of the active phase is joint pain and of the chronic recurrent phase, heart disease. Because the joints heal completely without residuum of function loss, it is the cardiac facet of rheumatic fever that makes it of such immense importance. It is the commonest cause of organic heart disease in patients under 40 and the greatest single cause of death in those under 20.

The pathogenesis of rheumatic fever is still not entirely clear and this text is not the place to indulge in a lengthy discussion of the numerous theories. We know that it is related to infections with the Group A beta hemolytic streptococcus and probably represents a sensitivity state to this organism or its products. In most initial attacks of rheumatic fever, a bout of streptococcal infection can be determined one to three weeks earlier. This infection is usually manifested as a sore throat or acute tonsillitis.

At the outset of the rheumatic fever the patient, usually a child, though the disease may develop at any age, complains of migratory joint or muscle pains and easy fatigue. There is often a marked degree of pallor. Fever, tachycardia and excessive perspiration are usual. Joint involvement may be solitary or multiple. Any joint or group of joints may be affected but usually the disease announces itself in a single, large, weight-bearing articulation. The joint becomes painful and excruciatingly tender, red, swollen and hot. There is obvious effusion early in the disease. The inflammation persists for 2 to 10 days and then subsides, leaving the joint completely healthy. Before complete healing in one joint, another may become involved, and thus a number of joints may be attacked during the course of the active initial phase or during recurrence. About one third of the cases of well defined rheumatic fever with joint disease sooner or later develop cardiac involvement.

Pathology. The pathology of rheumatic fever is probably the same whether it occurs in the collagen of the heart, the joints or elsewhere in the body. We had the opportunity of studying a case in which fairly characteristic lesions occurred in the meninges.[30] Scarring occurs in the cardiac structures and plays an important role in rheumatic heart disease. Yet it is never reported in joint tissues, not because of important differences in the lesions but rather because of differences in the environment and functional stresses of the collagen involved. Microscopic areas of necrosis that heal with shrinking scar tissue in the mitral valve leaflet produce dramatic functional alterations, whereas they are unnoted in the joint synovia.

The lesion of rheumatic fever is a microscopic focus of inflammation in the perivascular tissue of a small blood vessel. The cell type most prominently displayed is the histiocyte but lymphocytes and plasma cells are also present. In cardiac tissues these tiny cell aggregates are called Aschoff bodies and are pathognomonic of the disease. In other tissues these lesions show a variety of modifications in size, pattern and cell arrangement. They have been reported in a wide variety of body tissues. The nidus of the nodule eventually becomes necrotic and collagen proliferation follows in an attempt to repair it. It is the contracting scar tissue that causes failure in cardiac valve function. Small masses of scar tissue are less important elsewhere in the body.

MISCELLANEOUS TYPES OF ARTHRITIS

Intermittent Hydrarthrosis

This is a rare and curious joint disease characterized by periodic episodes of effusion which for extended periods of time do not advance to the destructive phase of rheumatoid arthritis. The attacks usually last only a few days, they are rarely painful, heat and tenderness are lacking and the joint retains full function except for the minor inconvenience of enlargement and stiffness due to effusion. The periodicity of the attacks may become rhythmic and they have been reported persisting for more than 10 years. Some cases now are reported to have evolved into more classic rheumatoid arthritis. Analysis of joint fluid has shown it to be similar to that in the effusion state of rheumatoid arthritis. Biopsy has shown infiltration with lymphocytic follicles similar to those seen in the early stage of true rheumatoid arthritis. Many observers believe that intermittent hydrarthrosis is a forme fruste of the more serious disease. An explanation of why the process is so remarkably similar to the early stage of rheumatoid arthritis, yet usually does not advance to destruction of the articular plate, might clear up much of the obscurity that beclouds the pathogenesis of the latter disease.

Palindromic Rheumatism

This entity is another exotic and enigmatic joint disease that probably is related to rheumatoid arthritis. The attacks usually come on suddenly, in some cases at about the same time of day. The attack may last a few hours or a few days and then it subsides, leaving a completely normal joint. Different joints are apt to be involved in the next attack.

Swelling of the joint is the outstanding clinical feature. There are pain, heat and redness of the area. Sometimes the attack is associated with fever. Data concerning the morphology of the tissue reaction are fragmentary, but the synovial fluid apparently contains more granulocytes and fibrin than that of typical rheumatoid arthritis and the disease usually does not progress to articular plate destruction. A few patients have been reported to develop typical rheumatoid arthritis several years after the initial disease. Many have tried to explain palindromic rheumatism as the joint manifestation of an allergic reaction, but no antigen has been found to precipitate the attacks and the usual antisensitivity drugs are ineffective in therapy. Many think that this is a variant forme fruste of rheumatoid arthritis.

Arthritis Mutilans

This rare and interesting disease has been described as a variant of both osteoarthritis and rheumatoid arthritis. It

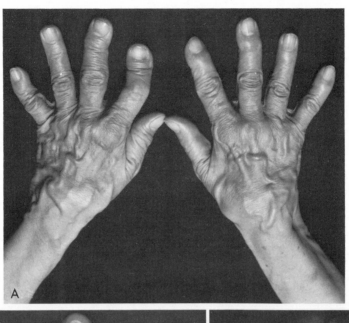

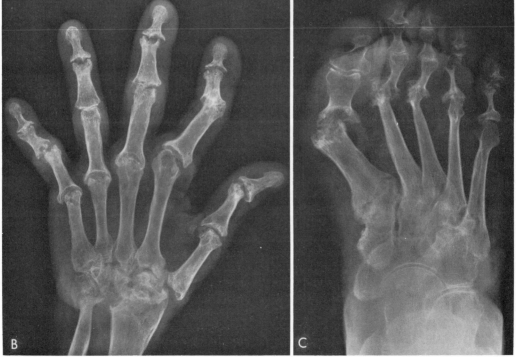

Figure 21–58 Arthritis mutilans. The fingers are short and the skin is loose around the joints (A). There is marked destruction of bone at most of the joints in the hands and feet, but swelling of the periarticular soft tissues is not present.

probably belongs to neither category though presenting certain features common to both. It is more common in women than men, and it usually occurs in the last trimester of life. The pattern of joint involvement is like that of rheumatoid arthritis. The disease starts within the joint and quickly causes lysis of the articular plates, thus resembling rheumatoid arthritis. But it extends beyond the cartilage to cause resorption of the juxtapositional bone ends like a severe osteoarthritis. The periarticular tissues usually escape and fibrous and bony ankyloses do not occur. There is little or no atrophy of the overlying skin so that the member is markedly shortened owing to loss of joint and bone-end structures and ensheathed in loose skin (Fig. 21–58). Thus the involved members may be extended by traction, providing the descriptive name that the French have given the disease, "Mains ou doigts en lorgnette."

At times non-articular cartilage, that of the trachea, nasal septum and ears, may share in the resorption suggesting that the disease is primarily a lytic process affecting all body cartilage and bone. Insufficient material has been studied by microscopic section to make a discussion of pathogenesis more than a hazardous guess. Rogers and Lansbury[31] reported a case in which treatment with chorionic gonadotropins apparently precipitated massive lysis of extra-articular cartilage and suggested the possibility that, because one frequently encounters exacerbations of degenerative joint disease in menopausal women with high output of pituitary secretion, these or related hormones may play a causative or precipitating role. We pose the question of the relationship of this form of arthritis to cortisone therapy arthropathy.

Cysts of the Menisci

Focal accumulations of mucoid material may occur within the menisci of the knee joint. The pathogenesis of these lesions is not clear. Because the cysts are usually multilocular it is assumed that a group of small cystic areas coalesce.

The lateral meniscus is more commonly affected than the medial. A history of trauma is frequently obtained but traumatic alteration (tears) is usually lacking. Typically, the patient is troubled by a nagging ache, which may occur on either side of the knee. This is usually accompanied by swelling. Sometimes the function of the joint is impaired by locking, buckling or snapping. Effusion is not characteristic.

The cysts measure a few millimeters to several centimeters in diameter. Occasionally they can be aspirated with relief of symptoms but recur as the fluid reaccumulates. The source of the fluid is unknown. Some think that it is the product of mucinous degeneration of cartilage. Others have reported a fragmentary synovial lining. It appears probable that these cysts represent metaplastic errors in which synovial cells become enclosed in the fiber-cartilage of the meniscus. They secrete mucin, the small cysts coalesce and pressure may cause atrophy and degeneration of the lining cells. The fact that these cysts recur with such constancy if the walls are not entirely removed suggests that the lesion is not the product of a purely degenerative process.

Baker's Cyst

Any cystic structure formed by a herniation of the lining synovial membrane through the capsule of a joint or wall of a bursa is usually called a Baker's cyst, though Baker's original paper described liquefaction degeneration of a variety of dissimilar tissues. The lesion most commonly occurs as a herniation of the synovial lining of the knee joint through the posterior capsular wall into the popliteal space (Fig. 21–59). Chronic inflammation caused by this foreign mass among the moving structures of the area causes the development of a fibrous wall the thickness of which depends upon the duration and size of the mass. If the herniation canal remains open the cyst fluid may closely resemble the synovial fluid of the joint. If the canal becomes closed by fibrous proliferation the fluid may become highly mucinous in character. As pressure builds up within the cyst the lining synovia may undergo atrophy and disappear. Various tensions from within and without the cyst may cause it to become multilocu-

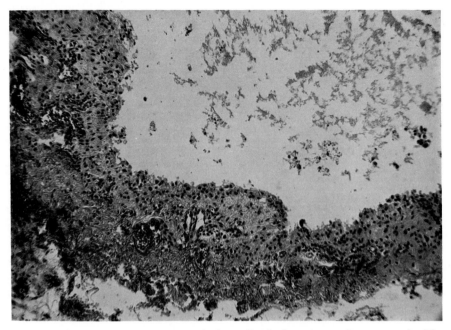

Figure 21-59 Baker's cyst. Cross section through the wall. The lumen is at the upper right. The synovial lining has atrophied. (× 150.)

lated. Synovial villi within the cyst may metaplase to chondroblasts and form rounded masses of cartilage, which may become detached to form free bodies within the cyst cavity. Because the cartilage is capable of maintaining life in synovial fluid, it may continue to grow and even ossify in its central portion. These osseous nidi calcify and become radiopaque. Such multiple opacities in the periarticular tissues must be differentiated from tenosynovial chondrometaplasia. (See p. 748.) Baker's cyst of the periarticular soft tissues is analogous to the subchondral or ganglion cysts that occur in the cancellous tissue of the ossified epiphysis (see p. 440).

DISEASES OF PERIARTICULAR TISSUES

Fibrositis

Fibrositis has been defined as "an acute, subacute or chronic painful state of muscles, subcutaneous tissues, ligaments, tendons or fasciae caused by a number of agents such as trauma, strain, occupation, exposure, posture, infection, arthritis or stimuli that may be considered toxic or psychogenic." It is an exceedingly common condition in Great Britain, of much lower incidence in the United States. Many clinicians have attempted to describe the pathology of this condition but their descriptions are couched in terms too nebulous for interpretation by a pathologist. We have no material whatsoever that can be classified under this heading. We can only presume that the symptoms of pain, tenderness and stiffness, which are said to characterize the disease, are too indefinite or too vaguely localized to permit biopsy. We suggest that the term be relegated to the same status as "stiffneck and lumbago" until something pathologically more definitive can be offered.

Bursitis

Acute and chronic bursitis is an inflammatory process in a bursa, almost always an extension of a lesion, usually calcification, less frequently trauma, infection or arthritis, from nearby tissues. Of the nearly 150 bursas of the body the subdeltoid is the one most frequently involved. It

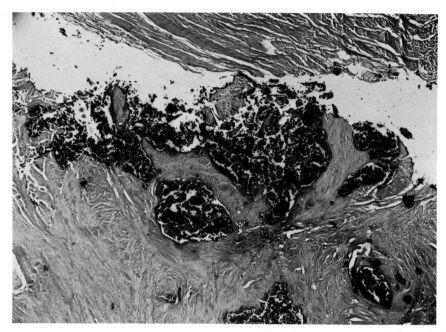

Figure 21–60   Chronic bursitis. Section through the thickened wall of a bursa. The dark areas represent deposits of calcium salts embedded in a densely collagenous matrix. (× 40.)

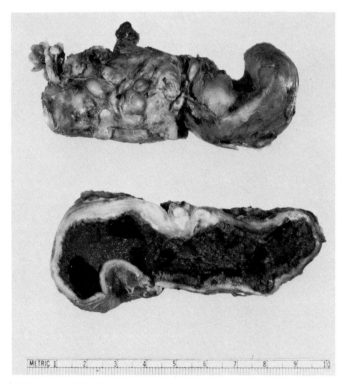

Figure 21–61   Chronic bursitis. The bursa has been sectioned. The exterior surface is shown above, the interior below. The wall is greatly thickened and fibrous.

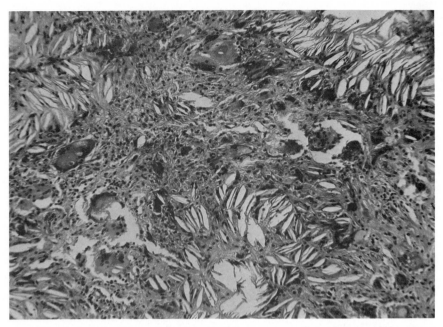

Figure 21–62   Chronic bursitis. Hemorrhage into the bursa may result in cholesterol deposits in the wall (fusiform clefts). The lipid sets up a foreign body reaction with histiocytes and giant cells. (× 150.)

is the most common cause of the painful shoulder.

Acute bursitis often has a sudden onset. Pain is the most prominent symptom and it may be excruciating. The lesion is exquisitely tender and motion accentuates it so that the involved part is rigidly splinted. In acute attacks there may be fever, in-

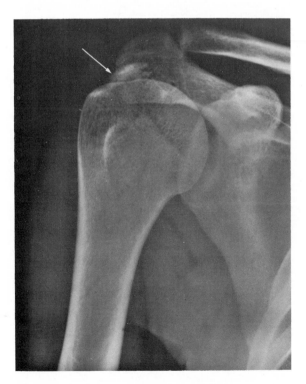

Figure 21–63   Bursitis. Calcification is evident in the supraspinatus tendon (arrow). Multiple projections are necessary to localize calcification in other tendons of the rotator cuff of the shoulder.

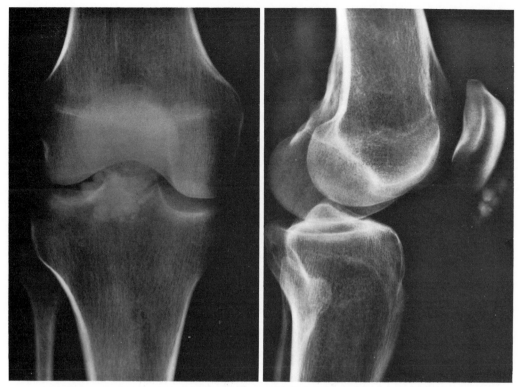

Figure 21–64   Bursitis. There is a group of calcifications in the prepatellar bursa.

creased sedimentation rate and even leukocytosis. Muscle spasm complicates the picture and adds to the patient's discomfort and inability.

The most common type of subdeltoid bursitis is secondary to calcification of the supraspinatus tendon. This tendon runs through the floor of the subdeltoid bursa and the deposits of calcium apparently set up an inflammatory reaction in the wall of the latter (Fig. 21–60). In acute states there is distention with fluid and exudative inflammatory reaction about the calcium deposits like the inflammatory reaction about the tophi of gout. Indeed, the two conditions, different in pathogenesis, may be quite similar clinically and pathologically.

If the bursitis is chronic and longstanding the wall becomes greatly thickened with collagenous tissue (Fig. 21–61). The synovial lining that was present in the early stage atrophies and disappears.

Cholesterol crystals are frequently formed, possibly from degenerating fat in the region, and a foreign body inflammatory reaction is commonly encountered

(Fig. 21–62). Massive deposits of calcium salts are precipitated and have the appearance and consistency of thick toothpaste. Muscles may atrophy because of disuse. The calcareous deposits may rupture into the bursal lumen. Eventually dense fibrotic scar may efface the normal architecture of the bursa and surrounding tissues.

The reason for the original calcification of tendon tissue is poorly understood. Some alteration in collagen makes it develop an affinity for calcium salts similar to that of osteoid. The chemical nature of this alteration is unknown. As long as circulation to the area is not too greatly impaired, the calcium deposits remain reversible. Often, fairly large masses of calcium in tendons and in bursal walls disappear with rest and proper therapy.

Ganglia

The ganglion is a sacklike structure that usually arises subcutaneously on the extensor surface of the wrist, at times on the flexor surface and less commonly on the dorsum of the foot or rarely about the knee. It usually consists of a rather thin fibrous wall surrounding an irregular lumen containing mucinous fluid. The cyst often dissects between tendons to approach the surface and elevate the skin. It is often painful, sometimes symptomless.

The pathogenesis of the ganglion still remains controversial though it is agreed now that it is not tuberculous, as was once thought. Most observers believe that it is a herniation of a tendon sheath, which may eventually become isolated from the parent sheath lumen by constriction and postinflammatory fibrosis. Others believe that it is a myxomatous degeneration of collagenous tissue that has proliferated because of inflammation.

It is certain that fragments of synovial lining can occasionally be found in some ganglia and it seems likely that the process is a herniation of this membrane, which develops a fibrous wall, becomes isolated from its source and then undergoes atrophy of its lining. Sections through the wall sometimes reveal a granulomatous reaction with numerous giant cells, a picture that probably inspired the idea of the tu-berculous pathogenesis. More often the wall consists of a layer of fibrous connective tissue without lining, giving no hint of its origins (Fig. 21–65).

Synovial Chondrometaplasia

Free bodies within the joint space—joint mice or rice bodies—may be formed whenever fragments of viable cartilage are freed there. They may represent the cartilaginous portion of a detached osteochondritis dissecans or a cartilage fragment torn away by trauma. They may represent the detached cap of an inflammatory spur. More frequently they are the result of a metaplastic error of synovial cells. Microscopic masses of chondroid begin to appear, usually in the tips of the synovial villi. The surrounding cells have become altered to resemble chondroblasts. As the cartilage mass grows it forms a spheroid body, the villous process serving as its pedicle. Eventually, it becomes detached and falls free into the joint space (Fig. 21–66 A). The chondroblasts are nourished by the synovial fluid and continue to proliferate and form cartilage so

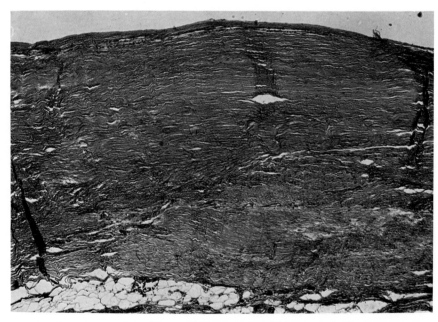

Figure 21–65   Ganglion. Section through a greatly thickened and fibrotic wall. The lumen is pictured above. The synovial lining has atrophied. The ganglion is surrounded by fatty tissue, below. (× 55.)

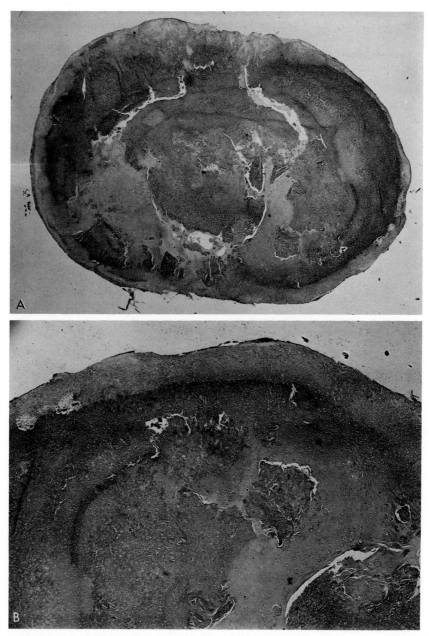

Figure 21-66   Joint body. *A*, The body was sectioned and photographed to show the cut surface. The center is bony with irregular areas of cartilage. The body is covered with a layer of cartilage like an articular plate. (× 17.) *B*, Higher magnification showing bone nidus and cartilage covering. (× 40.)

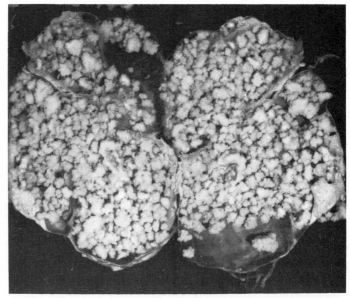

Figure 21–67   Synovial chondrometaplasia. A bursa, filled with loose bodies, was fixed and sectioned. The photograph shows the lumen filled with discrete, cartilage-covered nodules.

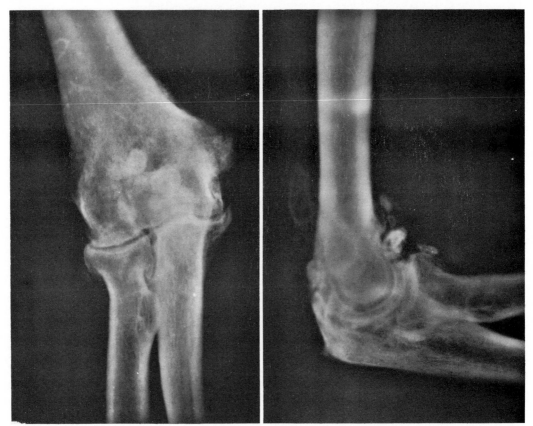

Figure 21–68   Synovial chondrometaplasia. Roentgenogram of an elbow. About the joint the synovial linings of tendon sheaths have formed numerous cartilaginous bodies that have ossified to produce round and ovoid areas of opacity.

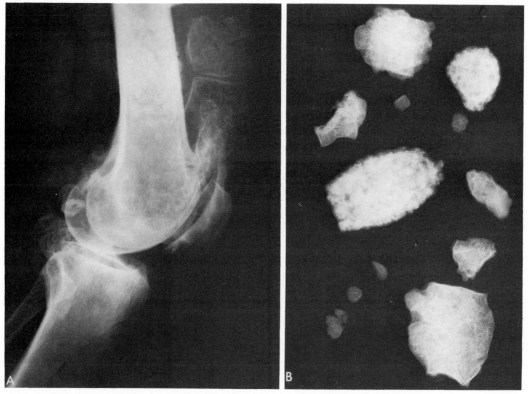

Figure 21–69   Chondrometaplasia. In this instance, most of the loose bodies are in fact predominantly osseous in nature (*B*).

that the spheroid structure continues to grow. The cells within the mass may now metaplase to osteoblasts to form a nidus of bone that is surrounded by a layer of cartilage, the structure mimicking an articular plate over subchondral bone (Fig. 21–66 *B*). These may be formed by the hundreds by the synovia so that the joint cavity, or in some cases a bursa, may be greatly distended and crowded with fairly uniform glistening white bodies (Fig. 21–67).

In the past, this condition has been quite generally called osteochondromatosis. Because it is entirely non-neoplastic this is a poor descriptive term. Also, because the true osteochondroma may be multiple, the term "osteochondromatosis" should be reserved for that condition.

At times tendon sheath or bursal synovia may assume the same peculiar metaplastic activity. Spheroid cartilage masses then appear in the periarticular tissues. If the centers of these masses ossify they become radiopaque and appear on the roentgeno-

gram (Fig. 21–68). They often have been misinterpreted as chondrosarcoma. The synovia may continue to produce these bodies after the initial set has been removed. This suggests recurrence and malignant behavior. We have collected 29 cases of this condition, which we choose to call periarticular tenosynovial chondrometaplasia. Most of our cases occurred after the age of 40, predominantly in males. Whereas the knee is the joint most commonly affected in synovial chondrometaplasia, the wrist and hand are most often involved in tenosynovial chondrometaplasia. In our material there are four affecting the tendons of the wrist, 11 of the fingers, four about the knee, three the ankle and three the foot.

References

1. Hollander, J., Ed.: Arthritis and Allied Conditions. Ed. 7. Philadelphia, Lea and Febiger, 1966.
2. Bluhm, G.: Bull. Pathol., April, 1969, p. 91.

3. Kulka, J. and Schumacher, H.: J. Arth. Rheum., *11*:106, 1968.

4. Forrester, D. M. and Nesson, J. W.: The Radiology of Joint Disease. Philadelphia, W. B. Saunders Co., 1973.

5. Pugh, D. G.: The Roentgenologic Diagnosis of Diseases of Bone. Baltimore, Williams and Wilkins, 1952 and 1954.

6. McCarty, D., Kohn, N. and Faires, J.: Ann. Intern. Med., *56*:711, 1962.

7. La Du, B., Zannoni, V., Laster, L. and Seegmiller, J.: J. Biol. Chem., *230*:251, 1958.

8. Smith, J.: J.A.M.A., *120*:1282, 1942.

9. Young, H.: J. Urol., *51*:48, 1944.

10. Brinkhous, K.: Hemophilia and Hemophilioid Diseases. Chapel Hill, University of North Carolina Press, 1957.

11. Lack, C.: J. Bone Joint Surg., *41B*:384, 1959.

12. Aegerter, E. E. and Long, J. H.: Am. J. Med. Sci., *218*:324, 1949.

13. Bennett, G. A., Waine, H. and Bauer, W.: Changes in the Knee Joint at Various Ages. New York, Commonwealth Fund, 1942.

14. Sokoloff, L., et al.: Syllabus to Set of Lantern Slides. New York, Arthritis and Rheumatism Foundation, 1956.

15. Landells, J. W.: J. Bone Joint Surg., *35B*:643, 1953.

16. Silverman, F. and Gilden, J.: Radiology, *72*:176, 1959.

17. Alarcón-Segovia, D. and Ward, L.: J.A.M.A., *193*:1052, 1965.

18. Fisher, D., Bickel, W. and Holley, K.: Mayo Clin. Proc., *44*:252, 1969.

19. Jaffe, H., Lichtenstein, L. and Sutro, C.: Arch. Pathol., *31*:731, 1941.

20. Smith-Petersen, M.: N. Engl. J. Med., *230*:409, 1944.

21. Clark, W.: N. Engl. J. Med., *245*:112, 1951.

22. Carr, C., Berley, F. and Davis, W.: J. Bone Joint Surg., *36A*:1007, 1954.

23. Stengel, B., Watson, R. and Darling, R.: J.A.M.A., *198*:125, 1966.

24. Lowney, E. and Simons, H.: Arch. Dermatol., *88*:853, 1963.

25. Page, J.: J. Mich. Med. Soc., *60*:888, 1961.

26. Edeiken, J. and Hodes, P. J.: Roentgen Diagnosis of Diseases of Bone. Vol. 2. Ed. 2. Baltimore, Williams and Wilkins, 1973.

27. Smith, J. H. and Pugh, D. G.: Am. J. Roentgenol., *87*:1146, 1962.

28. Martel, W. and Page, J. W.: Arthritis Rheum., *3*:546, 1960.

29. Martel, W., Holt, J. F. and Cassidy, J. T.: Am. J. Roentgenol., *88*:400, 1962.

30. High, R. H. and Aegerter, E. E.: J. Pediatr., *27*:343, 1945.

31. Rogers, F. B. and Lansbury, J.: Am. J. Med. Sci., *229*:55, 1955.

32. Murray, R.: Am. J. Roentgenol., *77*:729, 1961.

Chapter 22

DISEASES OF SKELETAL MUSCLE

Perhaps 90 per cent of all diseases affecting voluntary striated muscle fall within three categories: (1) neuromyopathy, muscle paralysis and atrophy secondary to denervation, most commonly due to poliomyelitis, (2) muscular dystrophy or (3) one of the types of polymyositis. There are several other types of myopathies that are important only because they must be differentiated from the more common varieties. A complete discussion of these diseases cannot be undertaken in a book of this magnitude but a classification and a moderately detailed description of the microscopic features should be helpful to the orthopedist in understanding these conditions and to the pathologist who must reach a diagnosis on the basis of what he sees in the sections. Both should have available the very fine volume *Diseases of Muscle* by Adams, Denny-Brown and Pearson[1] for a discussion in depth of any specific muscle disease.

THE MYOPATHIES

I. Muscular dystrophy
    Progressive muscular dystrophy (Duchenne)
    Facioscapulohumeral and limb-girdle types
    Distal muscular dystrophy
    Ocular myodystrophy
    Myotonic dystrophy
II. Neuromyopathy
    Congenital hypotonia
      Werdnig-Hoffman type
      Rod disease
      Central core disease
    Progressive muscular atrophy
      Amyotrophic lateral sclerosis
      Bulbar palsy
      Progressive neuromuscular atrophy
    Viral neuromyopathy
    Miscellaneous neuromyopathies

III. Arthrogryposis
IV. Allergic myopathy
    Polymyositis
    Polymyositis associated with other mesenchymal diseases, Sjögren's syndrome or cancer
V. Infectious myositis
VI. Congenital myotonia (Thomsen)
VII. Stiff-Man Syndrome
VIII. Myasthenia gravis
IX. Familial periodic paralysis

The Muscle Biopsy

For decades pathologists have recognized the muscle biopsy as a tricky and deceptive tool in the diagnosis of muscle disease. Certain innate features of muscle tissue make artifacts so common and

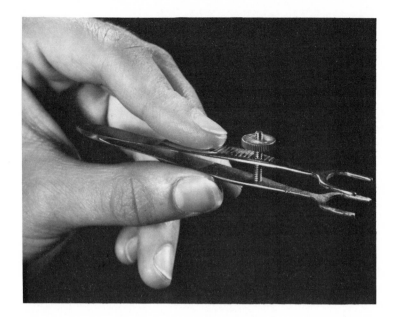

Figure 22–1 Clamp used in biopsying muscle. The fascicle is gently dissected free, the clamp applied and the fascicle sectioned on either side of the clamp. Specimen and clamp are then immersed in fixative.

varied that sections may be impossible to interpret. Today we know that passive stretching in removal or violent contraction caused by dropping live muscle tissue into fixative causes alterations that have jeopardized the integrity of morphologic interpretation. These pitfalls can be avoided if a rigid technique of biopsy and tissue processing is followed. It is suggested that all muscle biopsies, regardless of the service that claims the patient, be performed by a single, experienced surgeon. Also the sectioning and staining of the specimen obtained should be carried out by a single technician, thus keeping all variables at a minimum.

In general, samples of proximal muscles, pectoral, deltoid or quadriceps femoris, yield more satisfactory samples than those of the distal portions of the extremities. A muscle in the early stages of involvement is preferable to one that is completely atrophied. When the muscle has been selected, the biopsy site is determined by electrical stimulation, the area responding to the lowest possible voltage. Infiltration of the muscle with analgesic agents must be avoided. The fascia is incised in the direction of the muscle fascicles. A fascicle is selected and gently dissected free. A special U shaped muscle biopsy clamp is then applied to maintain orientation and prevent contraction (Fig. 22–1). The fascicle

is sectioned on either side of the clamp and placed directly in a glutaraldehyde solution to terminate enzymatic activity. After an hour the biopsy specimen, still in its clamp, is placed in freshly buffered formalin solution. After fixation it is treated as any ordinary soft tissue specimen, staining routinely with hematoxylin and eosin and Masson trichrome stains.

As soon as the clamped specimen has been removed, another fascicle is injected with a 0.03 per cent saline solution of methylene blue warmed to 38° C. This sample need not be clamped because this technique is designed to give nerve rather than muscle detail. The specimen is divided into thin slices (2 to 3 mm.) to facilitate oxygenation. The latter is accomplished by placing the specimen on gauze moistened with saline in a Petri dish in an oven at 38° C. A funnel is placed over the specimen and the latter is exposed to a high oxygen tension for one hour. Immediately after oxygenation it is placed in a cold aqueous saturated solution of ammonium molybdate in a refrigerator at 4° C. for 24 hours. It is washed in running water for one hour and then placed for an equal time in 10 per cent formol-saline fixative. It is then dehydrated in various solutions of alcohol and cleared in xylene. The tissue is then placed on a slide, covered and crushed.

Anatomy and Physiology of the Muscle Cell

The muscle fiber is a syncytium, an elongated mass of protoplasm enclosed in a membrane, containing up to several hundred nuclei. The diameter and length of the fiber vary greatly depending upon its anatomic site (and function) and the age of the organism. The ocular muscles are narrow and short; those of the thigh and buttock are coarse and long. Some fibers at birth increase their diameter tenfold in maturation. Variation ranges from 10 to 100 μ in cross section and from a few to 25 mm. in length.

The multiple nuclei are normally at the periphery of the fiber just beneath the fiber membrane (Fig. 22–2). Migration of the nucleus to the center of the fiber usually means that the fiber is diseased. The membrane of the fiber is too thin to be appreciated by the light microscope. It is combined with the fibrous supportive tissue that ensheaths each fiber called the endomysium. The combined endomysium and fiber membrane is called the sarcolemma. The membrane alone is sometimes referred to as the plasmalemma. Normally the endomysium is not visualized by the light microscope. In instances in which it is seen, the connective tissue content is abnormal and the muscle is said to be sclerotic. Fibers are grouped in bundles by a coarser fibrous structure called the perimysium and the muscle is surrounded by a sheath named the epimysium. The perimysium ensheaths the fasciculi. Each fasciculus extends through only a fraction of the length of the muscle; they are staggered so that a cross section of the muscle cuts across several fasciculi at different levels.

Occasionally one may be able to demonstrate a muscle fiber nucleus nested in a cove in the side of a mature fiber. The cell is short and spindled. Because it is not apparently a part of the endomysium it was originally called a satellite cell. More recently it has been suggested that it is a myoblast or reserve muscle cell. It probably plays a role in muscle regeneration. It is intriguing to consider the possibility of it being the stem cell for the primitive rhabdomyosarcomas.

Each muscle fiber is actually a bundle of muscle fibrils; each fibril measures 0.5 to 1.0 μ in diameter. The fibrils are parallel to the long axis and run the entire length of the fiber. Each fibril has alternating dark and light bands and the bands of all the

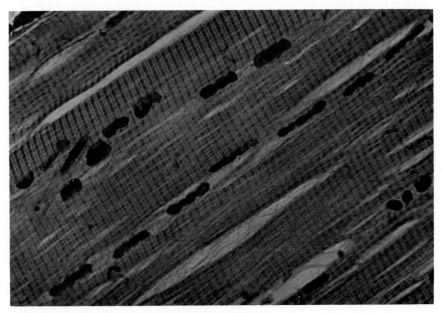

Figure 22–2   Normal striated muscle. The nuclei are multiple and arranged peripherally beneath the plasmalemma. ($\times$ 200.)

fibrils of the fiber and all fibers of the fascicles are arranged synchronously so that the muscle is said to be striated (Fig. 22–3). The dark zone, often called the A band, is divided by a narrower light zone, sometimes called the H zone, and the light stripe, often referred to as the I band, is divided by a narrower dark zone, called the Z line (Fig. 22–4). The designations vary among different investigators and discussion in greater detail, except in illustrating the current hypothesis of muscle contraction, would serve no useful purpose here.

Tendons and ligaments are collagenous prolongations of the muscle fibers. Bands of this substance are elaborated by collagenoblasts and merge with the fibrillar prolongations of the sarcoplasm. Secreting collagenoblasts mature to form spindled, pyknotic fibrocytes lying in rows between bundles of tendon collagen (Fig. 4–38, page 73).

The sensory organ of the muscle is located within the muscle spindle (Fig. 22–5). Each muscle has perhaps 100 of these organs, which are found in the perimysium and must be recognized as a normal mus-

cle component. They have been mistaken for encysted parasites. They are spindle shaped and 0.5 to 3.0 mm. long consisting of a fibrous capsule surrounding a compartmentalized area containing one or more small muscle fibers and the sensory apparatus.

Skeletal muscle is a highly vascularized organ. Each muscle fiber is ensheathed in a plexus of capillary channels. On section these cannot be visualized because the channels are compressed. When extended under pressure they become obvious. It is apparent that muscular contraction demands large amounts of oxygen and nutrient material made possible only by this rich blood supply.

The well known symptom of intermittent claudication results from a transient ischemia of skeletal muscle. This may be caused by damage (arteriosclerosis, etc.) to the vessels, impairing delivery, or by excessive demand on the muscles, energy expenditure outstripping normal oxygen and nutrient supply. An interesting example of the latter is the anterior tibial syndrome in which, because of exertion and lack of conditioning, the anterior tibialis

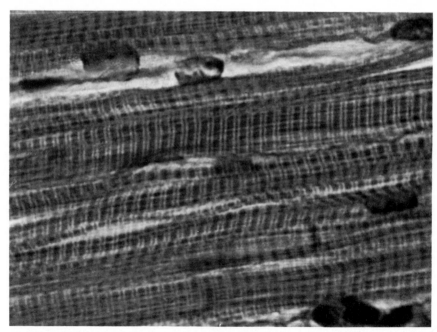

Figure 22–3   Normal skeletal muscle showing striations. The dark stripes are the A bands. Careful scrutiny reveals a light stripe within this band, the H zone. The wide light stripe is called the I band and the dark stripe that divides it, the Z line. (× 1000.)

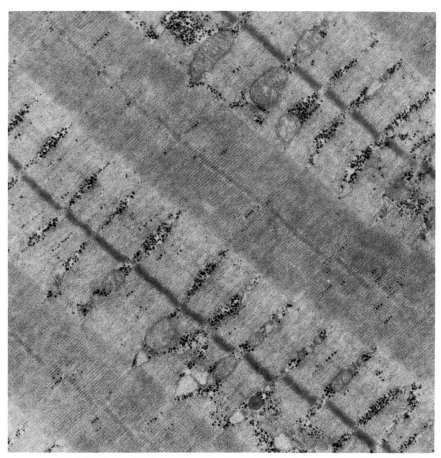

Figure 22–4   Electron photomicrograph of striated muscle. The striations cross the field obliquely. The darker zone crossing the field from upper left to lower right is the A band. The H zone appears dark here. The dark granules extending in aggregates vertical to the Z line are spherules of glycogen. Close scrutiny of the original print discloses fine striations crossing the A band. These are chains of myosin. Even finer striations cross the I band. These are chains of actin. These chains probably interdigitate, several of the latter between each two of the former, thus causing contraction. ($\times$ 33,000.)

muscle may actually undergo necrosis. It is treated by surgical decompression of the anterior tibial compartment by incision of the overlying fascia.[2]

The finer ramifications of the nerves that supply muscle cannot be appreciated by ordinary processing techniques. With the vital methylene blue stain used to such advantage in the descriptions by Coers and Woolf[3] the finest arborizations can be studied. Each motor neuron has only one axon, which branches to send a single nerve fibril to each of 100 to 200 muscle fibers. This group of fibers and its neuron are called a motor unit. As each nerve fibril (Fig. 22–6) approaches its muscle fiber its supportive sheath of Henle merges with the supportive sheath of the latter, the en-domysium. Each fibril then arborizes into two to six filaments, each ending in a loop called a telodendron (Fig. 22–7). The sarcoplasm (cytoplasm) of the muscle fiber is heaped into a mound at this area usually with a cluster of nuclei and the plasma-lemma is invaginated into this mound of sarcoplasm to form pockets into which the telodendria dip. The entire complex is covered by the endomysium to form a structure resembling a bulge on the surface of the muscle fiber measuring about 50 μ in diameter. This structure is known as the motor end plate.

Contraction, the function of the muscle fiber, is a complex chemicophysical process initiated by a nerve (electrical) impulse. The impulse from the motor neuron

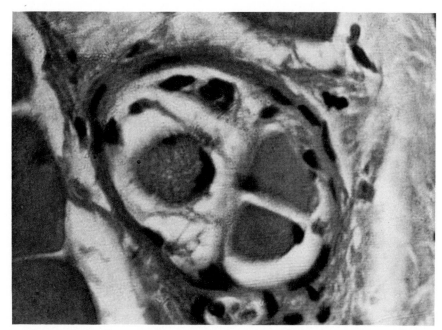

Figure 22–5   A sensory spindle. It is compartmentalized, containing three muscle fibers and a sensory apparatus. (× 1000.)

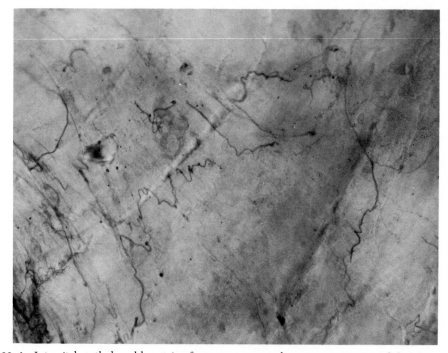

Figure 22–6   Intravital methylene blue stain of nerve axons seen here as wavy or curved dark lines on a light background. The wavy contours are artifactual because of crushing of the muscle fibers. (× 370.)

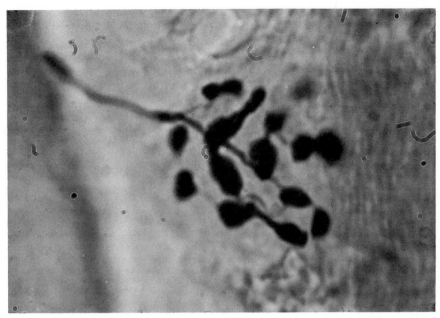

Figure 22–7   Axonal arborization of a motor neuron. The axon divides into several filaments each of which terminates in an ovoid expansion called a telodendron. (× 370.)

descends the motor axon and arriving at the end plate causes the release of a small amount of acetylcholine. This substance probably renders this portion of the membrane permeable to sodium and potassium ions. Depolarization results in the establishment of an end plate potential. A store of cholinesterase has been demonstrated in the membrane beneath the end plate. This hydrolyzes the acetylcholine to form choline, thus neutralizing the activity initiated by the impulse.

The most prominent protein constituent of the muscle fiber sarcoplasm is myosin. It is associated with a second protein known as actin. The interaction of these two proteins causes the muscle fiber to shorten. The exact mechanism of this shortening is still hypothetical but it is thought by some that chains of actin molecules concentrated about the Z line slide between strata of myosin molecules concentrated in the A zone (the sliding film theory). Thus the sarcoplasm protein constituents actually telescope into each other, causing shortening (Fig. 22–4).

Energy for contraction is supplied by the release of high energy stores by dephosphorylation and transphosphorylation of adenosine triphosphate and phospho-creatine within the sarcoplasm. When the muscle fiber degenerates the transaminase enzymes are released into the serum where their levels can be measured. The muscle cell must be replenished with energy for the next contraction during the resting phase. Blood glucose is converted to muscle glycogen. With a plentiful supply of oxygen this is hydrolyzed to carbon dioxide and water. In the absence of oxygen, glycogen is converted to pyruvate and lactic acid. The former is utilized in the tricarboxylic cycle; the latter is released into the blood and transported to the liver where it is reused in the synthesis of glucose. Thus the muscle fiber is enabled to contract in states of low oxygen tension creating an oxygen debt. But when concentrations of lactates reach a critical level the fiber shows signs of fatigue.

THE MUSCULAR DYSTROPHIES

The muscular dystrophies constitute the group of diseases manifested by an idiopathic, primary degenerative process within the muscle fibers. The motor neuron, its axon and end plates remain normal. There is no evidence of an allergic, toxic or infectious factor and the muscle vasculature is consistently intact.

This curious degenerative process expresses itself in a variety of ways but with the single exception of one rare type, myotonic dystrophy, the microscopic features of sections of involved muscle tissue do not allow differentiation.

A variety of types and classifications have been based on the age of onset, rate of progression, muscle groups involved and hereditary features but a division into five basic clinical types will suffice for this discussion: (1) progressive muscular dystrophy (pseudohypertrophic type, Duchenne), (2) facioscapulohumeral (Landouzy and Déjerine) and limb-girdle dystrophies, (3) distal muscular dystrophy, (4) ocular myodystrophy and (5) myotonic dystrophy.

Progressive Muscular Dystrophy

Progressive pseudohypertrophic muscular dystrophy is the most important of the dystrophy group from the standpoint of both incidence and mortality. It accounts for about 65 per cent of all dystrophies. This type affects males five times more frequently than females; it almost always begins within the first five years of life. The disease is steadily progressive and the victim rarely survives to maturity. Muscle weakness usually begins centrally and spreads to the extremities; it is first noted in the muscle groups of the shoulder girdle, the pelvis and the lumbosacral region of the spine. Involvement of the latter groups results in a waddling gait and an insecure stance with a wide base and lordosis. In rising from a seated position on the floor the patient is compelled to climb his legs with his hands (Gower's sign) to maintain his knees in extension and to augment the action of the extensor muscles of the trunk.

Muscle involvement is eventually widespread but the ocular, facial and bulbar (tongue and pharynx) groups are spared or uninvolved until late. Weakness develops slowly but progressively until the patient is confined to his chair and then his bed.

One of the curious features of this type of dystrophy is the enlargement of some of the involved muscles. Though the actual muscle mass is reduced, an infiltration with mature fat cells between the degenerating muscle fibers causes the muscle diameter to increase resulting in a pseudohypertrophy. These fat cells are an important microscopic feature. Pseudohypertrophy characteristically affects some muscles and not others. Involvement of the gastrocnemius in conjunction with wasting of the thigh muscles, and enlargement of the deltoid and atrophy of the biceps present a distinctive clinical picture. Contractures are not common until disability forces the patient to chair or bed confinement (Fig. 22–8).

Recent serum enzyme studies have shed some light on the natural history of the disease.[4, 5] Serum glutamic-oxalacetic transaminase and glutamic-pyruvic transaminase levels are elevated in the early and active phase of the process. Because skeletal muscle has a considerable compensatory reserve, the disease may be asymptomatic at this stage. Paradoxically in the advanced and symptomatic stages, degenerative activity is slowed or completed and the enzyme levels may now be normal. It is apparent therefore that the disease starts much earlier than we have heretofore appreciated and the terminal phase is like that of rheumatic endocarditis, a manifestation of functional loss due to the residual scars of the earlier active phase. A more recent test based on serum levels of creatine phosphokinase (CPK) is said to be more sensitive and useful in following the course of the muscle degeneration disturbances.

A decreased urinary output of creatinine and an increase in the urine creatine level are found in the symptomatic stages of the diffuse muscular dystrophies. Because healthy skeletal muscle, in contraction, utilizes creatine and excretes creatinine the reason for the reversal is obvious. There is also a lowered creatine tolerance because total muscle mass is decreased. Unfortunately these findings are not of great diagnostic significance because in the other muscle diseases metabolic activity is likewise impaired.

When adequate series of progressive muscular dystrophy are analyzed it becomes obvious that the cases fall into two

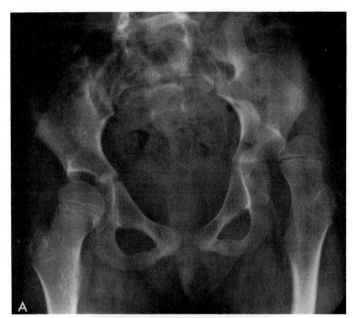

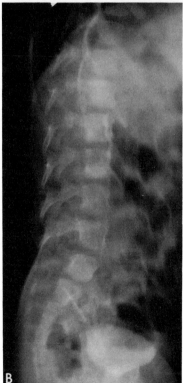

Figure 22–8 Absence of the stress of weight-bearing and absence of normal muscular activity influence the configuration of the femoral necks as well as the configuration of the vertebral bodies. In *A*, there is valgus deformity of the femurs with subluxation of the left hip. The vertebral bodies become square as a consequence of an increase in their height (*B*).[23, 24]

main groups, the autosomal recessive and the sex-linked recessive types. The latter occurs much more commonly in boys and again can be divided into two types, the aggressive variety, which has been described, and a much more slowly developing disease with a considerably more favorable prognosis. This type usually does not manifest itself until the third decade and runs its course into the fifth.

Facioscapulohumeral and Limb-Girdle Dystrophies

A second variety of muscular dystrophy is sometimes called the facioscapulohumeral dystrophy of Landouzy and Déjerine when the muscles of the face and shoulder girdle are predominantly involved and the limb-girdle type when those of the pelvis and thigh are most concerned. Though onset may be as early as in the Duchenne type, it is apt to be much later and may appear in the elderly. Progress is usually much slower than in juvenile pseudohypertrophic dystrophy and though the end stage may result in considerable disability, it is usually not fatal. Muscles of the face may escape but when involved there may be inability to pucker the lips and close the eyes when under gentle resistance. The scapula and other bones of the shoulder become prominent. Pelvic instability and lordosis develop consequent to involvement of muscles of the pelvic girdle. Though the disease is usually confined to the skeletal muscles, myocardial involvement has been reported.[6] Such involvement may be the most prominent feature of the disease causing arrhythmias or even sudden arrest with skeletal muscular weakness as a seemingly unimportant concomitant finding.

Distal Muscular Dystrophy

There is a clinical type of muscular dystrophy that begins in the peripheral muscles of the extremities. This type is usually referred to as distal muscular dystrophy. Uncommonly it may spread to involve muscle groups of the trunk thus reversing the usual direction of progression seen in the more common progressive muscular dystrophy. Because the leg muscles are often involved, differentiation from peroneal muscular atrophy may be a problem. The onset of distal muscular dystrophy is in adults of almost any age and it progresses slowly over a period of many years. The most commonly involved muscle groups are those of the hands. The disease is inherited as an autosomal dominant.

Ocular Myodystrophy

Ocular myodystrophy or progressive dystrophic ophthalmoplegia is a slowly progressive type of dystrophy that is usually confined to the levator muscles. Other facial muscles are involved in some cases. Ptosis and ophthalmoplegia are usually the prominent features.

Myotonic Dystrophy

A peculiar and progressive though fortunately rare type of muscular dystrophy is called myotonic dystrophy. Myotonia is a symptom rather than a disease entity. It is manifested by a prolongation of the period of muscle relaxation time due to a series of impulse discharges rather than a single one. The response is most dramatically seen following forceful contraction. This symptom is found in both myotonic dystrophy and congenital myotonia of Thomsen but the two diseases are otherwise unrelated.

The onset of myotonic dystrophy is usually in young adults. It is inherited as an autosomal dominant and often occurs in families without a history of the disease as a dominant mutation. It is familial.[7] In each successive generation the manifestation of the process becomes more severe until propagation is impossible and the family dies out.

Muscle groups most prominently involved are those of the forearm and hand, dorsiflexors of the feet, and those of the neck and face. Atrophy of the last group causes the so-called "taper mouth." In cases in which the hand muscles are involved the patient may shake hands but has difficulty in relaxing his grip. This feature is more prominent when the muscles are cold.

Accompanying the muscle degeneration and myotonia there is multiglandular involvement. The thyroid may be enlarged and the basal metabolic rate low. There is apt to be testicular atrophy, loss of libido and impotence. The pituitary may contain numerous large, basophilic Crooke's cells of castration and the adrenal cortices are frequently atrophic. Lack of body hair, presenile baldness and gynecomastia are usual findings. Mental deterioration is sometimes seen and presenile cataracts are a constant and characteristic finding.

Radiologic findings have been described in this condition. The cranial bones are thickened; the mandibular angle is larger than normal; the volume of the sella is significantly small; the interorbital distance decreased from normal and the basal angle decreased. Pectus excavatum deformity and straightening of the cervical and thoracic curves have been observed. The alterations are most marked in the older patients.

Hypercholesterolemia is usual and atherosclerosis develops at an early age. A great many patients with this disease have died of coronary occlusion in the third or fourth decade.

Microscopy of the Dystrophies. Examination of microscopic sections of samples of skeletal muscle tissue from patients suffering with the various types of muscular dystrophies makes it obvious that the muscle fibers are undergoing degeneration. Great variation in the rate of this process depending upon the type and phase of the disease results in considerable variation in the microscopic picture. To compound the difficulty muscle fiber degeneration is found in the inflammatory and neuromyopathies as well so that differences are largely quantitative. Thus a degree of experience is often important in making the distinction on the basis of microscopy alone and in some instances such distinction may be impossible, even for the veteran. An overall knowledge of the subject, of the clinical features of the specific case, the results of electromyographic and serum enzyme analyses coupled with the knowledge obtained by good biopsy technique in almost every event lead to a firm and clear-cut diagnosis. The importance of a sound biopsy method cannot be overemphasized. Poor technique by the surgeon and casual handling of the specimen by the technician result in sections that are worthless for interpretation. Because the surgical procedure is not considered difficult or complex, it is too often relegated to the least experienced of the house staff. This procedure is considered so important in our hospital that all muscle biopsies, whatever service the patient may be on, are performed by one experienced orthopedic surgeon. The tissue is processed in a special laboratory by a technician with special skills in this field. Muscle biopsy is more fully discussed in the introductory section of this chapter.

In sections of muscles with minimal changes one is apt to find only some variation in staining intensity and some disparity in fiber diameter. Staining variation is frequently encountered in normal muscle tissue that has been improperly biopsied and fixed. Rough handling, stretching by pulling with forceps in removal and sudden contraction because of fixation before the enzyme systems are inactivated may produce this feature. If biopsy and processing techniques are rigidly controlled, variations in staining intensity are probably significant. The fibers that stain darkly with eosin are the ones revealing early degenerative change (Fig. 22–9). Variation in fiber diameter at this stage of the disease is due solely to atrophy. As yet there are no hypertrophied fibers. Sections of the thigh muscles of a healthy, vigorous, mature male at a magnification of × 400 reveal approximately five fibers in cross section in each wide-angle eyepiece field. Variations in diameter in muscular dystrophy range from normal to diameters of less than 10 μ (Fig. 22–10). In cross section the fibers are round, oval or polygonal. In longitudinal section the striations are usually well preserved. Striation alteration is as often artifactual as it is due to muscle disease. One encounters fibers showing every feature of extreme atrophy with almost no alteration of the striation pattern. On the other hand poor biopsy technique or staining may cause complete loss of striation in normal muscle.

Following these earliest changes the fibers become vacuolated and the nuclei develop characteristic changes. Small vacuoles, especially about the nuclei, are found in normal fibers even with careful processing technique. Larger vacuoles may be artifactual or the result of muscle disease. They must be carefully interpreted. The nucleus that is undergoing early degenerative change becomes larger and takes the basic stain more intensely. This is in contrast to the nuclei of regenerating fibers, which are large but take the

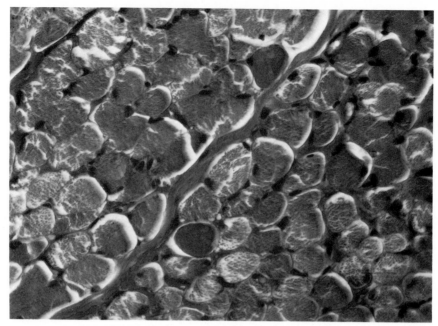

Figure 22–9   Muscular dystrophy. A band of perimysium crosses the field from lower left to upper right. At upper center above this band and lower center below it appear two fibers with condensation of their sarcoplasm and nuclear shrinkage. These are very early changes, probably significant. (× 470.)

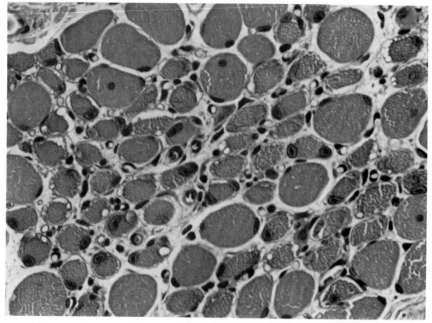

Figure 22–10   Muscular dystrophy, illustrating the variation in diameter of the muscle fibers. The largest are probably hypertrophied. The smaller fibers are degenerating. The increase in the number of nuclei is due partly to regeneration, mostly to collagenoblastic proliferation. (×500.)

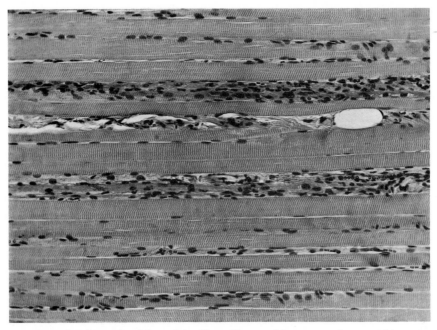

Figure 22-11 Muscular dystrophy. Most of the fibers illustrated here are quite normal in appearance. Two bands of proliferating collagenoblasts cross the field horizontally. Between them there is a degenerating fiber with regenerating nuclei. (× 200.)

basic stain lightly. In these the chromatin is most dense just within the nuclear membrane (penciled delineation) and the nucleolus is unusually prominent. As degeneration advances the nuclear chromatin is fragmented and finally the nuclear membrane is lost. Normally the nuclei lie peripherally within the sarcoplasm beneath the plasmalemma but in muscle disease they often migrate to the interior of the cell. Nuclear position is best judged on cross section; centralization of nuclei is especially prominent in myotonic dystrophy.

"Nuclear proliferation" is significant but sometimes difficult to interpret (Fig. 22-11). Abnormal numbers of nuclei in a microscopic field may be the result of a number of mechanisms. The nuclei of a diseased muscle fiber may proliferate in an attempt at muscle regeneration. These nuclei are large, plump, pale staining and have large nucleoli. The related sarcoplasm is more basophilic than normal. Nuclei may only seem to be proliferating because atrophy and disappearance of the internuclear fiber substance may concentrate the cells. It is also probable that myoblastic cells do not participate in the early degenerative phase and these too may be concentrated and mistaken for muscle fiber nuclei. The nuclei of histiocytes and less often other infiltrating exudative inflammatory cells may be mistaken for muscle nuclei. Finally the muscle fiber may atrophy completely leaving only a chain of nuclei between healthier muscle fibers or strands of collagen.

As atrophy progresses the cross section silhouette becomes more and more irregular. It may be crescent shaped with a more markedly atrophied fiber nested in its concavity. Sometimes the fiber is seen to split so that there appears to be two fibers within one endomesial sheath.

Degenerative change of the peripheral myofibrils in a zone just beneath and contiguous with the plasmalemma presents the appearance of a homogenous eosin staining ring. These have been called "ringbinden." They are not specific for any particular type of muscle degenerative process.

Because the muscle spindles do not share in the degenerative process, they may be found within and completely sur-

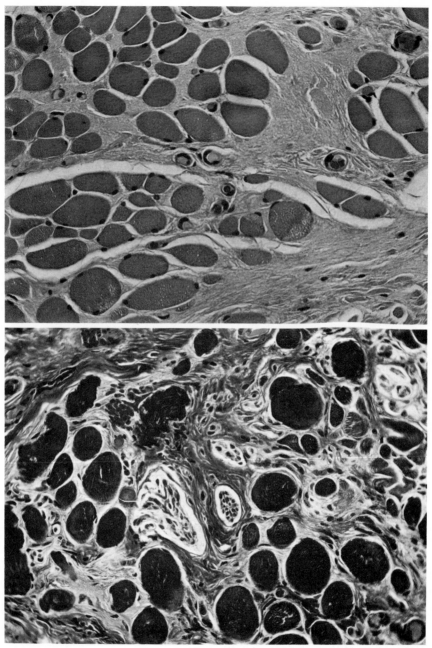

Figure 22–12   Muscular dystrophy. Upper illustration shows an increase in endomysial collagen. H and E stain. (× 290.) Lower illustration is of same case. Masson stain. (× 350.)

rounded by large fields of collagenous scar tissue; they are often concentrated by the loss of the muscle fibers that normally separate them.

By this time the degenerative process may have been florid enough to have engendered a mild inflammatory reaction. Small loosely scattered aggregates of lymphocytes, plasma cells and sometimes histiocytes may be found. Sometimes these have a perivascular distribution and then the vessel often reveals a sclerotic thickening of its walls. By now variation in muscle size may have become quite dramatic. Some fibers have atrophied to 10 μ in diameter, while others have hypertrophied to 250 μ.

Normally the endomysium cannot be appreciated with the light microscope and hematoxylin and eosin staining. If the endomysium is visible under these conditions it is probably abnormal. Fibrosis is a relatively late phenomenon but in the last phase of the disease it is one of the most prominent features. Early fibrosis is most easily appreciated with the several stains for collagen (Fig. 22–12), Masson trichrome, Mallory's and Gomery's reticulin stains.

Perhaps the most dramatic microscopic feature in pseudohypertrophic muscular dystrophy is the presence of fat. Because the volume is increased by the presence of mature fat cells it can hardly be contended that this is merely a muscle fiber replacement. The fat cells appear between the muscle bundles and between the muscle fibers (Fig. 22–13). Eventually the entire field may be converted to fat and collagen. Sometimes one can find irregular fragments of muscle fibers within these fields

or the nuclear and sarcolemmal remnants of a fiber that has undergone complete atrophy.

Even when the muscle fibers are found to be severely damaged, the specially stained neurons and end plates that supply them remain quite normal in appearance. When the muscle fiber appears to be completely destroyed the axon may produce a new sprout and arborization in the replacement collagen tissue as though the nerve were seeking a new fiber to supply with impulses. Study of the cord and brain in cases of far advanced muscular dystrophy has failed to show pathologic alterations.

The pathologist is most often asked to differentiate, on the basis of microscopic sections, five muscle diseases—progressive muscular dystrophy, amyotonia congenita, poliomyelitis, polymyositis and congenital myotonia. A clear-cut and firm opinion cannot always be given, but large amounts of fat and endomysial collagen usually denote muscular dystrophy. Evidence of regeneration is usually greater than in the neuromyopathies, amyotonia and poliomyelitis and not as obvious as in polymyositis. A prominent exudative inflammatory reaction is

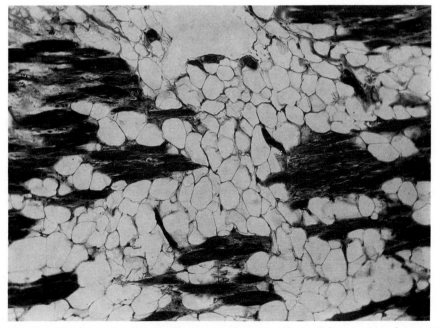

Figure 22–13 Muscular dystrophy. Muscle fibers are undergoing advanced degenerative change. Mature fat cells now dominate the section. (× 140.)

much more indicative of polymyositis and the evidence for rapid degenerative alteration of muscle fibers is apt to be most prominent in this disease. Microscopic sections usually appear normal in congenital myotonia and myasthenia gravis.

THE NEUROMYOPATHIES

The neuromyopathies constitute an important group from the standpoint of their frequency because not only are there the congenital childhood types (congenital hypotonia) and idiopathic adult varieties (the amyotrophies) but also the paralysis secondary to brain, cord or nerve damage due to poliomyelitis and other traumatic, toxic and perhaps allergic agents fall into this category. The classification in the outline at the beginning of this chapter is used in this discussion.

Congenital Hypotonia

Amyotonia congenita of Werdnig-Hoffman is the most important clinical type of this group of muscle atrophies. In all types of neuromyopathies the cause is a failure of development or a degeneration of the motor neurons of the central nervous system or damage of the pathways through which their impulses flow. The muscle pathology is basically an atrophy of the muscle fiber due to loss of impulses. In amyotonia congenita the muscle loss is secondary to a failure of proper development and maturation of motor neurons.

Amyotonia congenita is often obvious at birth or within the first few weeks of life. The child is flaccid. He lies on his back, the head turned to one side, the arms abducted laterally from the chest wall, the forearms flexed, the thighs rotated outward and partially flexed and the legs flexed on the thighs. The cry is weak. The tendon reflexes are reduced or absent. When onset is early, the course is progressive and most, perhaps 90 per cent, die before their fifth year. When onset occurs later in childhood, the progress is somewhat slower and most of these children die of chronic pulmonary infections between their seventh and tenth years. A few patients survive

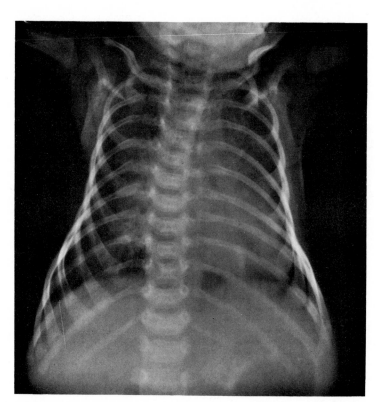

Figure 22–14 Amyotonia congenita (Werdnig-Hoffman). The thorax is bell-shaped; there is paralysis of the intercostal muscles. The diaphragm was observed to move at the time of fluoroscopy. The pulmonary parenchymal disease is secondary to aspiration of swallowed material.

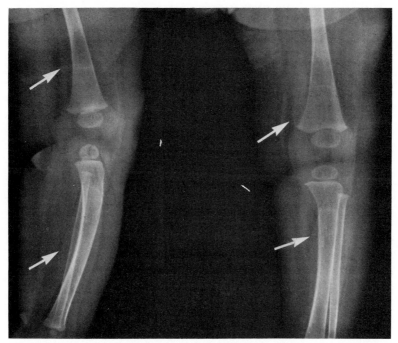

Figure 22–15   Amyotonia. The muscle groups are small; there is abundant subcutaneous fat as well as an obvious increase in fat between the muscle groups (arrows). The bones are poorly mineralized.

into adolescence or adult life. Contractures are encountered even less frequently than in the dystrophies. The "myotonia congenita" of Oppenheim now appears to be only a symptom complex that may occur in muscular atrophy, muscular dystrophy or myositis. The term should be discarded.

Congenital hypotonia is familial and appears to be autosomal recessive. Males and females are affected with equal frequency.

Sections of the cord and brain show a numerical reduction in the motor neurons of the anterior horns of the cord, medulla, pons and midbrain. There are several reports of degenerative changes in many of the surviving motor cells.

Microscopic study of the involved muscles reveals great disparity in cross section diameter (Fig. 22–16). Most fibers are extremely small and this is said to be because the disease has a congenital onset, before the fibers have reached the size of normal maturity. Some fibers are represented merely by chains of nuclei and the distorted remnants of the sarcolemmal sheath (Fig. 22–17). In the more intact fibers the striations are often preserved. Here and there throughout the sections

one may find much larger fibers. Whether these are normally matured or hypertrophied is debatable. Increase in the endomysial and perimysial collagenous tissue is obvious in the more advanced cases but rarely does it approach the degree of fibrosis seen in muscular dystrophy. Mature fat cells too are found but, again, not to the extent seen in the dystrophies.

The lack of evidence of regeneration and exudative inflammatory reaction is notable. Though some evidence of the latter may be encountered, neither is characteristic of the disease. Should either occur prominently in the sections the possibility of a juvenile myositis should be seriously considered.

The most characteristic finding in the muscle sections of the patient with amyotonia congenita is the loss or failure of development of the end plates on the arborizations and beading of the motor axons (Fig. 22–18). If the vital methylene blue staining technique is carried out these alterations in the impulse carrying apparatus may be helpful in establishing a diagnosis. Practically, however, the terminal nerve fibrils and end plates often do not

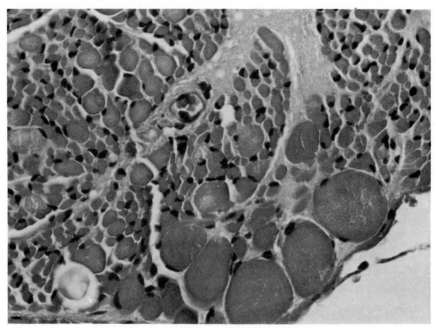

Figure 22–16 Amyotonia congenita, illustrating the remarkable disparity in muscle fiber diameter. The large fibers at lower right are hypertrophied. Elsewhere the fibers reveal various degrees of atrophy. (× 500.)

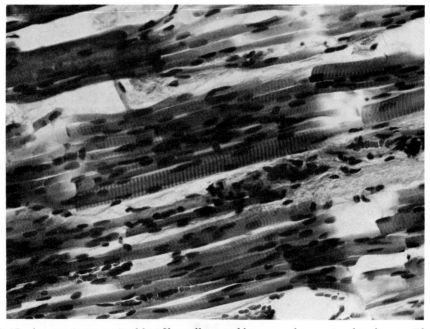

Figure 22–17 Amyotonia congenita. Most fibers illustrated here reveal some atrophic changes. There is some nuclear regeneration though fiber loss has exaggerated this appearance. (× 350).

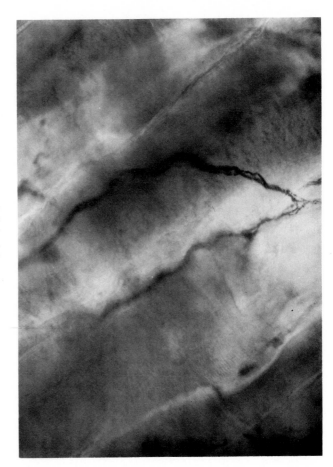

Figure 22–18 Amyotonia congenita. Two bundles of axons cross the field from left to right. They are probably somewhat thickened and on the right they show the typical beading that indicates an attempt at sprouting. Vital methylene blue. (× 370.)

appear in preparations of normal muscle. Their absence, therefore, may not be significant.

Because a group of muscle fibers is supplied by a single nerve axon the degeneration has an irregular group pattern. Hence it is usual to see extensive degeneration in one group and complete lack of involvement in a contiguous group. Because these groups interdigitate and are not at the same level, serial step sections may be required to bring out this feature.

Because the muscle mass is decreased by a slow wasting due to denervation the serum transaminase and aldolase levels are rarely elevated. This is in sharp contrast to polymyositis and may even be helpful in differentiating neuromyopathy from dystrophy.

Rod disease is usually classified as a rare subtype of congenital hypotonia. It can be identified by examination of microscopic sections of freshly formalin fixed tissue stained with phosphotungstic acid hematoxylin or methyl green pyronine. The rods or nemalin (thread) bodies are found grouped in the sarcoplasm (Fig. 22–19). Central core disease is probably another variety of congenital hypotonia. Its clinical features are very similar to those of the more common varieties but when colloidal silver stains are used a core of densely staining myofibrils is found within the sarcoplasm.[9] With hematoxylin and eosin the central portion of the fiber appears to be hyalinized. Proximal muscles are most prominently involved and though weakened, they do not progress to the stage of paralysis. Tendon reflexes remain active. The disease is familial (Fig. 22–20).

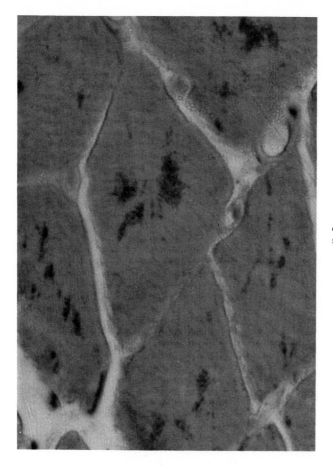

Figure 22-19 Amyotonia congenita. Rod disease. The dark objects are the "rods" stained with pyronine green. (× 900.)

Progressive Muscular Atrophy

There are three clinical varieties of this disease but the pathogenesis, though possibly not the etiology, is the same for all. There is muscle atrophy secondary to degeneration of the motor nerve system. The onset is usually in middle age, though it often appears in the aged and occasionally in young adults.

The commonest type is called amyotrophic lateral sclerosis. This usually begins with atrophy and weakness of the muscles of the hands. Though it may begin on one side it always becomes bilateral. Prominence of the intermetacarpal spaces is often an early finding. Weakness spreads to more proximal muscle groups involving successively those of the arm, shoulder and finally those of the bulbar group, laryngeal and pharyngeal. At the same time or some time after involvement of the upper extremities a spastic paralysis is noted involving the muscles of the legs. Thus it becomes apparent that not only the motor neurons of the anterior horns are involved but degenerative changes also begin to appear in the corticospinal tracts. The disease progresses steadily over a period of 2 to 10 years, until difficulty in swallowing leads to inhalation pneumonia and death.

When the bulbar groups are initially and prominently involved the condition is usually called bulbar palsy.

In a third type known simply as progressive neuromuscular atrophy or peroneal muscular atrophy of Charcot-Marie-Tooth, corticospinal degeneration apparently does not occur so that there is no spasticity and no hyperactive tendon reflexes. The paralysis is completely flaccid.

The microscopy of the progressive muscular atrophies both in the central nervous system and in the skeletal muscles is the same as that for the congenital amyotonias (Fig. 22-21). It is apparent that a

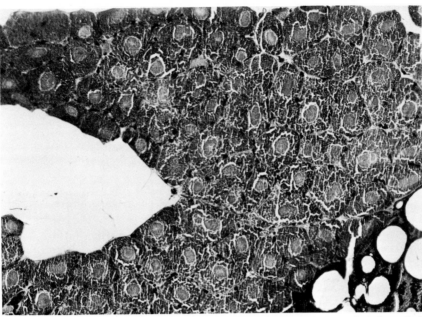

Figure 22–20   Central core disease. Cross section. Note central core in each fiber of condensed, deeply staining myofibrils. Colloidal silver stain.

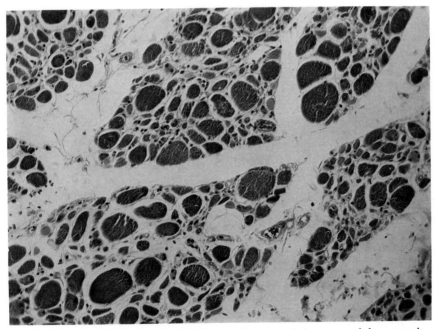

Figure 22–21   Progressive muscular atrophy. The larger fibers are of about normal diameter; the smaller are atrophied. There is some increase in endomysium. (× 370.)

progressive, idiopathic degeneration of the motor elements of the central nervous system causes a neuromuscular atrophy of the associated muscles. It has been shown[10] that sectioning the motor nerve (denervation) causes more rapid atrophy of its muscle fiber than simple disuse. Mitochondrial modifications suggest that the fiber reverts to the simpler metabolic processes of embryonic muscle.

Viral Neuromyopathy

The most important type of muscle atrophy secondary to motor neuron disease is poliomyelitis. This is not the place for a detailed discussion of the epidemiology of this disease. It is now quite certain that the disease is caused by one of three types of related viruses. The portal of entry is probably the gastrointestinal tract; at least the virus can be cultured from the saliva and rectal contents. The onset of the disease is usually announced by one or two days with varied but mild symptoms, malaise, sore throat, fever and upper respiratory congestion. There usually follows an asymptomatic period of one to several days during which antibody titers rise. If these are sufficient to neutralize the virus the patient escapes neurologic damage. If they are insufficient the virus attacks the motor neurons, principally in the cord, at times at higher levels. These cells are damaged directly by the virus and indirectly by the edema and hemorrhage in their supportive glial tissue.

Neural damage is reflected in the sudden paralysis of the related muscle groups. Paralysis often ushers in the period of active illness which lasts up to a week. This period is expressed as fever, headache and drowsiness; cerebrospinal fluid pressure is elevated and the cell count rises to as high as 200/cu. mm. Though initially there may be granulocytes in the exudate, these are eventually replaced by lymphocytes. The protein level of the fluid is also elevated. There is often stiffness and pain of the muscles of the neck and back and involved limb muscles may become tender. Symptoms are not necessarily commensurate with the degree of paralysis. Because the nerve cells may recover, paralysis may be transient. Paralysis is flaccid in type. It may be complete or manifested by subclinical weakness. It may involve a single muscle, groups of muscles or all the muscles of one or more extremities. Because apparently the virus spreads through the neural tissue, groups of muscles whose neurons are contiguous are affected. Paralysis is most common in the lower limbs, second in the upper extremities and least in the trunk muscles.

Some degree of muscle recovery is usually noted within 10 days. For one to three months the recovery may be fairly rapid and then it slows down over a period of the following one to three years. A muscle that is still severely paralyzed at the end of three months cannot be expected to recover to functional usefulness.

Residual deformity is due to eventual scarring and shortening of the involved muscles and the unopposed contraction of normal muscles. Surgical therapy must be designed to counteract these factors and a successful result may depend upon the utmost ingenuity and skill of the operator. This is not a task for the novice who may do considerably more harm than good by injudicious surgery.

Microscopic changes within the cord and brain tissues have been carefully plotted[11] and recognized for many years. The motor neurons of the anterior horns swell and their cytoplasm becomes granular. Neuronophagia by aggregates of gitter cells results in removal of the dead cells (Fig. 22–22). Edema is marked and microhemorrhages are usually found. Often there is perivascular cuffing of the small vessels to the involved areas.

The microscopic changes within the muscles can be noted within three weeks of the onset of paralysis. These changes are the same as those for other neuromyopathies (See p. 703). Infiltration with exudative inflammatory cells has been described but this is probably never marked and due entirely to the rate and degree of degeneration of the muscle fibers (Fig. 22–23). Fat cells are said to be somewhat more prevalent than in other types of neuromyopathies. If this be true it is only long after the onset of muscle degeneration and probably due to factors not related to it. The extensive fibrosis that is occasionally

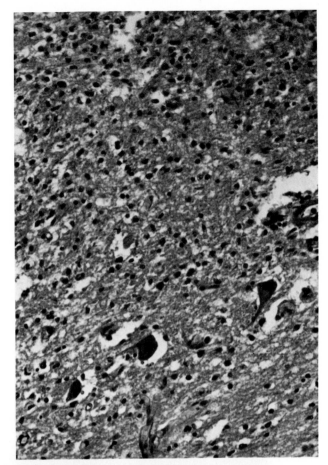

Figure 22-22 Section of spinal cord in poliomyelitis, acute phase. There is considerable edema and several small foci of hemorrhage. Motor neurons are undergoing degeneration and neuronophagia. Most of the cells here are gitter cells, microglia, the inflammatory cells of the central nervous system. (×300.)

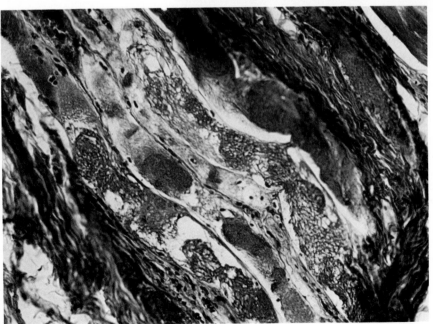

Figure 22-23   Poliomyelitis, muscle, degenerative phase. Muscle fibers reveal fracturing, vacuolization and loss of nuclei. (× 470.)

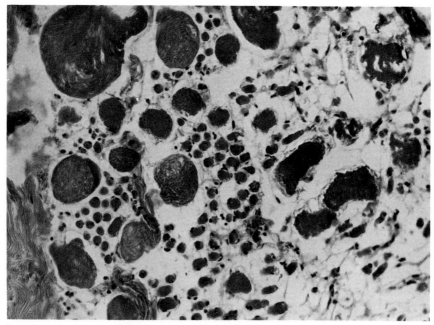

Figure 22-24   Poliomyelitis, muscle, late phase. Some fibers have undergone hypertrophy, others atrophy. There is fat infiltration and some fibrosis. It may be impossible to differentiate the end stage of poliomyelitis from the dystrophies and neuromyopathies on sections alone. (× 240.)

encountered in contracted muscles must be explained in the same manner. We have found the greatest difficult in differentiating the sections of muscle in poliomyelitis from those of other neuromyopathies (Fig. 22-24) and occasionally the sections of a badly scarred muscle of a distant poliomyelitis infection may closely resemble those of the dystrophies.

Miscellaneous Neuromyopathies

Any disease or lesion that damages the motor nerve complex or interrupts the transport of impulses therefrom may result in muscle fiber atrophy. These range from traumatic transverse myelitis to syringomyelia, infectious, toxic and deficiency types of neuritis and degenerative processes caused by metabolic diseases such as diabetes mellitus. The most important condition of this group is that called "toxic neuromyopathy." It results from the nerve damage caused by a number of agents such as diphtheria toxin, alcohol and a number of other drugs and chemicals. Enumeration and discussion of these causes belong

in the textbook of neurology and will not be included here.

ARTHROGRYPOSIS (AMYOPLASIA CONGENITA)

Arthrogryposis multiplex congenita is probably a clinical syndrome rather than a pathologic entity. It is characterized by multiple, symmetric contractures that develop in utero. These contractures often interfere with parturition. The condition was known in the nineteenth century but the first definitive description was by Sheldon in 1932.[13]

Early accounts suggested that this was a disease of the joint structure but as knowledge was collected it became obvious that though the joint tissues may be thickened and fibrotic the contractures in most cases are due to a shortening of the flexor muscles. Congenital ankylosis has been reported in rare instances but it is uncertain whether this is a primary or secondary event.

The disease is manifest at birth or signs

begin to develop in the first few months of life. The postpartum cases have usually, possibly always, been associated with a myopathy that simulates progressive muscular dystrophy with unusual muscle shortening and contracture. The infant lies supine, the head turned to one side, the shoulders rotated internally, the hips rotated externally and the arms and legs in partial flexion. The muscles are hypotonic, deep tendon reflexes are absent, electrical reactions are weak and the muscles are small. The decreased muscle mass causes the limbs to appear spindly with large, fusiform joints. The skin over the involved areas is often loose and wrinkled. It feels thickened and sections reveal an increase in the depth of the collagenous corium. Sections of the muscles show the fibers to be diminished in size and number. In early stages the sections are composed predominantly of muscle fibers but they are all very small and appear immature. Later there is considerable disparity in fiber diameter and in advanced stages, muscle fibers are almost entirely lacking and replaced by collagenous scar tissue and fat.

For several decades the pathogenesis of arthrogryposis has been the subject of debate and conflicting accounts of pathologic findings. One attempts a discussion of this condition with considerable trepidation because biopsy material is scarce and pathologic reports are apparently not wholly reliable. At present it is probably best to divide this symptom complex into two groups: those that are neuropathic in origin and those that are myopathic. It has been suggested that most or all of the former are the result of intrauterine neuromyopathy, perhaps the Werdnig-Hoffman type.[14] Supporting this thesis is the report of two cases by Turns, in twins, one with arthrogryposis, the other with Werdnig-Hoffman amyotonia, and several pathologic reports revealing a paucity of anterior horn neurons and demyelinization of motor tracts. Against the theory is the observation that the amyotonic aspect of the disease is not progressive and this condition does not explain the fibrous thickening of the skin, the joint tissues and, in truth, the muscles themselves. Conceivably other developmental de-

fects in the motor nervous system might be at fault. It has been stated that one half of the patients with arthrogryposis have a narrow cord and deficient neural canal.

The myopathic type is purported to represent the result of intrauterine progressive muscular dystrophy. It is almost certain that at least some of these cases are indeed such. It is not beyond the realm of comprehension to believe that the unaccountable features are the result of environmental influences. At present it is probably best to admit that the pathogenesis is still unknown to discourage a complacent attitude that might defer further investigation.

THE ALLERGIC MYOPATHIES

Polymyositis

Polymyositis is a collagen, or better, mesenchymal disease with kaleidoscopic symptomatology. Like all the other diseases of this group (formerly called the collagen diseases) the symptoms depend upon the rate of progress, the anatomic site and the stage of the disease. Because there is a fulminant and a chronic form of the disease, one type scarcely may be recognized as a form of the other. In addition, polymyositis is often accompanied by involvement of other systems such as the skin and is then known as dermatomyositis, the vessels and is known as polyarteritis, the reticuloendothelial derivatives and called systemic lupus erythematosus. Finally it is frequently associated with carcinoma, an association that is much greater than coincidence and that may depend upon the role of allergy in its pathogenesis.

Even a decade ago one might have been condemned for including these maladies under the heading of allergic disease.[15] Though conclusive data are still lacking, so many irregular pieces of the puzzle have turned up to suggest this probable conclusion that this category now appears to be a reasonably conservative hypothesis.

Pure, acute polymyositis attacks children and young adults, though older people are occasionally victims. This form is a serious disease with a mortality rate of approximately 30 per cent. Perhaps a third of this number run a fulminant course of several weeks, a few recover, and more have periodic remissions and undergo transition into the chronic type. About two thirds of patients with the acute form develop a skin rash and perhaps a third may develop Raynaud's phenomenon. Because these features never occur in the dystrophies or neuromyopathies they may be helpful road signs to direct the way to a correct diagnosis.

The rash characteristically appears on the knuckles, elbows and knees, the skin folds, the face and upper eyelids. It is often desquamative. Symptoms of muscle involvement usually appear proximally. The muscles become swollen, indurated and painful. There is usually edema of the overlying subcutaneous tissue. In the more florid types there is fever and leukocytosis. Muscle contraction is dramatically weakened. A fatal terminus may be precipitated by involvement of the thoracic groups. Mucous membranes as well as skin may be involved, manifested by a stomatitis and pharyngitis. As muscle involvement continues, the tendon reflexes disappear. Gradually the inflammatory reaction subsides but by this time the bulk of the muscle may have been destroyed leaving only a mass of scar tissue, which contracts causing shortening.

The subacute and chronic types of polymyositis are characteristically remittent in character. Fairly long periods of relatively good health may intervene between attacks though weakened, scarred and contracted muscles do not regain functional efficiency and permanent pigmentation may mark the site of skin involvement. Remissions in this disease are helpful in differentiating it from the dystrophies.

The acute fulminant variety of polymyositis is like no other disease of muscles and when it is uncomplicated by other types of mesenchymal disease, accurate diagnosis should rarely be a problem. But the subacute and chronic varieties of this condition are insidious in onset and much more subtle in expression. Then it may be difficult or impossible, for a while at least, to differentiate this type from some of the dystrophies.

The onset of the chronic type is more common in adults. Often the first symptom is weakness, sometimes with a vague complaint of malaise. All the signs and symptoms of the acute type may eventually appear but over months or years and the degree is dramatically subdued. But the end result may be the same; i.e., the patient may eventually succumb to paralysis of thoracic or bulbar muscles or involvement of the myocardium. Other facets of the mesenchymal diseases may occur also and dramatically change the course of the process, usually for the worse.

Contractures in the chronic form are even more common than in the acute. A type of calcinosis may be superimposed in the areas of muscle and skin involvement.

Sections of involved muscle tissue from patients with acute disease in the active phase usually offer little difficulty in interpretation. Sometimes the edema, necrosis and exudative inflammatory reaction are so prominent that the possibility of an acute bacterial or parasitic myositis arises. Because it is edematous the muscle tissue is pale and firm to the touch. Through the microscope the degenerative changes are most striking. The myofibrils are often hyalinized and dense, taking the eosin stain intensely, or broken and cloudy in appearance. The most pathognomonic feature is invasion of the sarcoplasm by histiocytes and obvious phagocytosis of fibrillar debris (Fig. 22-25). Sometimes only the sarcolemma remains, its contents replaced by exudative inflammatory cells among which one can usually identify granulocytes.

All stages of nuclear degeneration are found, the swollen, darkly staining forms often presenting an arresting appearance. Centralization of nuclei is frequently seen. Evidence of regeneration is usually prominent. The nuclei of these cells are also large but they take the hematoxylin stain much less intensely and they have prominent nucleoli. Because of the rapid synthesis of ribose nucleic acids in these cells, the cytoplasm takes a slightly more basophilic tint.

Vacuolization and fragmentation of muscle fibers are common (Fig. 22-26). Variation in fiber diameter is not as prominent as in the dystrophies or the neuromyopathies because the process here is usually

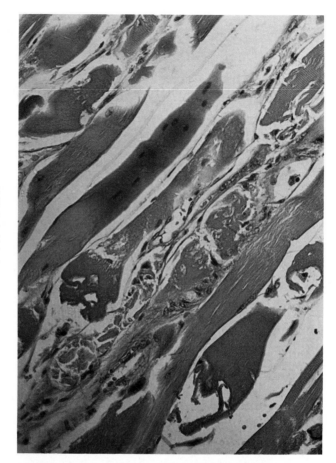

Figure 22–25 Polymyositis. Muscle fibers are undergoing advanced inflammatory and degenerative alteration. There is fractioning, vacuolization and nuclear degeneration. The fiber shown running from lower left to upper right has been invaded by macrophages and other exudative inflammatory cells. (× 270.)

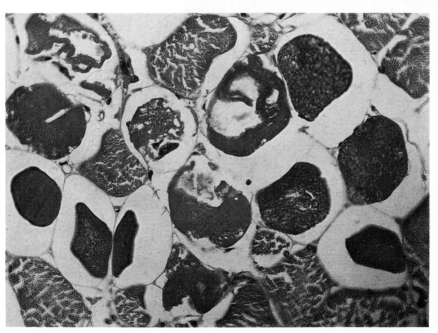

Figure 22–26 Polymyositis, acute phase. Cross section of muscle fibers reveals vacuolization and loss of nuclei. There is considerable edema of the bundle. (× 370.)

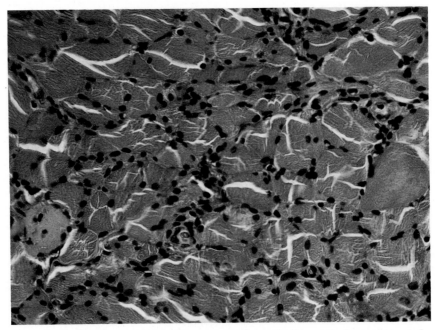

Figure 22-27   Polymyositis, active phase. Cross section of muscle fibers reveals exudative inflammatory reaction. (× 400.)

a rapid degeneration rather than a slow atrophy. The pattern of involvement in this disease is usually patchy and highly irregular rather than grouped in motor nerve units as in neuromyopathy or involving sporadic fibers as is sometimes seen in the dystrophies. Outside the fiber there is usually ample evidence of an inflammatory reaction. In places this may occur as large irregular aggregates of inflammatory cells (Fig. 22-27). Elsewhere these cells may be sprinkled more diffusely throughout the supportive tissue. Perivascular cuffing is usual.

As the edema and inflammatory exudate subside, muscle fiber degeneration reaches its climax and the debris is partially cleared by histiocytic phagocytosis. Collagenization is frequently dramatic and the entire muscle may be converted to scar tissue. More commonly one finds obvious sclerosis of both endo- and perimyesium. Vital staining with methylene blue reveals degeneration of the myoneural end plates and alterations in the axon arborizations. It appears that this is not a primary and etiologic feature of the disease but only a part of the general inflammatory reaction, which affects all of the tissues of the area.

The microscopic alterations found in biopsy material from patients with subacute and chronic polymyositis are the same as those seen in the acute type but they are less obvious, they develop more slowly and they appear in crops. Thus problems in diagnosis frequently occur in the differentiation of an insidious polymyositis and a florid type of progressive muscular dystrophy. Sometimes it is wiser not to attempt a distinction on the basis of the sections alone.

Polymyositis with Other Mesenchymal Diseases

In dermatomyositis there is a constant association of skin and muscle lesions. Perhaps a third of the cases of polyarteritis are accompanied by inflammatory and degenerative reactions in the skeletal muscle. The association of the two diseases appears to be somewhat less frequent in systemic lupus erythematosus. Inflammatory reactions with lymphocytic infiltration occur sporadically in the muscles in rheumatoid arthritis and inconspicuous foci of muscle degenerative and inflammatory alteration are now known to occur occasionally in rheumatic fever. The exact nature of these lesions, their meaning and whether they are related in pathogenesis are still unknown. Because pure polymyositis and dermatomyositis are unquestionably related in etiology and pathogenesis, it is tempting to assume that some relation occurs in the other mesenchymal diseases. Various authors have described these muscle lesions and there has been a tendency to emphasize the detailed differences rather than their similarities. This may be a healthy attempt to avoid premature conclusions concerning the relation of these diseases. On the other hand this philosophy may be harmful in postponing the day of enlightenment when we are able to demonstrate the common denominator in these fascinating processes.

The muscle reactions in those conditions classified as the "mesenchymal diseases" are usually described as nodular interstitial myositis. It is not completely groundless to suggest that the inflammatory reaction in all instances is not confined to the interstitial supportive tissue and that it may represent a subdued variation of the same process found in pure polymyositis.

Polymyositis with Sjögren's Syndrome

Rarely polymyositis may be associated with Sjögren's syndrome. This unusual disease is a disturbance in multiglandular function with infiltration of lymphocytes and sometimes plasma cells and histiocytes into the gland tissues. Most commonly affected are the lacrimal and salivary glands so that dryness of the eyes (keratoconjunctivitis sicca) and mouth (xerostomia) are usually the outstanding features. This combination is sometimes called the sicca syndrome. The disease was originally described by Mikulicz in 1888 and is still called Mikulicz's disease in some areas. Sjögren[16] described the condition and its pathology more definitively in 1933. An excellent modern review was published by Talal[17] in 1966.

The disease is usually, though by no means always, associated with one of the mesenchymal (collagen) diseases, most frequently rheumatoid arthritis. It usually affects middle aged females, all of the mucous membranes may be involved and a chronic thyroiditis simulating Hashimoto's disease is common. Antithyroid antibodies are present in about one third of the cases and hyperglobulinemia occurs in about one half. Antinuclear factors are also present relating the disturbance to systemic lupus erythematosus. It is apparently a bizarre type of mesenchymal disease and thus bears the same relation as previously noted to polymyositis.

Polymyositis with Cancer

It has been estimated that sometime in the course of one fifth of the cases of chronic dermatomyositis and rarely in cases of pure polymyositis, a cancer is discovered arising in one of a great variety of tissue systems. In almost all instances the dermatomyositis has been well established before the manifestation of the cancer. The cancers have been of a wide variety of types, more often carcinomas than sarcomas. The relation is more than coincidence because it is about five times that of the calculated figure based on incidence of the two diseases. The reason for the association is unproved but most assume that the neoplasm is the forerunner and that it somehow promotes an antigen that in turn is responsible for an antibody that destroys muscle.

INFECTIOUS MYOSITIS

Muscle tissue is apparently remarkably resistant to infection. Occasionally a muscle abscess may develop secondary to blood infection, a penetrating wound, compound fracture or a spreading osteomyelitis. The organism is almost invariably one of the staphylococcic or the streptococcic group. There is nothing particularly unique about these abscesses to make them different from focal infections in other tissues. Clostridial infection causes gas gangrene, which usually includes skeletal muscle in its field of activity. The only mycotic organism that infects muscle is *Actinomyces*. Again muscle in-

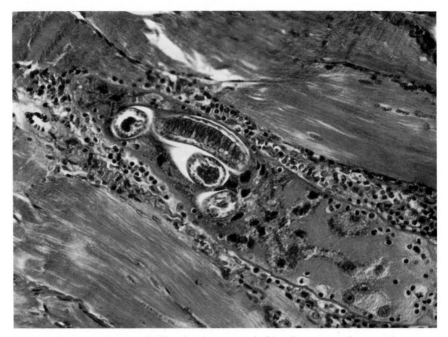

Figure 22–28   Trichinosis. The muscle fiber has been invaded by the parasite larvae. There is an exudative inflammatory reaction about the fiber. (× 300.)

volvement is only a part of the general process.

There are a number of parasitic infestations of striated muscle. These include trichinosis, echinococcosis and rarely sarcosporidiosis in this country and cysticercosis in India. Of these the first is the only one of importance for American physicians. The embryo trichinae are born in the gut wall and transported to muscle via the lymphatics and blood. This form of the parasite, measuring up to 150 μ in length, penetrates the sarcolemma and encysts itself within the muscle fiber (Fig. 22–28). The presence of the organism sets up an inflammatory reaction, which at first is predominantly eosinophilic and later develops components of an ordinary exudate with neutrophilic granulocytes and lymphocytes. Frequently there is a telltale eosinophilic leukocytosis. The inflammatory reaction may spread some distance from the parasite so that the section may not include the latter. Whenever an exudative inflammatory reaction is encountered in muscle tissue the block should be serially step sectioned, a blood leukocyte count done and a skin test carried out with specific antigen.

Trichinosis may be a serious disease but rarely leads to a fatal conclusion. It is accompanied by fever, chills and muscle pains. Trunk muscles are more commonly involved than those of the extremities with a particularly high incidence in the diaphragm and extraocular muscles. A peculiar suborbital edema is found in a high percentage of cases. In heavy infestations the brain may be involved and rarely the myocardium. When death occurs it is usually due to the last.

On the Eastern seaboard a preponderance of cases occurs among Italians who have a taste for sausage made with uncooked and often unapproved pork.

Though the encysted embryo may remain alive for a number of years it eventually dies. The inflammatory reaction heals with fibrous replacement and eventually the lesion calcifies. The points and striations of scar tissue and calcific deposits can be seen with the naked eye.

CONGENITAL MYOTONIA (THOMSEN)

Congenital myotonia is a rare disorder of voluntary muscle characterized by difficulty in initiating movement after rest and movement that is slow in performance and delayed in cessation. It is a rare disease.

This condition is sometimes called Thomsen's disease and rightly so because Julius Thomsen, a Danish physician, not only originally defined the disease but also was a victim of it as had been 20 members of his family. At least a quarter of the cases appear to be inherited as an autosomal dominant.

The phenomenon of myotonia is the cardinal feature of this condition. The affected muscles may eventually become hypertrophied. Congenital myotonia almost always begins in the first decade of life, sometimes during infancy, though it usually manifests itself most severely during adolescence. The symptoms of myotonia first expressed in young adult life are more apt to be due to myotonia dystrophica, a disease that is usually classified with the dystrophies. The myotonia in congenital myotonia is more pronounced than that in dystrophic myotonia but the general prognosis is much better. Though the muscles of the lower extremities are the ones usually most severely involved, those of the upper extremities and the head and neck are also affected. Involvement is symmetric. Contraction is difficult to initiate; once started it is slow and deliberate but smooth. Relaxation time is prolonged. Thus it may require a full minute to release a firm grasp of the hand. The more sudden and powerful the effort the more prominent the symptoms. Once the muscles are "warmed up" by exercise the myotonia gradually disappears but after a period of rest it reappears. Cold exaggerates the symptoms. Hypertrophy may be prominent, sometimes giving the patient a "muscle man" appearance. Contractures do not occur.

As might be expected there is an increased creatine tolerance because the muscle mass is greater than normal and its contractile power is not impaired. Creatinine levels are usually within normal limits.

Sections of the muscles in congenital myotonia show nothing more than hypertrophy. Abnormal branching of the motor end plates has been reported when the methylene blue technique was used.

STIFF-MAN SYNDROME

Moersch and Waltman[18] first reported this syndrome in 1956. This condition, which incidentally may occur in females as well as males, is characterized by tonic contracture of one or more muscle groups. Upon this tonic rigidity are superimposed paroxysms of painful muscle spasms precipitated by various physical and emotional stimuli. The electromyogram reflects the tonic contraction in a constant firing of impulses which continues even at rest and is unaffected by attempts at relaxation. Several cases have been effectively treated with diazepam,[19] a drug with anticonvulsant properties.

MYASTHENIA GRAVIS

Myasthenia gravis is a relatively common disorder of muscle function that was recognized and described as early as the seventeenth century. It is characterized by muscle weakness, which becomes more profound as the muscle is used.

The muscles of the head and neck, palpebral and extraocular, and those of chewing and swallowing, are usually the first to be involved and often the most severely affected. In advanced cases the weakening of respiratory muscles may lead to fatal complications with chronic pneumonia and crises of asphyxia. Eventually the muscles of the back, abdomen and extremities are involved in well defined cases. Symptoms of cardiac involvement are lacking though microscopic lesions in the myocardium have been reported.[20]

At the outset, muscle contraction becomes less forceful with repetitive stimuli, until contractile ability is completely lost. After a period of rest, original power is regained. Though the muscle becomes progressively weaker, it does not become painful as in physiologic fatigue. As the disease progresses, the capacity for contraction may be lost entirely even on initial stimulation.

Onset may be at any age though children are rarely affected. The disease is seen in both sexes with about equal frequency. The disability may be announced by weakness and inability to perform accustomed tasks or difficulty in properly focusing vision, closing the eyelids or simply in chewing and swallowing. These symptoms may spread to involve other muscles or the process may remain static so that they are the sole manifestations throughout the patient's lifetime. In the majority of cases there are long periods of remission though each succeeding attack may become more severe. In some cases the disease is steadily progressive. Thymic tumor is reportedly more common in these cases. This tumor occurs in about one third of the fatal cases of myasthenia gravis.[21] The pathogenetic significance of this association is still unknown but recent linkage of thymic function with the establishment of the immune state lends credence to the recently proposed hypothesis of myasthenia gravis as an autoimmune disease. A myasthenia-like state has frequently been reported accompanying bronchiogenic carcinoma.

The pathogenesis of myasthenia gravis is still unknown, but ever since the physiology of nerve-muscle impulse transmission has been known, it has been assumed that the disease is a disturbance in this mechanism. Thus it has been stated that failure of normal contracture must be due to inadequate acetylcholine production or excessive acetylcholine destruction, presumably by cholinesterase. The fact that the myasthenic muscle behaves like that poisoned with curare and the myasthenia is relieved by physostigmine and other cholinesterase inhibitors has strengthened this assumption. However, today it is universally agreed that both acetylcholine and cholinesterase are normal in quantity and quality and no other agent with a cholinesterase or curare-like action has been extracted. Moreover weak contractions are probably not due to an innate inability of the muscle fibers to react to normal amounts of acetylcholine because newborns with myasthenic mothers may themselves be myasthenic but usually evolve to a normal state in the course of a few weeks as though they were born with some substance of maternal origin that was eventually metabolized or neutralized in a normal organism.

Choline is an intermediate product in the hydrolysis of acetylcholine. It has been shown that an excess of choline at the end plate muscle interface may interfere with impulse transmission. The most recent suggestion that choline or some related protein in this metabolic chain may become antigenic associates myasthenia gravis with the autoimmune diseases and neatly ties this phenomenon in the same packet with thymic involvement.

Involvement of the thymus in perhaps one third of the cases of myasthenia gravis is a puzzling association. Removal of the thymic tumor may be associated with remission of myasthenia gravis or there may be no change in the progress or severity of the disease. Moreover a first attack of myasthenia has occurred more than once following thymectomy and myasthenic crises have apparently been precipitated by thymectomy. There are so many variables including the type and degree of involvement of the thymus that at present an explanation with the facts at hand is hopelessly impossible.

Pathology. Often sections of muscle in myasthenia gravis reveal nothing of pathologic significance. More often focal infiltrations with mature lymphocytes can be found if multiple sections are examined. Microscopic foci of muscle fiber necrosis have been reported. Muscle atrophy is probably no more than can be accounted for on the basis of disease wasting. Coers and Woolf,[3] using vital methylene blue stain, have demonstrated abnormal arborization of the terminal axons, which may be significant. Lymphocytic infiltrations also have been reported in the viscera and in endocrine glands, particularly the thyroid and the adrenals.

FAMILIAL PERIODIC PARALYSIS

One of the least common muscle disorders is known as familial periodic paralysis. This disease is characterized by sudden periodic attacks of flaccid paralysis. The period of paralysis lasts a few hours to several days. During the attack, tendon reflexes and electrical excitability are totally lacking. Onset is usually announced by the muscle groups of the pelvic and shoulder girdles but the paralysis spreads rapidly to involve those of both upper and lower extremities. Respiratory muscles, fortunately, are not affected. The myocardium is sometimes involved. Between attacks, muscle strength and function are completely normal. These periods of paralysis may recur every few days or they may be separated by months or even years. Attacks may be precipitated by vigorous treatment of diabetes with insulin or of Addison's disease with desoxycorticosterone. They may follow a high carbohydrate intake.

Manifestations of the disease usually appear during adolescence or a few years before or after. It is much more common in males. Attacks are apt to come on during periods of rest and thus frequently begin during sleep. This fact is cited in support of the potassium toxicity hypothesis. The potassium ion is excreted in contraction. Muscles that are continuously active do not concentrate the material thus explaining the exclusion of respiratory muscle involvement. Also many patients learn that they may abort a threatened attack by exercise.

It has long been known that the potassium ion is used in carbohydrate metabolism and excreted under the influence of desoxycorticosterone. Because, during the paralytic period the serum potassium level is low, it was long assumed that muscle paralysis was the consequence of potassium depletion of the interstitial fluid. When the condition known as aldosteronism was defined as an excessive elaboration of this hormone by the cells of adrenal cortical hyperplasia or tumor causing sodium retention and potassium loss with striking muscle weakness, these data were thought to support this hypothesis. Then it was learned that muscle paralysis occurs as a result of potassium poisoning but not from potassium depletion. Next it was found that the lowered serum level was not the result of urinary excretion but that the ion was "segregated" somewhere in the body—the interstitial fluids or perhaps the muscle fibers themselves. The reports of muscle analysis are conflicting, some indicating high potassium levels and normal or low sodium concentration. Others have found no alterations in ion content but excess water within the muscle fiber, a finding that might explain the vacuolization reported by microscopists. It is probably safest to admit that as yet we are not certain of the pathogenesis of paralysis in this disease.

Familial periodic paralysis is usually inherited as a simple autosomal dominant though many cases appear to arise as a spontaneous mutant. As the name implies there is usually a familial incidence.

Transient episodes of muscle weakness or even paralysis have been noted in a number of conditions other than typical familial periodic paralysis. As already noted, it can be induced in insulin and desoxycorticosterone therapy. It is seen in primary aldosteronism and paralysis without reduced serum potassium level occurs in what now appears to be a separate disease entity called paramyotonia by Adams, Denny-Brown and Pearson.

In the past, various reports have described fiber atrophy, fiber hypertrophy, fiber necrosis and mild exudative inflammatory reactions. Most workers now agree that there is no consistent microscopic picture. A number of workers agree that vacuolization of muscle fibers is a common occurrence. The identity of the material that inhabits the vacuoles has been the cause of some dispute. Most microscopists believe that it is probably water.[24]

References

1. Adams, R., Denny-Brown, D. and Pearson, C.: Diseases of Muscle. Ed. 2. New York, Harper and Bros., 1962.
2. Kennelly, B. and Blumberg, L.: J.A.M.A., 203:487, 1968.
3. Coers, C. and Woolf, A.: Innervation of Muscle. London, Blackwell, 1959.
4. White, L.: Calif. Med., 90:1, 1959.
5. Pearson, C.: N. Engl. J. Med., 256:1069, 1957.
6. Zatuchni, J., Aegerter, E., Molthan, L. and Shuman, C.: Circulation, 3:846, 1951.
7. Waring, J. and Ravin, A.: Arch. Intern. Med., 65:763, 1940.
8. Lee, K. F., Lin, S. and Hodes, P. J.: Am. J. Roentgenol., 115:179, 1972.
9. Sky, G. and Magee, K.: Brain, 79:610, 1956.
10. Muscatello, U. and Patriarca, P.: Am. J. Pathol., 52:1169, 1968.
11. Landon, J. and Smith, L.: New York, The Macmillan Co., 1941.

12. Blattner, R.: J. Pediatr., *68*:823, 1966.
13. Sheldon, W.: Arch. Dis. Child., 7:117, 1932.
14. Westermark, B.: Acta Paedeatr., *55*:117, 1966.
15. Aegerter, E. and Long, J.: Am. J. Med. Sci., *215*:324, 1949.
16. Sjögren, H.: Acta Ophth., *11*:1, 1933.
17. Talal, N.: Bull. Rheum. Dis., *16*:404, 1966.
18. Moersch, F. and Waltman, H.: Proc. Mayo Clin., *31*:421, 1956.
19. Cohen, L.: J.A.M.A., *195*:160, 1966.
20. Mendelow, H. and Genkins, G.: J. Mt. Sinai Hosp., *21*:218, 1954.
21. Rowland, L., Hoefer, P., Aranow, H. and Merritt, H.: Neurology, *6*:307, 1956.
22. Girdany, B. and Danowski, T. S.: Am. J. Dis. Child., 9:339, 1956.
23. Houston, C. S. and Zaleski, W. A.: Radiology, *89*:59, 1957.
24. Sky, M., Wanko, T., Rowley, P. and Engel, A.: Exp. Neurol., 3:53, 1961.

Chapter 23

TUMORS OF SOFT PARTS

A heterogeneous group of tumors, hamartomas, choristomas and tumorlike processes affect the regions that are often referred to as "the soft parts," i.e., tissues exclusive of the skeleton and the viscera. Actually, these areas include the skin, the mediastinum and the retroperitoneal tissues. Because the orthopedist is not primarily concerned with these regions he has refined the term to mean the extremities, shoulders and buttocks exclusive of the skin. Because there are no glandular

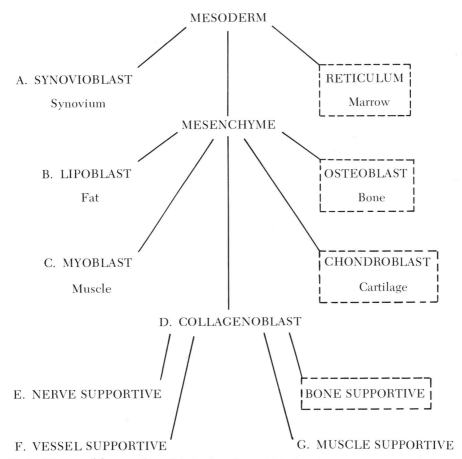

Figure 23–1   Diagram of the mesodermal derivatives from which the soft part tumors arise. The boxed derivatives represent the primary bone tumors discussed in previous chapters.

structures in these areas, these processes are all, with the exception of some of the peripheral nerve tumors, of mesenchymal origin. Some of the mesenchymal soft part tumors rarely occur in areas other than the skin, mediastinum and retroperitoneal regions and these need not be included in this discussion because the orthopedist is rarely called upon to diagnose and treat them. In brief, the lesions to be considered here are simply those mesenchymal masses of the non-osseous portions of the extremities and the regions to which the latter are attached.

Because the number of cell types is considerable and the terminology complex and often nondescriptive, many clinicians find great difficulty in organizing this group. For this reason an attempt will be made here to group them, hoping that by association the various entities will remain distinct in the minds of those who encounter these conditions.

In dealing with the class of lesions called tumors of bone, we went into considerable detail in attempting to differentiate between the true tumors, the hamartomas and those lesions that for lack of a better designation were called proliferative reaction to injury. The same distinction must be made between these classes of lesions in describing the "tumors" of the soft parts, because here too one finds grouped together under this heading, true neoplasms, hamartomas and reactive proliferations. We shall first include an orthodox classification that covers all these lesions and then, in more detail, give a classification of each of the lesional types.

A glance at Figure 23–1, a diagram of the mesodermal derivatives, reminds us that we have already considered the lesions arising from four important tissue types in this class. They have been placed in rectangles to exclude them from the remaining mesodermal derivatives. Each of the latter contributes certain lesions to the soft part "tumor" group and we shall consider them in the progression of their designating letters. The following is an outline of the soft part "tumors" that come to the attention of the orthopedist. This is the classification used in most texts on the subject. It is well to remember in using it that it includes many lesions, hamartomas and proliferative reparative reactions that are not neoplasms. Indeed, it is nothing more than a catalogue of the tissue masses of all types that are formed in soft parts. We prefer to break down this general classification into the more definitive groups of neoplasms, hamartomas and proliferative reactions.

"TUMORS" OF SOFT PARTS

I. Lesions of mesothelial origin
  Synovioma
    Chronic tenosynovitis (villonodular tenosynovitis, fibrous xanthoma, giant cell tumor of tendon, benign synovioma)
    Ganglion
    Tenosynovial chondrometaplasia (osteochondromatosis)
    Tumoral calcinosis
II. Lesions of lipoblastic origin
  Lipoma
  Hibernoma
  Liposarcoma
  Fat necrosis
III. The muscle "tumor" group
  Leiomyoma
  Leiomyosarcoma

Rhabdomyosarcoma
Myositis ossificans (fibrositis ossificans)
IV. Lesions of collagenoblastic tissue
  From simple connective tissue
    Keloid
    The fibromatoses
    Desmoid
    Pseudosarcomatous fasciitis (nodular fasciitis)
    Juvenile aponeurotic fibroma
    Fibrosarcoma and aggressive fibromatosis
  From nerve supportive tissue
    Neuroma
    Neurilemmoma
    Malignant schwannoma
    Neurofibroma

Neurofibrosarcoma (neurogenic sarcoma)
From vessel supportive tissue
Granuloma pyogenicum
Hemangioma
Hemangiosarcoma
Hemangioendothelioma
Hemangiopericytoma

V. Lesions of uncertain tissue origin
Granular cell myoblastoma
Alveolar soft part tumor
Epithelioid sarcoma
Clear cell sarcoma
Malignant giant cell tumor
VI. Tumors of mixed tissue origin
Mesenchymoma

When the hamartomas and reactive hyperplasias are removed from the preceding classification there remains a group of lesions characterized by progressive hyperplasia, destructive invasion and the capacity to metastasize, in short a group of malignant tumors that arise from the various derivatives of mesoderm.

TRUE NEOPLASMS OF SOFT PARTS

I. From the synovioblast
Synovioma
II. From the lipoblast
Pleomorphic liposarcoma
Differentiated liposarcoma
Myxoid liposarcoma
III. From the myoblast
Leiomyosarcoma
Pleomorphic rhabdomyosarcoma
Alveolar rhabdomyosarcoma
Embryonal rhabdomyosarcoma

IV. From the collagenoblast
Fibrosarcoma
V. From nerve supportive tissue
Neurofibrosarcoma
Malignant schwannoma
VI. From vessel supportive tissue
Angiosarcoma
VII. Miscellaneous
Alveolar soft part tumor
Epithelioid sarcoma
Mesenchymoma

TUMORS OF MESOTHELIAL ORIGIN

The mesothelium is that mesodermal derivative which is specialized for the lining of body cavities and fluid-conducting channels. The mesothelial cells are closely related to the fibroblasts. Indeed, when a fluid-filled cavity or channel is formed in collagenoblastic tissue there appears to be a transition in the lining collagenoblasts to the mesothelial structure, and in situations leading to mesothelial proliferation one can often find small amounts of collagen appearing in the cell aggregates, an atavistic reminder of its earlier status. The pleura gives rise to an important group of mesotheliomas but the mesothelial type that is pertinent to this discussion is the synovia. It lines the joint cavities except for the weight-bearing articular surfaces, the bursal walls and the sheaths of moving tendons and ligaments. It is concerned with the elaboration of hyaluronates, which act as a lubricant for parts in motion where friction would otherwise cut down efficiency.

Two lesions of the synovia are commonly classified as tumors. The synovioma is a true malignant tumor. Villonodular synovitis and tenosynovitis are curious lesions whose exact nature is unknown; they appear to be a proliferative reaction to some type of inflammation or more probably a hamartomatous metaplasia, the result of some hidden metabolic error.

Synovioma

This tumor is unusual elsewhere than the extremities,[1] and more often in the legs

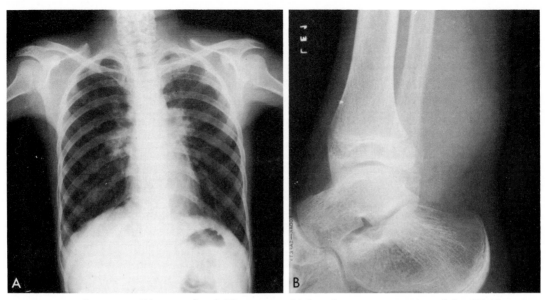

Figure 23–2 Synovioma (11 years of age). There are multiple pulmonary metastatic nodules (A). There is a large mass noted in relation to the distal end of the fibula (B). Erosion of the cortex is most apparent posteriorly. Calcification is present within the tumor.

than the arms. It is most commonly encountered in the vicinity of a joint and usually appears to arise from a tendon sheath, though in many instances it has been impossible to demonstrate an origin from a normal synovial structure. In some series there has been a preponderance in females; in others there has been a male preponderance. The tumor may develop at any age but usually occurs between the ages of 18 and 25.

The commonest site of occurrence is about the ankle and foot, the second commonest site, the periarticular soft tissues of the knee. Indeed, about 80 per cent occur in the lower extremity distal to the mid-thigh. The next site in frequency is the shoulder area. Perhaps a dozen have been reported in the soft tissues of the chest and abdomen. Perhaps half that many are reported arising from deep tissues in the neck[2] and presenting in the pharynx. We have examined sections from one such

case. They have been called cervical synovial sarcoma.

The early accounts of synovioma were misleading because its slow growth led these writers to the conclusion that the tumor is benign. In the initial reports[3] many treated patients were thought to have been cured by conservative excision. Later these patients returned with recurrent tumor and many of them eventually succumbed to their disease after they had been reported as cured. Recurrence after excision is as characteristic as the slow growth. One patient in our material had eight such recurrences before the tumor metastasized widely.

In our series (73 cases) 31 were in females and 42 in males. Fifty-four were located in the region of the knee or in the lower extremity distal to the knee, 16 in the foot. Thirteen were in the elbow or distal to it. Fifty-three patients were under the age of 30. There were but five tumors arising from joint synovia, and all involved the knee. Seven were treated by local excision, with six deaths in from a few months to several years. Seven were treated by amputation, with five deaths. It is obvious that the diagnosis of synovioma is associated with a very grave prognosis. It is our belief that if, in resection, there is the slightest doubt on the part of the surgeon that the tumor has been completely and widely eradicated, the limb should be sacrificed. Indeed, the vast majority of patients with synovioma eventually come to amputation. The clinical and cytologic features are disarmingly innocent in character. Because of this, radical treatment is too often delayed until the tumor is no longer curable.

Microscopy. Diagnosis of the synovioma on the basis of microscopy is often exceedingly difficult because of the kaleidoscopic variation in cell form and pattern. These forms may show little or no structural resemblance to each other. This capacity for variation may relate to the morphologic inconstancy of the synovial cell from which the tumor arises. This cell, even in non-neoplastic lesions, may vary in shape from an elongated spindle to palisaded cylindrical cells closely mimicking secreting gland cells.

Three microscopic types are generally described and accepted as synoviomas. In the commonest variety, the sacromatous type, the cells are spindled or fusiform, quite uniform and have little fibrous supportive structure (Fig. 23–3). Slit spaces occur, usually lined by tumor cells. The channels may contain an eosin-staining material that is said to be hyaluronate; it is positive with the PAS stain. In a second variety, the biphasic type, the cells are more cylindrical and often arrange themselves radially about spaces to form a pseudoacinar pattern (Fig. 23–4). In a third group the cells are quite uniform in type, round or oval resembling histiocytes or endothelial cells with little or no appreciable supportive stroma (Fig. 23–5). Cleft spaces are apt to be lacking. This is called the endothelial type.

We have examined the sections of three tumors whose cells, except that they were larger, resembled those of the endothelial cell type synovioma. Long term follow-up has shown them to be primary tumors. Their locations, age group and propensity for repeated recurrence and final metas-

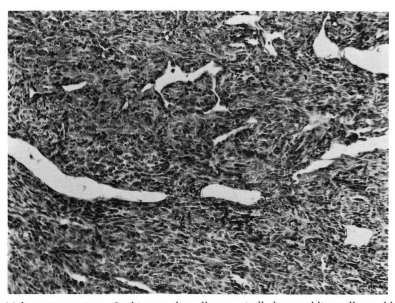

Figure 23–3   Malignant synovioma. In this type the cells are spindled, resembling collagenoblasts. The most characteristic feature is the formation by the tumor cells of irregular, elongated, empty spaces. These may have contained hyaluronate in the living tissue. ($\times$ 130.)

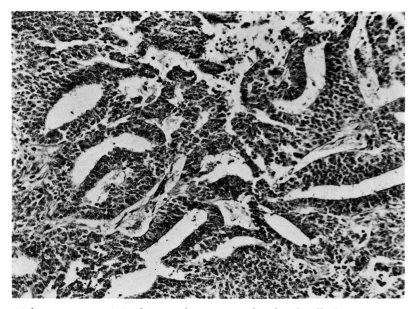

Figure 23–4 Malignant synovioma. In this type the spaces are lined with cells that suggest an epithelial origin. These tumors may be mistaken for metastatic adenocarcinoma. (× 130.)

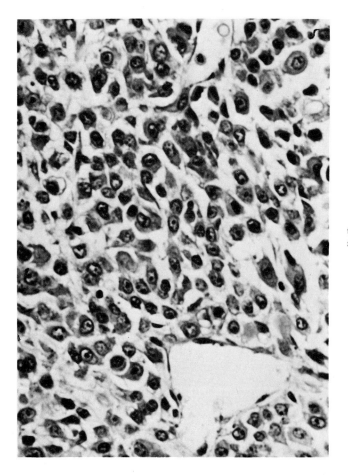

Figure 23–5 Synovioma, endothelial type. Cells are rounded, and supportive stroma is scant. (× 370.)

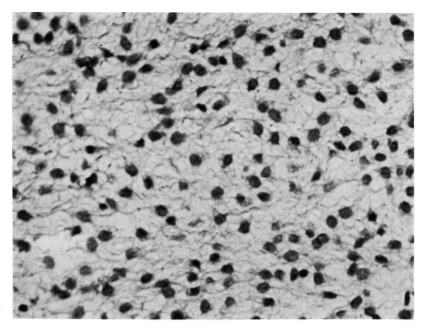

Figure 23–6   Clear cell sarcoma. This tumor had its origin in synovia. It is probably a subtype of synovioma.

tasis to lymph nodes and then lungs were the same as in synovioma. We suspect they were a subtype of the endothelial cell variety.

Recent reports have indicated a 50 per cent five year survival rate for the sarcomatous and biphasic types but only 25 per cent for the endothelial type.

The clear cell sarcoma has been described recently[4] as a distinct pathologic entity. We have studied one case of what was universally accepted as a typical example of this lesion affecting the popliteal tissues. On closer scrutiny of this case we found that a tumor had been removed from the synovia of the nearby knee joint approximately three years earlier. It appeared to us to be a synovioma and in it were clear cell areas identical to the periarticular tumor removed later (Fig. 23–6). We are inclined to the conclusion, therefore, that the clear cell sarcoma is another variety of synovioma. Kubo[5] has studied one of these tumors by electron microscopy and come to the same conclusion. In most clear cell sarcomas one can find areas that resemble the more common spindle cell variety. There even may be rather typical cleft spaces.

There are four clear cell type tumors in our material. There is a tendency for the cells to be arranged in an alveolar pattern. They are rounded or spindled. The cytoplasm is largely clear or vacuolated, sometimes granular. Mitoses are scarce. Their age and site incidence is the same as for synovioma, as are their propensity for multiple recurrence and eventual metastasis. The mortality data are also similar. For these reasons and because one of these tumors in our collection was primary in synovial tissue we believe that the clear cell sarcoma is in reality a subtype of the endothelial type of synovioma.

A few so-called malignant giant cell tumors of tendon sheaths have been reported.[6] Careful analysis of these tumors will, we believe, show most of them to be instances of villonodular tenosynovitis in which there is an unusually florid proliferation of stromal and giant cells (Fig. 23–7). However, in very rare examples there may be aggressive neoplastic behavior. It seems to us of little consequence whether we classify these as neoplastic alteration in tenosynovitis or synovioma with giant cells. For the sake of uniformity we prefer to consider them the latter because their behavior is identical with synovioma and because there is no proof that earlier in

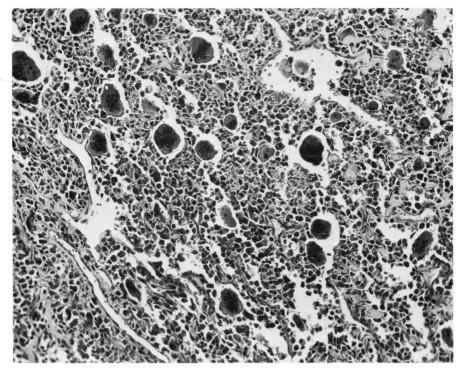

Figure 23–7 Malignant giant cell tumor of tendon sheaths. There are a cellular stroma and numerous giant cells. This is probably a subvariety of synovioma. (× 150.)

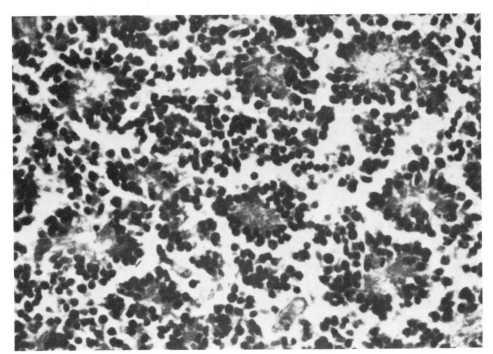

Figure 23–8 Malignant neuroepithelioma. This tumor is characterized by rosettes of cells. It may be a subtype of synovioma. (× 350.)

their genesis they were non-neoplastic lesions. They must be exceedingly rare. We have encountered but one instance in our material.

Dr. A. P. Stout, long ago, described what he called "malignant neuroepithelioma of soft tissues." As one reads his description one gathers that the separate categorization is made because of the presence of rosettes in the sections (Fig. 23–8). Later Dr. Stout expressed doubt as to the existence of malignant neuroepithelioma of soft tissues as a separate entity. We have encountered but a single instance of this tumor. Because other than the rosettes, the microscopy and the behavior are acceptable for synovioma, we prefer to think of it as a subtype of that group.

In summarizing this chameleon of microscopy, the synovioma, we can say there are three generally accepted types—the sarcomatous, the biphasic and the endothelial. However, we believe that it is now permissible to add that there are three microscopic types of tumors whose behavior is similar to that of synovioma, i.e., a propensity for repeated recurrence and finally metastasis to the regional lymph nodes and then the lungs. These are tumors whose cell origins are unknown but which might conceivably arise from synovial cells lining tendon sheaths. Until we have more knowledge about these three rare tumors (the clear cell sarcoma, the malignant giant cell tumor of soft parts and the malignant neuroepithelioma of soft tissues) we consider it justifiable to classify them as variations within the synovioma group. Until this thesis is disproved we recommend they be treated in the same manner as their more renowned relatives.

TUMORS OF LIPOBLASTIC ORIGIN

Young fat cells and primitive fibroblasts cannot be differentiated until the former begin to accumulate lipid within their cytoplasm. Then the cell enlarges to many times its original size, the minute fat droplets coalescing to form a spheroid globule, which stretches the cytoplasmic membrane about it and pushes the nucleus to one side, flattening it against the cell wall. Fields of these adult fat cells appear through the microscope as a network of delicate cell walls enclosing spaces from which the fat has been dissolved by the processing agents. When fat cells are injured, new fat cells may be formed from what appear to be primitive fibroblasts. As these enlarge their cytoplasm acquires a peculiar, ground glass opacity, which gives them a characteristic appearance. These are called embryonic fat cells.

It is insufficiently understood that the fat cell and the other mesenchymal derivatives, particularly the collagenoblast, when undergoing neoplastic change, suffer profound alterations in their metabolic routines. Their stored fat may be quite different from that of the normal fat cell and, more important, the fatty acids of their ground substance may be protein linked, producing a myxoid matrix. Since the ground substance influences the cell shape we suspect this may explain why the cells of the so-called "myxoma" are often stellate. Thus the myxoma and myxosarcoma are not of independent tissue types (there is no myxoblast) but rather lipoblastic (and perhaps fibroblastic) tumors that produce a myxoid ground substance.

Physiologists have been able to tell us little about the reasons for and the mechanisms of intracellular fat accumulation. When the organism is exposed to an excess of lipids, it stores this material in certain depots. The distribution of these deposits is controlled, to some extent at least, by endocrine influence, being somewhat different in males than females. Excessive deposits of fat in abnormal places constitute the lipomas. Proliferation of the vestigial fat storage organ cells results in a hamartomatous mass known as a hibernoma. True neoplastic proliferation of fat cells results in the liposarcoma.

Liposarcoma

The liposarcoma is an important tumor from the standpoint of its incidence and its prognosis. It occurs most often in the fat-containing tissues of the buttock, the thigh and the lower leg but may be seen in the arm and shoulder region. It is often a bulky tumor and is usually invasive with very little evidence of border delineation. It almost always begins as a liposarcoma rather than a transition from a lipoma, but we have seen one perfectly characteristic, common, encapsulated lipoma of the leg in the center of which there was an undeniably obvious liposarcoma.

Liposarcoma rarely occurs before the age of 30 and is most frequently encountered in the fifth decade. It usually grows slowly, the history stating that it has been present for a considerable time. About one half of these tumors are known to have recurred within three years and about one third have metastasized. Five year cures are reported as high as 85 per cent in some series. This figure appears somewhat optimistic to us.

Enterline et al.[7] have divided liposarcomas into five types: the well differentiated myxoid, the poorly differentiated myxoid, the lipoma-like, the myxoid mixed and the nonmyxoid. Their paper should be consulted when unusual types are encountered. Most pathologists are content to divide them into the undifferentiated or pleomorphic and the differentiated types.

Most liposarcomas have a characteristic vascular pattern. The cells are often arranged about broad channels which may mislead the microscopist into a diagnosis of angioma or angiosarcoma.

In its usual form, the pleomorphic type, the liposarcoma is not hard to diagnose on its microscopic appearance. It is composed of bizarre cells whose nuclei reveal all the characteristics of malignancy. Distorted giant cells are usual. The identifying features are the embryonic and even adult fat cells that are scattered among the more obvious tumor cells (Fig. 23–9). Sometimes the more mature forms are lacking and the tumor cells are quite uniform. Then one must search for evidence of fat-storing cells. In these undifferentiated tumors a fat stain may be of little help because the tumor cells may contain no more fat than tumors of other cytogenesis. Fat stains should always be done, however, if liposarcoma is suspected.

The liposarcoma must be removed widely or it will recur and often metastasize in the usual sarcoma pattern. Stout has described what he calls a "differentiated liposarcoma." Among lipoblasts and lipocytes (Fig. 23–10) one finds areas composed of stellate cells in a myxomatous

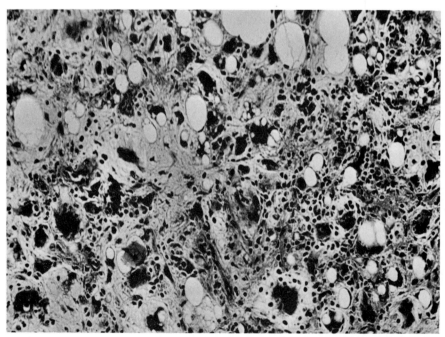

Figure 23–9 Liposarcoma. The sections have a pleomorphic appearance. There are many bizarre, multinucleated giant cells, primitive spindled lipoblasts, embryonic fat cells and mature lipocytes. (× 200.)

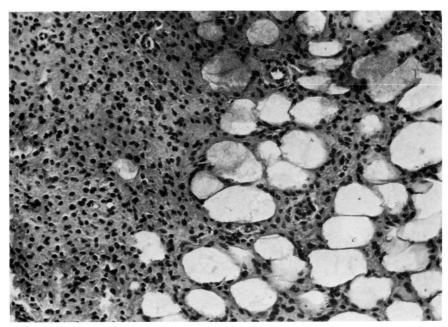

Figure 23–10   Differentiated liposarcoma. Lipoblasts, the small opaque cells, are mixed with mature lipocytes, the large clear spaces. Granular embryonal fat cells can be seen in the section but are difficult to recognize in the illustration. (× 300.)

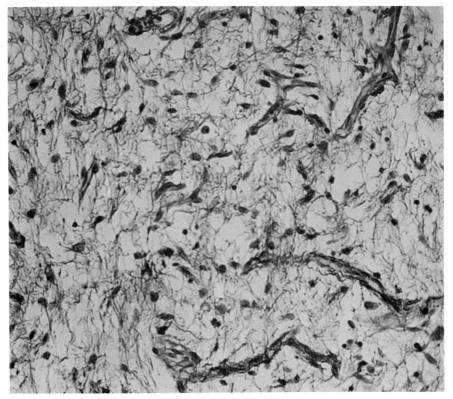

Figure 23–11   Myxoid liposarcoma. Stellate cells in a myxoid ground substance are grouped around blood channels. Little or no fat is found within the cells. (× 230.)

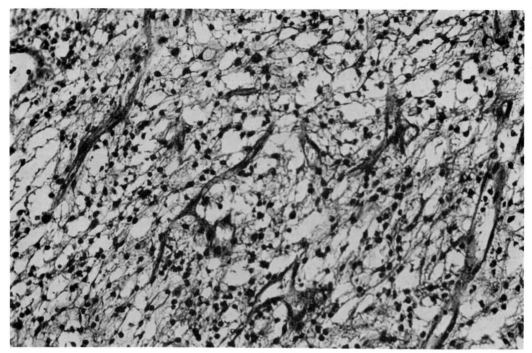

Figure 23–12   Myxoid liposarcoma. This is a recurrence of the myxoid liposarcoma shown in Figure 23–11. The cells are now more rounded and contain lipid. Note prominence of vessels.

ground substance. These tumors are apparently invasive but they do not metastasize.

The liposarcomas are apt to be myxoid. Usually the presence of mature and embryonic fat cells and pleomorphic forms makes the diagnosis possible but in some, especially the primary and first few recurrences, these elements are lacking. The sections may reveal only an infiltrating tumor composed of stellate cells in a myxoid ground substance (Fig. 23–11). Eventually, sometimes after numerous recurrences, the cells take on the features of neoplastic lipoblasts (Fig. 23–12). Though recurrence is the rule and complete removal may be a formidable surgical task, only a few of these tumors metastasize to the lungs.

THE MUSCLE TUMOR GROUP

This group contains several entities, the leiomyoma, the leiomyosarcoma and the rhabdomyosarcoma. The rhabdomyoma probably occurs only in the heart so is not considered here. Besides these lesions of known muscle origin a few authors still include two others, the granular cell myoblastoma and the alveolar soft part tumor, whose origins are actually unknown. The former was described as coming from the myoblast and this hypothesis has not been unequivocally disproved. The latter is thought by some to be the malignant analogue of the granular cell myoblastoma. These lesions will be discussed under the heading "lesions of uncertain tissue origin."

Leiomyosarcoma

The sarcoma of nonstriated muscle rarely occurs in the deep tissues of the extremities. We have seen only one in the material from Temple Health Sciences Center. These tumors occur somewhat more often in the skin and in the soft tissues of the trunk. A diagnosis is usually made by excluding leiomyoma, fibrosarcoma, liposarcoma and rhabdomyosarcoma. The greatest difficulty may arise in

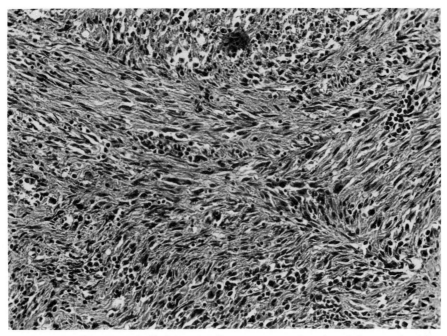

Figure 23–13 Leiomyosarcoma. Spindled tumor cells are woven in broad, undulating trabeculae. Note that the nuclei show considerable pleomorphism. (× 200.)

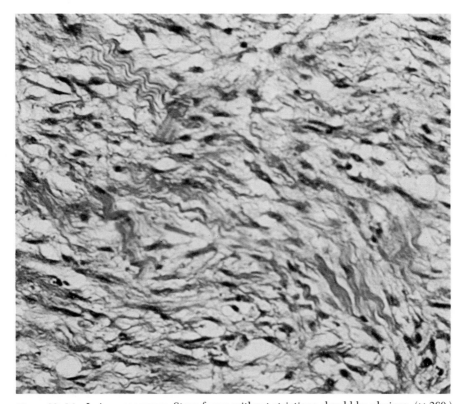

Figure 23–14 Leiomyosarcoma. Strap forms without striations should be obvious. (× 260.)

determining whether a smooth muscle tumor is benign or malignant. It has been said that if a deeply situated, smooth muscle tumor of an extremity is over 5 cm. in diameter it is probably malignant. Because benign smooth muscle tumors (leiomyomas) are rarely found in the soft parts, if the tumor cells are unquestionably nonstriated muscle (a rare instance, indeed) then the tumor is leiomyosarcoma. Gross evidence of invasion, hemorrhage and necrosis suggest malignancy. In the sections, the degree of cellularity, nuclear pleomorphism, mitotic figures and occasional irregular giant cell forms, when present, make the distinction (Fig. 23–13).

Rhabdomyosarcoma

The malignant tumor of striated muscle occurs often enough to be of real importance.

The rhabdomyosarcomas are usually divided into three morphologic groups: the pleomorphic, the alveolar and the embryonal types. The pleomorphic type is probably the most common and more than half of these occur in the buttock, groin or leg. They grow rather slowly to form a large mass. The mortality rate is greater than 50 per cent, and unless they are eradicated early they metastasize by way of the blood, usually to the lungs. It is unusual

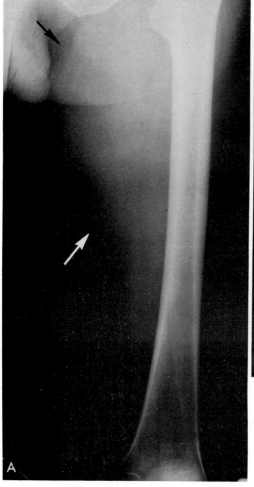

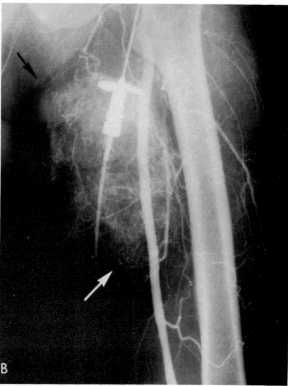

Figure 23–15 Rhabdomyosarcoma (male, 66 years of age.) A large mass without underlying osseous abnormalities is present in the medial aspect of the thigh near the groin arrows, (*A*). An arteriogram demonstrates the vascularity of the tumor; there are numerous areas of capillary blush and larger abnormal vessels (*B*).

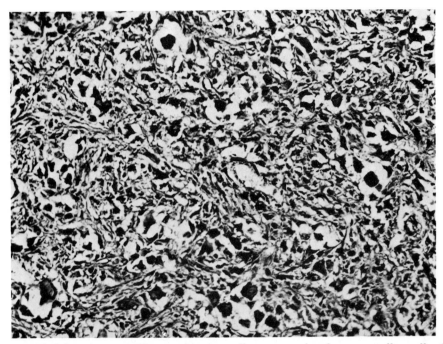

Figure 23–16   Rhabdomyosarcoma. Pleomorphic giant cells may occur but they are usually smaller than those of liposarcoma. Elongated (strap) forms are helpful features. The staining quality of the cytoplasm is not illustrated in this photograph. (× 200.)

for them to occur in patients younger than 50. They are usually found within the substance of the skeletal muscles and it may be impossible to determine the margins of the tumor. For this reason recurrence is usual unless a very wide excision is carried out. As in most malignant mesenchymal tumors, hemorrhage and necrosis are common. Usually, the tumor type is not suspected until sections are examined through the microscope.

Disparity in cell size and shape characterizes the pleomorphic rhabdomyosarcoma just as in liposarcoma (Fig. 23–16). It is frequently difficult to differentiate the two. In the former, however, the cytoplasm of many or even most of the cells takes a deep rose eosin stain that is reminiscent of the sarcoplasm of normal muscle cells. This may be due to the presence of myoglobin. The less differentiated the cells, the less likely this staining characteristic is to appear. The next helpful diagnostic feature is the appearance of elongated straplike forms (Fig. 23–17). When these appear they may contain more

than one nucleus, sometimes arranged eccentrically beneath the sarcolemma. These appear in the better differentiated tumors. If one can find cross striations in these the diagnosis is certain. Phosphotungstic acid staining helps to bring out these striations. Giant cells, often with numerous bizarre nuclei, are common and these help to differentiate this tumor from fibrosarcoma and leiomyosarcoma. Occasionally the nucleus and a narrow rim of cytoplasm are situated in what appears to be a large vacuole traversed by threadlike processes radiating from the cell to the outer wall (Fig. 23–18). These forms have stimulated the imagination of some microscopists to call them "spider cells." They occur more often in the rhabdomyoma of the heart than in the rhabdomyosarcoma of soft parts. Some writers contend that the clear portions of the cell contained glycogen before the cell was processed. The appearance has suggested to us that the very large cell contained a considerable amount of water and water-soluble substances that left the cytoplasm in the

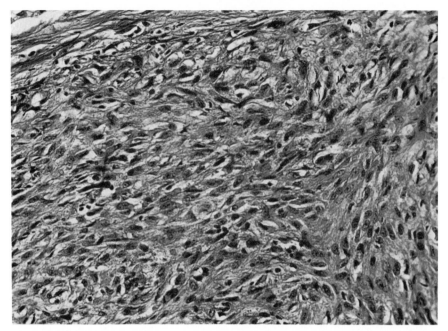

Figure 23–17   Rhabdomyosarcoma. Strap forms and racquet-shaped cells are helpful in distinguishing this tumor. Nuclear pleomorphism is prominent. (× 250.)

course of dehydration, causing the residuum to shrink away from a cell membrane that was held in shape by the more rigid surrounding tissues.

The alveolar rhabdomyosarcoma has been well described by Enterline and Horn.[8] Most of these are found involving the skeletal muscle tissues of the extremi-

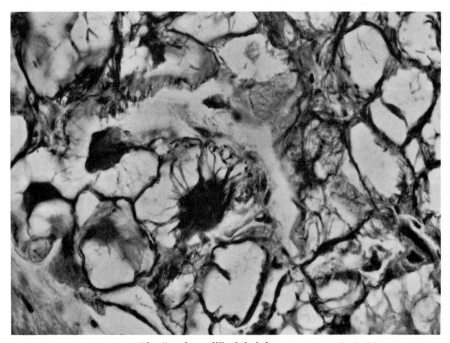

Figure 23–18   The "spider cell" of rhabdomyosarcoma. (× 440.)

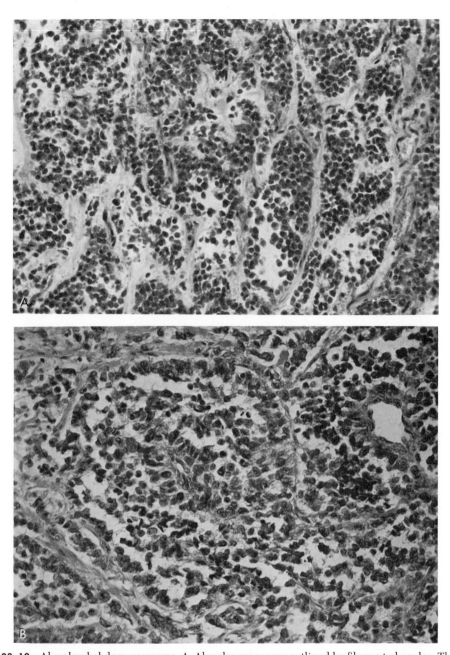

Figure 23–19   Alveolar rhabdomyosarcoma. *A*, Alveolar spaces are outlined by fibrous trabeculae. The spaces so delineated contain embryonic muscle cells loosely organized, lining the walls and sometimes filling the spaces. (× 200.) *B*, Spaces are outlined by fibrous septums. Tumor cells appear to line the space and drop loose into the lumen. (× 400.)

ties, predominantly in children and young adults. They occur more often in males; about three quarters of them appear in the soft tissues of the extremities, more frequently the lower extremity. This tumor is associated with a high mortality rate, perhaps 100 per cent. Irradiation appears to be of little value.

Grossly the tumor may show areas of liquefaction necrosis, hemorrhage or a gelatinous consistency. It is composed predominantly of large, rounded cells floating freely in alveolar spaces or loosely lining alveolar walls (Fig. 23–19). Myofibrils are sometimes found and striations can usually be seen in some of the racquet forms. The curious "floating cells" and cells loosely attached along thin stromal walls that delineate the alveolar pattern are the diagnostic features of the section.

The embryonal rhabdomyosarcoma has been described by Strobbe and Dargeon.[9] It usually occurs in the head or neck structures or in the urogenital tract. In the latter positions it is usually botryoid (rounded masses on pedicles in grapelike clusters). Occasionally it may be encountered in skeletal muscle. It occurs in infancy through adolescence. It is composed predominantly of small, round, undifferen-

tiated cells with pyknotic nuclei and short, spindled cells with deep red cytoplasm arranged in interlacing bands (Fig. 23–21). Intermixed are cells resembling lymphocytes. Longitudinal fibers and usually striations can be found. The cell ground substance is almost always myxomatous. The mortality rate is high. Most patients are dead within one year.

TUMORS OF COLLAGENOBLASTIC TISSUE

The collagenoblast, i.e., the cell that as it matures is associated with the formation of an intercellular substance known as collagen, is the chore boy of the other body tissues. It supplies the support for the more highly specialized cells of the glands, the viscera, the nerves, the vessels, the muscles and even the skeletal structures. This type we call simply "supportive collagenous tissue." In each location its structure and pattern is modified to accomodate and complement the function of the tissue it supports. Another type binds each of the specialized units into a whole so that their function is organized for the welfare of the total organism. This we call

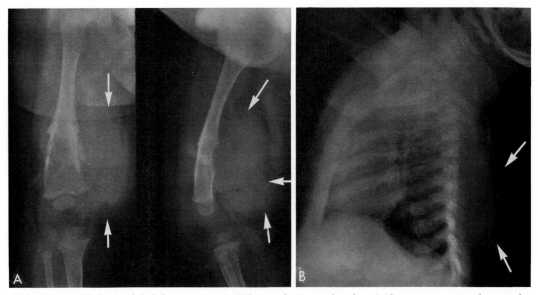

Figure 23–20 Embryonal rhabdomyosarcoma. (White male, 6 months of age.) The tumor arose in the muscles of the thigh and secondarily involved the femur. The mass of the tumor was huge (arrows, *A*). Within a short period of time, there were metastases to the soft tissues of the thorax (arrows, *B*), as well as to the lungs.

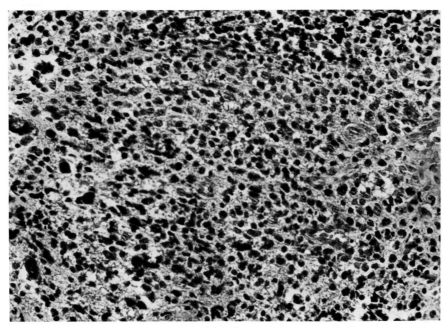

Figure 23–21   Embryonal rhabdomyosarcoma. The cells are very young in character. Tadpole or racquet-shaped cells are easier to recognize in the section than in the illustration. The cytoplasm of these cells stains intensely with eosin but it has a bluish cast suggesting the presence of myoglobin. (× 250.)

"connective tissue." Recent emphasis on the study of collagen has revealed that it, in its subtle way, plays a very important role in body physiology, not only from the standpoint of association, support and protection but also in the diffusion of most of the fluids and minerals that are so meticulously metabolized and so important to the parenchymal cells.

Abnormal proliferations, hamartomas and true tumors may develop from each collagenic type. They form a nebulous group difficult to classify, because one lesion merges imperceptibly into another without clear lines of distinction. In no other tissue type are the neoplasms and pseudoneoplasms so difficult to categorize.

These fall into four groups though the gross and microscopic characteristics of each may not always be depended upon to distinguish it from members of another group. At times, only the behavior of the lesion may be relied upon to determine its exact nature. The term "fibroma" will be avoided because it connotes a benign tumor of connective tissue. If there is such a thing as a benign tumor of this tissue type it is the desmoid or a member of the fibromatoses. The lesion that has been

called a fibroma is probably nothing more than a reactive proliferation of collagenoblasts. It is not progressive because the cells mature and stop growing. It does not predispose to fibrosarcoma. In short, it may be likened to a spontaneous keloid that occurs elsewhere than in the skin. It is a most uncommon lesion in the deep soft parts of the extremities. Most of the so-called fibromas that affect the extremities occur in relation to the skin as congenital, localized overgrowths of the corium (true hamartomas), as the result of injury (keloids), as a part of neurofibromatosis (fibroma molluscum) or as a response to cholesterol-containing macrophages (xanthomas). None of these should be mistaken for a true tumor.

There is one very important characteristic of the immature collagenoblast which the embryologists and histologists have failed to appreciate adequately. This is the capacity of these young cells to phagocytize. Only recently have we been hearing about "facultative fibroblasts," i.e., histiocytes that become converted to collagen-producing cells. It is more logical to assume that the histiocyte and collagenoblast are derived from the same stem cell and that they are interchangeable depending upon environmental circumstances. If we accept the fact that the young collagenoblast, normal or neoplastic, can phagocytize lipids then we can avoid the polemics of the xanthoma and the malignant fibroxanthoma. These are simply collagenoblastic lesions whose cells have ingested lipid. Close scrutiny of a number of these lesions has brought us to this conclusion.

In summary there is only one neoplastic lesion of the collagenoblast, the fibrosarcoma. This includes the malignant fibroblastoma or histiocytoma. There are a number of idiopathic, non-neoplastic, collagenoblastic proliferations. These are best grouped under the heading of "hamartoma." These are the desmoids and the aggressive fibromatoses. Finally, the proliferative reactions to injury, known or unknown, include the keloid, the nodular fasciitis, the aponeurotic fibroma, the fibrous histiocytoma and xanthoma.

Fibrosarcoma

Fibrosarcoma occurs in the supportive structures of muscles, tendons and liga-ments, in fascia and periosteum, in subcutaneous tissue and in the corium. It is rather uncommon in the soft parts of the extremities.

The great preponderance of fibrosarcomas are very slow growing. If they metastasize it is late. Perhaps the outstanding characteristic of fibrosarcoma is its history of recurrence or, to state it more exactly, its tenacious persistence following attempts at removal. This means simply that it is infiltrative and that fine ramifications of the tumor process extend farther than the unaided vision can appreciate, farther indeed than is expected. Because it rarely kills except by repeated recurrences and eventual invasion of vital structures, the surgeon is apt to decide on conservative measures of treatment. Such measures are often inadequate. A relatively small group of these tumors manifests a moderately rapid and progressive growth with blood metastasis and death with deposits in the lungs and elsewhere. Once the diagnosis is unequivocally established, and this can be achieved only by biopsy, the excision should be designed, with the aid of frozen sections, to eradicate the entire process even though it necessitates muti-

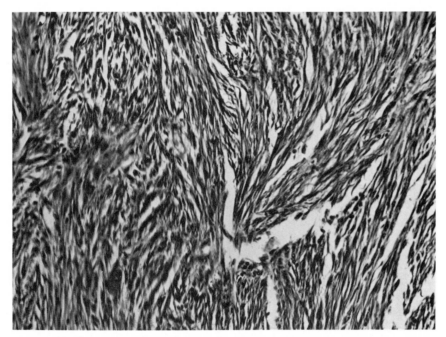

Figure 23–22   In the fibrosarcoma the nuclei are of neoplastic type. They form poorly defined trabeculae, which weave through the section. (× 200.)

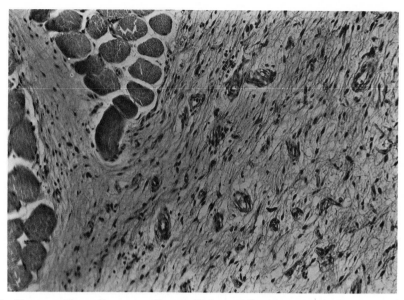

Figure 23–23   Myxoma. The cells are small, spindled or stellate in a myxomatous ground substance of plural hyaluronates. Invasion of muscle is highly characteristic. (× 130.)

lating surgery. The results of radiotherapy have not been encouraging.

The common type of fibrosarcoma is made up of spindled cells terminating in fine fibrils that take the silver stain. The more mature the cell type, the more tendency there is for the cells to grow in fascicles that interweave in undulating patterns (Fig. 23–22), produce a herringbone arrangement or form whorls. Varying amounts of collagen are formed and large amounts of intercellular collagen do not necessarily insure benignity. Indeed, some tumors with large fields of dense sclerosis and few cells have proved highly aggressive. In threadlike fibers it stains black with silver; in broader bands it stains brown. The nuclei are usually larger and more rounded than those of normal young collagenoblasts but in some cases the distinction is exceedingly difficult to make. The number of mitotic figures is a fairly good indicator for the rate of growth. In general, the absence of trabecular or whorl pattern, the lack of collagen and the presence of nuclear pleomorphism suggest a more malignant behavior. It must be added, however, that tumors with the most innocent microscopic features occasionally manifest a frankly malignant course. In 1967 Stout[10] reported 23 fibrosarcomas and added 31 more to a total of 54 followed

for five years or longer. Only four of these metastasized.

It is still uncertain in our minds whether the true fibrosarcoma can develop a myxoid ground substance. The few "myxosarcomas" that we have encountered have eventually converted to more typical myxoid liposarcomas and we are inclined to believe they were fat tumors from their beginning. It is probably best to avoid dogmatism in the matter and presume that either the collagenoblast or the lipoblast can undergo the neoplastic metabolic alteration that produces a myxomatous ground substance.

We believe that the malignant histiocytoma or fibroxanthoma is nothing more than a fibrosarcoma in which the cells have retained their earlier capacity to phagocytize lipids (facultative fibroblasts). The xanthomatous or histiocytic tumors are characterized by tumor cells whose cytoplasm is finely vacuolated by lipids, usually cholesterol esters. Rarely the cells are quite pleomorphic. Often they are multinucleated. At times the nuclei are arranged in a rosette about the periphery of the cell, the Touton giant cell. In these rare tumors we have been unable to distinguish a difference in mortality rates from that of the more ordinary low grade fibrosarcoma.

Tumors of Nerve Supportive Tissue Origin

The pseudoneoplastic and neoplastic lesions of the nerves of the extremities form a group about which there is considerable disagreement concerning cytogenesis. These lesions arise from the supportive cells of the nerve fibril, the latter playing little or no part in the production of the mass. The argument stems from the disagreement concerning the origins of these supportive cells. Some eminent writers believe that all structures within the outer nerve sheath are derived from the neural crest and are, therefore, ectodermal. Others believe they are all of mesenchymal derivation. Still others agree that the cells of the Schwann sheath are ectodermal but believe that the supportive cells between the ensheathed fibrils are collagenic. In order to avoid the involved polemics of one stand or the other it may be wiser to present the subject with a foot in each camp. Thus there can be four varieties of supportive tissue proliferation: (1) the neurilemmoma,* a hamartomatous growth from Schwann sheath cells, (2) the malignant schwannoma, its malignant counterpart, (3) neurofibroma, a hamartoma of the endoneural fibrous connective tissue, and (4) its malignant analogue, the neurofibrosarcoma. A fifth lesion is the traumatic neuroma, which is a reactive, non-neoplastic proliferation of all the supportive elements in an attempt to reestablish the continuity of a divided nerve.

MALIGNANT SCHWANNOMA

The malignant tumor of Schwann cell origin is rarely seen in the extremities except in neurofibromatosis. Its growth is said to be more rapid than that of neurilemmoma and it metastasizes widely through the blood. Because its cells are less mature than those of neurilemmoma, it may be impossible to differentiate this tumor from a fibrosarcoma of nerve or

*The term neurilemmoma is derived from the Greek "alifo" (to coat). The letter F when followed by M is changed to M for euphony. Neurilefmoma = neurilemmoma.

other soft tissue structure. Cellularity and nuclear pleomorphism are the features on which the diagnosis of malignant tumor must depend. A palisaded pattern suggests its origin from the Schwann sheath.

NEUROFIBROSARCOMA

This lesion has been responsible for much controversy among oncogeneticists. Most writers agree with Stout that it is usually impossible to determine whether a fibrosarcoma is arising in the supportive structures of a nerve or in extraneural connective tissue. There is a tumor with a fairly constant microscopic appearance and clinical behavior that is believed by many pathologists to arise from nerve supportive tissue, whether the nerve is demonstrable or not. Its most common site of origin is the medial aspect of the thigh though it may occur elsewhere, usually within large muscle groups. It grows slowly, is infiltrative and has the same penchant for recurrence as does fibrosarcoma. It is set apart from the ordinary fibrosarcoma by a tendency for its cells to palisade (Fig. 23–24). When a tumor of this microscopic pattern is associated with a nerve, many microscopists would call it a malignant schwannoma. This particular tumor, the neurofibrosarcoma, however, tends to recur in the proximal nerve stump and it rarely metastasizes.

Tumors of Vessel Supportive Tissue

In the embryonic formation of the finer ramifications of the vascular system the venous channels split off longitudinally from the arteries. Incomplete division may result in fistulous passages between the two systems. These have been called arteriovenous fistulas or, less appropriately, arteriovenous aneurysms. They may occur in any tissue or organ and if they are large they may result in excessive work for the heart and eventual cardiac failure. When very small vessels are involved they are apt to be multiple. Microfistulas have been suggested as the cause of Paget's disease. They may cause hypertrophic osteoarthropathy. They are probably the cause of the

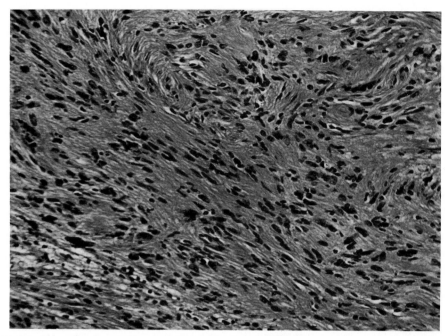

Figure 23–24 The cells of neurofibrosarcoma are like those of fibrosarcoma wherever it is found, except that there is a greater tendency for nuclear palisading. Some would call this a malignant schwannoma. (× 200.)

disturbance in the dynamics of blood flow that results in aneurysmal bone cyst.

Hamartomatous proliferations of small vessels are called angiomas. They may involve blood vessels (hemangiomas) or lymph channels (lymphangiomas, Fig. 23–25). Proliferation of various vessel components produces hemangioendotheliomas

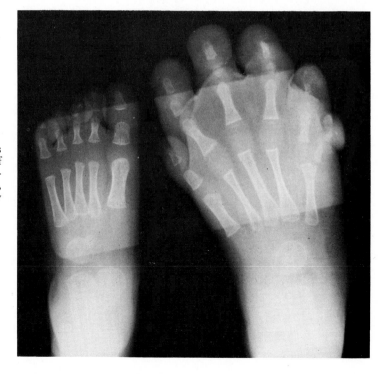

Figure 23–25 The right foot is quite large as a result of lymphangioma. The bones are enlarged but not directly involved, i.e., invaded. A supernumerary digit is present.

when the lining cells are principally involved, hemangiopericytomas when the pericytes are involved and sclerosing hemangioma when the outstanding component is the collagen-producing fibroblast of the media. The true neoplasm of this group is the hemangiosarcoma.

HEMANGIOSARCOMA

Kaposi's disease begins as an inflammatory reaction in vessels, usually of the skin. Poorly formed capillary channels leak blood into the surrounding supportive tissue. It is interesting to speculate upon the effect of this extravasated blood on the tissue, which may eventually lead to malignant behavior. Early lesions may disappear spontaneously but some, probably less than one quarter, eventually progress, invade and ultimately metastasize (Fig. 23–27). Death may occur because of widespread metastatic deposits or hemorrhage from an eroded lesion within the intestinal mucosa.[11] A few cases have been primary in the pericardium. These lesions are probably true hemangiosarcomas though there is some debate concerning their exact nosologic position. Occasionally one is tempted to diagnose a hemangiosarcoma that cannot be included under the heading of Kaposi's disease. These tumors demonstrate more nuclear pleomorphism and they are apt to have an explosively rapid and wide metastatic dissemination.

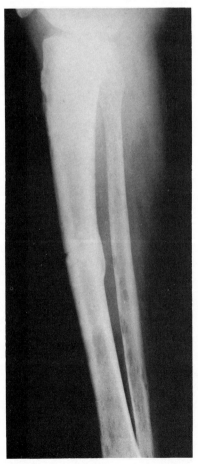

Figure 23–26   Kaposi's disease. There are poorly defined masses in the soft tissues as well as destructive areas in the bones, particularly of the cortices.

TUMORS OF UNCERTAIN TISSUE ORIGIN

Alveolar Soft Part Tumor (Malignant Granular Cell Myoblastoma, Granular Myoblastoma)

This tumor is less than one quarter as common as granular cell myoblastoma. Many writers contend that it is unrelated to the latter. Others[12] believe that it is probably the malignant analogue of the benign granular cell myoblastoma. About half of these tumors run a rather benign course, at least for a number of years. They may invade and recur but seem to be controlled if completely excised. The other half have probably metastasized by the time the original tumor is discovered and removed. The patient has an interim of several months' freedom of any signs of tumor and then a metastasis appears. One patient in our material had eight such episodes before the tumor metastasized widely and caused death. The first four metastases occurred in striated muscle groups in various areas. Later the tumor went to lymph nodes and eventually ended as a sarcomatosis. Most alveolar soft part tumors arise within muscles of the extremities (Fig. 23–28), though some appear to be derived from the sheath. They are

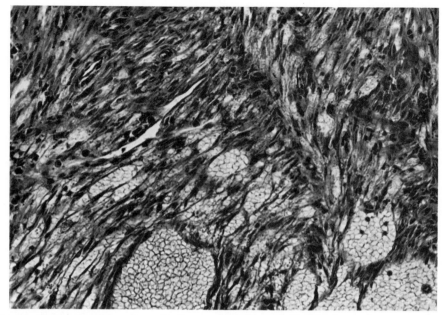

Figure 23-27   Hemangiosarcoma. Kaposi's disease. In the lower half of the figure there are numerous blood channels of various sizes. Intermixed with these are tumor cells, which appear to be derived from fibroblastic and endothelial cells. (× 280.)

usually obviously invasive from the beginning.

Microscopically, they are made up of cells that are quite reminiscent of those of the granular cell myoblastoma. They are large and granular though they show much greater disparity in size, shape and staining quality. The most outstanding feature of the microscopy is the grouping of the cells in aggregates surrounded by narrow

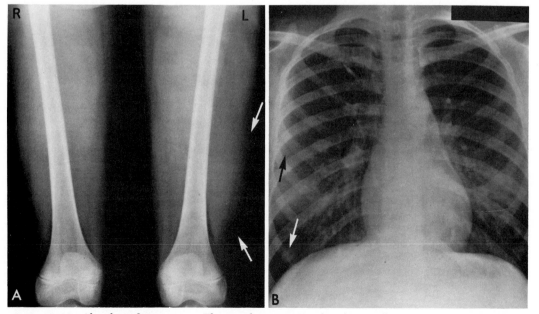

Figure 23-28   Alveolar soft part tumor. The neoplasm originated in the muscles of the left thigh (arrows, *A*). Approximately one year after diagnosis, pulmonary metastases appeared *(B)*.

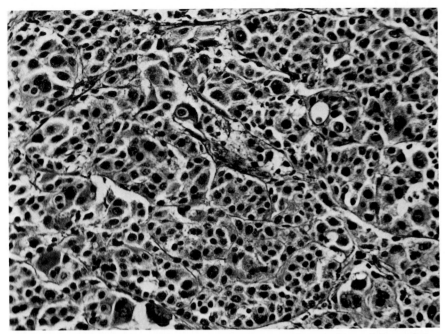

Figure 23–29 Alveolar soft part tumor. The cells are much more pleomorphic and the nuclei are more irregular and hyperchromatic than those of granular cell myoblastoma. The alveolar grouping by thin partitions is the most characteristic feature. (× 200.)

trabeculae of fibrous connective tissue (Fig. 23–29). This pattern has given rise to the term "alveolar" soft part tumor. The microscopist experiences the greatest difficulty in predicting the course this tumor will take. Some of the most innocent appearing will manifest the most malignant behavior.[13]

Epithelioid Sarcoma

In 1920, Enzinger[14] reported 62 cases of what he chooses to call "epithelioid sarcoma" because intermixed with the spindled sarcoma cells one finds what appear to be epithelial cancer cells. These tumors usually occur about the joints of the extremities, in his series more frequently in the arm and hand, but they may arise in aponeuroses and other sites where synovia does not normally exist. These are malignant tumors with a remarkable propensity for recurrence quite like that of synovioma. Indeed, many microscopists prefer to consider these a cellular subtype of synovioma and we feel there is consider-

able justification for this contention though there are insufficient data to confirm it.

Epithelioid sarcoma usually grows in nodules, the centers of which are frequently necrotic with an accompanying inflammatory reaction. These features frequently have led to the misdiagnosis of necrotizing granuloma. Often there are groups of cells with intensely eosin cytoplasm in an arrangement suggestive of squamous cell carcinoma. But there are always some spindled cells and these, plus the young age group, the site of involvement and the lack of a primary tumor, usually result in a correct diagnosis.

TUMORS OF MIXED TISSUE ORIGIN

Mesenchymoma

Stout reserves the term "mesenchymoma" for a tumor that is composed of malignant components of two or more me-

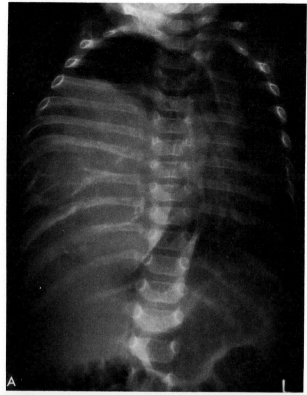

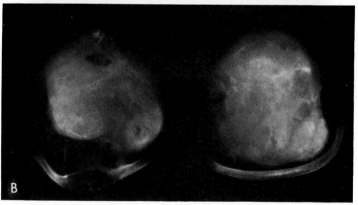

Figure 23–30 Mesenchymoma. (White male, 4 months of age.) This bulky tumor is primary in the soft tissues of the thorax. The ribs are secondarily involved. Calcification and ossification are present and are seen best in the radiograph of the resected specimen, B.

senchymal derivatives.[15] Because fibrosarcomatous elements are commonly found in liposarcoma, rhabdomyosarcoma, chondrosarcoma and osteosarcoma, the second element must consist of some other than fibrosarcoma in these types. Areas of osteosarcoma or chondrosarcoma may be encountered in rhabdomyosarcoma or liposarcoma and various other combinations have been reported. This tumor runs a malignant course consistent with the types of tumor that are involved. Only a few bona fide mesenchymomas have been reported and most of these have occurred in the large muscles of the buttock and lower extremity.

HAMARTOMAS OF SOFT PARTS

I. From the synovioblast
  Tenosynovial chondrometaplasia
II. From the lipoblast
  Lipoma
  Hibernoma
III. From the myoblast
  Rhabdomyoma
  Leiomyoma
IV. From the collagenoblast
  The desmoid, aggressive fibromatosis, etc.
  Juvenile aponeurotic fibroma
  Dupuytren's contracture and plantar fibromatosis
  The myxoma
V. From nerve supportive tissue
  Neurilemmoma
  Neurofibroma
VI. From vessel supportive tissue
  Hemangioma
  Hemangioendothelioma
  Hemangiopericytoma
VII. Miscellaneous
  Granular cell myoblastoma

TENOSYNOVIAL CHONDROMETAPLASIA

The synovial cells lining tendon sheaths may form cartilage just as does the synovial lining of joints (see p. 682). This condition is usually called osteochondromatosis, a name which is not only inappropriate but very confusing because that condition in which there are multiple osteochondromas should have this descriptive title. In examining microscopic sections of this lesion (Fig. 23–31) one gets the impression that there is a metaplasia of the tenosynovial cells into chondroblasts. We have suggested that the condition be called tenosynovial chondrometaplasia. Since no cause for this curious metaplasia has ever been demonstrated and since once started it appears to be self-propagating we place it among the hamartomas.

This process is the production of multiple nodules of innocuous cartilage in and within the tendon sheath. The cartilage masses vary in size from microscopic to over a centimeter in diameter. At times they lie within the wall of the sheath, covered by a layer of tenosynovial cells. At other times they are found as free bodies within the lumen of the sheath. As they age their centers mineralize and then they are radiopaque. Less frequently the centers ossify and then mineralize. This disease is almost entirely restricted to the periarticular tendons and so the radiogram reveals a shower of irregular opaque bodies in the soft tissues about the joint.

These chondroid masses usually cause no symptoms but sometimes they interfere with tendon function and cause pain. The surgeon usually encounters little difficulty in shelling them out but they may recur or because they are multicentric the "recurrence" may be the manifestation of a new lesion. The greatest danger associated with these lesions is their misinterpretation, usually by the microscopist. They are all too frequently misdiagnosed as chondrosarcoma. The uninitiated pathologist can hardly be blamed, because the proliferating chondroblasts may display every feature of malignant cartilage neoplasm. If those involved in making a diagnosis remember that chondrosarcoma arising in soft tissues and apart from normal cartilage is one of the rarest of all tumors, if it occurs at all (these writers have never encountered one), then the correct diagnosis is usually easy.

There are 29 cases of tenosynovial chondrometaplasia in our material. They most commonly occur in the latter half of life (over 40 years of age) and they are considerably more frequent in males. They are most often encountered in the soft tissues about the joints of the wrist and fingers, less frequently those of the ankle and foot, occasionally the knee. Several of our cases have recurred. None has undergone neoplastic alteration.

LIPOMA

The lipoma is a metabolic disturbance rather than a true neoplasm. In the extremities it is usually subcutaneous in location. It sometimes occurs within the mus-

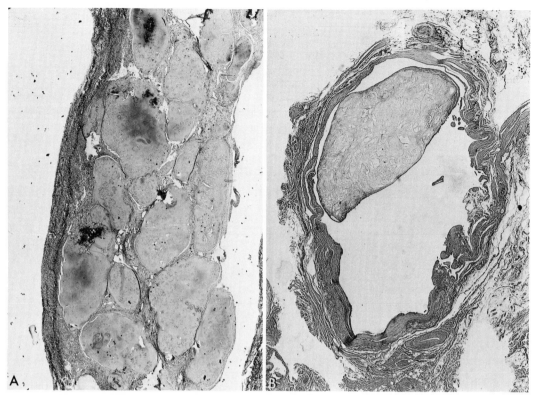

Figure 23–31   Tenosynovial chondrometaplasia. *A,* Low magnification (× 18) of a segment of tendon sheath (at left). Nodules of chondroid are clustered in the loose tissue of the inside layers of the sheath. *B,* A circular tendon sheath cut across to reveal a chondroid nodule within.

cles of the buttock. It produces a rounded, soft, poorly defined mass, which may grow to considerable proportions. Masses of several pounds were frequently reported before access to surgical clinics was attainable by all. The accumulations may be multiple (lipomatosis) and sometimes symmetric. Rarely they are painful.

The fat metabolism within the lipoma is governed by a different mechanism from that of normal fat depots. In the starvation state, fat may completely disappear from the usual storage depots and still the lipoma may continue to grow. This is the only aspect of the lesion that is similar to true neoplasm.

Most of the common lipomas consist merely of aggregates of adult fat cells with a rather scant trabeculated fibrous support (Fig. 23–32) and a capsule so thin and delicate that it may be difficult to follow surgically, particularly when the lipoma lies within normal fat tissue. Admixtures of other mesenchymal derivatives are rela-

tively common. When there is a considerable amount of proliferating fibrous tissue the lesion is sometimes designated a fibrolipoma, and when vascular channels are numerous it may be called angiolipoma. Often one can find fields in which embryonic fat cells predominate. Then the distinction between lipoma and well differentiated liposarcoma may depend upon lack of capsule, evidence of invasion and history of rapid growth.

HIBERNOMA

The hibernoma is a rare entity, usually occurring on the back or around the hips. It is thought by some to be a manifestation of a vestigial fat storage organ and comparable to the dorsal fat pads of hibernating animals. It has a striking microscopic appearance because it is made up of very large, polyhedral cells with a coarsely granular cytoplasm (Fig. 23–33).

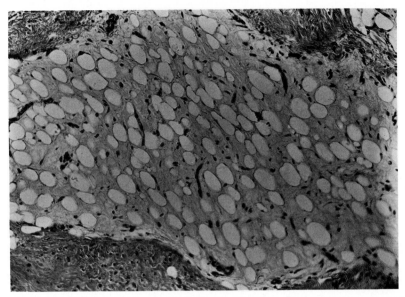

Figure 23–32 Lipoma. The lesion may consist entirely of mature fat cells. Some areas may contain numerous embryonic fat cells such as those seen here. They are smaller, the nuclei more central and the cytoplasm opaque. (× 130.)

RHABDOMYOMA

A few rhabdomyomas of the soft parts have been reported in the older literature.

This lesion does occur in the heart but most modern writers are of the feeling that the tumors reported in soft tissues must have been misdiagnosed. We have never encountered one in that location.

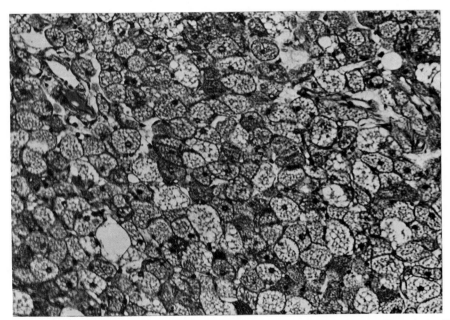

Figure 23–33 Hibernoma. The sections are composed of huge, coarsely vacuolated cells with small but central nuclei. (× 200.)

LEIOMYOMA

The leiomyoma is an unusual lesion in the soft parts of the extremities, though it may occur in the skin and rarely in the deeper tissues. Its most common sites, of course, are in the uterus and gastrointinal tract. In the deep tissues of the extremities the leiomyoma is apt to occur in a purer form than in other tissues where it is mixed with a rich component of fibrous connective tissue and then is frequently designated a fibroid. Most of the leiomyomas of the extremities probably arise from the muscle sheath of vessels, though their exact origins are usually impossible to determine.

By many pathologists the leiomyoma is classified as a hamartoma rather than a true neoplasm. There is much to be said for this reasoning because the proliferation of nonstriated muscle cells is usually not progressive; i.e., the mass reaches a certain size and then stops growing, and the muscle cells apparently become completely mature. It is slowly growing and, though probably not truly invasive, its margins are usually difficult to determine either by gross or microscopic examination. It is made up of bluntly terminating, extending, fusiform cells with long oval nuclei. It may be exceedingly difficult to differentiate these cells from those of a fibroblastic proliferation, but careful study usually makes the distinction. The cells of leiomyoma have a tendency to arrange themselves in parallel rows, a feature that is called palisading. This arrangement is characteristic of neurilemmoma and sometimes the distinction between these lesions is not easy. Leiomyomas arising from the muscle sheath of vessels often form numerous vascular sinuses in their substance. These may be so prominent that they are apt to be classified as true angiomas. A Mallory stain for collagen may be of great help. A leiomyoma in an extremity usually takes very little of the blue color whereas the other tumor types that produce more collagen may stain predominantly blue.

It is important to note the number of mitotic figures in a leiomyoma. If there are more than one to the field, one may be dealing with a leiomyosarcoma. Both lesions, however, are rarities in the soft parts. The diagnosis should be made only after the fibromatoses group and neurofibroma have been ruled out with certainty. We have never encountered a lesion which we were certain was a leiomyoma of the soft parts.

DESMOID

The desmoid was originally defined as a fibrosis of the rectus abdominal muscles, usually following pregnancy. More recently it has come to mean in many clinics a progressive fibroblastic proliferation in the striated muscle of any part of the body and sometimes the same process occurring in periosteum. This proliferation progresses slowly, microscopic fingers of cells insinuating themselves between muscle bundles and fibers. This gives the lesion the appearance of invasion. In reality, this appears to be less a matter of invasion than a spreading of the agent that stimulates collagenoblasts to overgrowth. In resecting the lesion it is difficult to make sure that all the offending tissue has been removed. Recurrent growth apparently springs from the remaining tags. Thus the lesion is characterized by slow growth, progression and recurrence. If inadequately treated over a long period it may eventually destroy large areas of normal tissue or, gaining access to the trunk, surround and even infiltrate parenchymal organs. One such lesion beginning near the inner surface of the ischium in an adolescent female penetrated into the pelvic interior and infiltrated the bladder wall and distal ureter. Eventually, in order to control the process, it was necessary to do a hemipelvectomy. After the process was entirely removed the patient recovered and is now completely without sign or symptom of the disease 17 years later. We know of two other such cases. All were in young women. Two followed pregnancy.

The insidious thing about the desmoid is the benign appearance of its cells (Fig. 23–34). In the early stages the lesion is relatively acellular, the nuclei are mature in appearance and considerable amounts of collagen are produced. The microscopist concludes that he is dealing with prolif-

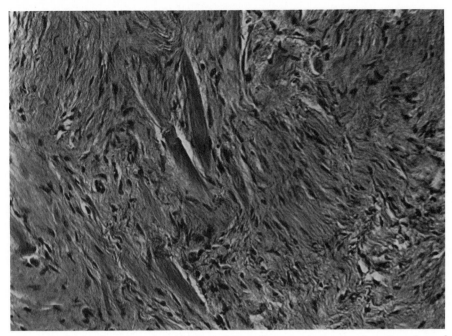

Figure 23–34 The desmoid is relatively acellular and the cells are quite mature. Invasion of muscle is quite characteristic. (× 200.)

erating scar tissue following an injury or, if he is more concerned because of the clinical findings, he may suspect he has been given an area of collagenous reaction at the periphery of a more serious lesion. Sometimes it may take repeated biopsies to convince him that the innocent appearing cells in his sections constitute an invasive lesion. Blocks carefully taken from the periphery of the process usually reveal evidence of this invasion, and this feature alone may be the only clue to the exact nature of the disease. If a reasonably early diagnosis is made and the lesion completely excised, a cure is certain. Desmoids never metastasize.

There is certainly a relationship between the desmoid and the process called aggressive fibromatosis. Usually they cannot be distinguished on the basis of their microscopic anatomy.

AGGRESSIVE FIBROMATOSIS

This rather unusual lesion has a number of names: extra-abdominal desmoid, fibromatosis, aggressive fibromatosis, invasive fibroma and well differentiated fibrosar-

coma. A consideration of its terminology reflects a fairly accurate concept of this fascinating process. Examination of microscopic sections of this lesion show them to be identical with the abdominal desmoid of the older literature. Since several have been reported arising in surgical scars[16] they are apparently closely related to the keloid. These lesions are not rare. They appear somewhat more often in males than females, the great majority of them in the second and third decades. They involve aponeuroses and like fibrositis ossificans they involve the supportive tissues of muscles; unlike that lesion, however, they do not produce cartilage or bone. A very similar lesion is the juvenile aponeurotic fibroma or calcifying aponeurotic fibroma except this lesion has a remarkable propensity for producing chondroid, which usually mineralizes.

It becomes apparent as we analyze this group of lesions that all of them are constituted of a proliferation of collagenoblastic cells of supportive tissue, usually of muscle, fascias, aponeuroses and subcutaneous tissues. Some are completely idiopathic, such as the aggressive fibromatoses; others appear to rely upon some type of injury, traumatic or otherwise, to the normal tissues wherein they arise, i.e., the desmoid, the keloid, nodular fasciitis and usually fibrositis ossificans. The former group, because they are completely idiopathic, we tend to relegate to the hamartomas. The latter group we classify as reactions to injury. Neither category helps much to explain their existence but it keeps them from being classified as neoplasms which they certainly are not.

Aggressive fibromatosis is most commonly encountered in the muscles of the thigh and those about the shoulder. The lesion is often large and infiltrative. In about half the cases one can elicit a history of trauma which may be significant. When the lesion is sectioned grossly it usually gives the appearance and consistency of scar tissue – firm, homogeneous, white and glistening. Through the microscope one finds that it is composed of rather mature spindled cells producing considerable amounts of collagen. In some areas the latter may be myxomatous. The nuclei are not heavily chromatized and mitotic figures are scarce, even rare. One has the impression that he is looking at a rather florid growth of scar tissue (Fig. 23–35).

The most characteristic feature of aggressive fibromatosis is, as its name implies, its capacity to infiltrate the tissues in which it arises. This probably explains its other feature – the ability to recur after excision. It may recur repeatedly, each time reducing the distance between itself and the vital organs of the trunk. In a few instances it has become necessary eventually to amputate the affected extremity. Early recognition and wide resection is the treatment of choice. It has been noted that the propensity for recurrence is greater the younger the patient. In middle aged patients a simple resection is usually adequate.

APONEUROTIC FIBROMA

This lesion has been called juvenile aponeurotic fibroma because it usually, though not always, occurs in children. It has been called calcifying aponeurotic fibroma because it often produces small, irregular masses of chondroid which usually mineralize. Its commonest site of occurrence is in the ligaments of the wrists and hands.[18] It may be seen in the plantar aspects of the feet and a sporadic few have been scattered throughout the aponeurotic tissues of the body. Its stromal cells are strikingly similar to those of the other fibromatoses, masses of spindled cells, often oriented in the same directions, producing a considerable amount of collagen (Fig. 23–36). Nuclei are regular in profile and lightly chromatized. Mitotic figures are uncommon. In places, the cells are apt to become more plump; they then begin to resemble chondroblasts. This resemblance is not fortuitous since one can usually find small irregular masses of chondroid scattered through the lesion. Often this chondroid mineralizes, causing a stippled appearance on the radiogram. This lesion, like aggressive fibromatosis, is apt to recur but since it appears to grow more slowly and is more localized it is more amenable to simple surgical removal.

DUPUYTREN'S CONTRACTURE AND PLANTAR FIBROMATOSIS

In several regions of the body in which normal fibrous connective tissue exists in considerable amounts, the fibroblasts, apparently spontaneously, begin to proliferate to form hard, bulky masses of collagenous tissue that interfere with the function of the part involved. These may occur in certain muscle groups such as those of the neck where they cause fibromatosis colli or congenital wryneck. Or they may be more diffusely scattered throughout several groups – progressive myositis fibrosa. They may develop in the supportive structure of parenchymal tissues as in penile fibromatosis (Peyronie's disease). The most important group involves the fasciae of the hands (palmar fibromatosis or Dupuytren's contracture) and the feet (plantar fibromatosis). As masses of connective tissue form and mature, considerable amounts of collagen are formed. Moving tendons become adherent and fixed. As the collagenous tissue ages it shrinks just as scar tissue does anywhere in the body, and the resulting contraction

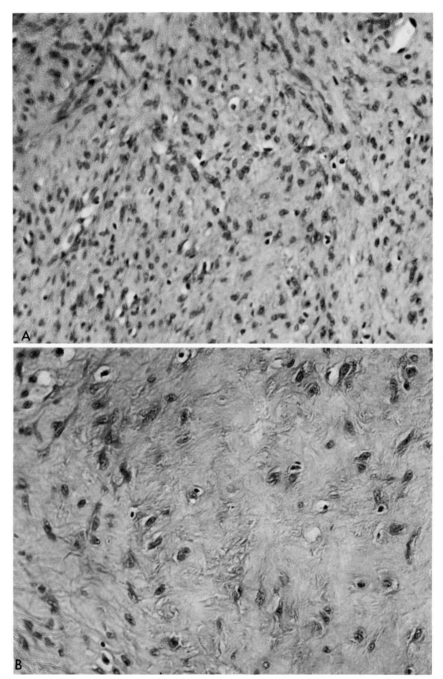

Figure 23–35   Aggressive fibromatosis. *A*, Aggregates of collagen producing spindled cells. The lesion resembles scar tissue. *B*, At times the collagen dominates the lesion. This does not necessarily denote lack of aggressiveness. (× 230.)

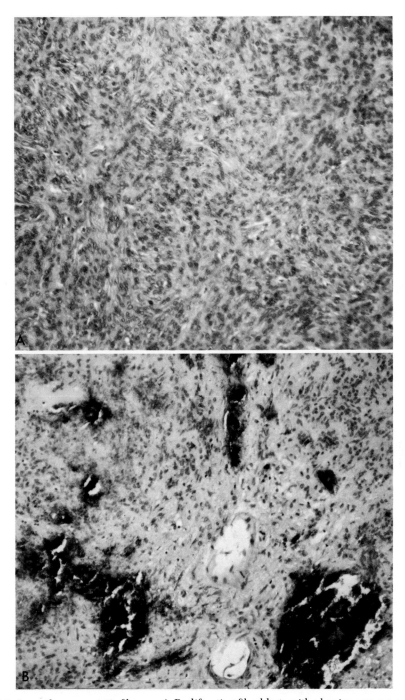

Figure 23-36 Juvenile aponeurotic fibroma. *A*, Proliferating fibroblasts with a benign appearance. *B*, Irregular masses of chondroid are formed, which then mineralize. (× 180.)

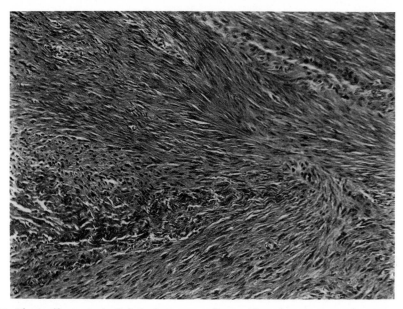

Figure 23–37 Plantar fibromatosis. Relatively mature collagenoblasts form a more or less organized pattern of trabeculae. (× 120.)

deforms the part and further inhibits function. Eventually, the corium of the overlying skin is involved. The result is a crippled, useless hand or foot. The exuberant growth may recur after removal. Because of the appearance of this tumorlike mass (Fig. 23–37), the appearance of invasion and the propensity for recurrence, these lesions are frequently misdiagnosed fibrosarcoma. Making the distinction between a well differentiated fibrosarcoma and a fibromatosis in the proliferative stage is by no means an easy task. Metastasizing neoplasms do arise in the fascias of the hands and feet but they are rare and usually their microscopic features are florid enough to betray their identity.

In the past, x-ray therapy has been given for these lesions occurring in the palms and soles. It is now realized that this type of treatment has little to recommend it. The problem is one for a good hand surgeon though in the early stage a fasciotomy in the case of Dupuytren's contracture may be effective, at least for a time.

MYXOMA AND MYXOSARCOMA

These terms have led to great confusion throughout the entire spectrum of connec-

tive tissue neoplasms. Originally, it was supposed that these tumors arose from something called the "myxoblast," a cell which was said to derive primarily from the cells of Wharton's jelly. For decades it has been known that the primitive fibroblast is multipotent. Depending upon environmental factors and functional need it can synthesize collagen, chondroid or osteoid and thus join the ranks of those cells so designated. However, many writers today have adopted the idea that these early cells are also motile and phagocytic and have suggested the title of "facultative histiocytes." All this seems rather academic to us who, for years, have believed that the fibroblast and histiocyte, in many sites and under many conditions, are interchangeable forms of the same cell. Moreover, under certain endocrine and possibly environmental influences these cells may become lipoblasts. These early cells when laden with phagocytized lipid or mucopolysaccharides, etc. were thought to represent a special cell line and were named "myxoblasts." When the metabolic routine of these cells is altered by reaction or neoplastic change, they produce a myxomatous or mucoid ground substance. Early pathologists insisted on a distinction — "myxomatous" if produced by mesenchymal cells, "mucoid" if by cells of epithelial origin, the distinction dictated by the reaction to certain stains. Today, providently, most of this rigamarole has been forgotten but we still place the myxomatous reactions and tumors in a special category. The myxomatous fibromatoses are called myxomas and the myxomatous lipomas and fibrosarcomas are called myxosarcomas, histiocytomas and malignant xanthofibromas. It is time we adopt a simpler and more modern terminology.

NEURILEMMOMA

A proliferation of cells that cover the myelin sheath produces a small mass attached to the nerve. It is usually encapsulated by a distended nerve sheath. The cells grow in palisaded groups of spindled cells (the Antoni type A) or as a patternless array of stellate forms in a clear, acellular substance (Antoni type B), doubltless representing myxomatous alteration. For illustration see Figure 6–101. In the former,

short rows of palisaded nuclei may oppose each other forming a vaguely delineated area called a Verocay body. The lesion probably never becomes malignant except perhaps in neurofibromatosis.

NEUROFIBROMA

The term "neurofibroma" is usually applied to the nodular growths along the course of peripheral nerves in neurofibromatosis. They are poorly delineated and usually the edges merge into the surrounding fibrous tissues. Because they are nonprogressive it is doubtful if they can be considered true tumors. It is probable that they are aberrations of growth with a hereditary background. Occasionally a solitary lesion may be encountered.

HEMANGIOMA

Hemangiomas occur in practically every body tissue. They are fairly common in

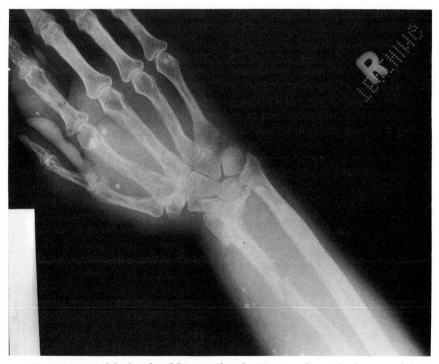

Figure 23–38 Hemangioma of the hand and forearm, female, 36 years of age. The lesion is characterized by a deep soft tissue mass that has resulted in changes in the contour of the bones by extrinsic pressure. Multiple phleboliths are present. There is a fracture of the radius.

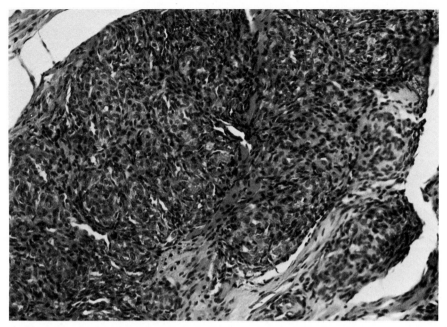

Figure 23–39   Benign hemangioendothelioma. Poorly delineated channels are surrounded by cells of endothelial origin. The cellularity of this lesion frequently leads to the mistaken diagnosis of malignant tumor. (× 250.)

the skeletal muscles. The vessels are distinctly formed and, depending upon the size of the lumina, they are called cavernous hemangiomas or capillary hemangiomas. They are congenital hamartomas because they grow in proportion to the structure they involve. A birthmark on the face grows during childhood and adolescence but at maturity, if it persists, it usually occupies about the same proportion of the face surface as it did at birth. The great majority of hemangiomas of the skin that appear during the first two years of life regress spontaneously before the seventh year. Occasionally growth is excessive and these hamartomas produce a vermiform mass of tangled blood channels, which may have an ominous appearance. In rare instances the hemangioma may develop into a hemangiosarcoma. Arteriovenous fistulas and hemangiomas are commonly encountered in the gastrocnemius muscle. Occasionally they grow to immense proportion and constitute a challenge to the technical ability of the surgeon in accomplishing their removal.

The microscopy of cavernous hemangioma makes diagnosis simple. The hamartoma is composed of masses of thin walled vascular channels, usually filled with blood. Rarely one needs to rule out vermiform varicosities, arteriovenous fistula or conceivably telangiectasis. The capillary and cellular endothelial types may be more difficult. Here one must not mistake reparative granulation or granuloma pyogenicum for hemangioma. More seriously, the benign hemangioendothelioma, juvenile hemangioma or hemangioma cellulare (Fig. 23–39) may be mistaken for a hemangiosarcoma. Though this lesion is quite cellular and the vascular channels poorly delineated, nevertheless the vascular pattern is still discernible and the cells are nonmalignant in appearance.

SCLEROSING HEMANGIOMA

When the proliferating component of the vessel is the collagen forming supportive tissue the lesion consists of a poorly delineated, highly vascularized mass that is usually difficult to differentiate from young scar tissue, healing granulation or, if it contains lipid-laden histiocytes, a xanthoma. They are innocuous lesions, important largely because they may be overdiagnosed.

HEMANGIOENDOTHELIOMA

If the proliferation is restricted to the endothelial lining cells in these vessel lesions, the result is a rather solid mass of large cells traversed by narrow blood channels about which the cells are arranged (Fig. 23–39). The pattern may not be obvious and because the cells resemble a number of the reticulum derivatives—serosal cells, synovial cells, histiocytes, epithelioid cells—the lesion is easy to misdiagnose on examination of microscopic sections. This benign hamartomatous form of hemangioendothelioma must not be confused with the malignant tumor (see p. 744). The hemangioendothelioma is a rare tumor occurring most commonly in young children. It is diagnosed much more often than it occurs. Several lymphangiosarcomas caused by a neoplastic proliferation of the endothelial lining of lymphatic channels of the arm, following interference with lymph drainage by radical mastectomy, have been described.

HEMANGIOPERICYTOMA

Stout has described a tumor that apparently arises from the Rouget cell or pericytes of Zimmermann. These are elongated cells that are obliquely wrapped about the capillaries outside the basement membrane. They are modified muscle cells.

They produce hamartomatous masses composed of spindled cells with a rich vessel network (Fig. 23–40). The nuclei are usually quite uniform and the sections may resemble those of a rather cellular, young fibrosarcoma. Sometimes they are arranged in rosette fashion about a vascular lumen. The hemangiopericytoma is related to the glomus tumor but it has no neve elements like the latter.

The behavior of these lesions has not been unequivocally established. Some writers contend that a few hemangiopericytomas have described a malignant course. Others insist that these were not bona fide hemangiopericytomas. We have

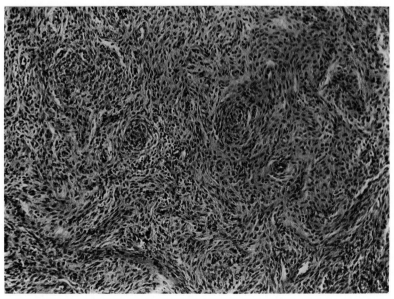

Figure 23–40   Hemangiopericytoma. Spindled cells grow in a perivascular pattern. With special stains the cells are found to be outside the endothelial basement membrane. (× 120.)

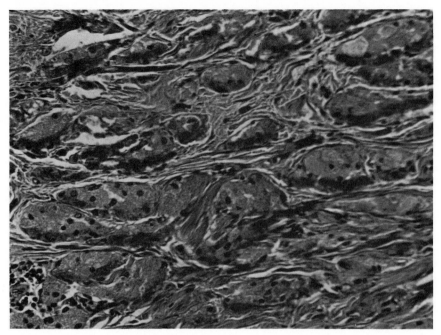

Figure 23–41   Granular cell myoblastoma. The cells are large, the nuclei relatively small and central, the cytoplasm granular. The cells are grouped in alveoli. (× 200.)

never encountered a member of this group that has shown malignant behavior.

GRANULAR CELL MYOBLASTOMA

This peculiar entity is uncommon but not rare. It has been reported in most tissues of the body but about one half develop in relation to striated muscle. Because of this relationship and the fact that the cells of which it is composed have a resemblance to the cross section of a young muscle fiber, it is said to be derived from the myoblast, hence the name. Actually, many granular cell myoblastomas are found in tissues where no normal muscle components exist, and embryologists claim that its cells do not resemble the rhabdomyoblast. Fust and Custer[19] analyzed a large number of these lesions and believed that all or most arose in the supportive cells of peripheral nerve filaments. This concept of cell origin is the one most widely supported today.

The lesion grows slowly to form a small encapsulated mass, usually not greater than a centimeter in diameter. Though it may occur in almost any of the soft tissues, about one third occur in the extremities, one third in the trunk, neck and head and one third in the tongue. Several have been reported recently in the vulva. They may be present for a year or much longer before they are brought to the attention of the physician.

Seen through the microscope they present uniformly similar fields of very large, polyhedral cells with relatively small nuclei. The cytoplasm is filled with rather coarse, moderately eosinophilic granules, which give the tissue its outstanding characteristic (Fig. 23–41). The lesion, at least in this form, never demonstrates a malignant behavior.

REACTIVE LESIONS OF SOFT PARTS

I. From the synovioblast
   Villonodular tenosynovitis
   Ganglion
   Tumoral calcinosis
   Calcinosis circumscripta
II. From the lipoblast
   Fat necrosis
III. From the myoblast
   Proliferative myositis
IV. From the collagenoblast
   The keloid
   Nodular fasciitis
   Fibrous histiocytomas, xanthomas, etc.
V. From nerve supportive tissue
   Post-traumatic neuroma
VI. From vessel supportive tissue
   Granuloma pyogenicum
VII. From muscle supportive tissue
   Fibrositis ossificans

CHRONIC TENOSYNOVITIS (VILLONODULAR TENOSYNOVITIS, GIANT CELL TUMOR OF TENDON, BENIGN SYNOVIOMA)

This curious lesion is not a neoplasm. In many instances it appears to be the final outcome of an idiopathic synovitis. It has been called giant cell tumor of tendon, tendon xanthoma, tendon fibroma and sclerosing hemangioma. It probably originates as a pigmented villonodular tenosynovitis, and then by an exaggerated proliferation of synovia-derived cells produces a solid tumorlike mass. In the tendon sheaths there is less evidence that it begins as a synovitis but we have found a few instances of the lesion in the frankly inflammatory stage. In some instances the lesion probably exhibits the proliferative phase from the outset.

Chronic villonodular tenosynovitis is a very common lesion in the periarticular soft tissues. It occurs much less frequently in the joint synovia, usually in the knee and less often the hip. It is somewhat more common in females. It grows slowly, reaching a size of 0.5 to 2 or 3 cm., and occurs most commonly in the hands. When it rests against cortical bone it may cause erosion of the latter (Fig. 23–42), sometimes arousing the suspicion of malignant tumor. It has a tendency to recur after local excision[20] probably because ramifications of the process are left behind.

When chronic synovitis occurs within a large joint it may produce a bulky mass that gives the surgeon the impression that he is dealing with a sarcoma. If the biopsy material is unusually active and cellular, the pathologist also may overdiagnose the lesion. The tissue mass may break through the articular plate and invade the meta-

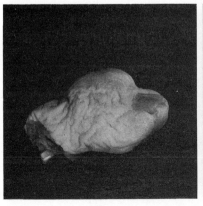
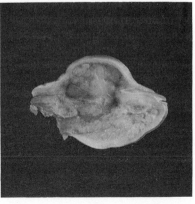

A   **B**

Figure 23–42   *A,* Chronic villonodular tenosynovitis on the dorsal aspect of an amputated finger. *B,* Sagittal section illustrating the well defined borders and erosion of the phalanx from without.

physis, and in rare instances no perforation can be found, suggesting that the metaphyseal tissues are subject to the same proliferating stimulus as the synovia. Symptomless metaphyseal lesions have been discovered accompanying chronic tenosynovitis in tendons, suggesting that this association may be more common than we have suspected. If such is the case, because the histologic appearance of chronic synovitis and the more innocuous variety of what has been called benign giant cell tumor may be identical, it is quite certain that we have included this non-neoplastic entity in some of our series of giant cell tumors.

The term benign synovioma is an unfortunate one because it confuses this relatively innocent lesion with true synovioma, a highly malignant tumor. The only thing these lesions have in common is the genesis of the cells of which they are composed and, therefore, they are no more closely related than pulmonary tuberculosis and bronchogenic carcinoma.

We analyzed a series of 144 cases. Nearly nine tenths of them were located in the hand, usually the fingers. Twenty-four were found in the knee. The ages varied from 11 to 72 years. The incidence was twice as great in females as males. One lesion was located in the ankle and recurred three times, causing considerable soft tissue destruction before it was controlled.

The cause of chronic villonodular synovitis is unknown. Because at least some of the lesions are known to undergo transition from the inflammatory phase to the proliferative, "tumor" phase (we have seen progression of one lesion into the other in a case with repeated biopsies), it appears to be a proliferative reaction to some inflammatory or possibly antigenic agent. Reaction to intercellular hemorrhage has been an attractive hypothesis because the cellular constituents include giant and xanthoid cells, and hemosiderin is often a prominent feature, all of which factors are caused by extravasated blood. But the lesion is not common in hemophiliacs who commonly bleed into their joints, and some experimenters have been unable to produce the lesion in animals by injections of blood or blood and cholesterol. Recently it has been suggested that the hemosiderin or one of its breakdown products may become antigenic and establish an allergic inflammatory reaction. The process is not a part of systemic xanthoma-

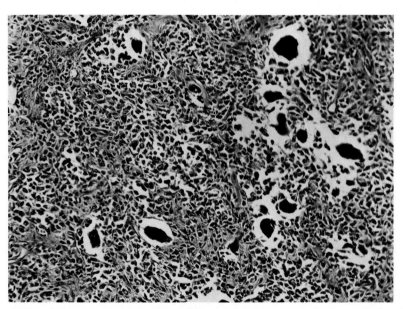

Figure 23–43 Villonodular tenosynovitis. The cellular matrix is composed of spindled and polyhedral synovial cells. The giant cells are found in spaces. This lesion is often confused with the giant cell tumor of bone, particularly when it occurs within the metaphysis. (× 130.)

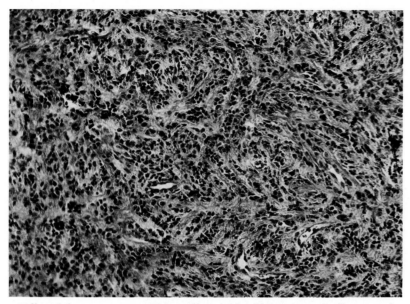

Figure 23–44 Villonodular tenosynovitis. Eventually considerable amounts of collagen are formed, replacing both matrix cells and giant cells. One must use care in differentiating this form from the Class III osteosarcoma. Spaces may be formed in either type, suggesting the possibility of malignant synovioma. (× 130.)

tosis and hypercholesterolemia has not been reported in a fairly large number of cases in which it has been looked for.

Morbid Anatomy. Grossly the lesion as it occurs in relation to tendons is rarely large, seldom achieving a diameter greater than 3 cm. It is usually brown, reddish brown or yellow, the color contributed by the hemosiderin and cholesterol ester. It is usually ovoid and often definitely encapsulated with a smooth surface. Sometimes projections extend from the main mass and dissect between nearby tendons, thus accounting for an unexcised residuum that may later give rise to recurrence.

When sections are viewed through the microscope the lesion is seen to consist of masses of spindled, cylindrical or less frequently polyhedral cells. Slit spaces and irregular channels are found in the younger lesions, suggesting the synovial origin of its cells (Fig. 23–43). In many of the spaces giant cells are seen. These vary considerably in size but usually they are not large and do not contain more than 10 or 12 nuclei. They appear to be the product of the cells that line the spaces. As the process ages a network of collagen bands is found, dividing the stromal cells into irregular fields. One gets the impression in

looking at large numbers of these lesions that sclerosis progresses as the lesion ages (Fig. 23–44). Eventually it becomes a mass composed larely of collagen and scattered spindle cells. The xanthoid cells and hemosiderin granules are usually more prominent in the younger lesions.

Alteration of this apparently reactive lesion to malignant neoplasm (synovioma) has never been proven. Though the presence of giant cells in the sections is strong evidence that the lesion is not a synovioma, this finding is not absolutely dependable. There are a variety of histologic types of synovioma and one of the rarest of these may exhibit occasional giant cells. When such is encountered the morphology of the stromal cells can usually be depended upon to make the distinction.

THE GANGLION

The ganglion has been described in Chapter 21 (see p. 681). It is believed by many to represent the end stage of a proliferation of mesenchymal cells that have elaborated a myxomatous material and eventually become cystic. This concept has arisen from the fact that usually no communication can be found between the ganglion lumen and the joint or tendon sheath cavity. Such communications have been described, however, and it is entirely possible that both modes may be correct.

A synovial lining often can be found lining parts of the cavity. Just as often a granulomatous inflammatory reaction is encountered. It is important to recognize that this reaction is not infectious in nature.

TUMORAL CALCINOSIS

A rare condition in which calcium salts are deposited in localized[21] masses in the collagenous tissue about joints has been called tumoral calcinosis.[22] It appears to be an entity apart from calcinosis universalis, in which there is generalized calcification of skin, subcutaneous tissues and muscles in children, and calcinosis circumscripta, a

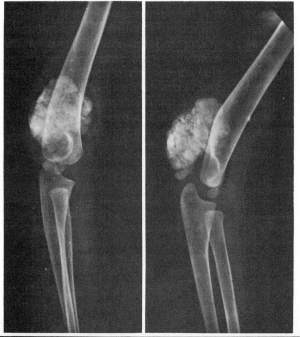

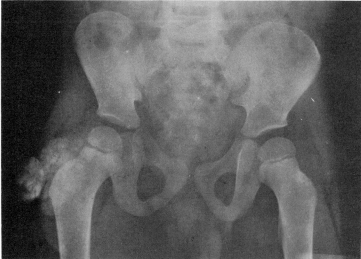

Figure 23–45 Tumoral calcinosis. Well circumscribed, irregularly opaque masses are evident in relation to the elbow and hip joints. A soft tissue component cannot be identified. The bones of the elbow are undermineralized. (Courtesy of Dr. J. W. Hope, Philadelphia.)

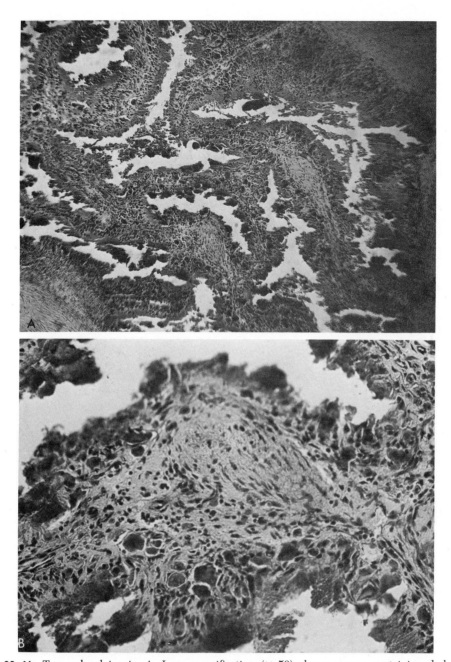

Figure 23–46   Tumoral calcinosis. *A*, Low magnification (× 50) shows spaces containing dark staining amorphous calcium salts surrounded by collagenized tissue. *B*, Higher magnification (× 250) reveals the giant cell reaction surrounding the calcium deposits. (Courtesy of Dr. William Yakovac.)

less severe type in adults in which localized deposits of calcium are associated with Raynaud's phenomenon or scleroderma.

Tumor calcinosis usually first manifests itself in childhood or adolescence. Firm, tumorlike masses develop in the soft tissues about joints, particularly the large joints. The shoulders are most often involved, then the elbows and then the hips. The masses are usually painless and interfere with function only if they develop to large size. They have been recorded up to 20 cm. in diameter.

The surgeon finds an encapsulated, cystic mass embedded in the collagenous tissues in the vicinity of the joint. The cavity of the cyst may contain a fluid or semifluid content of calcium salts. When sectioned, the lesion is found to consist predominantly of masses of amorphous, powdery calcium salts in which are embedded crystals of the mineral. In one case examined by us these crystals were ovoid and vaguely resembled the ova of parasites. There is a striking giant cell reaction about these deposits (Fig. 23–46) forming a scalloped and convoluted border. About this there is a lymphocytic infiltration and fibrous proliferation.

Baldursson et al.[23] reported a family of four siblings. All had high levels of serum phosphate, a feature which had been noted previously. They believe that the pathogenesis is related to a genetic error in phosphorus metabolism and is not related to vitamin D toxicity, the milk alkali syndrome or renal osteodystrophy. They reviewed the world literature since 1899, finding 35 cases.

Prognosis. If a solitary lesion of tumoral calcinosis is discovered one can expect that other lesions will develop in other joints as the patient ages. In a few severely involved cases many joints eventually became involved over many years with eventual distortion of the limbs and crippling of the patient. Only those lesions that cause disfigurement or limitation of function should be excised because they are quite apt to recur.

CALCINOSIS CIRCUMSCRIPTA

This condition is apparently a completely different entity from the one described above. In this condition there are multiple focal, cutaneous, allergic, inflammatory lesions that for some reason undergo calcification. It is apparently a part of the more disseminated diseases of scleroderma and Raynaud's phenomenon.

FAT NECROSIS

Focal areas of fat necrosis occasionally occur in the subcutaneous tissue and rarely deeper. A poorly defined nodule is formed that is usually firmer than the surrounding structures. It is usually reddish brown, sometimes gray. When sectioned, the lesion is found to be composed of a fibroblastic proliferation, often with an exudative inflammatory reaction.

Sometimes the proliferating cells elaborate a myxomatous ground substance. These lesions may be difficult to differentiate from myxomatous lipomas or even liposarcomas. They frequently calcify. Lipid-bearing histiocytes are usual; sometimes there are multinucleated giant cells. Pointed cleft spaces may testify to the presence of extracellular cholesterol esters. The lesion is usually precipitated by local trauma.

PROLIFERATIVE MYOSITIS

Another mesenchymal reactive process or a variation of the ones discussed above has been described by Kern[24] and again by Enzinger.[25] There is considerable doubt in the minds of many whether this lesion represents a separate and specific entity or whether it is a variety of intramuscular nodular fasciitis, myxomatous fibromatosis (intramuscular myxoma) or even a myxomatous fibrositis ossificans. These lesions have always involved muscle and are seen mostly in the latter half of life. A history of trauma is probably significant. The lesion usually has a short history, grows rapidly and is infiltrative. Sections reveal a myxomatous ground substance in which are imbedded rather mature spindled cells, apparently young fibrocytes. In addition one should find larger cells that are said to resemble myoblasts (Fig. 23–47). A plentiful number of mitoses is an index of the growth rate but does not mean malignant neoplasm for there is no account of a metastasis. Conservative resection is said to be the treatment of choice.

THE KELOID

The keloid is a curious proliferation of scar tissue whose pathogenesis has aroused considerable debate. Its growth is stimulated by trauma, accidental or ia-

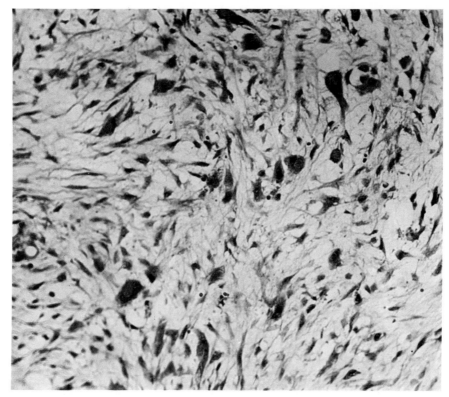

Figure 23–47 Proliferative myositis. There is a myxomatous ground substance in which are imbedded fibroblasts among which are large racquet forms resembling myoblasts. (× 220.)

trogenic, and it produces nodular masses of dense collagenous tissue far in excess of the physiologic amount. It has been called the nightmare of the plastic surgeon. It is more common and more florid in those with dark skin and tends to recur when removed. It occurs more often in women. It has been suggested that the excessive proliferation is in fact a foreign body reaction to inconspicuous agents such as hair, keratin debris, dust, etc. If this be true it is difficult to explain its hereditary and racial pattern and the high incidence following burns.

NODULAR FASCIITIS (PSEUDOSARCOMATOUS FASCIITIS)

This curious lesion was mentioned in numerous reports and seminars in the decade before a definitive name and description was supplied by Konwaler et al. in 1955.[26] The lesion is essentially a reactive proliferation of fibroblasts, which occurs almost always in the subcutaneous fat, usually in association with fascia. A history of trauma can be elicited in a high proportion of the cases and because extravasated blood is commonly found in sections of the lesion, it may be a peculiar reaction to hemorrhage.

The lesion is nodular, rarely measuring more than 2 cm. in diameter. The skin is usually movable over it and it is often tender. More than one half occur about the upper arm and shoulder area. Others are found on the volar aspect of the forearm. They appear suddenly and grow rapidly. The history is usually not longer than three weeks.

Because the cellular proliferation is so florid the most important aspect concerning pseudosarcomatous fasciitis is the danger that it may be diagnosed as malignant neoplasm. It has frequently been mistaken for fibrosarcoma, angiosarcoma or

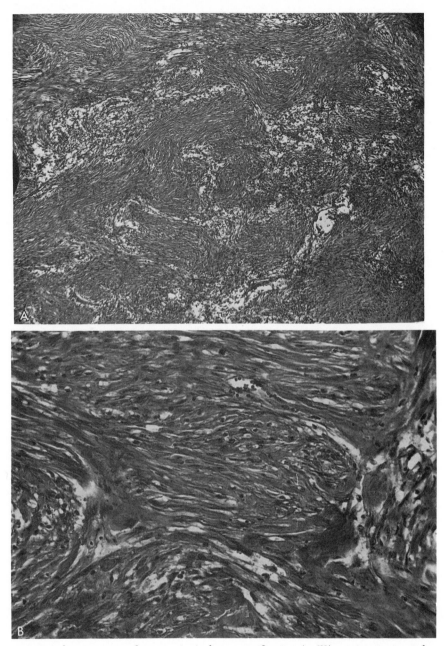

Figure 23–48 Pseudosarcomatous fasciitis. *A*, At low magnification (× 50) one appreciates the pattern of whorls of proliferating spindled cells about vascular channels. *B*, At higher magnification (× 250) the character of the cells can be seen.

liposarcoma.[27] The lesion is composed of a very cellular mass of fibroblasts in a highly vascular matrix (Fig. 23–48). The profusion of young, rapidly growing cells suggests fibrosarcoma. When the vessels predominate the lesion may suggest the possibility of hemangiosarcoma. At the edges where the cells appear to be invading fat the lesion may be mistaken for a liposarcoma.

Nodular fasciitis is quite common. It is best treated by simple excision but it may recur, in which case, if the pathologist has had misgivings about his original diagnosis he may yield to clinical persuasion to call it cancer.

FIBROUS HISTIOCYTOMAS, XANTHOMAS

Just as the young fibroblast may elaborate an abnormal intercellular material, myxomatous ground substance, instead of normal collagen, it may also, like the histiocyte, have the capacity to phagocytize particulate matter such as hemosiderin and globules of lipid. The latter is usually cholesterol and cholesterol esters. These lipoid materials appear as vacuoles within the cytoplasm. When the vacuoles are numerous they produce what is known as a foam cell. The cell may become overstuffed, die and disintegrate. The concentration of lipids thus produced in collagenous tissue causes a "foreign body" reaction. Very young fibroblasts (histiocytes) join together (or undergo replication without cytoplasmic separation) to form multinucleated giant cells. Sometimes the nuclei arrange themselves in a rosette in the center of the cell. This cell is usually called a Touton giant cell. The proliferating fibroblasts sometimes form an arresting pattern of multiple small whorls. This arrangement has been named the storiform pattern.

Combinations of these features—proliferating fibroblasts sometimes in a storiform pattern, foam cells (histiocytes), ordinary giant cells and Teuton giant cells—occur in a number of lesions in the presence of a "foreign body" lipid. When they occur as an expression of a systemic disease such as diabetes or hypercholesterolosis they are called xanthomas. When they appear in the corium of the skin and subcutaneous tissues as the reaction to some idiopathic trauma they are usually called fibrous histiocytomas. In rare instances the true neoplasm, fibrosarcoma, may be for some reason associated with the presence of lipids. Much the same features appear in the sections of these lesions but the stromal cells are apt to be pleomorphic and other features of malignant neoplasm may be obvious. These tumors have been called malignant fibrous histiocytomas.

There is much disagreement among writers in this particular field of oncology. Though the above account may be oversimplified, it probably approaches accuracy as nearly as the other explanations now in fashion, and, moreover, it has the advantage of being rational.

NEUROMA

The term neuroma or post-traumatic or postoperative neuroma is now commonly used to designate the nodule of tissue that grows out from the proximal end of a nerve that has been severed by accident or surgery. It may be painful. It consists of a tangled mass of Schwann cells attempting to form sheaths for the growing nerve fibrils and the collagenic supportive cells. In cross section multiple tiny circles are found in which one can sometimes locate the nerve processes (Fig. 23–49). The lesion is non-neoplastic and warrants surgical intervention only when painful.

GRANULOMA PYOGENICUM

This curious lesion usually occurs in the corium and subcutaneous tissues; therefore, it most often claims the attention of the dermatologist rather than the pathologist. The name is misleading because it is in no sense a granuloma but rather a mass of granulation tissue (or capillary hemangioma) covered by epidermis and elevated above the skin surface. Whether it is a vascular reaction to injury or a hamartomatous angioma cannot be stated at this time. Because it eventually ulcerates and develops an inflammatory reaction it is classified here with the reactions.

FIBROSITIS (MYOSITIS) OSSIFICANS

Fibrositis ossificans is a heterotopic formation of bone, usually in the collagenous supportive tissue of skeletal muscle, in tendons, ligaments, fascias and aponeuroses. There are two distinct types of osseous heterotopia. In fibrositis ossificans circumscripta the lesion is usually solitary

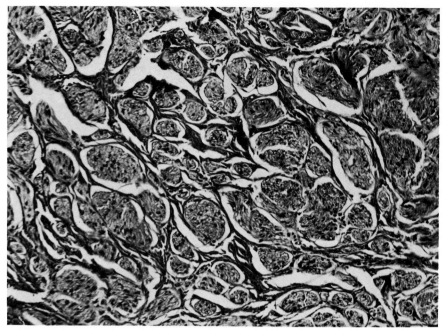

Figure 23–49 Neuroma. Cross section of the tangled mass of nerve filaments and their supportive tissue. (× 180.)

and in the majority of cases follows trauma, which appears to trigger the mechanism that results in the formation of bone. Certain cases of fibrositis ossificans circumscripta are idiopathic; no history of trauma can be obtained. It had been stated[28] that about 4 per cent of paraplegics develop the lesion spontaneously in the region of the knee, thigh or hip. Myositis ossificans progressiva is a congenital, hereditary and sometimes familial disease in which group after group of muscles, tendons and joint ligaments is involved until ability for all active movement is lost. Life may continue until inhibition of respiration or deglutition causes prolonged respiratory infection and eventual death.

The cause and mechanism of heterotopic bone formation is unknown. It appears to be a chain of events that is initiated by an excessive proliferation of collagenoblasts. Interstitial hemorrhage is thought to play an important role in the post-traumatic type. Muscle necrosis may also stimulate this activity. Because the respiratory pigments, hemoglobin and myoglobin, are a common denominator one might conjecture that the complex protein moieties of

these substances may serve as activators, possibly as antigenic agents.

Microscopic examination of the lesions in the early stages has revealed an edematous inflammatory reaction, often with an exudative cellular infiltration. This type of reaction is frequently encountered in sites of allergic tissue response. Could hypersensitivity play a role in the idiopathic and progressive types? Large masses of collagen are produced by this edematous cellular proliferation and this collagen is apparently different from normal collagen inasmuch as it accepts the deposition of calcium salts. This is known as dystrophic calcification. Wherever and whenever heterotopic mineralization of collagen occurs in the body, it is apt to be followed by a metaplasia of the collagenoblasts into osteoblasts and chondroblasts. Islands of osteoid and cartilage appear within the collagen and soon dominate the microscopic scene (Fig. 23–51). When osteoblastic activity is florid with numerous young and hyperchromatic osteoblasts amid irregular masses of crude osteoid, it may be impossible, on the basis of microscopy alone, to make the distinction between fibrositis os-

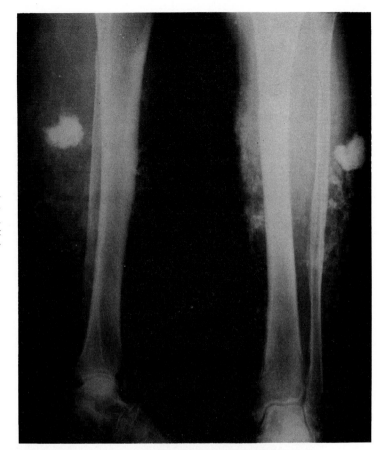

Figure 23–50 Fibrositis ossificans circumscripta. There are fine streaks and flecks of ossification as well as one large confluent opaque mass within the soft tissues of the calf.

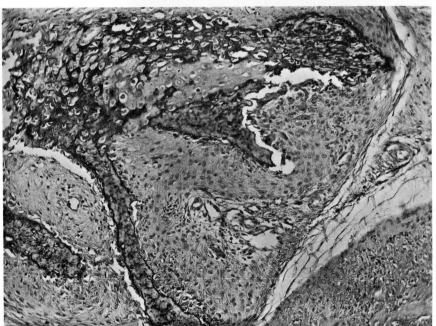

Figure 23–51 Fibrositis ossificans. The first stage is characterized by edema and inflammatory reaction. In the second stage there is collagen formation, which is then converted to chondroid such as that seen in this illustration. (× 197.)

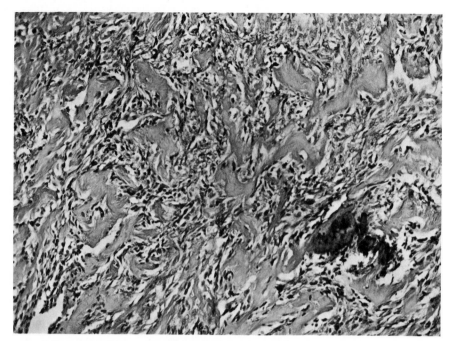

Figure 23–52   Fibrositis ossificans. Osteoblastic proliferation with osteoid formation may closely mimic the picture of osteosarcoma. (× 197.)

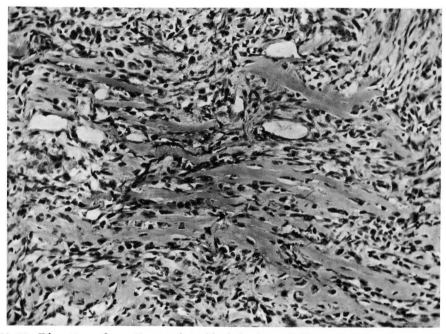

Figure 23–53   Fibrositis ossificans. Frequently viable skeletal muscle fibers may be found persisting amid the jumble of proliferating osteoblasts. This is a helpful feature in differentiating the case from one of osteosarcoma. (× 197.)

sificans and osteosarcoma (Fig. 23–52). Differentiation from malignant neoplasm is even more difficult when the lesion occurs in juxtaposition to bone where it gives the roentgenographic picture of parosteal sarcoma. Fine and Stout[29] have reviewed this subject and called these lesions pseudotumors. They report that these pseudotumors usually occur in a younger age group (under 30) than does extraosseous osteosarcoma, that the cellular components are less irregular, that the formed bone is more normal in appearance and regular in disposition, that cellular activity at the periphery of the lesion is more like that of reaction than neoplasm, and that the lesion is more apt to be well circumscribed. We have found that the presence of viable muscle cells among the proliferating osteoblasts and spicules of bone is of great help in establishing a microscopic diagnosis (Fig. 23–53). Tumor has a tendency to destroy muscle as it advances.

Eventually the lesion is transformed into a mass of mature bone often with a cortical shell surrounding cancellous tissue containing marrow. It may involve the periosteum and then appears to be a mass of appositional bone, thickening and distorting the cortex. It involves tendons and is probably responsible for most of the pointed exostoses that are not osteochondromas. Bony struts may be formed between two bones producing a synostosis. The disease often involves the ligaments about joints to cause an external ankylosis. It progresses along muscle sheaths and the collagenous supportive tissue within muscle bundles, gradually causing atrophy and replacement of the latter. In the progressive type the victim gradually "freezes" with loss of one movement after another until he is eventually transformed into a being within a rigid, calcareous shell (Fig. 23–54). Some of these patients have earned their livings in their terminal years by exhibiting themselves as freaks in side shows. Such a person is usually billed as the "petrified man."

Myositis ossificans progressiva is a curious and rare disease. Most cases are diagnosed during the first few years of life and a few have been found in infancy. Though siblings usually are not affected

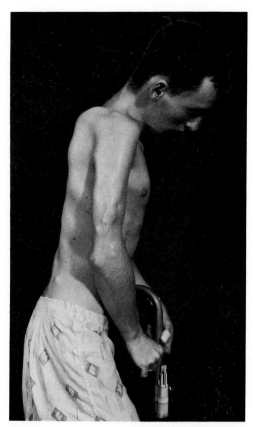

Figure 23–54 Myositis ossificans progressiva. Note the irregular contours of the arms and back caused by heterotopic masses of bone. The neck muscles are involved, causing tilting of the head. Muscle function is inhibited making movement difficult.

there is an increased incidence among those of the same genetic linkage. The disease has been reported in two sets of homozygous twins.[30] First manifestations of the process are usually found about the dorsal neck region and shoulders. Firm or doughy, subcutaneous masses appear. They may be painful, hot and tender.[31] At this stage they may be accompanied by fever. These masses gradually shrink in size as they collagenize. They become firm and fixed and the acute symptoms disappear. A roentgenogram may show them to contain calcium salts. Gradually they ossify and new masses appear and go through the same cycle. The neck, spine and shoulders are most commonly affected and the lower extremities may not be involved. Muscles of the heart, diaphragm,

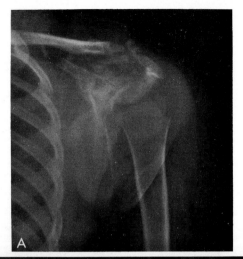

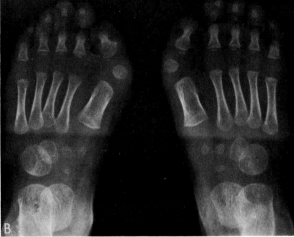

Figure 23–55 Myositis ossificans progressiva. There is ossification of the soft tissues of the shoulder *(A)*. The examination of the feet reveals bilateral hallux valgus secondary to hypoplasia of the proximal phalanx of the great toes *(B)*.

tongue, larynx and the sphincters are spared. As the disease progresses the head is often tilted to one side by involvement of the sternocleidomastoid muscles and a dorsal kyphosis develops. The intervertebral discs in the cervical region ossify so that the cervical spine becomes a solid mass of bone.

Associated with this disease and now considered a part of the syndrome there is usually microdactyly of the large toes and sometimes of the thumbs. There is often a bilateral hallux valgus (Fig. 23–55). The middle phalanx of the fifth finger is often lacking. There may be ankylosis of the interphalangeal and metatarsophalangeal joints. A "moon face" has been reported in several patients. About one quarter of cases show no accompanying anomalous alterations.

Minor trauma in these patients appears to set off an exacerbation of the process. For this reason it is hazardous to biopsy the lesions. It would be most interesting to know whether these patients have a sensitivity to the globulins that are components of hemoglobin and myoglobin.

Fine and Stout have reviewed the incidence of extraosseous osteosarcoma as a complication of fibrositis ossificans. They found 12 such cases. Because they did not state otherwise it is assumed that these were cases of fibrositis ossificans circumscripta. The osteosarcoma has the same microscopy, course and prognosis as that of osteosarcoma of bone.

Many types of therapy have been used in myositis ossificans progressiva. to little or no avail. Corticotropins and cortisone are probably useful in the acute, inflammatory stage. Used at this time they may minimize the reaction and thus modify the course that follows. They are of no purpose in altering the effects of the process after the stage of ossification.

References

1. Park, G. and Arill, J.: Surgery, 28:1045, 1950.
2. Attic, J., Steckler, R. and Platt, N.: Cancer, 25:758, 1970.
3. Smith, L.: Am. J. Pathol., 3:355, 1927.
4. Enzinger, F.: Cancer, 18:1163, 1965.
5. Kubo, T.: Cancer, 24:948, 1969.
6. Gravanis, M.: Bull. Pathol., 9:130, 1968.
7. Enterline, H., Culbertson, J., Rocklin, D. and Brady, L.: Cancer, 13:932, 1960.
8. Enterline, H. and Horn, R.: Am. J. Clin. Pathol., 29:356, 1958.
9. Strobbe, G. and Dargeon, H.: Cancer, 3:826, 1950.
10. Stout, A.: Cancer, 15:1028, 1962.
11. Aegerter, E. and Peale, A.: Arch. Pathol., 34:413, 1942.
12. Christopherson, W., Foote, F. and Stewart, F.: Cancer, 5:100, 1952.
13. Lieberman, P., Foote, F., Stewart, F. and Berg, J.: J.A.M.A., 198:121, 1966.
14. Enzinger, F.: Cancer, 26:1029, 1970.
15. Nash, A. and Stout, A. P.: Cancer, 14:524, 1961.
16. Enzinger, F. and Shiraki, M.: Cancer, 20:1131, 1967.
17. Rios-Dalenz, J., Kim, J. and McDowell, F.: Am. J. Clin. Pathol., 44:632, 1965.
18. Allen, P. and Enzinger, F.: Cancer, 26:857, 1970.
19. Fust, J. and Custer, R.: Am. J. Clin. Pathol., 19:522, 1949.
20. Wright, C.: Br. J. Surg., 38:257, 1951.
21. Barton, D. and Reeves, R.: Am. J. Roentgenol., 86:351, 1961.
22. Sobel, H.: Bull. Pathol., 10:238, 1969.
23. Baldursson, H., Evans, E., Dodge, W. and Jackson, W.: J. Bone Joint Surg., 51A:913, 1969.
24. Kern, W.: Arch. Pathol., 69:209, 1960.
25. Enzinger, F.: Am. J. Clin. Pathol., 43:104, 1965.
26. Konwaler, B., Keasbey, L. and Kaplan, L.: Am. J. Clin. Pathol., 25:241, 1955.
27. Kay, S.: Am. J. Clin. Pathol., 33:433, 1960.
28. Miller, L. and O'Neill, C.: J. Bone Joint Surg., 31A:283, 1949.
29. Fine, G. and Stout, A. P.: Cancer, 9:1027, 1956.
30. Eaton, W. L., Conkling, W. S. and Daeschner, C. W.: J. Pediatr., 50:591, 1957.
31. Lockhart, J. D. and Burke, F. G.: Am. J. Dis. Child., 87:626, 1954.
32. Singleton, E. B. and Holt, J. F.: Radiology, 62:47, 1954.

INDEX

Note: Page numbers in *italic* indicate illustrations.

Abscess(es), Brodie's, 261, *262*
  cold, in tuberculosis of spine, 265, *267*
Achondroplasia, 101
  clinical features of, 102, *102, 103*
  etiology of, 101
  heredity in, 102
  microscopy of, 108, *111*
  prognosis in, 109
  roentgenographic manifestations of, 105, *106–110*
  vs. metaphyseal dysostosis, 112
  vs. spondyloepiphyseal dysplasia, 132
Acid(s). See specific names.
Acinar cell(s), and thyrocalcitonin, 30
Acrocephalosyndactylism. See *Apert's syndrome.*
Acromegaly, 378, *380*
Acro-osteolysis, 502
Acropachy, thyroid, 385, *385*
Actinomyces infection, of bone, 279, *280*, 715
Adenoma, parathyroid. See *Parathyroid adenoma.*
Agammaglobulinemia, joint disease in, 637, *638*
Albers-Schönberg disease. See *Osteopetrosis.*
Albright's syndrome, 167
Alkaptonuria, 632
  and tenosynovial chondrometaplasia, 634
Alveolar soft part tumor, 744, *745, 746*
Amino acid(s), in bone growth, 24
Aminoaciduria, with hypophosphatemic–vitamin D refractory rickets, 366
Amyloidosis, in plasma cell myeloma, 577
Amyoplasia congenita, 710–711
Amyotonia congenita, 702
  clinical features of, 702
  heredity in, 703
  microscopy of, 703, *704, 705*
  roentgenographic manifestations of, *702, 703*
Amyotrophic lateral sclerosis, 706
Anemia(s), chronic hemolytic, 318–324. See also specific names.
  in Paget's disease, 409
  in plasma cell myeloma, 575
Aneurysmal bone cyst, 424–433
  in hamartoma, 467, 507–509
  clinical features of, 425

Aneurysmal bone cyst (*Continued*)
  etiology of, 430
  incidence of, 424
  microscopy of, 431, *431*
  morbid anatomy of, 429
  pathogenesis of, 432
  prognosis in, 433
  roentgenographic manifestations of, *426, 427, 427, 428*
  vs. giant cell tumor, 610, 617
Angiolipoma, 749
Angioma, of bone, 467, 501–507
  microscopy of, 505, *506*
  morbid anatomy of, 505
  prognosis in, 506
Angiosarcoma, of bone, 562–565
  incidence of, 563
  microscopy of, 563, *564*
  roentgenographic manifestations of, 563, *563, 564*
Anterior tibial syndrome, 690
Apert's syndrome, 190–193
  clinical features of, 190, *191–193*
  roentgenographic manifestations of, *191, 192*
Apneurotic fibroma, 753, *755*
Arachnodactyly. See *Marfan's syndrome.*
Arteriography, 75
Artery, anatomy of, 48, *49*
Arthritis, 623–686
  alkaptonuric, 632
  blastomycotic, 659, *660*
  classification of, 623
  gonococcal, with osteomyelitis, 656, *657*
  hemophilic, 634
  hypertrophic. See *Degenerative joint disease.*
  in agammaglobulinemia, 637, *638*
  in dermatomyositis, 674
  in disseminated lupus erythematosus, 673
  in erythema nodosa, 674
  in gout, 626
  in polyarteritis, 674
  in pseudogout, 631
  in rheumatic fever, 674
  in scleroderma, 674, *674*
  in serum sickness, 673
  in ulcerative colitis, 637

Arthritis (*Continued*)
  infectious, 655–660
  miscellaneous types of, 675–678
  nonsuppurative, 657
  of collagen diseases, 673
  of hypersensitivity group, 660–675
  proliferative. See *Rheumatoid arthritis.*
  psoriatic, 637, *637*
  rheumatoid. See *Rheumatoid arthritis.*
  secondary, 626–638
  suppurative, 655, *656*
  synovial fluid in, 625
  syphilitic, 659
  traumatic, vs. degenerative joint disease,
    638
  tuberculous, 657
Arthritis deformans. See *Degenerative joint
  disease.*
Arthritis mutilans, 676, *676*
Arthrography, 76, *76, 77*
Arthrogryposis, 710–711
Arthropathy, cortisone, 650
  neurogenic, 646
    diabetic, 648
    incidence of, 646
    joints involved in, 648
    pathogenesis of, 646
    roentgenographic manifestations of, 646,
      646–648
    treatment of, 649
Articular cartilage, 11
Articular plate, 624, 625
Ascorbic acid, deficiency of, and scurvy, 333
  in bone growth, 24
Asphyxiating thoracic dystrophy, 196, *198*
Autosomal trisomy, 454–457

Baker's cyst, 677, *678*
Bamboo spine, 668, *671*
Barlow's disease, 333
Battered child, 244–245, *244, 245*
Bence Jones protein, and rickets, 364
  in plasma cell myeloma, 576
Beryllium, and osteosarcoma, 514
"Big head" disease, 411
Biopsy, in osteosarcoma, 515
  of muscle, technique for, 687
Blastomyces dermatiditis, and bone infection,
  279, *280, 281*
Blastomycotic arthritis, 659, *660*
Bleeding, in plasma cell myeloma, 575
Blount's disease, 130, *138, 139*
Boeck's sarcoid, in bone, 282–284, *283–286*
Bone, development of, 17, *17, 18*
  fracture of. See *Fracture(s), repair of.*
  infectious diseases of. See *Infectious dis-
    ease(s), of bone.*
  metabolic diseases of. See *Metabolism,
    diseases of.*
  tumors of. See *Tumor(s).*
Bone cyst(s), classification of, 440
Bone destruction, basic patterns of, 81
Bone infarct. See *Infarct, of bone.*
Bone lysis, 371
  normal, 31

Bone marrow. See *Marrow.*
Bone mineral, formation of, 15
Bone modeling, 31, *33, 34*
Bone repair. See *Fracture(s), repair of.*
Bone resorption, increased rate of, diseases
  due to, 371
Bone salt(s), deposition of, 15–16
Bone scanning, 76, 77
Bowing, prenatal, vs. pseudarthrosis, 185, *185*
Bowleg deformity, in Blount's disease, *138*
Brodie's abscess, 261, *262*
Brown tumor(s), in hyperparathyroidism,
    388, *389, 390*
  in renal osteodystrophy, *357*
  microscopy of, *397*
  vs. giant cell tumor of bone, 392
  vs. osteoclastoma, 619
Brucella, and chronic osteomyelitis, 277, *279*
Bulbar palsy, 706
Bursitis, 678, *680, 681*

Café-au-lait spot(s), in neurofibromatosis, 175
Caffey's disease, 440–443. See also *Infantile
  cortical hyperostosis.*
Caisson disease, 289
Calcification, dystrophic, 496
Calcinosis, tumoral, 764–766, *764, 765*
Calcinosis circumscripta, 766
Calcium, kidney function and, 30
Calcium absorption, in rickets, *28*
Calcium deficiency, and skeletal abnormali-
  ties, 27
Calcium loss, and osteomalacia, 361
Callus, in bone healing, 231, 234, 237
Callus formation, in osteogenesis imperfecta,
  142, *142,* 340
Calvarium, in Paget's disease, 408, *409*
Cambium, 19, 62, *63*
Camurati-Engelmann-Ribbing disease, 161,
  161, 162
Cancer, cause of, theories of, 462
  polymyositis with, 715
Carcinoma, of breast, metastatic tumor sec-
  ondary to, 472
Cardiovascular disease, in Paget's disease,
  410
Cartilage, calcification, of in stippled
    epiphyses, *139*
  hyalin, 625, *625*
  normal lysis of, 31
Cartilage-hair hypoplasia, 109
Causalgia, 339, *339*
Cells. See also specific names.
  development of, 4–6, *5*
  differentiation of, factors in, 3–4, *4*
  in cancer development, 462
  malignant vs. benign, 462
Cement line, 60, *61*
Central core disease, 705
Cerebroside reticulocytosis. See *Gaucher's
  disease.*
Chalk bone(s). See *Osteopetrosis.*
Charcot's joint, 646
  cortisone therapy and, 650
  in congenital indifference to pain, 649

Charcot-Marie-Tooth, peroneal muscular atrophy of, 706
Cholesterol reticuloendotheliosis. See *Hand-Schüller-Christian disease.*
Chondroblast(s), columnation of, *53*
  epiphyseal, proliferation of, and skeletal dysplasias, 115–129
  maturation of, 7
    idiopathic disturbances of, 101–115
Chondroblastoma, 538, *539–545*
  bones involved in, 539
  cell maturity in, 510
  clinical features of, 541
  incidence of, 539
  malignant variation of, *544*, 545
  metastasis in, 545
  microscopy of, 541, *542–544*
  morbid anatomy of, 541
  prognosis in, 545
  roentgenographic manifestations of, 540, 541, *541, 542, 544*
  vs. chondromyxoid fibroma, 466, 546
Chondrocalcinosis, 631, *631, 632*
Chondrocyte, 6, *12*
Chondrodystrophia fetalis calcificans, 139–140
Chondrodystrophy(ies), 87
Chondroectodermal dysplasia, 195–196, *195, 196, 197*
Chondroid, composition of, 11, *12*
  elaboration of, and dysplasias, 89–129
Chondroitin sulfate, in connective tissue, 10
Chondroma, 538
Chondromalacia, 645, *645*
Chondrometaplasia, synovial, 682–685, *684, 685*
  tenosynovial, 748, *749*
    alkaptonuria and, 634
    periarticular, 685
Chondromyxoid fibroma, 538, 545–551
  bones involved in, 546
  cell maturity in, 510
  clinical features of, 546
  incidence of, 546
  malignant variation of, *551*
  microscopy of, 547, *549, 550*
  morphology of, 547
  prognosis in, 550
  roentgenographic manifestations of, 546, *547, 548*
  vs. chondroblastoma, 466, 546
  vs. chondrosarcoma, 548, 551
Chondro-osteodystrophy. See *Morquio's disease.*
Chondrosarcoma, 538, 551–561
  as true neoplasm, 465
  cell maturity in, 510
  central, 552, 554
  characteristics of, 539
  clinical features of, 553
  "collar button" silhouette in, 552, *553*
  enchondromatosis and, 121, *121*
  in Paget's disease, 415, *418*, 552
  incidence of, 551
  mesenchymal, 559
  microscopy of, 554, *559, 560*
  osteochondroma and, 552
  pathology of, 554

Chondrosarcoma (*Continued*)
  periosteal. See *Parosteal sarcoma.*
  peripheral, 552, 554
  prognosis in, 561
  roentgenographic manifestations of, 553, *554–557*
  vs. chondromyxoid fibroma, 548, 551
  vs. enchondroma, 500
  vs. osteosarcoma, 551
Chromosome(s), abnormalities of, 451–453
Circulation, disturbances in, 289–330
  bone infarct, 289–294
  chronic hemolytic anemia, 318–324
  epiphyseal ischemic necrosis, 294–302
  focal osteolysis, 328–329
  hypertrophic osteoarthropathy, 305–308
  non-osteogenic fibroma, 308–314
  osteochondritis dissecans, 302–305
  post-hematoma cysts, 324–328
  subperiosteal cortical defect, 314–318
Clasmatocyte(s), 42
Claudication, intermittent, 690
Clear cell hyperplasia, 400
Clear cell sarcoma, 727, *727*
Cleidocranial dysostosis, 193–195, *194*
Clubbing of digits, in hypertrophic osteoarthropathy, 305
Clutton's joint, 660
Coccidioides immitis, and bone infection, 279
Codman's triangle, in Ewing's tumor, 590
  in osteosarcoma, 516, *517*
Cold abscess(es), in tuberculosis of spine, 265, *267*
Colitis, ulcerative, joint disease in, 637
Collagen, composition of, 9–11, *10*
Collagenoblast(s), maturation of, 6, 7
  young, 44, *45*
Collagenoblastic tumor(s), 738–744
  types of, 739
Collagenoblastoma, giant cell, 611
"Collar button" silhouette, in chondrosarcoma, 552, *553*
Congenital indifference to pain, 649
Connective tissue, collagenous, 44, *45*
  components of, cellular, 3–8
    intercellular, 9–16
      formation of, 14–15
  function of, 11
  general consideration of, 3–84
Contraction, of muscle fiber, 691
Cooley's anemia, roentgenographic manifestations of, *319*, 320
Cortical defect, subperiosteal. See *Subperiosteal cortical defect.*
Cortisone arthropathy, 650
Coxa plana, 294, 295
Coxa vara, epiphyseal. See *Epiphysiolysis.*
Craniofacial dysostosis, 161
Craniometaphyseal dysplasia. See *Metaphyseal dysplasia.*
Cretinism, 381
Cryoglobulin, in plasma cell myeloma, 576
Cushing's syndrome, 338, *338*
Cyst(s). See also specific names.
  of menisci, 677
Cysticercosis, 716
Cystine storage disease, with rickets, 364, 366

Deafness, in osteogenesis imperfecta, 142
Degenerative joint disease, 638–650
  clinical features of, 639
  cysts in, 642
  Heberden's nodes in, 641, 642
  incidence of, 639
  microscopy of, *639*, 640, *640, 641*
  pathogenesis of, 642
  pathology of, 640
  roentgenographic manifestations of, 642,
    643, 644
  treatment of, 645
Demineralization, of mature bone, 60, *61*
Dentinogenesis imperfecta, 142, 340
Deossification, osteoclast and, 34
Dermatomyositis, 711
  arthritis in, 674
Desmoid, 751–752, *752.* See also *Parosteal
    sarcoma.*
  extra-abdominal, 752
  periosteal, vs. periosteal fibrosarcoma, 566
de Toni-Debre-Fanconi syndrome, 363
Diabetes mellitus, osteopenia of, 339
Diaphyseal sclerosis, 161, *161–163*
Diaphysis, cortex of, 64, *65*
  formation of, 18
Diastrophic dwarfism, 130–132
Diet, in organic matrix formation, 23
Dieting, and osteopenia, 332
Disappearing bone, 371, 502
Disease(s). See specific names.
Disseminated lupus erythematosus, arthritis
    in, 673
Disuse atrophy, 339
Down's syndrome, 454, *455*
Dupuytren's contracture, 753
Dwarfism, diastrophic, 130–132
  in cartilage-hair hypoplasia, 112
  in Old Order Amish, 109
  metatrophic, 105, *105*, 196
  Peter Pan, 380
  pituitary, 380
  thanatophoric, 104, *104*, 196
  thyroid, 381
Dyschondroplasia, 116
Dyschondrosteosis, 187, *188*
Dysostosis, metaphyseal. See *Metaphyseal
    dysostosis.*
Dysplasia(s). See also specific names.
Dysplasia epiphysealis hemimelica, 128–129,
    128
Dysplasia epiphysealis punctata, 139–140
Dystrophy, asphyxiating thoracic, 196, *198*
  muscular. See *Muscular dystrophy.*

Echinococcosis, 716
Elastin fibrils, 9
"Elfin face," in idiopathic hypercalcemia, 447
Ellis–van Creveld syndrome, 195–196, *195–
    197*
Ellsworth-Howard test, in hyperparathy-
    roidism, 386
  in hypoparathyroidism, 403
Embryology, skeletal, 17–36
Embryonic fat cell(s), 729

Enchondral ossification, *50–55*
Enchondral plate, 52, *53*
Enchondroma, 466, 499–501
Enchondromatosis, 115, 116–121
  clinical features of, 116, *117*
  microscopy of, 119, *120*
  prognosis in, 121
  roentgenographic manifestations of, 117,
    118, 119
Endobone, in osteopetrosis, *153*
Endocrine dysfunction, disturbances due to,
    376–406
  in fibrous dysplasia, 169
Endocrine osteopenia, 338
Endomysium, 691
Eosinophil(s), 40, *41*
Eosinophilic granuloma, 207–208
  microscopy of, *209*
  roentgenographic manifestations of, 214,
    214–216
  vs. Hand-Schüller-Christian disease, 205,
    206
Epiphyseal dysplasia, multiple, 130, 137–139
  vs. Morquio's disease, 139
Epiphyseal hyperplasia, 128–129, *128*
Epiphyseal ischemic necrosis, 294–302
  microscopy of, 300, *301*
  pathologic morphology in, 299
  prognosis in, 302
  roentgenographic manifestations of, 297,
    297–300
  stages of, 296
Epiphyseal line, 50, *51*, 54, *55*
Epiphysiolisthesis. See *Epiphysiolysis.*
Epiphysiolysis, 420–424
  incidence of, 420
  microscopy of, 423
  pathogenesis of, 423
  pathologic morphology of, 422
  roentgenographic manifestations of, 421,
    421–423
Epiphysis, composition of, 20
  formation of, 18
  infarcts in, 290
  osseous nucleus of, 66, *67*
  ringing of, in scurvy, 334, *335*, 337
  slipped. See *Epiphysiolysis.*
  stippled, 139–140
Epithelioid cell(s), 42, *43*
  in tuberculosis of bone, 268
Epithelioid sarcoma, 746
Erlenmeyer flask deformity, in Gaucher's dis-
    ease, 220
  in metaphyseal dysplasia, 157
Erythema nodosa, arthritis in, 674
Erythroblastoma, 586
Estrogen, and skeletal abnormalities, 27
Eunuchoid giantism, 378
Ewing's tumor, 587–597
  bones involved in, 587
  clinical features of, 589
  derivation of, 572
  differential diagnosis of, 592
  gross pathology of, 592
  incidence of, 587
  microscopy of, 592, *594–596*
  prognosis in, 597

Ewing's tumor (*Continued*)
  roentgenographic manifestations of, 589,
    590–593
  treatment of, 597
  vs. Hand-Schüller-Christian disease, 205
  vs. lymphosarcoma of bone, 596
  vs. metastatic neuroblastoma, 596
  vs. osteomyelitis, 590, *590*
  vs. primitive multipotential sarcoma of
    bone, 526
  vs. reticulum cell sarcoma, 595
Exostosis(es), hereditary multiple. See *Osteochondromatosis.*
Exudate, suppurative, neutrophils in, 40, *41*
Exudative cell(s), *41*

Facioscapulohumeral dystrophy, 696
Fairbank's disease, 137–139
Familial neurovisceral lipidosis, 224–227
Familial periodic paralysis, 718–719
Fanconi syndrome, 363
  vitamin D and, 28
Fasciitis, 767–769
Fat cell(s), 5, 6
Fat necrosis, 766
Fat tissue, 48, *49*
  roentgenography of, *83, 84*
Felty's syndrome, 668
Fiberbone, 21
  primitive, 58, *59*
Fibroangioma, giant cell. See *Villonodular
  synovitis.*
Fibroblast(s), 6–8
  in formation of osteoblasts, 56, *57*
  in organizing hematoma, 38, *39*
  young, 44, *45*
Fibrolipoma, 749
Fibroma, 467. See also specific names.
  non-osteogenic. See *Non-osteogenic
    fibroma.*
  ossifying. See *Osteoblastoma.*
  osteogenic. See *Osteoblastoma.*
Fibroma molluscum, in neurofibromatosis,
    175, *176*
  microscopy of, *183*
Fibromatosis, aggressive, 752–753, *754*
  generalized congenital, vs. neurofibromato-
    sis, 184
  plantar, 753, *756*
Fibro-osseous metaplasia, 510
Fibrosarcoma, 565–571, 740, *740*
  cell maturity in, 510
  clinical features of, 566
  gross anatomy of, 566
  in Paget's disease, 415
  incidence of, 565
  microscopy of, 568, *570, 571,* 741
  prognosis in, 570
  roentgenographic manifestations of, 566,
    567–569
  sites involved in, 740
  treatment of, 571
  types of, 565
  vs. osteoclastoma, 611
  well differentiated, 752

Fibrosis, in muscular dystrophy, 701
Fibrositis, 678
Fibrositis ossificans, 769–775
Fibrous dysplasia, 167–174
  clinical features of, 168, *168, 169*
  endocrine dysfunction in, 169
  microscopy of, 171, *172–174*
  prognosis in, 173
  roentgenographic manifestations of, 169,
    170
  vs. non-osteogenic fibroma, 313
Fibroxanthoma, 741
Floating cell(s), in alveolar rhabdomyosarcoma, 738
Fluoroscopy, 74
Foam cell(s), in Gaucher's disease, 220
Fouchet sign, 645
Fracture(s), buckle, *233*
  callus formation in, 231, 234, 237
  Colles, *232*
  comminuted, *232*
  hematoma in, 231, 235, *236*
  in osteogenesis imperfecta, 142, 145
  in osteopetrosis, 149
  of hip, osteoporosis and, 372
  of rib, *243*
  pathologic, 245, 247, *247, 248*
  repair of, 231–250
    microscopy of, *236, 238–240*
    osteomyelitis complicating, 242
    principles of, 242
    pseudarthrosis in, 235
    sequence of events in, 235
  stress, 247–250, *248, 249*
  transverse, *232*
  through epiphyseal line, *234*
Fraenkel, white line of, in scurvy, 337
Fröhlich's adiposogenital dystrophy, 420
  lathyrism in, 424
Freiberg's disease, 294
Fungal infection, of bone, 279

Galactosamine, 10
Gamma A globulin, 576
Gamma B globulin, 576
Gamma globulin, 574
Ganglion(a), 681, *682,* 763–764
Ganglion cyst, vs. subchondral cyst, 440
Gardner's syndrome, 127
Gargoylism. See *Hurler's disease.*
Garré, osteitis of, 284, *286*
Gas gangrene, *80*
Gaucher's disease, 217–223
  clinical features of, 218
  gross pathology of, 219
  microscopy of, 220, *223*
  prognosis in, 222
  roentgenographic manifestations of, 219,
    219–222
Geographic destruction, of bone, 81
Giant cell(s), 42, *43*
  of giant cell tumor, 607, 609
  of granuloma, 42, *43*
  of inflammation, 42, *43*
Giant cell collagenoblastoma, 611

Giant cell epulis, 612
Giant cell osteosarcoma, 526, 610
Giant cell reaction(s), of bone, 619
Giant cell tumor, 467, 562, 607. See also
    Osteoclastoma.
  benign, 610
  calcifying. See *Chondroblastoma.*
  chondromatous. See *Chondroblastoma.*
  malignant, 727, *728*
  of tendon, 761–763
  of tendon sheath. See *Villonodular syno-*
    vitis.
  vs. aneurysmal bone cyst, 610, 617
  vs. brown tumor, 392
  xanthomatous. See *Villonodular synovitis.*
Giantism, focal, in neurofibromatosis, 175, *176*
  pituitary, 376
    vs. eunuchoid giantism, 378
Globulin, 572
Glucagon level(s), in pancreatitis, 388
Glucosamine, 10
Gorham's disease, 328, 502
Gout, 626
  clinical features of, 626
  heredity in, 626
  laboratory tests for, 629
  pseudo-, 631, *631, 632*
  renal involvement in, 629
  roentgenographic manifestations of, 629,
    630
  secondary, 629
  tophus in, 627, *627–629*
  treatment of, 631
  urate salts in, 628
Gower's sign, in muscular dystrophy, 694
Growth arrest line(s), 22
Ground substance, of collagen, 10
Granulation tissue, 18, 38, *39*
Granuloma(s), eosinophilic, 207–208
  of Boeck's sarcoid, *286*
  of tuberculosis, 272
Granuloma pyogenicum, 769
Granulomatosis, lipoid. See *Hand-Schüller-*
  Christian disease.
Ground glass appearance, in scurvy, 334
Gumma, in syphilis of bone, 274

Hale reaction, 11
Hallux valgus, in myositis ossificans, 774, *774*
Hamartoma(s), 462, 510
  of bone, 496–509
  of soft parts, 748–761
    classification of, 748
Hand-foot syndrome, in sickle cell anemia,
  322, 324
Hand-Schüller-Christian disease, 201, 202–
  207
  clinical features of, 203, *204*
  etiology of, 202
  microscopy of, 204, *206*
  prognosis in, 207
  roentgenographic manifestations of, 214
  vs. eosinophilic granuloma, 205, *206*
Harris' line(s), 22

Harrison's groove, in rickets, 343
Haversian canal(s), 21, 62, *63*
Haversian system, 21, 60, *61*
Heavy chain disease, 572
Heberden's node(s), in degenerative joint dis-
  ease, 641, 642
Hamangioblastoma, 562
Hemangioendothelioma, 501, *758, 759*
Hemangioma, of bone, *502, 503, 505, 506*
  of soft tissue, 757–758, *757*
  sclerosing, 758
Hemangiopericyte(s), of Zimmermann, 501
Hemangiopericytoma, 501, 759–760, *759*
Hemangiosarcoma, 501, 744, *744, 745*
Hemarthrosis, in hemophilia, 634
Hematoma, of fracture, 231, 235, *236*
  organizing, 38, *39*
Hemophilia, 634
  and solitary bone cyst, 439
  hemarthrosis in, 634
  pseudotumors of, 324, *324*
  roentgenographic manifestations of, 635,
    634–636
  treatment of, 635
Hemorrhage, subperiosteal, in battered child,
  244
Hepatosplenomegaly, in Hurler's disease, 97
Hereditary factor(s), 3
Hereditary multiple exostoses. See *Osteo-*
  chondromatosis.
Hereditary opalescent dentin, 142
Hernia, umbilical, in Hurler's disease, 97
Hibernoma, 749, *750*
Hip fracture, osteoporosis and, 372
Histiocyte(s), 42
  facultative, 756
Histiocytoma, fibrous, 769
  malignant, 741
Histiocytosis(es). See also *Hand-Schüller-*
  Christian disease.
  classification of, 202
  lipid, vs. non-osteogenic fibroma, 313
  non-neoplastic, roentgenographic mani-
    festations of, 214
Histiocytosis X, 201
Histology, of musculoskeletal system, 37–73
"Hitch-hiker's thumb," in diastrophic
  dwarfism, 130
Hodgkin's disease, 603–606
  classification of, 604
  derivation of, 572
  incidence of, 603
  microscopy of, *605, 606*
  pathology of, 604
  prognosis in, 606
  roentgenographic manifestations of, 604,
    604, 605
  treatment of, 606
Homogentisic acid, in alkaptonuria, 632
Hormonal disturbance(s), and skeletal abnormalities, 25
Hormone(s). See also specific names.
  and osteoid production, 331
  parathyroid, and bone calcification, 28
  somatotropic growth, 25
  steroid, 26
Hotchkiss-McManus stain, 10

Human growth hormone, 25
  in giantism, 376
  in pituitary dwarfism, 380
Humerus, length growth of, 22
  modeling of, *33*
Hunter-Hurler syndrome, 201
Hunter's syndrome, 100
Hurler's disease, 95
  clinical features of, 96, *96*
  incidence of, 95
  microscopy in, 99, *100*
  prognosis in, 100
  roentgenographic manifestations of, 96,
    97–99
  vs. Morquio's disease, 95
  vs. neurovisceral lipidosis, *225*
Hurler's syndrome, vs. hypothyroidism, 383
Hurler-variant, 224
Hutter's tumor, 590
Hyalin cartilage, 11, 625
Hyaluronate, in connective tissue, 10
Hydrarthrosis, intermittent, 675
Hydronephrosis, internal, in plasma cell
  myeloma, 578
Hypercalcemia, idiopathic, 447–448
Hypercalcemic crisis, in hyperparathyroidism, 389
Hyperglycinuria, with hypophosphatemic-
  vitamin D refractory rickets, 366
Hypernephroma, metastatic, *476*
Hyperostosis, infantile cortical. See *Infantile
  cortical hyperostosis.*
Hyperostosis corticalis generalisata, 407, 420
Hyperparathyroidism, 385
  brown tumor in, 392, *393*
  classification of, 399
  hypercalcemic crisis in, 389
  microscopy of, 391, *396–398*
  peptic ulcer in, 388
  renal failure in, 389
  roentgenographic manifestations of, 390,
    391–395
  vs. Boeck's sarcoidosis, 282
Hyperphosphatasia, 369, *370*
Hyperplasia, clear cell, 371, 400
  epiphyseal, 128–129, *128*
  idiopathic parathyroid, 399, *400*
  idiopathic spontaneous, 359
  metastasizing, 462
  of bone marrow, 318
  secondary parathyroid. See *Renal osteo-
    dystrophy.*
  wasserhelle, 400
Hyperthyroidism, 383
  in fibrous dysplasia, 169
Hypervitaminosis A, 448–450
Hypervitaminosis D, 28, *29*, 444–446
Hypoparathyroidism, 401, *402*
  chronic, 401
  pseudo-, 403, *404, 405*
  pseudo-pseudo-, 404
  symptoms of, 402
Hypophosphatasia, 368, *368*
Hypophosphatemic–vitamin D refractory rickets, 28, 362
  cystine storage disease with, 366
  hyperglycinuria with, 366
  microscopy of, 367

Hypophosphatemic–vitamin D refractory
  rickets (*Continued*)
  renal involvement in, 365
  roentgenographic manifestations of, 367,
    367, 368
  types of, 364
  with aminoaciduria, 366
  with myeloma kidney, 578
Hypoplasia, cartilage-hair, 109
Hypothyroidism, 381
  roentgenographic manifestations of, 382,
    383, 384
Hypotonia, congenital, 702

Idiopathic hypercalcemia, 447–448
Idiopathic parathyroid hyperplasia, 399, *400*
Immobilization, effect of, on ossification, 31,
  32
Infantile cortical hyperostosis, 440–443
  clinical features of, 443
  microscopy of, *443*
  pathology of, 442
  roentgenographic manifestations of, *441*,
    442, *442*
  vs. diaphyseal sclerosis, 162
Infarct, of bone, 289–294
  microscopy of, 291, *292, 293*
  prognosis in, 291
  roentgenographic manifestations of, *291,
    292*
  vs. non-osteogenic fibroma, 313
Infectious disease(s), of bone, 251–288
  nonsuppurative osteomyelitis, 264–288
  suppurative osteomyelitis, 251–264. See
    also *Osteomyelitis.*
Infraction(s), metaphyseal, *249, 250*
Intracranial pressure, in Apert's syndrome, 190
Involucrum, *254, 258, 258*
Iron deficiency anemia, roentgenographic
  manifestations of, *323*
Irradiation therapy, and osteosarcoma, 514
Ischemic necrosis, epiphyseal. See *Epiphy-
  seal ischemic necrosis.*

Jansen's disease, 112
Jaw(s), osteoclastoma in, 612
Joint(s), Charcot's, 646
  Clutton's, 660
  diseases of. See *Arthritis* and *Degenerative
    joint disease.*
  hemophilic, 634
  infections of, 659
    bacterial, 655
  synovial, 624–626, *624*
  types of, 624
Joint body, 682, *683*
Joint space, 66, *67*
Joint tissue(s), in tuberculous infection, 266

Kaposi's disease, 744, *744, 745*
Karyotype, normal, *451–453*

Keloid, 766–767
Kidney(s), in gout, 629
    in renal osteodystrophy, 359
    in vitamin D refractory rickets, 365
    myeloma, 578, 579
Kidney function, and calcium level, 30
Klinefelter's syndrome, 453–454
Knee, anatomy of, 83
Knockknee deformity, in metaphyseal
    dysplasia, 158
    in Morquio's disease, 92, 93
Köhler's disease, 294

Lacuna(ae), 19
Lamella(ae), interstitial, 21
Lamina(ae), 19
Lamina dura, in hyperparathyroidism, 389
Laminagraphy, 75, 75
Lathyrism, 424
Lead poisoning, bone growth in, 81
Legg-Calvé-Perthes disease, 294.
    vs. sickle cell disease, 318
Leiomyoma, 751
Leiomyosarcoma, 732
    microscopy of, 733
Length growth, of cylindrical bones, 21
Lesion(s), reactive, in bone, 478–496
Letterer-Siwe disease, 208–217
    clinical features of, 210, 210
    microscopy of, 210, 211
    prognosis in, 212
    roentgenographic manifestations of, 213,
        214, 216
Leukemia, lymphatic, 603
    and metastatic tumors, 473, 474
Levo-hexuronic acid, 333
Limb-girdle dystrophy, 696
Lipidosis, familial neurovisceral, 224–227
Lipoid granulomatosis. See Hand-Schüller-
    Christian disease.
Lipoma, 79, 748–749, 750
Liposarcoma, 729
    differentiated, 730, 731
    incidence of, 730
    myxoid, 731, 732, 732
    types of, 730
    sites involved in, 729
Liver, in Hurler's disease, 100
Looser zone(s), in osteomalacia, 350, 351, 352
    in rickets, 344, 346
Lowe's disease, 364, 367
Luetic infection, of joints, 659
Lymphangioma, 743, 504
Lymphocyte(s), 40, 41
Lymphocytoma, of bone, 586
Lymphosarcoma, of bone, vs. Ewing's tumor,
    596
Lysis, of bone and cartilage, 31, 33
Lysol poisoning, and osteomalacia, 350

Macroglobulinemia, Waldenström's, 572
Macrophage(s), 42, 43
Madelung's deformity, 187, 188

Maffucci's syndrome, 116, 501
Mains ou doigts en lorgnette, 677
Mandible, in Hurler's disease, 97
Marble bone(s). See Osteopetrosis.
Marfan's syndrome, 187–190
    clinical features of, 188, 189
    roentgenographic manifestations of, 189,
        189, 190
Marie-Strumpell disease, 668
Maroteaux-Lamy syndrome, 101
Marrow, 68, 69
    hyperplasia of, 318
    in Gaucher's disease, 218
    in Letterer-Siwe disease, 210
    in plasma cell myeloma, 575
Mast cell disease, 451
Melorheostosis, 162–165
    microscopy of, 165
    prognosis in, 165
Meniscus(i), cysts of, 677
Menstruation, precocious, in fibrous dys-
    plasia, 169
Mesenchyme, 5
    derivatives of, 6
Mesenchymoma, 510, 746, 747
Mesoderm, primitive, 4, 5
Mesothelium, primitive, 4
Metabolism, diseases of, 331–375
    osteolysis, 371
    osteomalacia, 340–371
    osteopenia, 332–340
    osteoporosis, 371–374
Metacarpal sign, in Turner's syndrome, 453
Metachromasia, 10
Metaphyseal dysostosis, 112
    clinical features of, 114
    roentgenographic manifestations of, 113,
        114, 115
    Schmid's type of, 112
    Spahr type of, 113
    vs. achondroplasia, 112
Metaphyseal dysplasia, 157–161
    roentgenographic manifestations of, 158–
        160
Metaphysis, cortex of, 64, 65
    elongated, in osteopetrosis, 149
    subepiphyseal, 55
Metaplasia, definition of, 4
    fibro-osseous, 19
Metatrophic dwarfism, 196
Microdactyly, in myositis ossificans, 774
Microradiography, in study of bone, 12, 14
Mikulicz's disease, 715
Milkman's syndrome, 28, 350
Mineral salt, in organic matrix, 27
Modeling, of bone, 31, 33, 34
Mongolism, 454, 455
Monostotic Paget's disease, 407
Morquio's disease, 90
    clinical features of, 91, 91, 92
    differential diagnosis in, 95
    heredity in, 91
    incidence of, 90
    microscopy of, 92, 94
    prognosis in, 95
    roentgenographic manifestations of, 91, 93
    vs. epiphyseal dysplasia, 139
    vs. spondyloepiphyseal dysplasia, 132

Morquio-Brailsford's disease, 90
Motheaten destruction, of bone, 81
Motor end plate, 691
Motor neuron, 691
  axonal arboration of, *693*
Mucolipidosis(es), 226
Mucopolysaccharide(s), in connective tissue, 10
Mucopolysaccharidosis(es), 90–101
  Hunter's syndrome, 100
  Hurler's disease, 95
  in classification of skeletal dysplasias, 88
  Maroteaux-Lamy syndrome, 101
  Morquoi's disease, 90
  Sanfilippo's syndrome, 101
  Scheie's syndrome, 101
Multiple epiphyseal dysplasia, 130, 137–139
Muscle(s), skeletal, 70, *71*
  diseases of, 687–720
Muscle biopsy, clamp in, *688*
  technique for, 687
Muscle cell(s), anatomy of, 689
Muscle fiber, 689, *689–691*
  contraction of, 691
  myosin in, *693*
Muscular atrophy, progressive, 706, *707*
Muscular dystrophy, 693–702
  biopsy in, 697
  classification of, 694
  distal, 696
  fibrosis in, 701
  microscopy of, 697, *698–701*
  progressive, 694, *695*
    fat in, 701
Musculoskeletal system, histology of, 37–73
Myasthenia gravis, 717–718
Myelocytoma, 586
Myeloma, benign, 584
  multiple. See *Plasma cell myeloma.*
  plasma cell. See *Plasma cell myeloma.*
  types of, 573
Myeloma kidney, 578, *579*
Myelomatosis. See *Plasma cell myeloma.*
Myelosclerosis, 572
Myoblastoma, granular cell, 760, *760*
  malignant, 744
Myodystrophy, ocular, 696
Myoglobin, 5
Myopathy(ies), allergic, 711–715
  classification of, 687. See also specific names.
Myosin, in muscle fiber, 693
Myositis, infectious, 715–716, *716*
Myositis, proliferative, 766, *767*
Myositis ossificans, 769–775
  microscopy of, 770, *771, 772*
  roentgenographic manifestations of, *771*
  vs. malignant neoplasm, 773
Myositis ossificans progressiva, 773, *773, 774*
  treatment of, 775
Myotonia, 696
  congenital, 716–717
Myotonic dystrophy, 696
Myxedema, 381
Myxoblast, 756
Myxoma, 756–757
  microscopy of, *741*

Myxomatous degeneration, in enchondromatosis, 119
Myxosarcoma, 741, 756–757

N hormone, and skeletal abnormalities, 27
Necrosis, epiphyseal ischemic. See *Epiphyseal ischemic necrosis.*
Nephrocalcinosis, hyperparathyroidism and, 387, *388*
  in hypervitaminosis D, 445
  in metastatic tumors, 471
Nephrolithiasis, in parathyroid adenoma, 389
Nerve(s), 48, *49*
Nerve axon, *692*
Neoplasm(s), of soft parts, 723. See also *Tumor(s).*
Neurilemmoma, 742, 757
  microscopy of, *182*
Neuroblastoma, metastatic, *472*
  vs. Ewing's tumor, 596
Neuroepithelioma, malignant, 728, *729*
Neurofibroma, 757
  in long bones, *177*
  in pelvis, *179*
Neurofibromatosis, 174–184
  clinical features of, 175, *176*
  microscopy of, 181, *182, 183*
  prognosis in, 183
  roentgenographic manifestations of, 175, *177–181*
  vs. congenital generalized fibromatosis, 184
Neurofibrosarcoma, 742, *743*
Neurogenic arthropathy. See *Arthropathy, neurogenic.*
Neuroma, 769, *770*
Neuromyopathy(ies), 702–710
  toxic, 710
  viral, 708, *709, 710*
Neurovisceral lipidosis, familial, 224–227
Neutrophil(s), 40, *41*
Nickerson-Kveim test, in sarcoidosis, 282
Niemann-Pick disease, 224
Nocardia intracellularis, and tuberculosis of bone, 273
Nodular fasciitis, 767–769
Non-osteogenic fibroma, 308–314, 492–495
  clinical features of, 309
  differential diagnosis in, 313
  incidence of, 493
  microscopy of, 311, *311–313, 493, 494*
  morbid anatomy of, 493
  prognosis in, 314
  roentgenographic manifestations of, 493, *493*
Nuclear proliferation, in muscular dystrophy, 699, *699*

Ochronosis, 632, *633*
Ocular myodystrophy, 696
Oculocerebrorenal syndrome, 364, 367
Ollier's disease. See *Enchondromatosis.*
"Onion skin" appearance, in Ewing's tumor, 589, 590, 592

Opalescent dentin, 142
Ophthalmoplegia, progressive dystrophic, 696
Organic matrix, deposition of mineral salt in, 27
  formation of, 23
    diet in, 23
    hormonal disturbances in, 25
Osgood-Schlatter disease, 294
Ossification, abnormal epiphyseal, and skeletal dysplasias, 129–140
  enchondral, 19–23
  intramembranous, 19
  stress stimulus in, 31, 32
Ossification center, primary, 18, 18
  secondary, 21
Osteitis, sclerosing, 284, 286
Osteitis condensans ilii et pubii, 140
Osteitis deformans. See Paget's disease.
Osteitis fibrosa cystica, 385
Osteitis fibrosa disseminata, 385
Osteoarthritis. See Degenerative joint disease.
Osteoarthropathy, hypertrophic, 305–308
    microscopy of, 307
    prognosis in, 308
    roentgenographic manifestations of, 307
Osteoblast(s), formation of, 56, 57
  maturation of, 7, 13
  origin of, 607, 608
Osteoblastoma, 465, 487–492
  microscopy of, 490, 491, 492
  pathology of, 489
  prognosis in, 492
  roentgenographic manifestations of, 488, 489, 489, 490
Osteochondritis, Parrot's syphilitic, 660
Osteochondritis deformans juvenilis. See Epiphyseal ischemic necrosis.
Osteochondritis dissecans, 302–305
  clinical features of, 303
  etiology of, 305
  incidence of, 302
  microscopy of, 304
  morbid anatomy of, 304
Osteochondroma, 465, 498–499
  and chondrosarcoma, 552
  and osteosarcoma, 514
  and parosteal sarcoma, 127, 533, 535
  from solitary enchondroma, 500
  microscopy of, 125, 126
  sagittal section of, 123
Osteochondromatosis, 115, 121–128
  clinical features of, 122, 123
  etiology of, 123
  heredity in, 122
  in synovial chondrometaplasia, 685, 748
  incidence of, 122
  microscopy of, 125, 125, 126
  prognosis in, 125
  roentgenographic manifestations of, 122, 124, 126, 127
Osteochondrosis. See Epiphyseal ischemic necrosis.
Osteochondrosis deformans tibiae, 130, 138, 139
Osteoclast, 46, 47
  and deossification, 34
  origin of, 607, 608

Osteoclastoma, 510, 607–620
  aneurysmal bone cyst vs., 432, 618
  clinical features of, 612
  differential diagnosis of, 617
  giant cell in, 607, 609, 609
  history of, 611
  incidence of, 612
  microscopy of, 614, 615–617
  roentgenographic manifestations of, 612, 613, 614
  treatment of, 619
  vs. brown tumor, 619
  vs. fibrosarcoma, 611
  vs. giant cell fibrosarcoma, 570
  vs. villonodular synovitis, 618
Osteocyte, 6
  formation of, 19, 58, 59
  in intramembranous ossification, 19
Osteodystrophy, renal. See Renal osteodystrophy.
Osteogenesis imperfecta, 141, 339
  clinical features of, 141, 142
  deafness in, 142
  fractures in, 142, 145
  microscopy of, 145, 146
  prognosis in, 147
  roentgenographic manifestations of, 143, 142–145
  scar formation in, 143
  teeth in, 142
Osteoid, 8
  composition of, 11–14, 13
  formation of, 56, 57
  in mineral infiltration, 31
Osteoid fibroma. See Osteoblastoma.
Osteoid mineralization, inadequate, diseases due to, 340–370
Osteoid osteoma, 465, 479–487
  clinical features of, 479
  giant. See Osteoblastoma.
  incidence of, 479
  microscopy of, 481, 484–486
  morbid anatomy of, 480
  pathogenesis of, 486
  prognosis in, 487
  roentgenographic manifestations of, 480, 480–483
  subperiosteal, 483, 484, 486
  vs. neoplasm, 487
  vs. osteoblastoma, 490
  disturbances in, and skeletal dysplasias, 129–186
  hormones and, 331
Osteoid synthesis, inadequate, diseases due to, 332–340
Osteolysis, deficient, and skeletal dysplasias, 147–167
  essential, with nephropathy, 329, 329
  focal, 328–329
  idiopathic hereditary, 329
  massive, 502
Osteoma, 465, 496–498
  fibrous. See Osteoblastoma.
  osteoid. See Osteoid osteoma.
  parosteal. See Parosteal sarcoma.
Osteomalacia, 340–370
  etiology of, 348
  microscopy of, 353, 353

Osteomalacia (*Continued*)
  prognosis in, 353
  puerperal, 349
  renal, 361, *362–364*
  roentgenographic manifestations of, 351,
    351, 352
  vs. osteopenia, 348
Osteomyelitis, complicating fracture, *242*
  nonsuppurative, 264–288
    acid-fast bacilli and, 272–273
    Boeck's sarcoid in bone, 282–284
    Brucellar infection and, 277–279
    congenital rubella syndrome, 286–288
    fungal, 279
    sclerosing osteitis, 284–286
    syphilitic, 273–277
    tuberculous, 264–272
    viral, 279–282
  suppurative, 251–264
    acute and chronic, 251–261
    Brodie's abscess, 261
    chronic granulomatous disease in, 254,
      255
    clinical features of, 252, *252, 254*
    microscopy of, 258, *260*
    prognosis in, 264
    roentgenographic manifestations of, 256
      256–259
    Salmonella and, 261–264
    squamous cell carcinoma in, 254, *255*
    Staphylococcus aureus and, 252, *262*
  vs. Ewing's tumor, 590, *590*
  vs. non-osteogenic fibroma, 313
  with gonococcal arthritis, 656, *657*
Osteopathia condensans disseminata, 166
Osteopathia striata, 165, *165*
Osteopenia, 332–340
  congenital, 339
  dietary, 332
  endocrine, 338
  of disuse, 339
  post-traumatic, 339, *339*
  stress deficiency, 339
  vs. osteomalacia, 348
Osteopetrosis, 147–154
  clinical features of, 149, *150*
  elongated metaphysis in, 149
  etiology of, 148
  fractures in, 149
  incidence of, 148
  microscopy of, 150, *153*
  prognosis in, 154
  roentgenographic manifestations of, 150,
    151–153
Osteophyte, 496
Osteopoikilosis, 166
Osteoporosis, 371–374
  clinical features of, 374
  microscopy of, 373, *373*
  morbid anatomy of, 373
  pathogenesis of, 372
  postmenopausal, *26*, 371
  roentgenographic manifestations of, 572,
    572
  senile, 371, 374
    vs. generalized plasma cell myeloma, 374
  starvation, *24*
  with osteomalacia, 348, *349*

Osteoporosis circumscripta, in Paget's dis-
    ease, *412*
Osteopsathyrosis, 339
Osteosarcoma, 464, 510, 511–530
  beryllium and, 514
  biopsy in, 515
  bones involved in, 511
  clinical features of, 514, *515*
  cytologic classification of, 521
    Class I, 521
    Class II, 524
    Class III, 524
    Class IV, 526
    Class V, 526
  extraosseous, 513, *513*
  gross pathology of, 519, *520*
  in Paget's disease, 415, *418, 419*, 514
  incidence of, 511
  metastatic lesions of, *475*
  microscopy of, 521
  multiple, sclerosing type, 512, *512*
  osteochondroma and, 514
  osteoclastoma and, 620, *620*
  primitive multipotential sarcoma of bone,
    526, *526*
  prognosis in, 528
  radiation therapy and, 514
  roentgenographic manifestations of, 516,
    517–519, 522, 526
  sclerosing, 522
  serum phosphatase levels in, 515
  treatment of, 529
  vs. chondrosarcoma, 551
  vs. osteoblastoma, 490
  vs. osteogenesis imperfecta, 340
  vs. villonodular synovitis, *763*
Osteosclerosis fragilis. See *Osteopetrosis.*

Paget's disease, 407–419
  anemia in, 409
  cardiovascular disease in, 410
  chondrosarcoma in, 552
  clinical features of, 408
  incidence of, 407
  microscopy of, 411, *417, 418*
  mosaic pattern in, 411, *417*
  osteoporosis circumscripta in, *412*
  osteosarcoma in, *513*, 514
  pathogenesis of, 410
  prognosis in, 414
  roentgenographic manifestations of, 411,
    412, 416, 419
  sarcoma in, 415, *418, 419*
  serum calcium level in, 410
  therapy in, 414
  vs. hyperphosphatasia, 369
Pain, congenital indifference to, 649
  insensitivity to, 245, 246, *247*
Palindromic rheumatism, 675
Palsy, bulbar, 706
Pancreatitis, hyperparathyroidism in, 388
Pannephritic osteodystrophy. See *Renal*
  osteodystrophy.
Panner's disease, 294
Pannus, 72

Paralysis, familial periodic, 718–719
in poliomyelitis, 708
Paramyotonia, 719
Parathormone, 29, 386
Parathyroid activity, glucagon and, 388
Parathyroid adenoma, 385
and tetany, 387
clinical features of, 388
incidence of, 387
microscopy of, 395, *396–398*
nephrocalcinosis of, 387, *388*
roentgenographic manifestations of, 390, *391–395*
vs. renal osteodystrophy, 355, 359
Parathyroid dysfunction, bone changes of, 385–405
Parathyroid gland, normal, microscopy of, 386, *386*
secretion of, effect of, 390
Parathyroid hormone, actions of, 401
and bone calcification, 28
Parathyroid hyperplasia, idiopathic, 399, *400*
Parosteal osteogenic sarcoma, 530
Parosteal sarcoma, 464, 510, 530, 537
bones involved in, 531
clinical features of, 531
differential diagnosis of, 534
incidence of, 531
microscopy of, 533, *535, 536*
morphology of, 531
osteochondroma and, 499, 533, *535*
prognosis in, 536
roentgenographic manifestations of, 531, *532, 534, 535*
treatment of, 537
Parrot's syphilitic osteochondritis, 660
Pectus excavatum deformity, in Marfan's syndrome, *190*
Peptic ulcer(s), in hyperparathyroidism, 388
Periarticular tissue, diseases of, 678–685
Perichondrium, formation of, 18
Periodic acid–fuchsin reaction, 10
Periodic-Schiff reaction, 10
Periosteum, components of, 62, *63*
formation of, 18
Permeated destruction, of bone, 81
Peroneal muscular atrophy, 706
Perthes' disease, 294, 295
Peter Pan dwarfism, 380
Peyronie's disease, 753
Phagocyte(s), mononuclear, 42
Phantom clavicle, 371, 502, *505*
Phosphatase, alkaline, 16
Phosphorus deficiency, and skeletal abnormalities, 27
Phosphorylethanolamine, in hypophosphatasia, 369
Pituitary dwarfism, 380
Pituitary dysfunction, bone changes of, 376–381
acromegaly, 378
giantism, 376
pituitary dwarfism, 380
Plantar fibromatosis, 753, *756*
Plasma cell, 573
Plasma cell myeloma, 573–587
amyloid in, 577, *577*

Plasma cell myeloma (*Continued*)
and aneurysmal bone cyst, 574
anemia in, 575
Bence Jones protein in, 576
bleeding in, 575
bones involved in, 573
cell morphology in, 586, *586*
clinical features of, 574
derivation of, 572
generalized, vs. senile osteoporosis, 374
globulins in, 576
heredity in, 580
incidence of, 573
kappa type of, 586
lambda type of, 586
marrow aspiration in, 575, *575*
microscopy of, 580, *585, 586*
morbid anatomy of, 580
prognosis in, 586
renal insufficiency in, 578
roentgenographic manifestations of, 580, *581–585*
serum calcium levels in, 574
serum electrophoretic pattern in, *576*
serum protein in, 575, *576*
uric acid in, 577
Plasmacyte(s), 40, *41*
Plasmacytoma, extramedullary, 573, 586
Plasmalemma, 689
Poker spine, 668
Polar bear liver intoxication, 449
Polyarteritis, 711
arthritis in, 674
Poliomyelitis, 708, *709, 710*
Polymerization, of chondroid, 11
Polymorphonuclear leukocyte(s), 40
Polymyositis, 711
clinical features of, 712
microscopy of, 712, *713, 714*
with cancer, 715
with mesenchymal diseases, 714
with Sjögren's syndrome, 715
Polypeptide chain(s), 572
Posthematoma cyst(s), 324–328, 433
Postmenopausal osteoporosis, 371
Pott's disease, 265, 659
Primary bone tumor, 461
classification of, 462–468
Primitive bone, 21
Proliferative myositis, 766, *767*
Pseudarthrosis, 184
in bone repair, 235
microscopy of, 186, *186*
prognosis in, 186
vs. prenatal bowing, 185, *185*
Pseudogout, 631, *631, 632*
roentgenographic manifestations of, 632
Pseudo-Hurler disease, 224
Pseudohypertrophic muscular dystrophy, 694, *695*
fat in, 701
Pseudo-hypo-hyperparathyroidism, 405
Pseudohypoparathyroidism, 403, *404, 405*
Pseudo-pseudohypoparathyroidism, 404
Pseudo-rheumatoid nodule, 668
Pseudosarcomatous fasciitis, 767–769, *768*
Pseudotumor(s), of hemophilia, 324, *324*

Psoriasis, joint disease in, 637, *637*
Puerperal osteomalacia, 349
Pyknodysostosis, 154–157
  clinical features of, *155, 156*
  microscopy of, *157*
Pyle's disease, 157–161
  roentgenographic manifestations of, *158–160*
Pyrophosphate, 632

"Rachitic rosary," in rickets, 343, *343*
Radiographic magnification, 75
Radiography, physics related to, 78
Radiology, of skeletal system, 74–84
  protection of patient in, 74
Radius, length growth of, 22
Ranvier, ring of, 610
Reactive lesion(s), of soft parts, 761–775
  classification of, 761
Reed-Sternberg giant cell(s), in Hodgkin's
    disease, 605, 606
Reilly granule(s), in Morquio's disease, 95
Reiter's syndrome, 657
Renal failure, in hyperparathyroidism, 389
Renal function, and calcium level, 30
Renal insufficiency, in plasma cell myeloma,
    578
Renal osteodystrophy, 354
  bone changes in, 355
  clinical features of, 354, *356*
  etiology of, 354
  microscopy of, 359, *360, 361*
  parathyroid adenoma vs., 355
  pathogenesis of, 355
  prognosis of, 361
  roentgenographic manifestations of, *356–358, 392*
Renal osteomalacia, 361, *362–364*
Renal rickets. See *Renal osteodystrophy.*
Rendu-Osler-Weber disease, 501
Reticulocytosis(es), cerebroside. See
    Gaucher's disease.
  neoplastic, 217
Reticuloendothelial system, functional dis-
    turbances of, 201–228
Reticuloendotheliosis(es), 201
  nonlipid. See *Letterer-Siwe disease.*
Reticulin fibrils, 9
Reticulum, 5
Reticulum cell sarcoma, 597–603
  bones involved in, 598
  clinical features of, 598
  derivation of, 572
  incidence of, 598
  metastatic pattern in, 599
  microscopy of, 600, *601, 602*
  morbid anatomy of, 600
  prognosis in, 603
  roentgenographic manifestations of, 599,
    599, 600
  silver stains in, 601
  treatment of, 603
  vs. Ewing's tumor, 595
  vs. non-osseous reticulum cell sarcoma, 598
Rh factor, in rheumatoid arthritis, 661

Rhabdomyoma, 750
Rhabdomyosarcoma, 734
  alveolar, 736, *737*
  arteriogram of, *734*
  embryonal, 738, *738, 739*
  microscopy of, 735, *735–737*
  types of, 734
Rheumatic fever, 674
Rheumatism, palindromic, 675
Rheumatoid arthritis, 661
  clinical features of, 661
  incidence of, 661
  juvenile, 668
    roentgenographic manifestations of, 671
  laboratory findings in, 661
  L.E. cells in, 662
  microscopy of, 662, *663–667*
  muscle atrophy in, 668
  pathology of, 662
  Rh factor in, 661
  rheumatoid factor in, 661
  rheumatoid nodule in, 666, *667*
  roentgenographic manifestations of, 669,
    669–672
  synovial fluid in, 662
Rheumatoid factor, 661
Rheumatoid nodule, in rheumatoid arthritis,
    666, *667*
  pseudo, 668
Rheumatoid spondylitis, 668, *669*
  roentgenographic manifestations of, 671,
    673
Rhizomelia, in achondroplasia, 108
Ribbing's disease, 161
Rice body(ies), 682
Rickets, 341–348. See also specific names.
  calcium absorption in, 28
  clinical features of, 342, *343, 345*
  etiology of, 342
  microscopy of, 346, *347*
  pattern of healing in, 346, *346*
  prognosis in, 348
  renal. See *Renal osteodystrophy.*
  roentgenographic manifestations of, 344,
    344–346
Ringbinden, 699
Ringing of epiphysis, in scurvy, 334, *335, 337*
Rod disease, 705, *706*
Rubella syndrome, congenital, 286–288, *287,
    288*

"Saber shin," of congenital syphilis, *277*
Salmonella osteomyelitis, 261–264
Salt(s), bone, deposition of, 15–16
  in organic matrix, 27
Sanfilippo's syndrome, 101
Sarcosporidiosis, 716
"Saturn's ring," in osteogenesis imperfecta,
    142
Sarcoma, cervical synovial, 724
  chondroblastic, 559
  clear cell, 727, *727*
  endothelial, of bone. See *Ewing's tumor.*
  epithelioid, 746
  juxtacortical. See *Parosteal sarcoma.*

Sarcoma (*Continued*)
  osteogenic. See *Osteosarcoma.*
  parosteal. See *Parosteal sarcoma.*
  primary, 590
Scanning, bone, 76, 77
Schaumann body(ies), in Boeck's sarcoidosis, 284
Scheie's syndrome, 101
Scheuermann's disease, 294
Schwannoma, malignant, 742
Scleroderma, arthritis in, 674, *674*
Sclerosis, amyotrophic lateral, 706
  diaphyseal, 161, *161, 162*
Scorbutic zone, 336
Scurvy, 147, 333–338
  clinical features of, 334
  etiology of, 333
  in childhood, 24, *25*
  microscopy in, 336, *336*
  osteopenia of, 339
  prognosis in, 337
  roentgenographic manifestations of, 334, *335*
Seabright bantam syndrome, 403
Seam(s), osteoid, 56
Senile osteoporosis, 371
  vs. generalized plasma cell myeloma, 374
Sensory spindle, *692*
Sequestrum, 254, *254, 258*
Serum calcium, and parathyroid function, 29
  in Paget's disease, 410
  in plasma cell myeloma, 574
Serum chemistry, in metastatic tumors, 470
Serum globulin, 572
Serum phosphatase, in osteosarcoma, 515
Serum sickness, arthritis in, 673
Sex hormone(s), 338
Shagreen plaque(s), 183
Sickle cell anemia, hand-foot syndrome in, 322, 324
  roentgenographic manifestations of, *320, 321*
  Salmonella osteomyelitis in, 261
  vs. Legg-Calvé-Perthes disease, 318
Sjögren's syndrome, polymyositis with, 715
Skeletal dysplasia(s), 87–200
  abnormal epiphyseal ossification and, 129–140
  abnormal osteoid production and, 167–186
  classification of, 87
  deficient osteoid production and, 141–147
  deficient osteolysis and, 147–167
  disturbances in osteoid production and, 129–186
  due to abnormal metaphyseal and periosteal ossification, 140–186
  due to abnormal maturation of growth plate chondroblasts, 89–115
  elaboration of chondroid and, 89–129
  proliferation of epiphyseal chondroblasts and, 115–129
Skeletal development, disturbances in, 85–228
Skeletal muscle, diseases of, 687–720
Skeletal system, radiology of, 74–84
Skeleton, embryology and physiology of, 17–36

Skeleton (*Continued*)
  formation of, diet in, 23
  miscellaneous diseases of, 407–458
  of human organism, 22
Slipped epiphysis. See *Epiphysiolysis.*
Smallpox, and bone infection, 279
Soft part(s), hamartomas of, 748–761
  reactive lesions of, 761–775
  tumors of, 721–775
Solitary bone cyst, 433–440
  clinical features of, 434
  incidence of, 433
  microscopy in, 437, *438*
  pathogenesis of, 439
  prognosis in, 439
  roentgenographic manifestations of, *434, 436, 436, 437*
  vs. non-osteogenic fibroma, 313
Somatomedin, 376
Somatotropic growth hormone, 25
  in giantism, 376
Spherocytic anemia, 318
Sphingomyelin, in Niemann-Pick disease, 224
Spider cell(s), in rhabdomyosarcoma, 735, *736*
Spine, tuberculosis of, 265, *265, 267, 268*
Spondylitis, ankylosing, 668
  rheumatoid, 668
Spondylitis rhizomélique, 668
Spondyloepiphyseal dysplasia, 130, 132–137
  roentgenographic manifestations of, 133, *133–137*
Sporotrichum schenckii, and bone infection, 279
Spotted bone(s), 166
Squamous cell carcinoma, in suppurative osteomyelitis, 254, *255*
Staphylococcus aureus, and suppurative osteomyelitis, 252, *262*
Stereoscopy, 75
Stiff-man syndrome, 717
Still's disease, 668
Stippled epiphyses, 130, 139–140, *139, 140*
Stress, and osteopenia, 332
Stress deficiency osteopenia, 339
Stress fracture, 247
Stress stimulus, in ossification, 31, *32*
Stroma, cells of, in osteoclastoma, 615, 618
Sturge-Weber disease, 501
Subchondral cyst, 433, 440
Subperiosteal cortical defect, 314–318, 495–496
  incidence of, 314
  microscopy of, 316, *318*
  roentgenographic manifestations of, *315–317*
  vs. non-osteogenic fibroma, 314
Succinic dehydrogenase, in chondroblasts, 20
Sudeck's disease, 339
Sunburst appearance, in Ewing's tumor, 592
  in osteosarcoma, 516, *517*
Suppurative osteomyelitis. See *Osteomyelitis, suppurative.*
"Swan neck," in vitamin D refractory rickets, 365
Syndactylism, in Apert's syndrome, 192, *192, 193*

Syndrome(s). See specific names.
Synovia, in tuberculous arthritis, 658
Synovial chondrometaplasia, 682–685, *684, 685*
Synovial fluid, 625
    functions of, 626
    in rheumatoid arthritis, 662
Synovial joint(s), anatomy of, 624–626, *624*
Synovial membrane, 624
    in hemophilia, 634
    of joint, 72, *73*
Synovioma, 723
    amputation in, 725
    benign, 761–763
    incidence of, 724
    microscopy in, 725, *725, 726*
    sites involved in, 724
    types of, 729
Synovitis, villonodular. See *Villonodular synovitis.*
Syphilis, of bone, 273–277
    acquired, 274, *275, 279*
    congenital, 276, *276–278*
Syphilitic arthritis, 659
Syringomyelia, neurogenic arthropathy in, 648, *648*
Systemic lupus erythematosus, 711

Talipes equinus deformity, in diastrophic dwarfism, *132*
Taper mouth, in myotonic dystrophy, 696
Tay-Sachs disease, with visceral involvement, 224
Tendon(s), anatomy of, 72, *73*
    giant cell tumor, 761–763
Tenosynovial chondrometaplasia, 748, *749*
Tenosynovitis, chronic, 761–763
    villonodular, 761–763
Tetany, parathyroid adenoma and, 387
Thanatophoric dwarfism, 196
Thermography, 78
Thiemann's disease, 294
Thomsen's disease, 716–717
Thoracic dystrophy, asphyxiating, 196, *198*
Thrombosis, vascular, in suppurative osteomyelitis, 253, *253*
Thymic tumor, in myasthenia gravis, 718
Thyrocalcitonin, and osteolysis, 371
    and release of mineral salts, 30
    properties of, 401
Thyroid acropachy, 385, *385*
Thyroid dwarfism, 381
Thyroid dysfunction, bone changes of, 381–385
    hyperthyroidism, 383
    hypothyroidism, 381
Thyroid hormone, 26
    site of action of, 381
Thyrotoxicosis, osteopenia of, 339
Tibia, in child and adult, comparison of, *82*
    length growth of, 22
Tibia vara, 130, *138*, 139
Tide line, 66, *67*
Tissue, granulation, *38, 39*
    periosteal, in intramembranous ossification, 19

Tomography, 75
Tophus, in gout, 627, *627–629*
Torulosis, of bone, *281*
Touton giant cell, 741, 769
Trauma, in battered child, 244, *244, 245*
Treponema pallidum, and syphilis of bone, 273
Trichinosis, 716, *716*
"Trident hand," in achondroplasia, 108
Trisomy 13–15, 457, *457*
Trisomy 18, *455, 456,* 457
Trisomy 21, 454, *455*
"Trumpeting," in achondroplasia, *104*
    in rickets, 343
Tuberculosis, of bone, 264–272
    microscopy of, 268, *272, 273*
    roentgenographic manifestations of, 266, *267–271*
    of spine, 658, 659
Tuberculosis sica, 266
Tuberculous arthritis, 657
    treatment of, 659
Tuberculous osteomyelitis, 264–272
Tuberculous spondylitis, 264
Tumor(s). See also specific names.
    brown. See *Brown tumor(s).*
    chondrogenic, 465–466, 538–561
    classification of, 468–469
    collagenic, 466–468, 562–571
    general consideration of, 461–477
    malignant vs. benign, 462
    metastatic to bone, 469–477
        clinical features of, 470
        microscopy of, 474
        needle aspiration of, 474
        pathology of, 472
        roentgenographic manifestations of, 471, *471–476*
        serum chemistry in, 470
    myelogenic, 468, 572–606
    of collagenoblastic tissue, 738–744
    of lipoblastic origin, 729–732
    of mesothelial origin, 723–729
    of mixed tissue origin, 746–747
    of muscle origin, 732–738
    of nerve supportive tissue origin, 742
    of soft parts, 721–775
        classification of, 722, 723
    of uncertain tissue origin, 744–746
    of vessel supportive tissue, 742
    osteogenic, 464–465, 510–537
Tumoral calcinosis, 764–766, *764, 765*
Tumor-like process(es), 478–509
    hamartomas, 496–509
    reactive lesions in bone, 478–496
Turner's syndrome, 453, *454*

Ulcer, peptic, in hyperparathyroidism, 388
Ulcerative colitis, joint disease in, 637
Umbauzonen, in rickets, 346
Unicameral bone cyst(s), 324
Uric acid, and gout, 626
    in plasma cell myeloma, 577
Urine, in alkaptonuria, 632
Urticaria pigmentosa, 450–451

Van Buchem's disease, 407, 420
Vein, anatomy of, 48, *49*
Verocay body, 757
Villonodular synovitis, 650–655
  incidence of, 650
  intraosseous, 652, *652*
  microscopy of, 650, *651, 653*
  pathogenesis of, 652
  roentgenographic manifestations of, *652–654*
  vs. osteoclastoma, 618
Villonodular tenosynovitis, 727, 761–763, *761*
  microscopy of, *762, 763*
Viral osteomyelitis, 279, 282
Vitamin A, in bone growth, 24
Vitamin A poisoning, 448–450
Vitamin C, deficiency of, and scurvy, 333
Vitamin D, action of, 444
  and calcium absorption, 27
  in idiopathic hypercalcemia, 447
  insufficient, and osteomalacia, 348
  and rickets, 342
Vitamin D poisoning, 444–446
Vitamin D refractory rickets. See *Hypophosphatemic–vitamin D refractory rickets.*
Volkmann's canal(s), 21
von Bechterew's spondylitis, 668
von Hippel-Lindau disease, 501

von Recklinghausen's disease, 385. See also *Neurofibromatosis.*
Voorhoeve's disease, 165, *165*

Waldenström's macroglobulinemia, 572
Wasserhelle hyperplasia, 400
Werdnig-Hoffman disease, 702
Wilson's disease, and rickets, 364
Wimberger's sign, *278*
Woven bone, 21
  primitive, 58, *59*

Xanthoma, 769. See also *Villonodular synovitis.*
  in non-osteogenic fibroma, 308
Xanthofibroma, of bone, 308
Xanthogranuloma. See *Villonodular synovitis.*
Xerography, 78, *78*
X-ray diffraction, in study of bone, 12, *14*
X-ray therapy, and osteosarcoma, 514

Zimmermann, hemangiopericytes of, 501